Methodology for Analytical Toxicology

Methodology for Analytical Toxicology

Editor

Irving Sunshine

Chief Toxicologist
Cuyahoga County Coroner's Office
Cleveland, Ohio
Professor of Toxicology
Institute of Pathology, School of Medicine
Case Western Reserve University
Cleveland, Ohio

CRC

Published by

CRC PRESS, Inc.
2255 Palm Beach Lakes Blvd. · West Palm Beach, Florida 33409

Library of Congress Cataloging in Publication Data

Main entry under title:

Methodology for analytical toxicology.

At head of title: CRC.
Includes bibliographies and index.
1. Poisons — Analysis. 2. Toxicology — Laboratory manuals. I. Sunshine, Irving. II. Chemical Rubber Company, Cleveland.
RA1221.M44 615.9'07 74-30747
ISBN 0-8493-0716-3
Former ISBN 0-87819-716-8

2nd Printing, April 1978
CRC Press, Inc.
Revised from *CRC Handbook of Analytical Toxicology*

International Standard Book Number 0-8493-0716-3
Former International Standard Book Number 0-87819-716-8

Library of Congress Card Number 74-30747
Printed in the United States

PREFACE TO METHODOLOGY FOR ANALYTICAL TOXICOLOGY

The current and growing interest in determinations for anticonvulsant drugs, digoxin and digitoxin, procaine amide, lidocaine, and theophylline indicates that monitoring drug therapy is an increasing challenge to clinical laboratory scientists. Physicians are anxious to have this laboratory support which they can use to better understand a patient who has not achieved the expected results from a prescribed therapeutic regimen. Among the several questions related to this problem are these. Was the patient taking the drug? Was the prescribed dose sufficient? Was the patient taking some other medication which could affect his proper utilization of the prescribed drug? (Polypharmacology is practiced by many, and seldom do they deem it necessary to inform the physician that they are taking medications other than those he prescribed.)

One of the objectives of this volume is to present acceptable methods for the analysis of therapeutic agents in biological fluids. By utilizing these procedures, the chemist can provide the physician with objective laboratory data which can be used to answer some of the questions postulated above. In the several laboratories where these analyses have been instituted the demand for them has been overwhelming. One of the contributions of this volume is to present the analyst with several methods for the analysis of therapeutic agents and present the physician with reasonable interpretations of the results.

Procedures for many substances have been included in this volume so that methods for the analysis of the many products involved in acute poisonings are more easily available to those who want to use them. The described methods are the essence of the pragmatic experience of many active analysts. They will yield a reasonable result when carried out exactly as described in the text. Subsequently, some may wish to modify these methods to suit their local needs; however, this should be done only after establishing that the proposed modifications are preferable. The exception to this rule must be those methods which use gas chromatography. Many different columns are described, and no laboratory should have access to all of them. Hence, the reader is advised to become familiar with the columns he has available and expand their use for as many substances as he can. A table of McReynold's Constants has been included in the text. Using this, one should be able to determine which column packings are comparable and interchangeable.

In many instances a given procedure is really a prototype for many other chemically related substances. The expanded index, therefore, indicates all the so-called "interferences" to a given procedure. If a substance is listed as interfering with a given determination, it may be determinable by the same procedure, providing the prototype is not present. One should verify this and then proceed with the analysis.

The problem for some laboratories dealing with the analysis of specimens from patients involved in acute poisonings is that the causative agent may not be known. To help resolve this problem the second section of this volume presents several approaches to the systematic analysis of a biological fluid. The approach one chooses depends on local facilities. To encompass most, procedures are described which require a minimum of special equipment (TLC), some commonly available instruments (spectrophotometry), or gas chromatography (a technique rapidly growing in popularity and value). The more experimental liquid chromatographic techniques and the more elegant, sophisticated combination of gas chromatography and mass spectrometry are not presented. Too few laboratories now have this potential, but probably the next revision of this material will find these techniques commonplace.

Coupled with the revised or new procedures are updated assessments of the interpretation of the laboratory values. Significant data have been elaborated in recent years. These results are included in the presentation, as are recent literature citations so that the readers so inclined may seek them out and digest them at leisure.

I.S.
1975

PREFACE TO THE MANUAL OF ANALYTICAL TOXICOLOGY

Published by the Chemical Rubber Co., 1971.

A growing number of requests for toxicological analyses is being made by physicians in order to establish whether or not particular patients may have been poisoned. This is understandable, because the signs and symptoms seen in acutely ill patients are not pathognomonic of exposure to a specific exogenous chemical agent, and a reliable history of an exposure to a toxic chemical often cannot be obtained. Thus, a correct diagnosis of poisoning frequently depends on the result of a chemical analysis of a biological specimen obtained from a patient. Simple and reliable methods for these analyses are not readily available for use in clinical chemistry laboratories. This book proposes to assemble and present a number of such methods.

The comprehensive toxicological treatises that have been published to date present many methods for the analysis of toxic substances. Unfortunately, their multiplicity often leaves the clinical chemist perplexed. Which of the many methods should *he* use in *his* laboratory? This volume is designed to answer that question. The basic principles of the many published methods will not be discussed, but details of some carefully selected and tested procedures will be presented.

The choice of the described methods was based on many factors, including reliability, the availability of equipment and reagents, the simplicity of the procedure, and the relative speed with which an informative result can be obtained. These methods are mainly personal modifications of procedures originally developed by others. When applied exactly as described, they will produce meaningful and reliable data.

Three types of methods were planned for each substance: Type A, a simple, direct, and qualitative test; Type B, a quantitative procedure using facilities found in the average laboratory; and Type C, an elegant, precise procedure using whatever equipment may be required. This goal was not realized for many obvious reasons and remains as a challenge for subsequent volumes.

Because the interpretation of the results obtained from these analyses will not be within the common experience of many readers, a summary of the reported correlations between the clinical condition of the patient and the concentration of the toxic agent in a relevant specimen will be given. More detail can be obtained by referring to the bibliobraphy following each method. The interpretive data will interest not only toxicologists, clinical chemists, and clinical pathologists, but also all physicians who face the problem of treating a symptomatic patient purportedly poisoned by the most frequently offending drugs, household products, and economic poisons.

No extensive effort will be made to present methods that are primarily concerned with industrial toxicology and the evaluation of occupational hazards.

I.S.
1971

CONTRIBUTORS

This manual could never have been prepared without the help of the contributing authors. I and every reader of this volume are indebted to each of them for their time and effort. The procedures they contributed represent *their* considered judgment on an acceptable, reproducible, and reliable method for the substance involved.

John K. Abbott, B.A.
Chemist
Federal Aviation Administration, DOT
P.O. Box 25082
Oklahoma City, Oklahoma 25082

Vijay Aggarwal, B.A.
Toxicologist
Bureau of Forensic Science
1 North 14th Street
Richmond, Virginia 23219

Steve Andryauskas
Senior Chemist
Office of Chief Medical Examiner
520 First Avenue
New York, New York 10016

Joseph S. Annino, B.S.
Director
Clin-Chem Laboratories
1106 Commonwealth Avenue
Boston, Massachusetts 02215

David N. Bailey, M.D.
Clinical Fellow
Yale University School of Medicine
Box 1001
New Haven, Connecticut 06510

John R. Barnes, Ph.D.
Section Chief, Biochemistry Section
Haskell Laboratory of Industrial Medicine and Toxicology
Elkton Road
Newark, Delaware 19711

Frank E. Barnhart, B.S.
Forensic Toxicologist
San Diego County Coroner's Office Laboratory
5555 Overland Avenue
San Diego, California 92123

Milton L. Bastos, Ph.D.
Director of Toxicology
Office of the Chief Medical Examiner
520 First Avenue
New York, New York 10016

Raymond J. Bath, Ph.D.
Chief Toxicologist
Bureau of Forensic Science
1 North 14th Street
Richmond, Virginia 23219

David J. Berry, L.R.I.C.
Chief Technician
Poisons Unit, New Cross Hospital
Avonley Road
London, S.E. 14, England

Robert V. Blanke, Ph.D.
Professor of Pathology and Director of Toxicology Laboratory
Virginia Commonwealth University
Box 696, MCV Station
Richmond, Virginia 23298

Paul B. Bondo, M.S.
Research and Development Chemist
South Bend Medical Foundation
531 North Main Street
South Bend, Indiana 46601

Robin A. Braithwaite, A.R.I.C., Ph.D.
Senior Clinical Biochemist
Poisons Unit, New Cross Hospital
Avonley Road
London, S.E. 14, England

Robert D. Budd, B.S.
Toxicologist
Rancho Los Amigos Hospital
7601 East Imperial Highway
Downey, California 90242

Wing Chan, M.S.
Chemist
New York City Department of Health
125 Worth Street
New York, New York 10013

Claude Charette, Dipl. Technol.
Chemical Technologist
Department of National Health and Welfare
Health Protection Branch
Ottawa, Ontario, Canada K1A OL2

George Cimbura, M.Sc.Phm.
Head, Toxicology Section
The Centre of Forensic Sciences
8 Jarvis Street
Toronto, Ontario, Canada M5E 1M8

John Cooper, Dipl. Technol.
Biochemical Technologist
Department of National Health and Welfare
Health Protection Branch
Ottawa, Ontario, Canada K1A OL2

Charles Russell Crane, Jr., Ph.D.
Chief, Biochemistry Research
Civil Aeromedical Institute, DOT, FAA
P.O. Box 25082
Oklahoma City, Oklahoma 73125

Robert H. Cravey, B.S.
Toxicologist
Office of the Sheriff-Coroner
550 North Flower Street
Santa Ana, California 92702

Bernard Davidow, Ph.D.
Assistant Commissioner for Laboratories
City of New York Department of Health
455 First Avenue
New York, New York 10016

Walter A. Dechtiaruk, B.S.
Chemist, Senior Associate
Department of Laboratory Medicine
601 North Broadway
Baltimore, Maryland 21205

Kurt M. Dubowski, Ph.D.
Professor, Clinical Chemistry and Toxicology, and Director, Toxicology Laboratories
University of Oklahoma Health Sciences Center
P.O. Box 26901
Oklahoma City, Oklahoma 73190

Leslie Eidus, M.D.
Director, Bureau of Bacteriology
Laboratory Centre for Disease Control
Health and Welfare Canada
Ottawa, Ontario, Canada K1A 0L2

John Epton, M.Sc.
Biochemist
Regional Toxicology Laboratory
Dudley Road Hospital
Birmingham, England

Milton Feldstein, M.A., M.S.
Deputy Air Pollution Control Officer
Bay Area Air Pollution Control District
939 Ellis Street
San Francisco, California 94103

Frank J. Fernandez, B.S.
Applications Chemist
Perkin-Elmer Corporation
Main Avenue
Norwalk, Connecticut 06856

Bryan S. Finkle
Toxicologist
Center for Human Toxicology
University of Utah
Salt Lake City, Utah 84112

Arthur J. Fisk, B.S.
Director of Laboratories
Dade County Medical Examiner's Office
1700 N.W. 10th Avenue
Miami, Florida 33136

Robert Forney, Jr., Ph.D.
Instructor
Case Western Reserve University
2065 Adelbert Road
Cleveland, Ohio 44106

A. W. Freireich, M.D.
Consulting Toxicologist
Nassau County Medical Examiner
P.O. Box 160
East Meadow, New York 11554

James C. Garriott, Ph.D.
Chief Toxicologist
Dallas County Institute of Forensic Sciences
5230 Medical Center Drive
Dallas, Texas 75235

Franklin D. Griffith, Ph.D.
Toxicologist
3M Company
3M Center, Medical Department
St. Paul, Minnesota 55101

Jeffrey Grove, A.R.I.C.
Senior Biochemist
Nicholas Laboratories Ltd.
225 Bath Road
Slough, Berks, England SL1 4AV

J. V. Halliwell, B.Sc.
Chemist
Poisons Unit, Guy's Hospital
St. Thomas Street
London, S.E.1., England

Horace E. Hamilton, M.S.
Instructor, Department of Pathology
University of Texas Health Science Center
7703 Floyd Curl Drive
San Antonio, Texas 78284

Bette L. Hamman, M.S.
Chief Toxicologist
National Health Laboratory
653 North Glebe Road
Arlington, Virginia 22203

Keith B. Hammond, M.S.
Director and Senior Instructor in Pediatrics
University of Colorado Medical Center
4200 East 9th Avenue
Denver, Colorado 80220

Jesse A. Hancock, Ph.D. (Deceased)
Professor of Clinical Chemistry and Toxicology
The University of Texas at El Paso
P.O. Box 180
El Paso, Texas 79999

Anita Harnanansingh, B.S.
Chemist
Laboratory Centre for Disease Control
Health and Welfare Canada
Ottawa, Ontario, Canada K1A 0L2

Wayne H. Harrington, Ph.D.
Assistant Professor
Chemistry Department
Cleveland State University
Cleveland, Ohio 44115

Norman W. Henry III, B.A.
Chemist
Haskell Laboratory of Industrial Medicine
and Toxicology
Elkton Road
Newark, Delaware, 19711

Bradford R. Hepler, B.S.
Assistant Director, Special Chemistry Branch
Clinical Pathology Services
Wilford Hall Medical Center
Lackland AFB, Texas 78236

Jocelyn M. Hicks, Ph.D.
Acting Director
Clinical Laboratories, Children's Hospital
National Medical Center
2125 13th Street, N.W.
Washington, D.C. 20009

Mary M. Hodgkin, B.Sc.
Chemist
Laboratory Centre for Disease Control
Health and Welfare Canada
Ottawa, Ontario, Canada K1A 0L2

Naresh C. Jain, Ph.D.
Director of Toxicology
Rancho Los Amigos Hospital
7601 East Imperial Highway
Downey, California 90242

Peter Jatlow, M.D.
Associate Professor, Department of
Laboratory Medicine
Yale University School of Medicine
789 Howard Street
New Haven, Connecticut 06504

George Johnson, Ph.D.
Clinical Chemist
The Johns Hopkins Hospital
601 North Broadway
Baltimore, Maryland 21205

Susan H. Jones, B.A.
Technician
Dallas County Institute of Forensic Sciences
5230 Medical Center Drive
Dallas, Texas 75235

David G. Kaiser, Ph.D.
Research Head, Drug Metabolism Research
The Upjohn Company
301 Henrietta
Kalamazoo, Michigan 49001

Gerald E. Kananen, Ph.D.
Applications Chemist
Hewlett-Packard Corporation
Route 41 and Starr Road
Avondale, Pennsylvania 19311

Sidney Kaye, Ph.D.
Professor of Toxicology, Pharmacology, and Legal Medicine
School of Medicine
University of Puerto Rico
San Juan, Puerto Rico 00936

Leo Kazyak, M.A.
Chief Toxicologist
Walter Reed Army Institute of Research
Walter Reed Army Medical Center
Washington, D.C. 20012

Edgar W. Kivela, Ph.D.
Chief, Division of Crime Detection
Michigan Department of Public Health
3500 North Logan Street
Lansing, Michigan 48914

David Landau, M.S.
Toxicologist
Nassau County Medical Examiner's Office
P.O. Box 160
East Meadow, New York 11554

Charles J. Least, Jr., M.S.
Supervisor, Therapeutic Drug Monitoring Laboratory
The Johns Hopkins Hospital
601 North Broadway
Baltimore, Maryland 21205

Beverly Lorenzo, B.S.
Chemist
Cuyahoga County Coroner's Laboratory
2121 Adelbert Road
Cleveland, Ohio 44106

Robert Maes, Ph.D.
Professor of Toxicology
University of Utrecht
Voldelhaan 14
Utrecht, Holland

Robert S. Martin, B.A.
Biology, Biochemistry Assistant
The Upjohn Company
301 Henrietta
Kalamazoo, Michigan 49001

Arthur J. McBay, Ph.D.
Chief Toxicologist
Office of the Chief Medical Examiner
P.O. Box 2488
Chapel Hill, North Carolina 27514

Michael McGee, B.S.
Chemist
Bureau of Forensic Science
1 North 14th Street
Richmond, Virginia 23219

Ian J. McGilveray, Ph.D.
Head, Biopharmaceutics Section
Drug Research Laboratory, Health Protection Branch
Health and Welfare Canada
Ottawa, Ontario, Canada K1A OL2

John J. McHugh, J.D.
Chief of Laboratory
Department of Public Safety
1010 Commonwealth Avenue
Boston, Massachusetts 02215

John M. Meola
Assistant Director, Clinical Chemistry
Albany Medical Center Hospital
46 New Scotland Avenue
Albany, New York 12208

Kamal K. Midha, Ph.D.
Research Scientist
Drug Research Laboratory, Health Protection Branch
Health and Welfare Canada
Ottawa, Ontario, Canada K1A 0L2

Joseph R. Monforte, Ph.D.
Toxicologist
Wayne County Medical Examiner's Office
400 East Lafayette Street
Detroit, Michigan 48226

Sunil K. Niyogi, Ph.D.
Consultant
5247 North 10th Street
Philadelphia, Pennsylvania 19141

Robert J. Osiewicz, Ph.D.
Toxicologist
Bureau of Forensic Sciences
401 A. Colley Avenue
Norfolk, Virginia 23507

Robert J. Perchalski, B.S.
Research Chemist
Veterans Administration Hospital
Medical Research
Gainesville, Florida 32602

L. F. Prescott, M.A., M.D., F.R.C.P.
Consultant Physician
Department of Therapeutics
The Royal Infirmary
Edinburgh, Scotland EH39YW

Arnold O. Rathje, B.S.
Senior Industrial Hygienist
General Electric Company
Nela Park
Cleveland, Ohio 44112

Philip C. Reynolds, B.S.
Chief Toxicologist
Institute of Forensic Sciences
2945 Webster Street
Oakland, California 94609

Fredric Rieders, Ph.D.
Laboratory Director
National Medical Services, Inc.
2300 Stratford Avenue
Willow Grove, Pennsylvania 19090

William Robinson, B.Sc.Phm.
Toxicologist
The Centre of Forensic Sciences
8 Jarvis Street
Toronto, Ontario, Canada M5E 1M8

Denis O. Rodgerson, Ph.D.
Chief of Clinical Chemistry
The Center for the Health Sciences
University of California at Los Angeles
Los Angeles, California 90024

Joseph I. Routh, Ph.D.
Professor of Biochemistry and Pathology
University of Iowa
Iowa City, Iowa 52242

Donald C. Sanders, M.S.
Research Chemist
Civil Aeromedical Institute, FAA
P.O. Box 25082, AAC-114A
Oklahoma City, Oklahoma 73125

Phillip Santinga, B.S.
Chemist
Bendix Corporation
Box 80
Brandey Station, Virginia 22714

Bernard Searle, Ph.D.
106D Finderne Avenue
Grandview Gardens, New Jersey 08876

Paul Richard Sedgwick, B.A.
Associate Toxicologist
Orange County Sheriff-Coroner
550 North Flower Street
Santa Ana, California 92701

Richard F. Shaw, B.S.
Chief Toxicologist
San Diego County Coroner's Office
5555 Overland Avenue
San Diego, California 92123

Theodore J. Siek, Ph.D.
Toxicologist
Northern Virginia Branch, Bureau of Forensic Science
P.O. Box 486
Merrifield, Virginia 22116

Thomas C. Sneath, B.S.
Senior Toxicologist
Rancho Los Amigos Hospital
7601 East Imperial Highway
Downey, California 90242

Harvey M. Solomon, M.D.
Clinical Pathologist
The Johns Hopkins Hospital
601 North Broadway
Baltimore, Maryland 21205

F. William Sunderman, Jr., M.D.
Professor and Chairman, Department of Laboratory Medicine
University of Connecticut School of Medicine
P.O. Box G
Farmington, Connecticut 06032

Irving Sunshine, Ph.D.
Chief Toxicologist
Cuyahoga County Coroner's Office
2121 Adelbert Road
Cleveland, Ohio 44106

Marjorie Q. Swift, B.S.
Senior Chemist
Department of Public Safety
1010 Commonwealth Avenue
Boston, Massachusetts 02215

James B. Terrill, Ph.D.
Research Toxicologist
Haskell Laboratory, DuPont Company
Elkton Road
Newark, Delaware 19711

Jerry J. Thoma, M.S.
Research and Development Chemist
South Bend Medical Foundation
521 North Main Street
South Bend, Indiana 46601

Robert Turk, Ph.D.
Chief Toxicologist
Clinical Bio-Tox Laboratories, Ltd.
1436 Old Skokie Road
Highland Park, Illinois 60035

James C. Valentour, Ph.D.
Associate Toxicologist
Cuyahoga County Coroner's Office
2121 Adelbert Road
Cleveland, Ohio 44106

Michael Vanko, Ph.D.
Assistant Director
Albany Medical Center Hospital
120 Mohawk Drive
Schenectady, New York 12307

Clifford B. Walberg, Ph.D.
Clinical Chemist
Toxicology Lab, LAC-USC Medical Center
1200 North State Street
Los Angeles, California 90033

Jack E. Wallace, Ph.D.
Associate Professor
University of Texas Health Science Center
7703 Floyd Curl Drive
San Antonio, Texas 78284

John Wells, Ph.D.
Toxicologist
The Centre of Forensic Sciences
8 Jarvis Street
Toronto, Ontario, Canada M5E 1M8

Rhondda J. Wells, B.S.
Assistant Director
Pediatric Microchemistry Laboratory
University of Colordo Medical Center
Denver, Colorado 80220

H. R. Wetherell, Ph.D.
Crime Laboratory Scientist
Michigan Department of Public Health
3500 North Logan Street
Lansing, Michigan 48914

B. J. Wilder, M.D.
Chief
Neurology Service
Veterans Administration Hospital
Gainesville, Florida 32802

Louis A. Williams, B.S.
President
Clin-Chem Laboratories
1106 Commonwealth Avenue
Boston, Massachusetts 02215

William J. Wilson, Jr., M.Sc.
Chief Toxicologist
Office of Bexar County Medical Examiner
527 North Leona Street
San Antonio, Texas 78207

Bennie Zak, Ph.D.
Professor of Pathology
Wayne State University School of Medicine
540 East Canfield
Detroit, Michigan 48201

TABLE OF CONTENTS

Type A: a simple, direct qualitative test.
Type B: a quantitative procedure using facilities found in the average laboratory.
Type C: an elegant precise procedure using whatever equipment may be required.

*Use and Interpretation of Measurements, p. 86. Unit Conversion, p. 99.

Type A: a simple, direct qualitative test.
Type B: a quantitative procedure using facilities found in the average laboratory.
Type C: an elegant precise procedure using whatever equipment may be required.

Type A: a simple, direct qualitative test.

Type B: a quantitative procedure using facilities found in the average laboratory.

Type C: an elegant precise procedure using whatever equipment may be required.

ACKNOWLEDGMENT

I would like to thank Jerry Thoma and Paul Bondo for their assistance in reviewing and editing the numerous manuscripts submitted by the authors. Their diligence and expertise contributed significantly in compiling this volume.

I would also like to thank the editorial staff of CRC Press, Inc., in particular Sandy Pearlman, for their conscientious application to the many details involved in converting the first drafts of the contributors' manuscripts to a useful and practical book.

APOLOGIA

"To err is human, ..." Extensive efforts have been made to insure the reliability and lucidity of the material presented in this volume. The reader is encouraged to send his observation of errors of omission or commission to the editor so that subsequent volumes will be improved. Requests for additional information on procedural details will be welcomed by the editor.

Introduction

IS MY PATIENT POISONED?

Initially, someone must suspect that a potential toxicological problem exists. Unless the question "Is this person poisoned?" is raised, there is no need for chemical analysis. If, however, a diagnosis of poisoning is entertained, a chemical analysis may be requested. Analysis of biological samples taken from the victim of a suspected poisoning may include some determinations that are routinely performed in clinical chemistry laboratories. These determinations may be helpful in the evaluation of some poisonings. For example, blood pH and carbon dioxide combining power determinations are valuable guides in the treatment of victims of salicylate poisoning, and elevated BUN and creatinine concentrations, indicating severe renal damage, may suggest the possibility of mercurialism.. Abnormal concentrations of any of these substances, however, may also result from disease processes. Whether or not they reflect the consequences of a poisoning can best be ascertained by demonstrating the presence of a toxic agent in a biological sample.

To request a chemical analysis designed to establish the presence of a specific toxic agent in a biological sample is simple. To do the analysis is not always simple, even for an experienced toxicologist, and it may prove to be a very vexing problem for the average clinical chemist.

Far more troublesome are those requests in which no particular suspected toxic agent is specified. The number of chemical substances that may be involved is legion, the specimen size is limited, the time during which a result may be of any real use is often short, and the required skills and equipment may be lacking. Subsequent chapters in this book may provide remedies for a few of these many difficulties, but they cannot supply such basic information as to which substance or which types or categories of substance is most probably involved in a given poisoning. This essential information can only come from the physician responsible for treating the patient. Only when this information is supplied can one judiciously select an analytical scheme which will yield significant results in a reasonable period of time.

Several parallel investigations should be started by the attending physician as soon as he suspects poisoning may be the cause of a patient's illness. While he examines the patient to elicit signs and symptoms which may be indicative and to determine the initial therapy, he should direct others to examine the locale of the suspected incident and the personal effects of the victim for clues to the possible offending agent. Any containers of drugs or household chemicals, including the "empty" ones as well as unidentified material or containers found at the "scene," should be collected and brought to the attention of the physician. Any unusual odors should be noted and characterized. Although none of these may be the causative agent, their potential hazard and possible involvement should be evaluated. This physical survey should be accompanied by a thorough questioning of anyone who had any contact with the patient prior to his hospitalization.

It is essential that such information, coupled with the physician's personal observations, be summarized and sent to the chemist if the most appropriate analytical scheme is to be chosen. Specific answers can be provided to specific questions. These questions should be framed not only in terms of the examinations mentioned above, but also on the basis of local data on the prevailing incidence of fatal and nonfatal poisonings. Local customs often influence the nature of the agents encountered. Commonly used and available substances are likely to be frequently involved and substances uncommon to the area, infrequently (e.g., in a rural area DDT or parathion rather than strychnine, a barbiturate rather than a bromide). Publicity is also a factor to be considered. Printed details suggesting the death of a prominent person was caused by a particular poison, or that glue sniffing or LSD is in vogue, may produce a flurry of similar incidents.

Familiarity with local conditions may thus help determine which substance is the most probable offending agent in a given situation when no other data are available.

When the physician does not obtain or communicate the relevant data, the chemist may well be faced with the task of analyzing a small sample for any toxic substance. It is not uncommon, even at teaching hospitals, for the laboratory to receive a small specimen accompanied by a form requesting "Toxicology." Each chemist must decide which determinations he can perform on such a sample. Some suggested guides will be presented, but it is unlikely that an adequate answer will be obtained unless the sample size is very large; even then, the usefulness of the result may have been diminished because of the length of time required for the many determinations involved.

GUIDELINES FOR SUBMISSION OF SAMPLES

The establishment of proper communication between the physician and the chemist is only a first step toward providing the physician with the help he requests. In addition to information, the physician must also provide suitable samples to be analyzed. He must also see that they are obtained promptly, and he must be certain that they are sent to the laboratory at once. Too often the physician inadvertently assumes his responsibility has ended when he writes the order that the samples are to be obtained. In many hospitals the routines are such that a significant period of time elapses between the writing of a request for an analysis and the subsequent receipt of the specimens in the laboratory. If the toxicological analysis is needed and is to be meaningful, the physician must ascertain that samples are taken properly and that all procedures necessary to insure their prompt delivery to the laboratory are instituted.

What samples are to be sent to the laboratory? From the living patient, blood and urine are the specimens of choice in most instances, especially in cases of "common drug intoxication." Sometimes the concentration of the drug in the blood, even in a severe poisoning, may be beyond the limits of detection by available procedures. This is particularly true for those potent new drugs whose therapeutic or abuse doses range from less than 1 to 5 mg. In these instances the largest volume of urine that can be conveniently obtained should be submitted. If only a short time (e.g., 4 hr) has elapsed between the initial ingestion and the time the patient is seen by a physician, the stomach content, vomitus, or lavage fluids are desirable specimens. The samples that are submitted should be adequate for the analysis requested. The word "adequate" may only be defined in very general terms. Compromises involving quantities must often be made. When multiple toxic agents are to be investigated, the sample must be large. When the sample is not large, the number of substances to be investigated must be correspondingly limited. Desirable quantities of biological specimens are

Unclotted blood	10–20 ml
Urine	200–400 ml
Aspirate	all
Gastric lavage fluid	first 500 ml
Emesis	all

Substances requiring special samples will be cited in the text whenever relevant (e.g., hair and nail clippings in chronic arsenic poisoning).

Each sample should be placed in a chemically clean, sealed container and properly labeled. The label and/or accompanying request or order form should indicate the patient's name, the attending physician's name and telephone number, the date and time the sample was taken, the specific analyses requested, and the urgency of the analysis. Some history and statement of the patient's condition should be supplied on an accompanying note unless the physician has previously spoken to the chemist. If a "stat" analysis is required, the label, request form, or information slip should indicate to whom the immediate or interim report should be made and how and where the recipient may be reached.

If the samples are sent to the laboratory promptly, their preservation is no problem. If delay is unavoidable, the samples should be stored in a refrigerator. Do not add "preservatives" to urine samples, because this may complicate the subsequent analysis. Keep blood samples cold, but do not "deep freeze" them because this will cause hemolysis of the blood; however, an anticoagulant should be added to each blood sample.

The most suitable is sodium citrate or EDTA; heparin, potassium oxalate, and fluoride are not as desirable.

Subsequent to an autopsy in a known or suspected fatal poisoning, the pathologist should save all liver, kidney, brain, and spleen tissue, except that required for his histological preparations. In addition, samples of blood (100 ml), fat, all bile, stomach and duodenal content, and any urine present should be obtained. All specimen tissues included should be placed in separate sealed containers. Strong plastic bags are adequate and convenient for solid tissues. Screw-capped bottles, glass, or plastic can be used for fluid samples. All specimens from one subject should be collected, then placed in a large container and, properly labeled, sent to the laboratory. If they cannot be sent immediately, the specimens should be deep frozen to prevent deterioration; they may later be sent to the laboratory in frozen condition. If they are mailed, they should be packed in dry ice.

The laboratory to which the specimens are sent must, of course, be one that has the capability to undertake the requested analyses. In addition, in the case of living patients, the capability should be available at all times. At present this service is not available in the majority of large hospitals that otherwise provide excellent patient care. Often the laboratories are open only 40 hr per week, usually during the least hazardous daytime hours. This is a vexing problem, particularly for smaller communities and their hospitals, where "on-call" arrangements with personnel may be difficult to arrange. The joint support for the operation of one laboratory on a 24-hour-a-day basis by a number of geographically closely situated hospitals and communities is a solution that merits serious consideration.

MONITORING THERAPY

Many physicians have come to realize that the chemist can help resolve some of the dilemmas posed by patients who apparently are not benefiting from a prescribed therapeutic regimen. Chemical analysis of a patient's serum will indicate whether or not the patient is taking the prescribed medication, whether the amount taken is adequate to achieve therapeutic concentrations, and whether adjustment in the dose or counseling the patient is in order. Neurologists request assays for the anticonvulsant drugs, cardiologists for the cardiotonic drugs, pediatricians for theophylline, and the list is constantly growing. Described in the text are many procedures which, if followed as given, will enable any laboratory to elaborate answers pertinent to monitoring patients for their use of therapeutic drugs.

ANALYSIS

Supplied with adequate specimens and specific requests, the experienced toxicologist should be able to perform most of the required analyses. Very often, however, other chemists are also asked to perform these tests, because the number of available analytical toxicologists is limited. Most chemists can make the requested analyses if they have the necessary equipment, supplies, and detailed procedures at hand. This book will attempt to supply only the analytical methods. The methods given will be limited to determinations of those substances most frequently involved in therapeutic monitoring and/or accounting for 80 to 90% of acute poisonings. To encompass the remainder would entail an encyclopedic volume.

Three methods will be given for each substance whenever feasible. One will be a simple, rapid, qualitative screening test. The second will be a procedure requiring more elegant and careful techniques, using instruments commonly found in most laboratories. Finally, a procedure providing precise and accurate data will be given, which may require equipment and instrumentation not always available in every laboratory. The experimental details will include all of the essential information about the necessary equipment and reagents and will be followed by a step-by-step description of the procedure. These details will include important minutiae that are sometimes omitted in journal presentations. Information on proper control solutions will also be included, as well as exemplary calculations of quantities and concentrations, following application of the procedure. To help interpret the results, each presentation will include the potential and the limitations of the procedure with respect to its specificity, precision, and sensitivity. Known correlations between the quantities of the toxic agent found in the blood or other specimens and a patient's clinical condition will be briefly summarized.

Should the analysis indicate the presence of an exogenous chemical agent, careful evaluation of the qualitative and quantitative data by the physician is essential. Profound coma in the presence of 0.5 mg of barbiturate/100 ml of blood is unusual; this must be appreciated, and other causes must be sought to explain the coma. The quantitative data must be interpreted in terms of chronic or acute exposure, synergism with other drugs, tolerance, and the possible interaction of several drugs when more than one is detected.

In addition to providing separate and distinct procedures for the determination of many specific substances, the manual also devotes a section to the systematic analysis of biological samples for more than one substance. Positive results obtained by the procedures described in this section can be confirmed by analyzing other specimens related to the case for the substances thus detected, using the more specific methods given in the first section. Negative results can be meaningful because they may rule out the presence of many commonly used toxic agents; if that is the case, causes other than poisoning should be considered in the differential diagnosis.

CAVEAT INTERPRETOR

As man does not live by only bread, so the toxicologist cannot interpret his results by numbers only. Precise and accurate though they may be, they have meaning only as they refer to one person and his well-being. For example, a concentration of 0.10 mg of lead/100 ml of blood usually reflects significant absorption and accumulation of lead and is interpreted as an indicator of lead toxicity. This is true for most young children, but it is not true for many employees in the lead industry who have been exposed to lead for a long time. Certainly these employees have accumulated a high body storage of lead, but they are viable, asymptomatic, and seemingly have no detectable sequelae to their blood lead concentrations which range from 0.10 to 0.15 mg/100 ml. Similarly, a concentration of 10 mg of phenobarbital/100 ml of blood usually is compatible with a comatose patient. However, if an epileptic who has been taking phenobarbital in therapeutic doses for many months has this concentration of phenobarbital in his blood, he may be walking about.

Tolerance is the explanation usually offered to explain this phenomenon. It is only one of many pharmacological parameters that may be offered as an explanation for an unusual reaction to chemical agents. Tolerance has been noted for many drugs, particularly the opiates and the barbiturates. Cross-tolerance also exists; prolonged exposure to one drug may predispose an individual to tolerate another pharmacologically similar drug.

Individual idiosyncracy, not tolerance, may explain other hypo or hyper reactions.

"Death on the sigmoid" was a phrase used to explain this phenomenon. The sigmoid or "normal distribution" curve is applicable to drug reactions. It indicates that for any given concentration results are predictable for the vast majority of people, but that a certain few will react differently to a given drug concentration. Though the curve suggests that a few abnormal reactions will occur, it never predicts who these few unusual reactors will be.

The analytical data provided by the laboratory may not be the last piece in the poisoning puzzle. Too frequently the analyst finds one drug and stops there – because of pressures of time, lack of sample, limited staff, or for any one of a number of other reasons. Another drug may be present, not sought for, and hence not reported. Since polypharmacology is so common today, the presence of more than one drug is not an unreasonable possibility. The attitude most people have is that over-the-counter medications – aspirin, sedatives, cough syrups, etc. – are not drugs. They use them indiscriminately in conjunction with prescribed drugs; or they may consult two different physicians for two separate ailments and receive prescriptions for different medication from each. Whatever the reason for using more than one drug, the patient, or the person who brings the patient to medical attention, may not report the use of all drugs available to him. If the analyst reports a concentration of one drug, this result may not provide a reasonable explanation of the patient's condition. Another drug, originally undetected, may also be involved. Factors that need further clarification are the possibilities of interaction between two or more drugs, additive effects, antagonistic effects, and synergism. All these terms, except possibly the last, are self-explanatory. Synergism refers to the combined effect of two drugs, which is greater than that expected from each drug acting independently. The most frequently synergistic pair – ethanol and barbiturates – is very frequently encountered in adult poison victims. If only the barbiturate concentration is determined and the patient's central nervous system is depressed more than the blood barbiturate concentration indicates, more laboratory work may reveal the cause.

Beyond the immediate problem of "How does the determined concentration explain the patient's condition at the time the sample was taken?" is the question of "What will his subsequent clinical course be like?" Generally, predictions that a patient's clinical condition parallels the concentration of the drug in his blood are based on the half-life of the drug, if it is known. Of course, the half-lives of all drugs are not known. Those known are given in current pharmacology textbooks[1] or toxicology handbooks.[2,3] These reference books should be readily available to the analyst. Any prediction based on the established half-life of a drug assumes that absorption is complete and that normal metabolism, distribution, and excretion patterns prevail. This assumption must be evaluated.

Is absorption complete? Two analyses several hours apart will objectively determine this. For most drugs a period of 6 or 8 hr is required before a significant change in blood concentration takes place. Clinically, however, it is desirable to make a judgment earlier. Hence, suitable answers to the following question are needed. When did the ingestion (injection or inhalation) take place? When did the victim last partake of food and drink? Did vomiting occur? If food is present in the stomach, absorption will be affected, and its rate is unpredictable. Liquids may dissolve the drug and increase absorption because more surface area is covered, but they also affect the emptying time of the stomach and decrease absorption from the stomach because the drug passes on into the intestinal tract more quickly. Movement from the acid stomach environment to the alkaline one of the intestinal tract will also affect absorption. Thus, salicylates are rapidly absorbed from the stomach, whereas organic bases – morphine, quinine, or ephedrine – are quickly absorbed through the intestinal mucosa. Vomiting obviously will affect absorption, since the vomitus should contain unabsorbed material which, if left in the stomach, could jeopardize the patient. A word of caution is in order here. Too frequently the assumption is made that, because the patient vomited or because gastric lavage was initiated promptly, further absorption will no longer occur because all foreign matter has been removed. Both emesis and lavage have been shown to have limited therapeutic effectiveness. If absorption is incomplete, whatever the reason, predicting the future clinical course of a patient is well-nigh impossible. This projection is best made when one is certain that the patient is in a postabsorptive stage and, hence, on the declining portion of the time-concentration curve.

Should one be reasonably sure that absorption is complete, any prediction will assume normal metabolism and excretion patterns. For most drugs normal metabolism depends on normal liver function. If the patient's liver is impaired, many biotransformations essential to metabolism may be affected. Oxidation (hydroxylation, dealkylation, or deamination), hydrolysis (deesterification), and synthesis (conjugation – glucuronide, sulfate, or acetate) are essential metabolic reactions, which, if abnormal, will affect the patient's ability to get rid of the effects of a drug.

Impaired renal function can cause similar problems because it affects excretion patterns. These patterns are also altered by urinary pH changes brought about by disease, diet, or therapy. Excretion of phenobarbital and salicylic acid can be enhanced so that it could be life-saving if a high flow of alkaline urine is maintained in the patient. Excretion of amphetamine increases when the urine is acid.

This entire discussion is designed to warn the unwary against making categorical statements about laboratory findings. Within wide latitudes, tentative conclusions can be made, but they must be guarded and circumspect. Experience teaches far better than words.

Caveat interpretor!

REFERENCES

1. **Goodman, L. S. and Gelman, A.,** *The Pharmacological Basis of Therapeutics,* 4th ed., Macmillan, N.Y., 1970.
2. **Sunshine, I.,** *Handbook of Analytical Toxicology,* The Chemical Rubber Co., Cleveland, 1969.
3. **Clarke, E. G. C.,** *Isolation and Identification of Drugs,* Pharmaceutical Press, London, 1969.

GENERAL REFERENCES

Baselt, R. C., Wright, J. A., and Cravey, R. H., Therapeutic and toxic concentrations of more than 100 toxicologically significant drugs in blood, plasma or serum, *Clin. Chem.,* 21, 44, 1975.

Goldstein, A., Aronow, L., and Kalman, S. M., *Principles of Drug Action: The Basis of Pharmacology,* 2nd ed., John Wiley & Sons, N.Y., 1974.

La Du, B. N., Mandel, H. G., and Way, E. L., *Fundamentals of Drug Metabolism and Drug Disposition,* Williams and Wilkins, Baltimore, 1971.

Section I

Methods for Specific Substances

ACETAMINOPHEN

PRINCIPLE

Overdosage of acetaminophen can result in hepatic necrosis; hence, tests for the presence of this drug should be done very quickly. Procedure A describes a simple color test which can be performed in minutes on the urine. Acetaminophen and its metabolites are hydrolyzed in acid solution to *p*-aminophenol, which is then coupled with *o*-cresol to give a distinctive indophenol blue. Quantitation and confirmation of acetaminophen may be made by saturating plasma with ammonium sulfate and then extracting with ether. The ether extract is then evaporated to dryness and the acetaminophen in the residue is determined spectrophotometrically (Procedure B) by dissolving the residue in ethanol and measuring the absorbance at 250 nm. Alternatively, acetaminophen is extracted into ether from aqueous solutions. The solvent is evaporated and the drug and internal standard (*N*-butyryl-*p*-aminophenol) are acetylated prior to chromatographic analysis (Procedure C).

TYPE A PROCEDURE

D. J. Berry and J. Grove

REAGENTS

All chemicals should be analytical reagent grade.

1. Saturated *o*-cresol reagent
   Shake 10 ml of *o*-cresol with one liter of distilled water. Allow to stand for 24 hr before use.
2. Ammonium hydroxide, 4*N*
   Dilute 284 ml of 0.880 ammonia to one liter with distilled water.
3. Concentrated hydrochloric acid
4. Reference urine
   Use an aliquot of a urine sample obtained from a patient who took 1 g of acetaminophen in the previous 24-hr period.

PROCEDURE

1. Pipet 1 ml of sample (test urine, reference urine, and water as a reagent blank) and 1 ml of concentrated hydrochloric acid into separate test tubes and heat in a boiling water bath for 10 min.
2. Dilute 0.1 ml of this solution to 10 ml with *o*-cresol reagent and add 2 ml of 4*N* ammonium hydroxide.
3. Observe color. A blue color is an indication that paracetamol may be present.

INTERPRETATION (see p. 7)

The formation of the indophenol blue is extremely sensitive. A strong positive can be obtained with urines from volunteers who have taken 1 g of acetaminophen 24 hr previously.

INTERFERING SUBSTANCES

Acetaminophen and *p*-aminophenol are metabolites of phenacetin; hence, this reaction can give positive results after ingestion of phenacetin.

REFERENCE

Berry, D. J. and Grove, J., Emergency toxicological screening for drugs commonly taken in overdose, *J. Chromatogr.,* 80, 205, 1973.

TYPE B PROCEDURE

John Epton and Jeff Grove

APPARATUS

1. Recording spectrophotometer

REAGENTS

All chemicals should be analytical reagent grade.

1. Redistilled diethyl ether
2. Ammonium sulfate (ether washed)
3. Acetaminophen stock solution, 10 mg/dl
   Dissolve 10 mg of acetaminophen in ethanol and dilute to 100 ml with ethanol.
4. Acetaminophen reference solution, 1.0 mg/dl
   Dilute 10 ml of the stock solution to 100 ml with ethanol.
5. Ethanol

PROCEDURE

1. Saturate 1 ml of sample (plasma, reference solution) with solid ammonium sulfate in a 30-ml centrifuge tube and extract with 25 ml of diethyl ether. (The plasma forms a hard pad from which the ether can be decanted or aspirated.)
2. Centrifuge, aspirate the upper organic layer into a clean tube, and evaporate to dryness.
3. Redissolve the residue in 4 ml of ethanol and determine its UV absorption between 220 to 360 nm in 1-cm cuvettes using ethanol in the reference cuvette. Dilute the sample solution, if necessary.
4. Compare the absorbance of the sample at 250 nm with that of the 10 mg/dl acetaminophen reference solution analyzed simultaneously with the test sample.

CALCULATION

Acetaminophen concentration

$$C_S = \frac{A_S}{A_R} \times C_R \times \frac{D_S}{D_R}$$

where

C_S = concentration of the specimen
A_S = absorbance of the specimen at 250 nm
A_R = absorbance of the reference solution at 250 nm
C_R = concentration of the reference solution
D_S = volume of ethanol used to dissolve the sample extract
D_R = volume of ethanol used to dissolve the reference extract

INTERPRETATION (see p. 7)

Following the ingestion of 1 g of acetaminophen, the maximum plasma concentration ranges from 10 to 25 μg/ml and is attained within 0.5 to 2 hr. The normal plasma half-life is 2 hr. Following overdosage the plasma concentration must always be assessed in relation to the time after ingestion.

ACCURACY AND PRECISION

The mean recovery of paracetamol from plasma was 95% with a standard deviation of ±5%.

INTERFERING SUBSTANCES

A direct extraction of body fluids will result in a number of drugs interfering in the assay. In general, however, their levels are much lower than those found in paracetamol overdosage. If salicylate (maximum at 236 and 305 nm) and phenylbutazone (maximum at 240 nm) are present, erroneous results can be obtained, and alternative procedures (such as Type C) should be used.

TYPE C PROCEDURE

L. F. Prescott

APPARATUS

1. Pasteur pipets
2. Glass-stoppered test tubes, 15 ml
3. Centrifuge
4. Glass-stoppered centrifuge tubes, 15 ml
5. Rotary vacuum evaporator
6. Vortex mixer
7. Gas chromatograph equipped with a 1 mV recorder, with a glass column 4′ × ¼″ o.d., packed with 1 or 3% HI-EFF 8BP (cyclohexanedimethanol succinate) on 80/10 mesh Gas Chrom Q

   Operating Conditions

   Gas Flow Rates:
   - air – 300 ml/min
   - hydrogen – 40 ml/min
   - nitrogen – 60 ml/min

   Temperatures:
   - column – 230°C
   - injection port – 250°C
   - detector – 280°C

REAGENTS

All chemicals should be analytical reagent grade.

1. Phosphate buffer, 1*M*, pH 7.4
2. Sodium chloride
3. Ethyl ether, redistilled
4. Acetaminophen stock solutions, 50 mg/dl
   Dissolve 50 mg of acetaminophen in 100 ml of water and 100 ml of drug-free plasma.
5. Acetaminophen urine control solutions, 2.5 and 25 mg/dl
   Dilute 1.0 ml of the aqueous acetaminophen stock solution to 20 ml with water. Dilute 10.0 ml of the aqueous acetaminophen stock solution to 20 ml with water.
6. Acetaminophen plasma control solutions, 2.5 and 25 mg/dl
   Dilute 1.0 and 10 ml, respectively, of the plasma acetaminophen stock solution to 20 ml with drug-free plasma.
7. Internal standards, 1 mg/dl and 10 mg/dl
   Dissolve 50 mg of *N*-butyryl-*p*-aminophenol in ethyl ether and dilute to 500 ml with ethyl ether to give 10 mg/dl. Dilute 50 ml of this solution with ether to 500 ml to give 1 mg/dl.
8. Pyridine
9. Acetic anhydride

PROCEDURE

1. Add 2 ml of sample (plasma, urine, and plasma control solutions) to 1 ml of pH 7.4 phosphate buffer in a 15-ml glass-stoppered test tube. Appropriate dilutions are made of samples containing more than 25 mg/dl.
2. Add 5 ml of the appropriate internal standard solution according to the sample concentration. Extract by gently shaking on a mechanical shaker (horizontally at 150 strokes/min for 10 min).
3. Centrifuge to separate the phases.
4. Transfer the supernatant ether into a dry 10-ml tapered centrifuge tube and evaporate the solvent using a rotary vacuum evaporator at 30°C.
5. Add 1 μl of pyridine and 5 μl of acetic anhydride to the residue. Vortex the tube to help dissolve the residue. Stopper the tubes and incubate them at 100°C for 10 min. With concentrations above 5.0 mg/dl, use 2 μl of pyridine and 15 μl of acetic anhydride.
6. Add 15 μl of ethanol, vortex, and inject 1 to 3 μl into the gas chromatograph.
7. Determine the ratio of the peak heights of acetaminophen to that of *N*-butyryl-*p*-aminophenol (R).

CALCULATION

$$C_S = C_p \times \frac{R_s}{R_p}$$

where

C_S = the concentration of the sample
C_P = the concentration of plasma control solution
R_S = the ratio of the peak heights for the sample
R_P = the ratio of the peak heights for the plasma control solution

INTERPRETATION (see p. 7)

Following the ingestion of 1 g of acetaminophen, the maximum plasma concentration ranges from 10 to 25 μg/ml and is usually attained within 0.5 to 2 hr. The normal plasma half-life is 2 hr. Following overdosage the plasma concentration must always be assessed in relation to the time after ingestion (Figure 1). Liver damage may occur at levels above the line shown, and is invariably present at levels above 300 μg/ml 4 hr after ingestion.

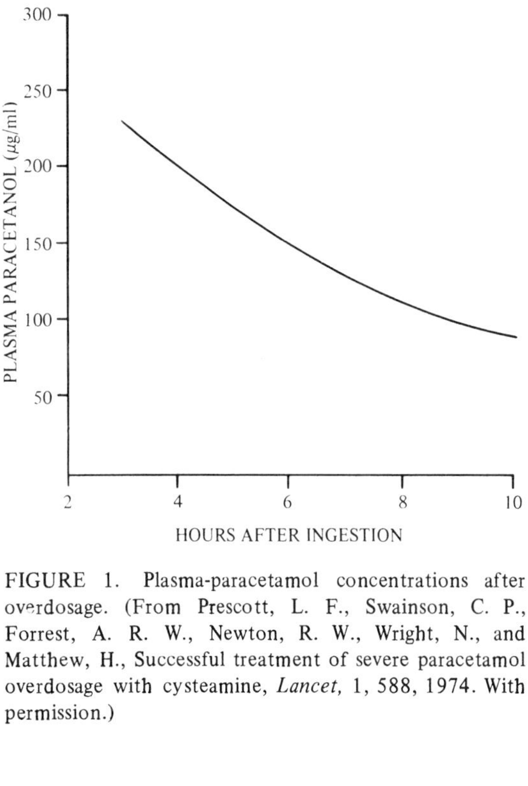

FIGURE 1. Plasma-paracetamol concentrations after overdosage. (From Prescott, L. F., Swainson, C. P., Forrest, A. R. W., Newton, R. W., Wright, N., and Matthew, H., Successful treatment of severe paracetamol overdosage with cysteamine, *Lancet,* 1, 588, 1974. With permission.)

SENSITIVITY AND PRECISION

The sensitivity of the method is 1 μg/ml. Over the ranges 5 to 25 and 50 to 500 μg/ml, the standard deviation of an analysis is 3 to 4%.

INTERFERING SUBSTANCES

p-Aminophenol will yield the same acetylated derivative as acetaminophen, but this is of little consequence since, in man, *p*-aminophenol is not detectable in biological fluids following ingestion of acetaminophen. A single large peak, whose retention time is longer than that of the internal standard's, may be encountered. Although its identity has not been established, it does not interfere with the quantitative result. Acetanilide and phenacetin both yield acetaminophen as a metabolite, and if taken by man will interfere.

REFERENCES

Mrochek, J. E., Katz, S., Christie, W. H., and Dinsmore, S. R., Acetaminophen metabolism in man as determined by high-resolution gas liquid chromatography, *Clin. Chem.,* 20, 1086, 1974.

Prescott, L. F., Gas liquid chromatographic estimation of paracetamol, *J. Pharm. Pharmacol.,* 23, 807, 1971.

Prescott, L. F., Swainson, C. P., Forrest, A. R. W., Newton, R. W., Wright, N., and Matthew, H., Successful treatment of severe paracetamol overdosage with cysteamine, *Lancet,* 1, 588, 1974.

Thomas, B. H. and Coldwell, B. R., Estimation of phenacetin and paracetamol in plasma and urine by gas liquid chromatography, *J. Pharm. Pharmacol.,* 24, 243, 1972.

AMITRIPTYLINE

PRINCIPLE

Amitriptyline is extracted from an alkaline solution of the biologic specimens with *n*-hexane and subsequent back-extraction into a solution of ceric sulfate in sulfuric acid. The aqueous acid extract is refluxed with *n*-heptane, oxidizing the drug to anthraquinone which, in contrast to unoxidized amitriptyline, has a unique and high molar UV absorbance. The anthraquinone can be measured both spectrophotometrically and by gas-liquid chromatography (Procedure B). In Procedure C amitriptyline and other basic drugs, including nortriptyline, are extracted into an organic solvent from an alkaline solution of the specimen. After the addition of trifluoroacetic anhydride the extract is concentrated and analyzed by gas chromatography.

TYPE B PROCEDURE

Jack E. Wallace and Horace E. Hamilton

APPARATUS

1. Separatory funnels, 250 ml
2. Filter paper, Whatman #541
3. Graduated cylinders, glass-stoppered
4. Round-bottom flasks, 50 to 125 ml
5. Magnetic stirrers and Teflon® stirring bars
6. Reflux condenser
7. UV spectrophotometer, recording
8. Rotary vacuum evaporator

REAGENTS

All chemicals should be analytical reagent grade.

1. Amitriptyline stock solution, 50 mg/dl (as free base)
   Dissolve the appropriate amount of the available amitriptyline salt in water and dilute to 100 ml with water.
2. Amitriptyline reference solution, 1 mg/dl
   Dilute 1.0 ml of the amitriptyline stock solution to 50.0 ml with water. Other dilutions of the stock solution may be made as needed.
3. Ceric sulfate-sulfuric acid reagent
   Add 76 ml of concentrated sulfuric acid, very slowly and with constant stirring, to a large beaker containing 6.25 g of ceric sulfate and 174 ml of water. The solution is facilitated by stirring the mixture for 30 min at 80 to 100°C. The solution is stable for 2 months at room temperature.
4. *n*-Hexane, spectrograde
5. *n*-Heptane, spectrograde

PROCEDURE

1. Adjust urine or tissue homogenates to pH 11 to 12. Whole blood, gastric content, and plasma are adjusted to pH 7.2 to 7.8.
2. Place 2 to 5 ml (g) of each sample in 250-ml separatory funnels, each containing 100 ml of *n*-hexane, and shake the mixtures vigorously for 3 min. Include one 5-ml water sample as a reagent blank. Allow the phases to separate.
3. Filter the hexane layer into a graduated cylinder, using Whatman #541 filter paper or its equivalent. Retain a 90-ml aliquot and discard the remainder.
4. Add 10 ml of the ceric sulfate-sulfuric acid reagent to the *n*-hexane and shake the mixture vigorously for at least 3 min. Allow the phases to separate.
5. Transfer 9 ml of the subsequent aqueous layer to a 250-ml round-bottom flask.
6. Add 5 ml of the *n*-heptane and a Teflon®-coated magnetic stirring bar to the flask.
7. Position the flask in a heating mantle and attach it to a reflux condenser.

8. Reflux the contents of the flask for 30 min at a high reflux rate.
9. Cool the mixture, then separate the *n*-heptane from the aqueous solution.
10. Determine the absorbance of the *n*-heptane from 240 to 280 nm. Use the *n*-heptane obtained from processing the water reagent blank as the reference solution. Note the absorbance maxima at 260 and 250 nm (Figure 1).
11. An aliquot of the *n*-heptane can be directly injected into the column of a gas-liquid chromatograph if a chromatographic analysis is desired (Figure 2).

CALCULATION

The absorbance of the reaction product has a linear relationship to the concentration of amitriptyline in the specimen at either 250 or 260 nm. A reference calibration curve may be used for rapid estimation. For more precise results, compare the absorbance of the specimen with that obtained by analyzing reference solutions of appropriate concentrations.

INTERPRETATION (see p. 7)

Therapeutic blood levels are in the range of 3 to 40 μg/dl. Several investigators indicate that blood amitriptyline concentrations in fatal poisoning exceed 1.0 mg/dl. Thus, the method as described is not suitable for detection of amitriptyline in blood, except for very toxic incidents. The procedure is suitable for determining levels of the drug in urine and tissue specimens.

INTERFERING SUBSTANCES

Captodiamine, azacyclonol, cyclizine, diphenhydramine, hydroxyzine, and pipradol produce a reaction product with absorbance at 250 nm. None of these, however, shows maximum absor-

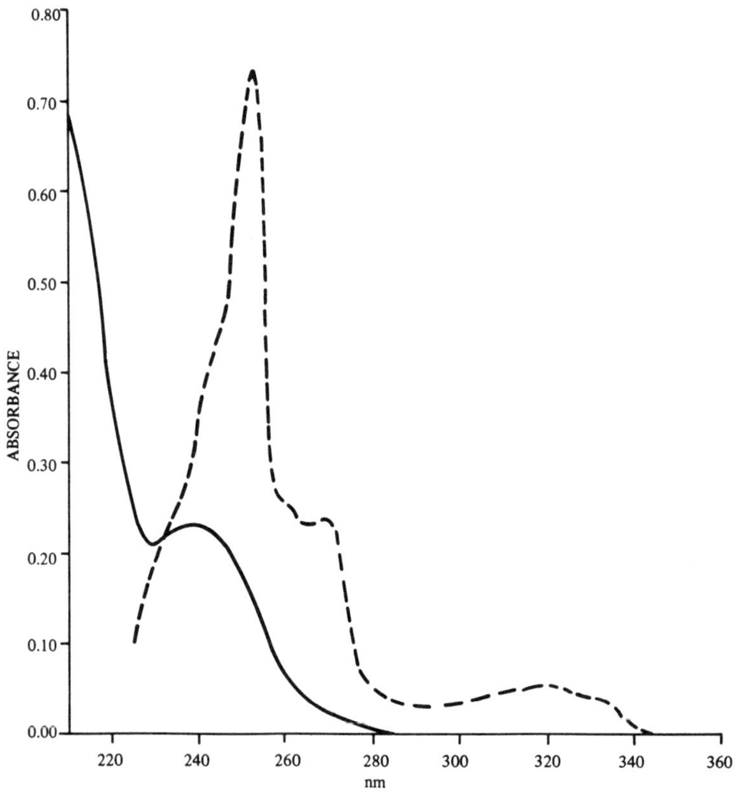

FIGURE 1. UV absorption spectra of amitriptyline in water (5 μg/ml of solid) and amitriptyline oxidation product corresponding to a sample of equivalent concentration in heptane (broken line).

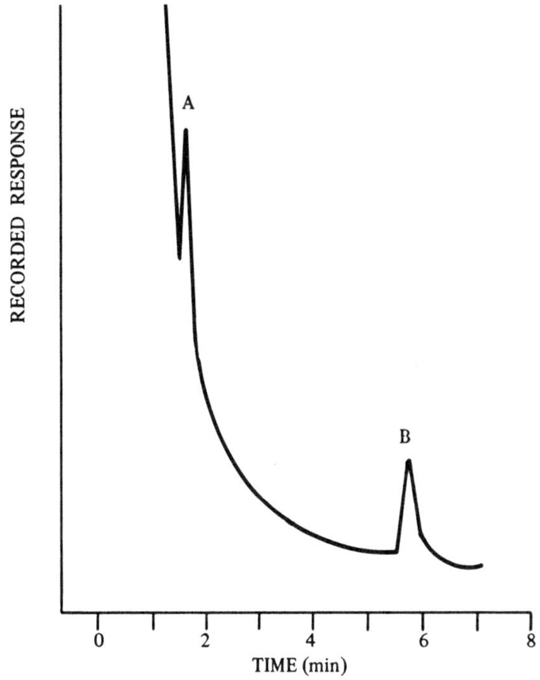

FIGURE 2. Gas chromatograph of (A) benzophenone and (B) anthraquinone, separated on 3% OV-17 (2.0 m × 4 mm i.d. glass column) at a column temperature of 240°C and nitrogen flow rate of 45 ml/min (Shimadzu 4BMPF, FID detector 300°C). Quantities injected were 0.0625 and 0.25 μg of benzophenone and anthraquinone, respectively.

bance at 250 nm, nor exhibits the absorption pattern characteristic of amitriptyline reaction products. With the exception of captodiamine, all the compounds cited yield a product whose maximum absorbance is at 247 nm (probably benzophenone). Although this method does not distinguish between amitriptyline and its chief metabolic products, *des-N*-methylamitriptyline and 10-hydroxy-amitriptyline, or between amitriptyline and nortriptyline, these distinctions are not likely to carry forensic or clinical importance.

REFERENCES*

Hamilton, H. E. and Wallace, J. E., Spectrophotometric and gas-liquid chromatographic determination of amitriptyline, *Anal. Chem.*, in press, 1974.

Royds, R. B. and Night, A. H., Tricyclic antidepressant poisoning, *Practitioner*, 204, 282, 1970.

Sunshine, I. and Baumler, J., A fatal case of poisoning with amitriptyline, *Nature*, 199, 1103, 1963.

Wallace, J. E. and Dahl, E. V., The determination of amitriptyline by ultraviolet spectrophotometry, *J. Forensic Sci.*, 12, 484, 1967.

TYPE C PROCEDURE

R. A. Braithwaite

APPARATUS

1. Centrifuge tube, glass-stoppered, 30 ml
2. Centrifuge tube, conical, 10 ml
3. Gas chromatograph, dual column (Pye 104 Model 24), equipped with a 1 mV recorder (Honeywell) and a silanized coiled glass column, 7′ × ¼″ i.d., packed with 1% PVP (polyvinyl pyrrolidinone) and 3% Versamid 900 on 80 to 100 mesh Chromosorb W HP

   Operating Conditions

   Gas Flow Rate:
   nitrogen (carrier gas) – 60 ml/min

   Temperatures:
   column – 215°C
   injection port – 240°C
   detector – 240°C

Both ends of the column are packed with a small plug of silanized glass wool. The packed column is conditioned for 48 hr at 245°C, with nitrogen flowing through the column at a rate of 60 ml/min. The column may be allowed to cool to room temperature, but the nitrogen flow must be maintained during this cooling period. It is also desirable to maintain the nitrogen flow when the column is not in use.

*For an updated list of reference material, see References, p. 21.

REAGENTS

All chemicals should be analytical reagent grade.

1. Sulfuric acid, 1*N*
   Dilute 3 ml of concentrated sulfuric acid with water, cool, then dilute to 100 ml.
2. Petroleum ether (40/60°)
3. Sodium hydroxide, 2*N*
   Dissolve 8 g of sodium hydroxide in water and dilute to 100 ml.
4. Sodium sulfate, anhydrous
5. Triphenylamine internal control stock solution, 15 mg/100 ml
   Dissolve 15 mg of triphenylamine in petroleum ether. Dilute this solution to 100 ml with petroleum ether. Stored at room temperature, this solution is stable for 2 to 3 months.
6. Triphenylamine internal control working solution, 0.15 mg/100 ml
   Dilute 1 ml of the triphenylamine stock solution to 100 ml with petroleum ether.
7. Chloroform, dry
8. Amitriptyline stock solution, 100 mg/100 ml
   Dissolve 114.5 mg of amitriptyline hydrochloride in water, alkalize the solution, then extract it twice, using 30 ml of petroleum ether each time. Dilute the combined extracts to 100 ml with petroleum ether.
9. Amitriptyline reference solutions
   Place 20.0, 10.0, 5.0, and 2.0 ml of amitriptyline stock solution in 100-ml volumetric flasks. Add 15 mg of triphenylamine to each flask, then dilute the resulting solutions to 100 ml with petroleum ether. Dilute 1 ml of each solution to 10 ml with petroleum ether. Stored at room temperature, the reference solutions are stable for several months.

PROCEDURE

1. Add 2.0 ml of 1*N* sulfuric acid to 10 ml of urine in a 30-ml glass-stoppered centrifuge tube.
2. Extract this mixture with 10 ml of petroleum ether.
3. Centrifuge the extract for 15 min at 3,000 rpm. Discard the petroleum ether.
4. Add 2.0 ml of 2*N* sodium hydroxide and 10 ml of petroleum ether, shake well, then centrifuge the mixture.
5. Remove an 8-ml aliquot of the petroleum ether extract and place it in a centrifuge tube containing 3 g of anhydrous sodium sulfate.
6. Add 10 ml of petroleum ether to the urine specimen in the first tube, shake, then centrifuge the mixture.
7. Remove a second 8-ml aliquot of the petroleum ether extract and add it to the first. Shake the combined extracts, then allow the tube to stand for 10 min.
8. Transfer the dried extract to a suitable container. Wash the sodium sulfate remaining in the tube with 5 ml petroleum ether, then add the washing to the dried extract.
9. Add 1.0 ml of triphenylamine working solution to the dried extract, then evaporate the mixture to approximately 5 ml. Transfer the concentrate quantitatively to a 10-ml centrifuge tube, then continue the evaporation to dryness, using a water bath at 60°C.
10. Dissolve the residue in 100 μl of dry chloroform.
11. Inject 5 μl of the dissolved residue into the gas chromatograph, making sure that the operating conditions stated above are met.
12. Inject 5 μl of each of the amitriptyline reference solutions. The relative retention time of amitriptyline with respect to triphenylamine should be 1.8 min.

CALCULATION

The ratio of the peak height of amitriptyline to that of triphenylamine is a linear function over the range from 0.01 to 0.1 μg of amitriptyline (equivalent to amitriptyline concentrations ranging from 0.02 to 0.2 μg/ml of urine).

INTERPRETATION (see p. 7)

Following oral ingestion of a 50-mg dose of amitriptyline, approximately 0.15% of the dose appears unchanged in the first 24-hr urine. In cases of amitriptyline overdosage, nortriptyline will be found in the urine.

ACCURACY AND PRECISION

When 0.5 to 2.0 μg of amitriptyline was added to urine, 90 ± 7% was recovered.

INTERFERING SUBSTANCES

Amitriptyline is well separated from other tricyclic antidepressants (Figure 1).

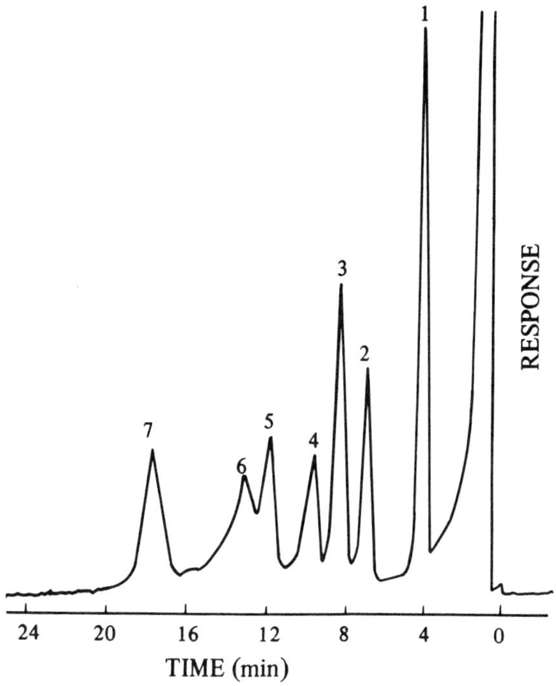

FIGURE 1. Separation of (1) triphenylamine, (2) amitriptyline, (3) imipramine, (4) nortriptyline, (5) desipramine, (6) protriptyline, and (7) prothiadene. (From Braithwaite, R. A. and Whatley, J. S., specific gas chromatographic determination of amitriptyline in human urine following therapeutic doses, *J. Chromatogr.*, 49, 303, 1970. With permission of Elsevier Publishing Co., Amsterdam.)

REFERENCES

Borga, O. and Garle, M., A gas chromatographic method for the quantitative determination of nortriptyline and some of its metabolites in human plasma and urine, *J. Chromatogr.,* 68, 77, 1972.

Braithwaite, R. A. and Whatley, J. A., Specific gas-chromatographic determination of amitriptyline in human urine following a therapeutic dose, *J. Chromatogr.,* 49, 303, 1970.

Braithwaite, R. A. and Widdop, B., A specific gas-chromatographic method for the measurement of "steady-state" plasma levels of amitriptyline and nortriptyline in patients, *Clin. Chim. Acta,* 35, 461, 1971.

Hucher, H. B. and Stauffer, S. C., GLC method for quantitative determination of amitriptyline in human plasma, *J. Pharm. Sci.,* 63, 297, 1974.

Norheim, G., Simultaneous determination of amitriptyline and nortriptyline in post mortem blood and urine using GLC, *J. Chromatogr.,* 88, 403, 1974.

AMPHETAMINE AND METHAMPHETAMINE

PRINCIPLE

As basic drugs, amphetamines are extracted from alkaline urine by an organic solvent. This solvent may be evaporated to dryness and the residue thin-layer chromatographed to determine if amphetamine is present (Procedure A). Back-extraction of the organic solvent extract into an acid, the addition of base to make the acid extract basic once again, and reextraction with a small volume of organic solvent sufficiently cleans the specimen for gas-chromatographic analysis. Free amphetamine drugs are separated by a 10% Apiezon-10% KOH column. Further confirmation is obtained by reacting the amphetamine drugs with trichloroacetyl chloride to obtain amphetamine *N*-trichloroacetamide derivatives which are separated by a 3% OV-17 column (Procedure B). Greater sensitivity may be obtained if an electron-capture detector (Procedure C) is used instead of a flame ionization detector. An Alternate Type C Procedure is available for the direct analysis of a biological specimen – immunoassay. The principles and procedures of this method are discussed subsequently.

TYPE A PROCEDURE

Irving Sunshine

APPARATUS

1. Culture tubes with Teflon®-lined screw caps
2. Rotator
3. Water bath
4. Thin-layer chromatography equipment: (a) silica gel G plates; (b) developing tanks; (c) spray bottles; (d) UV light source, 254 nm

REAGENTS

All chemicals should be analytical reagent grade.

1. Ammonium chloride buffer, pH 9.2
   To a saturated aqueous solution of ammonium chloride, add enough concentrated ammonium hydroxide to bring the pH of the mixture to 9.2.
2. Chloroform isopropanol extraction solution
   Mix 450 ml of chloroform and 50 ml of isopropanol.
3. Ethanolic acid mixture
   Carefully add 10 ml of concentrated sulfuric acid to 90 ml with ethanol.
4. Methanol
5. Developing solution
   Mix 85 ml of ethyl acetate, 10 ml of methanol, and 5 ml of ammonium hydroxide just prior to developing the plates. Do not use this solvent for developing more than two successive sets of plates.
6. Phosphate buffer, pH 10
   Adjust 500 ml of 0.4*M* KH_2PO_4 to pH 10 with 2*N* NaOH. Dilute to one liter with water.
7. Ninhydrin®, 4 mg/ml
   Dissolve 40 mg of Ninhydrin® in the pH 10 buffer and dilute to 10 ml with the buffer.
8. Phenylacetaldehyde, 40 m*M*
   Dilute 4.8 ml of phenylacetaldehyde to one liter with ethanol.
9. Amphetamine sulfate reference solution, 1 μg/ml
   Dissolve 17.0 mg of amphetamine sulfate, or 12.5 mg of amphetamine hydrochloride, in 95% ethanol. Dilute this solution to 10.0 ml with additional 95% ethanol. Add a drop of hydrochloric acid, if necessary, to affect complete solution. Prepare reference solutions for methamphetamine, phenylpropanolamine, or other amphetamine derivatives in a similar manner.

PROCEDURE

1. To a 35-ml screw-top tube, add 5 ml of sample, 2 ml of ammonium chloride buffer (pH 9.2), and 20 ml of the chloroform:isopropanol mixture. Be sure to include known amphetamine reference samples in each analysis.
2. Rotate this mixture for 30 min and then centrifuge the tubes.
3. Aspirate the aqueous (upper) layer, and filter the organic (lower) layer with Whatman #1 filter paper into a clean 35-ml screw-top tube.
4. Evaporate the extract just to dryness in a 60°C water bath under an air stream. When evaporation is half completed, add 2 drops of the ethanolic sulfuric acid.
5. Dissolve the residue in 25 μl of methanol, and spot 15 to 20 μl of the solution on a silica gel G thin layer plate.
6. Develop the plate for 15 to 18 min in the developing solution.
7. Dry the plate for 10 min at 70°C. Spray first with Ninhydrin® and then overspray with the phenylacetaldehyde solution. After about 15 min at room temperature, bluish-green fluorescent amphetamine spots under long wavelength UV light indicate that primary amines are present. An alternative to the Ninhydrin®-phenylacetaldehyde spray is fluram (Roche Diagnostics, Nutley, N.J.). The dried plate is oversprayed with triethylamine (10 mg/10 ml of acetone), immediately oversprayed with fluram (20 mg/100 ml of acetone), and then resprayed with triethylamine. After 15 min at room temperature, bluish-green fluorescent spots are observed if the plate is exposed to long wave UV light.
8. Compare the R_f of the spot with that due to the amphetamine control. If they are identical, amphetamine must be confirmed by another method; if not, amphetamine is absent.

INTERPRETATION (see p. 7)

The low therapeutic concentrations of these drugs make detection in blood difficult. Urine is, therefore, the recommended specimen for analysis in the procedure described above. Amphetamine can be detected in urine samples up to 24 hr after administration of a 10.0-mg therapeutic dose. It begins to appear in the urine shortly after oral administration and, after a large dose, continues to be excreted for as long as 7 days. At least 30 to 40% of a dose is excreted unchanged in the urine within 48 hr after ingestion.[1,2]

SENSITIVITY

The Ninhydrin®-phenylacetaldehyde spray test is sensitive to as little as 0.3 μg of amphetamine.

INTERFERING SUBSTANCES

The proposed method effectively distinguishes between amphetamine, methamphetamine, phenylpropanolamine, and a number of similar substances. If a positive reaction is obtained, a portion of the extract saved in Step 5 of the procedure can be used for further verification. This usually is done by some technique other than TLC. If TLC is the only technique available, preparation of the NBD-amphetamine fluorophor and its identification may be helpful. Details for this procedure will be found in an article by Monforte et al.[3]

REFERENCES*

1. **Alles, G. A. and Wisegarver, B. B.,** Amphetamine excretion studies in man, *Toxicol. Appl. Pharmacol.*, 3, 678, 1961.
2. **Dring, L. G., Smith, R. L., and Williams, R. T.,** The metabolic fate of amphetamine in man and other species, *Biochem. J.*, 116, 425, 1970.
3. **Monforte, J., Bath, R. J., and Sunshine, I.,** Fluorometric determination of primary and secondary amines in blood and urine after thin layer chromatography, *Clin. Chem.*, 18, 1329, 1972.

GENERAL REFERENCE

Wallace, J. E., Biggs, J. D., and Ladd, S. L., Determination of amphetamine by ultraviolet spectrophotometry, *Anal. Chem.*, 40, 2207, 1968.

*For an updated list of reference material, see References p. 29.

TYPE B PROCEDURE

Naresh Jain, Thomas Sneath, and Robert Budd

APPARATUS

1. Culture tubes, 16 × 150 mm, with Teflon®-lined screw caps
2. Culture tube racks to hold tubes
3. Variable speed reciprocating shaker (Eberback Corp. Model 6000)
4. Dispo-pipets, 6 in.
5. Medicine dropper bulbs
6. Serological pipets, 10 ml
7. Glass centrifuge tubes, 5 ml
8. Centrifuge tube racks
9. Vortex shaker
10. pH Paper, 0 to 14
11. Syringe, 10 μl
12. Gas chromatograph (Varian Model 2700), dual column, equipped with dual differential electrometer, two flame ionization detectors, and connected to a dual pen recorder. The gas chromatograph contains the following two columns. (A) 6′ × 2 mm i.d. glass column containing 10% Apiezon L-KOH on Hewlett-Packard Chrom W (NAW) 80/100 mesh. Dissolve 2.5 g of KOH in 100 ml of spectrograde methanol, mix with 25 g of Hewlett-Packard Chrom W (NAW), and rotary evaporate to dryness. Dissolve 2.5 g of Apiezon L grease (Arthur H. Thomas) in 100 ml of spectrograde chloroform and add. The mixture is again rotary evaporated to dryness. (B) 6′ × 2 mm i.d. glass column containing 3% OV-17 on HP Chrom W (AW + DMCS) 80/100 mesh (Varian Cat. No. 222).

Operating Conditions (for both columns)

Gas Flow Rates:
- nitrogen (carrier gas) – 45 ml/min
- hydrogen – 30 ml/min
- air – 300 ml/min

Temperatures:
- column – 150°C
- injection port – 220°C
- detector – 220°C

REAGENTS

All chemicals and solvents should be analytical reagent grade.

1. Sodium hydroxide, 1*N*
   Dissolve 40 g of NaOH in distilled water and dilute to 1,000 ml.
2. Sodium hydroxide, 1.5*N*
   Dissolve 60 g of NaOH in distilled water and dilute to 1,000 ml.
3. Sulfuric acid, 0.2*N*
   To 1,000 ml of distilled water, add 11.2 ml of concentrated H_2SO_4. Allow the mixture to reach room temperature and then dilute to 2,000 ml with distilled water.
4. Chloroform, spectrograde
5. Internal standard solution, β-phenethylamine in chloroform/isopropanol, 1.4 μg/ml
   To 950 ml of chloroform, add 50 ml of isopropanol and 1.4 mg of β-phenethylamine (free base) (Eastman Organic Chemicals, Cat. #2642).
6. Trifluoroacetic anhydride solution, 50% v/v
   Add 5 ml of trifluoroacetic anhydride (Matheson, Coleman, and Bell, Cat. #TX1285) to 5 ml of spectrograde chloroform. Store this reagent in a dark bottle at 4°C.
7. Standard reference solution of amphetamine, methamphetamine, and β-phenethylamine, 1 μg/ml
   Dissolve 0.135 g of amphetamine sulfate, 0.124 g of methamphetamine hydrochloride, and 0.100 g of β-phenethylamine in 100 ml of water. Adjust the pH of the solution to 10 with 1*N* NaOH. Extract the mixture twice with 25 ml of spectrograde chloroform. Filter both chloroform extracts into a 100-ml volumetric flask, then dilute to 100 ml with spectrograde chloroform. Discard the aqueous layer after the second extraction. Store in a glass-stoppered container; the reagent is stable and does not require refrigeration.

PROCEDURE

1. Label one 16 × 150 mm culture tube for each specimen and place in a rack.
2. Add 1.0 ml of 1*N* NaOH to each labeled tube.
3. Add 8 ml of the internal standard solution (Reagent 5) to each tube.
4. Add 7 ml of urine sample to the appropriately labeled culture tube.
5. Cap tubes and shake at 70 cpm in a horizontal position on a platform shaker for 15 min.
6. Aspirate and discard the top aqueous layer. *Do Not* remove any organic layer.
7. Add 1.0 ml of 0.2*N* H_2SO_4 to each tube.
8. Cap and shake at 70 cpm in a horizontal position on a platform shaker for 15 min.
9. While the tubes are shaking, label one 5-ml centrifuge tube for each specimen and place them in a rack.
10. Add 0.2 ml of 1.5*N* NaOH and 0.1 ml of spectrograde chloroform to each 5-ml centrifuge tube.
11. Using a 6 in. disposable pipet, transfer the acid extract (top layer) from Step 8 to the appropriately labeled centrifuge tube in Step 10. *Do Not* transfer any of the organic layer.
12. Shake each tube for 15 sec at medium speed on a Vortex. Specimens are now ready for gas-chromatographic analysis.
13. Inject 1 μl of the standard reference solution (Reagent 7) on both columns. The retention times (R_t) of the amphetamines are shown below:

Drug	R_t on Apiezon L-KOH column (min)	R_t on OV-17 column (min)
Amphetamine	1.27	1.01
Methamphetamine	1.70	1.57
β-Phenethylamine (internal standard)	1.06	1.12

14. Inject 1 μl of the chloroform layer of each specimen to be tested on the 10% Apiezon L-10% KOH column. Compare the peak retention times with those of the standards. Determine the peak heights to quantitate the positive samples (see Calculation below). For each specimen found positive for amphetamine or methamphetamine on the Apiezon L-KOH column, draw up 1 μl of the trifluoroacetic anhydride solution (50% v/v) and 1 μl of chloroform extract of the specimen. Inject the mixture onto the 3% OV-17 column. The trifluoroacetamide derivatives of the amines will be formed and appear on the column. Compare their peak retention times with those of the standards. Determine their peak heights to quantitate the positive samples (see Calculation below).

CALCULATION

Calculate the amphetamine and methamphetamine concentrations (μg/ml) in the specimen by the following formula:

$$C_x = C_s \times \frac{H_u}{I_u} \times \frac{I_s}{H_s} \times R$$

where

C_x = amphetamine or methamphetamine concentration in the specimen;
C_s = internal standard (β-phenethylamine) concentration in chloroform, 1.4 μg/ml (Step 3);
H_u = peak height of amphetamine or methamphetamine in the specimen;
H_s = peak height of amphetamine or methamphetamine in the standard reference solution;
I_u = peak height of the internal standard in the specimen;
I_s = peak height of the internal standard in the standard reference solution;
R = volume correction factor for internal standard concentration, i.e.

$$\frac{\text{ml chloroform (Step 3)}}{\text{ml sample (Step 4)}}$$

INTERPRETATION (see p. 7)

Chromatographic Criteria

Positive Specimen

A positive specimen for amphetamine or methamphetamine must contain, on gas-chromatographic analysis, peaks for the internal standard (β-phenethylamine) and amphetamine or methamphetamine of the same identity and concentration on both columns.

Negative Specimen

A negative specimen for amphetamine and/or methamphetamine must contain an internal standard (β-phenethylamine) peak and no peaks for either amphetamine or methamphetamine on the Apiezon L column. If a peak is found on the Apiezon L column which corresponds to either amphetamine or methamphetamine, but no corresponding peak is found on the OV-17 column, then this must be considered a negative. A peak produced only on one column could possibly be due to an interfering substance present in the specimen.

Improper Sample Preparation

A peak for the internal standard must appear on both columns, even when the specimen is negative for amphetamine and/or methamphetamine. If an internal standard peak does not appear on a column, it is an indication that the specimen has not been prepared properly, and the procedure must be repeated.

Blood concentrations ranging from 0.04 to 0.06 μg/ml are achieved 4 to 6 hr following 10- to 15-mg doses of amphetamine. Blood samples from persons suspected of abusing this drug have at least twice this concentration, depending on the amount of drug ingested. The maximum urine concentration following a single 10- to 15-mg dose is between 3 and 5 μg/ml; this is achieved within 24 hr following ingestion. The urines of subjects abusing amphetamine have a concentration at least ten times greater than the concentrations observed following therapeutic dosage. In these instances, concentrations are often in excess of 75 μg/ml, and occasionally as high as 200 to 300 μg/ml.

SENSITIVITY AND PRECISION

The method is sensitive to 0.1 μg/ml of amphetamine and methamphetamine. The quantitation is accurate to ±7%.

INTERFERING SUBSTANCES

The analysis of amphetamines by two different parameters, first analyzing them as free drugs, and secondly, as their trifluoroacetamide derivatives, virtually eliminates false positive results. In other methods which use only one parameter, other basic substances present in the urine may interfere. This procedure has been used to analyze about 10,000 specimens, and no substance has been found that interferes with the identification of amphetamine and methamphetamine.

REFERENCES*

Anggard, E., Gunne, L. M., and Niklasson, F., Gas chromatographic determination of amphetamine in blood, tissue, and urine, *Scand. J. Clin. Lab. Invest.,* 26, 137, 1970.

Barrett, M. J., An integrated gas chromatography program for drug screening in serum and urine, *Perkin-Elmer Corp. Clin. Chem. Newsletter,* 3, 1, 1971.

Bastos, M. L. and Hoffman, D. B., Comparison of methods for the detection of amphetamines, cocaine, and metabolites, *J. Chromatogr. Sci.,* 12, 4, 1974.

Beckett, A. K., Tucker, G. T., and Moffat, A. C., Routine detection and identification in urine or stimulants and other drugs, some of which may be used to modify performance in sport, *J. Pharm. Pharmacol.,* 19, 273, 1967.

Jain, N. C., Sneath, T. S., and Budd, R. D., A rapid gas chromatographic procedure for determining urinary amphetamine and methamphetamine, *Clin. Chem.,* in press.

Lebbe, J. and Lafarge, J. P., Determination of amphetamine in urine by gas-liquid chromatography, *Arch. Mal. Prof.,* 26, 221, 1965.

Lebish, P., Finkle, B. S., and Brackett, J. W., Determination of amphetamine, methamphetamine, and related amines in blood and urine by gas chromatography with hyrodgen flame ionization detector, *Clin. Chem.,* 16, 195, 1970.

Schweitzer, J. W. and Friedhoff, A. J., Amphetamines in human urine: Rapid estimation by gas-liquid chromatography, *Clin. Chem.,* 16, 786, 1970.

*For an updated list of reference material, see References, p. 29.

TYPE C PROCEDURE

Wayne Harrington

APPARATUS

1. Serological pipets, 2 ml
2. Screw-top test tubes with Teflon®-lined caps, 10 ml
3. Pasteur pipets
4. Lang-Levy micropipets, 10, 25, 50, and 100 μl
5. Perkin-Elmer PEP-1 data collection system
6. Gas chromatograph fitted with a ^{63}Ni electron-capture detector and a 6′ × ¼″ o.d. glass column, packed with 5% OV-7 on 80/100 mesh Chromosorb WHP

Operating Conditions

Gas Flow Rate:
argon and 5% methane (carrier gas) – 60 ml/min
Temperatures:
oven – 190°C (2 min), 190 to 260°C at 16°C/min
injection port – 220°C
detector – 300°C

Under the stated conditions, the retention time of amphetamine is 3.9 min and methoxyphenamine is 5.9 min.

REAGENTS

All chemicals should be analytical reagent grade unless otherwise indicated. Aqueous reagents should be prepared with glass distilled water.

1. Internal standard stock solution, 100 μg/ml
   Dissolve 10 mg of methoxyphenamine hydrochloride in water and dilute to 100 ml.
2. Internal standard working solution, 10 μg/ml
   Dilute 1 ml of the stock solution to 10 ml with water.
3. Amphetamine stock reference solution, 100 μg/ml
   Dissolve 13.6 ml of amphetamine sulfate in water and dilute to 10 ml.
4. Amphetamine working reference solutions
   Prepare the following dilutions of the amphetamine stock reference solutions:

Amphetamine concentration (μg/ml)	Stock solution (ml)	Final volume (ml)
Blood		
0.025	0.025	100
0.050	0.050	100
0.100	0.100	100
Urine		
0.5	0.5	100
1.0	1.0	100
5.0	5.0	100

5. Ammonium hydroxide
   Dilute 20 ml of concentrated ammonium hydroxide (28 to 30%) to 100 ml with water.
6. Trichloroacetyl chloride
7. Toluene, pesticide quality
8. Sodium hydroxide, 6*N*
   Dissolve 24 g of sodium hydroxide in water and dilute to 100 ml.

PROCEDURE

1. Blood analysis – To 2 ml of whole blood in a 10-ml screw-top test tube, add 10 μl of the internal standard working solution, 2 ml of ammonium hydroxide, and 1 ml of toluene. Parallel this and all subsequent operations with 2 ml of each of the blood amphetamine reference solutions. Proceed with Step 3.
2. Urine analysis – To 2 ml of urine in a 10-ml screw-top test tube, add 100 μl of the internal standard working solution, 2 ml of ammonium hydroxide, and 1 ml of toluene. Parallel this and all subsequent operations with 2 ml of each of the urine amphetamine reference solutions. Proceed with Step 3.
3. Rotate the mixtures for 30 min, and centrifuge the tubes to separate the layers.
4. Transfer the toluene (upper) layer to a clean 10-ml screw-top test tube, taking care not to include any of the aqueous (lower) layer.
5. Add 10 μl of trichloroacetyl chloride, mix by vortexing the tubes gently, then cap the tubes and allow them to stand at ambient temperature for 30 min.

6. Add 2 ml of 6*N* sodium hydroxide to the derivatized extract, vortex vigorously, and centrifuge to separate the two layers. The vortexing must be sufficiently vigorous to produce a water-white, crystal-clear toluene (upper) layer.
7. Inject a 3-μl aliquot of the toluene (upper) layer into the gas chromatograph under the operating conditions stated above.
8. For each sample and reference solution analyzed, calculate the ratio of the area of the amphetamine peak to that of the internal standard peak.

CALCULATION

To determine the amphetamine concentration in blood or urine sample, compare the calculated peak area ratio with one obtained from the parallel analysis of the amphetamine reference solutions.

INTERPRETATION (see p. 7)

Blood concentrations ranging from 0.04 to 0.06 μg/ml are achieved 4 to 6 hr following 10- to 15-mg doses of amphetamine. Blood samples from persons suspected of abusing this drug have at least twice this concentration, depending on the amount of drug ingested. The maximum urine concentration following a single 10- to 15-mg dose is between 3 and 5 μg/ml; this is achieved within 24 hr following ingestion. The urines of subjects abusing amphetamine have a concentration at least ten times greater than the concentrations observed following therapeutic dosage. In these instances, concentrations are often in excess of 75 μg/ml, and occasionally as high as 200 to 300 μg/ml.

PRECISION AND SENSITIVITY

This method of amphetamine analysis shows a coefficient of variation of 6.5% over the range 0.025 to 5.0 μg/ml. Recoveries over the range 0.1 to 5.0 μg/ml are 60 to 65%. Below 0.1 μg/ml they gradually decrease to a value of 40 to 45% at 0.025% μg/ml. Sensitivity is limited by both the decreasing recovery and the presence of solvent impurities. If a sample is known to contain amphetamine, it can usually be quantitated in concentrations as low as 0.005 to 0.010 μg/ml. If the analysis must identify as well as quantitate amphetamine, then 0.015 to 0.020 μg/ml is a reasonable limit of sensitivity.

Table 1

GAS–CHROMATOGRAPHIC RETENTION TIMES FOR PHENETHYLAMINES AND RELATED COMPOUNDS

Generic or chemical name	Relative retention time*
Tuaminoheptane	<0.5
Cyclopentamine	0.97
p-Hydroxyamphetamine	0.99
Mephentermine	1.13
Propylhexedrine	1.15
Methamphetamine	1.26
Tranylcypromine	1.28
Phenylpropanolamine	1.38
Methoxyphenamine	1.51
Nylidrin	1.54
Brompheniramine	1.56
Methoxamine	1.59
Phenmetrazine	1.60
Chlorpheniramine	>1.8
Diethylpropion	>1.8
Ephedrine	>1.8
Methylphenidate	>1.8
Amitriptyline	No response
Benzoic acid	No response
Benzephetamine	No response
Imipramine	No response
Isoproterenol	No response
Isoxsuprine	No response
Methadone	No response
Norepinephrine	No response
Phenformin	No response
Pheniramine	No response
Phenylephrine	No response

*Amphetamine retention time is 3.9 min.

INTERFERING SUBSTANCES

Of the substances listed in Table 1, only *p*-hydroxyamphetamine shows a retention time the same as that of amphetamine. *p*-Hydroxyamphetamine is an amphetamine metabolite, accounting for 3 to 6% of ingested drugs in man. Thus, measurement of combined *p*-hydroxyamphetamine plus amphetamine is not expected to introduce serious error.

The phenothiazines produce a large response from the electron-capture detector; under the program conditions used in this method, they emerge well-after methoxyphenamine; thus, they do not interfere with the detection of amphetamine. Because of their large detector response, if they are present, it is necessary to bake out the column to avoid an elevated baseline on succeeding samples. Elevated baselines are also observed when using other than Teflon®-lined test tube screw caps, nonpesticide grade toluene, or toluene which has come in contact with plastic or rubber.

REFERENCES

Anggard, E., Gunne, L. M., and Niklasson, F., Gas chromatographic determination of amphetamine in blood, tissue, and urine, *Scand. J. Clin. Lab. Invest.*, 26, 137, 1970.

Anggard, E., Jonsson, L. E., Hogmark, A. L., and Gunne, L. M., Amphetamine metabolites in amphetamine psychosis, *Clin. Pharmacol. Ther.*, 14, 870, 1973.

Bastos, M. L. and Hoffman, D. B., Comparison of methods for the detection of amphetamines, cocaine, and metabolites, *J. Chromatogr.*, 12, 4, 1974.

Campbell, D. B., A method for the measurement of therapeutic levels of (+)-amphetamine in human plasma, *J. Pharm. Pharmacol.*, 21, 129, 1969.

Klein, B., Sheehan, J. E., and Greenberg, E., Use of fluorescamine ("Fluram") to detect amphetamine in urine by TLC, *Clin. Chem.*, 20, 272, 1974.

Ramsey, J. and Campbell, D., An ultra rapid method for the extraction of drugs from biological fluids, *J. Chromatogr.*, 63, 303, 1971.

ALTERNATE TYPE C PROCEDURE IMMUNOASSAY

Details for the EMIT procedure will be found on p. 401. Details for the RIA procedure will be found on p. 403.

ARSENIC

PRINCIPLE

The classical Reinsch test (Procedure A) is an adequate presumptive procedure which can indicate whether arsenicals are present in samples of urine or stomach content. This procedure is based on the fact that copper will displace from solution elements below it in the electrochemical series. The copper remaining in the test area is coated by the displaced substance, and the resulting discolored copper wire is an indication of a positive result. The necessary precautions which must be taken to insure a valid conclusion are described in the procedure.

Should one wish to quantitate the arsenic present, a variation of the Gutzeit test is described in Procedure B. The organic matter in the sample is oxidized, as is any arsenical present. The resulting arsenical is then reduced to arsine, and the evolved arsine is trapped in a solution of silver diethyldithiocarbamate, the absorbance of which is a function of the arsenic content of the sample.

TYPE A PROCEDURE

Sidney Kaye

REAGENTS

All chemicals should be analytical reagent grade.

1. Copper strip, 5 × 10 mm, or a spiral of #20 copper wire wound tightly around a glass rod 10 times.
2. Nitric acid, 2.5*N*
   Dilute 15.0 ml of concentrated nitric acid to 100 ml with water.
3. Ethanol, 95%
4. Hydrochloric acid, concentrated
5. Sodium hydroxide, 10*N*
   Dissolve 40 g of sodium hydroxide in water and dilute to 100 ml.
6. Arsenic stock solution, 1 mg/ml
   Dissolve 1.32 g of arsenic trioxide in 10.0 ml of 10*N* sodium hydroxide and add 500 ml of water. Neutralize the solution with concentrated hydrochloric acid, then dilute it to one liter with water.
7. Arsenic reference solutions
   Dilute appropriate amounts of the arsenic stock solution to obtain solutions with concentrations ranging from 1 to 10 μg/ml.
8. Potassium cyanide, 10 g/100 ml
   Dissolve 10 g of potassium cyanide in water and dilute to 100 ml.

PROCEDURE

1. Wash the copper strip or spiral with 2.5*N* nitric acid, then rinse with 95% ethanol and dry.
2. Place 20.0 ml of urine or an aliquot of gastric lavage, vomitus, powders, tablets, or residues, dissolved or suspended in 20.0 ml of water, into a small Erlenmeyer flask. Add 4.0 ml of concentrated hydrochloric acid.
3. Add the freshly washed copper strip or spiral to the flask.
4. Heat the solution gently for about 1 hr.
5. Remove the copper and examine it. A silver deposit indicates that mercury may be present; a dark deposit indicates the presence of arsenic, bismuth, or antimony. A dull black deposit points to arsenic, whereas a shiny black deposit indicates bismuth, and a dark purple sheen indicates antimony. The dull black arsenic deposit is visible if as little as 0.010 mg of arsenic is present. An estimation of the arsenic content in the specimen may be made by comparing the deposit with those obtained from solutions of known arsenic content processed in the same manner.
6. Confirm that the dull black deposit is due to arsenic by placing the coated copper into 2.0 ml of the potassium cyanide solution. If the

black deposit is due to arsenic, it will dissolve; if due to bismuth or antimony, the black deposit will not be removed.

7. To further confirm the presence of arsenic, process a fresh copper strip or spiral as described above, but omit Step 6. Place the coated copper spiral into a small ignition tube. Heat the portion containing the copper very gently with the coolest portion of a Bunsen burner's flame. Allow the tube to cool, then examine it with a low-power microscope. Arsenic, if present, will sublime in the cool portion and can be recognized by the tiny white octahedral crystals typical of arsenic trioxide. Mercury, if present, sublimes into its typical tiny globules, and bismuth or antimony will not interfere.

CALCULATION

Since only approximately 50% of the arsenic present can be recovered by the deposition method, a factor of two should be used to compensate for the partial recovery. A fair estimate of the quantity present may be obtained by comparing the deposit of the unknown with those obtained from reference solutions.

INTERPRETATION (see p. 7)

A discolored black wire is an indication that an arsenical may be present in the sample. Normally there are traces of arsenic in urine, but these are very small and will not be detected in samples of the size suggested for the test described above. A positive test should be confirmed with a more precise quantitative procedure (see Procedure B).

SENSITIVITY

This test is specific for arsenic and sensitive to 0.010 mg.

INTERFERING SUBSTANCES

Parallel analysis of all reagents is necessary to rule out false positive results due to the reagents.

REFERENCE

Kaye, S., A rapid method for the detection and estimation of mercury, bismuth and arsenic in body fluids, *Am. J. Clin. Pathol.*, 14, 83, 1944.

TYPE B PROCEDURE

Irving Sunshine

APPARATUS

1. Kjeldahl flasks, 300 or 500 ml
2. Digestion rack and hood
3. Arsine generator (see Figure 1)
4. Photometer, photoelectric, with 540-nm filter, or a spectrophotometer

REAGENTS

All chemicals should be analytical reagent grade and low in arsenic.

1. Sulfuric acid, concentrated
2. Nitric acid, concentrated
3. Perchloric acid, concentrated
4. Hydrochloric acid, concentrated
5. Potassium iodide, 15 g/100 ml
   Dissolve 15 g of potassium iodide in water and dilute to 100 ml. Discard the solution when it turns yellow.
6. Stannous chloride, 40 g/100 ml
   Dissolve 40 g of stannous chloride in 50.0 ml of hot water. Cool and filter, then add 50.0 ml of concentrated hydrochloric acid.
7. Lead acetate, 10 g/100 ml
   Dissolve 10 g of lead acetate in water and dilute to 100 ml.
8. Sodium hydroxide, 10*N*
   Dissolve 40 g of sodium hydroxide in water and dilute to 100 ml.
9. Arsenic stock solution, 1 mg/ml
   Dissolve 1.32 g of arsenic trioxide in 10 ml of

10N sodium hydroxide. Add 500 ml of water to the solution, then neutralize it with hydrochloric acid. Dilute the solution to one liter with water.

10. Arsenic reference solutions
 Dilute appropriate volumes of the arsenic stock solution to obtain solutions with concentrations ranging from 1 to 10 μg/ml.
11. Color reagent
 Dissolve 1 g of silver diethyldithiocarbamate (Fisher Scientific Co.) in 200 ml of pyridine. Store the solution in a tightly stoppered amber bottle.* This solution is stable if kept refrigerated.
12. Soft glass wool
13. Zinc, granular, 20 to 30 mesh, low in arsenic

SPECIMEN REQUIREMENTS

Vomitus, stomach content, lavage fluids, and especially urine are desirable in connection with acute exposures. Urine is the specimen of choice many hours or days after onset of symptoms. Arsenical concentrations sufficient to permit detection seldom appear in the small blood specimens usually available in nonfatal cases.

Urine, hair, and nail clippings are the specimens of choice for the evaluation of chronic exposure. A considerable hair sample must be supplied, not two or three strands; such small hair samples may be dealt with by neutron-activation analysis, but not by chemical analysis.† Nail clippings from all the fingers and toes are necessary. Following an autopsy, at least 10 g of each tissue to be analyzed must be provided.

PROCEDURE

1. To Kjeldahl flasks containing the specimen, an aliquot of the arsenic reference solution, and another with water as a reagent blank, add 5.0 ml of concentrated sulfuric acid, 25.0 ml of concentrated nitric acid, and one or two boiling chips. After letting the mixture stand for a few minutes, apply gentle heat until the initial vigorous action subsides.
2. Increase the applied heat and digest the sample until it just begins to char. Allow the flask content to cool to room temperature, then add 10.0 to 20.0 ml of nitric acid and 1.0 to 2.0 ml of perchloric acid. *Be certain that the flask content is at room temperature before adding the perchloric acid.*
3. Reheat the flask content. Continue heating until white fumes just begin to appear. The digest should now be clear or straw-colored. If not, add increments of nitric and perchloric acid as above, heating after the addition until the solution clears.
4. Allow the flask content to cool. Add 10.0 ml of water and repeat the digestion until the solution clears.
5. After the digest is cool, transfer it quantitatively to a 50-ml volumetric flask, then dilute to volume with distilled water. Suitable aliquots of this digest containing between 0 and 12 μg of arsenic are then used for the arsenic assay.
6. Add this aliquot to the reaction flask (see Figure 1) and dilute it to 35.0 ml with water. Add 5.0 ml of concentrated hydrochloric acid and 2.0 ml of the potassium iodide solution.
7. After 1 min add the stannous chloride solution drop by drop until the yellow color disappears (about 0.5 ml).
8. Let the mixture stand for 15 min. In the interim put soft glass wool in the scrubber (see Figure 1), add several drops of the lead acetate solution to wet the glass wool, then shake out the excess.
9. Add 3.0 ml of the color reagent to the absorber tube (see Figure 1) and connect the latter to the scrubber with a pinch clamp.
10. Add 3 to 5 g of the granular zinc to the reaction flask containing the sample, then attach the reaction flask to the scrubber (see Figure 1). Allow the evolved gas (arsine) to pass through the color reagent.

*It is worthwhile to place a hood of Parafilm® over the stopper, securing it tightly with a rubber band to prevent contamination of other refrigerated materials with this powerful UV absorber.

† If the upper limit of "normal" hair arsenic is 6 μg per gram, it follows that at least 500 mg of hair would be required for a content of 3 μg of arsenic – the smallest quantity easily dealt with quantitatively. A convenient way to collect a sufficiently large sample is to tie a cord of hair, about twice the thickness of a kitchen match, at several places with thread; then, cut the hair cord as close to the scalp as possible. Segments weighing about 200 mg are suitable for analysis in cases of exposure where a crude dating of the event is to be made; for this purpose the analyst must locate the segment with the highest arsenic content, which is usually many times the highest "normal" content.

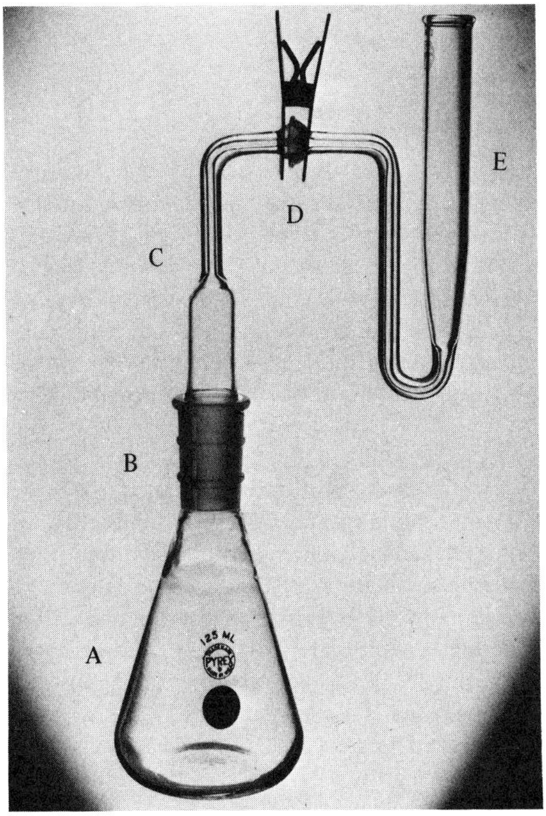

FIGURE 1. Arsine generator. (a) Reaction flask (125-ml Erlenmeyer flask); (b) Standard taper neck; (c) Scrubber (lead acetate on glass wool); (d) Ground glass ball-and-socket joint; (e) Absorber tube (contains silver diethyldithiocarbamate solution). (Reproduced with permission of Fisher Scientific Company, Pittsburgh, Pennsylvania.)

11. After 30 min disconnect the assembly and determine the absorbance of the trapping solution at 525 nm using the processed reagent blank solution as the reference solution.

CALCULATION

The absorbances resulting from analyzing the aqueous arsenic reference solutions are linear functions of their arsenic concentrations. If the reagents used are "arsenic-free," the reagent blank has no significant absorbance at 525 nm. The concentration in the specimen is determined by comparison of its absorbance with those of the arsenic reference solutions or by calculation from a linear plot of arsenic concentration versus absorbance.

INTERPRETATION (see p. 7)

Positive findings are significant, but must be considered in respect to the normal arsenic content. Normal blood arsenic may range from 3 to 7 μg/100 ml. Normal urine may occasionally contain up to 200 μg/liter. Hair and nail arsenic content normally ranges from 20 to 60 μg/100 g.[1,2] Since arsenicals are occasionally used as medications and are permitted in food up to 3.6 μg/g, such "normal" concentrations are to be expected.[3] Chronic or acute intoxication is accompanied by arsenic concentrations that are significantly higher than normal.

ACCURACY AND PRECISION

The described silver diethyldithiocarbamate method yields results within ±5% over a range of 0 to 10 μg/g.

REFERENCES

1. **Vallee, B. L., Ulmer, D. D., and Wacker, W. E. C.,** Arsenic toxicology and biochemistry, *A.M.A. Arch. Environ. Health,* 21, 132, 1960.
2. **Smith, H.,** Interpretation of the arsenic content of human hair, *J. Forensic Sci. Soc.,* 4, 192, 1969.
3. **Hoffman, L. and Gordon, A. D.,** Arsenic in foods. Collaborative comparison of the arsine-molybdenum blue and the silver diethyldithiocarbamate methods, *J. Assoc. Off. Agric. Chem.,* 46, 245, 1963.

BARBITURATES

PRINCIPLE

Barbiturates are still the drugs most frequently involved in adult poisonings. Every laboratory concerned with clinical toxicology must be prepared to analyze a biological specimen to ascertain whether or not any barbiturates are present. A reliable, simple, rapid, presumptive test has yet to be devised. Procedure A is probably the easiest to perform in any laboratory, but is not as reliable or sensitive as one would like. It depends on the formation of a mercury barbiturate salt which is extractable from a biological matrix into an organic solvent. The mercury in this salt is then complexed with dithizone to form an orange mercury dithizonate which is an indication of the presence of a barbiturate in the original sample. When *all* the analytical proscriptions given in Procedure A are followed rigorously, the result may be acceptable if no other alternatives exist.

A preferable procedure (B) requires that the barbiturate be extracted from the biological matrix by an organic solvent. It is then identified by its characteristic UV absorption spectra. This spectrum is obtained by reextracting the organic solvent with an alkaline solution and determining if the UV absorption spectrum of that alkaline solution is similar to one produced by the barbiturates. If so, it indicates that a barbiturate may be present in the sample. Buffering this solution to pH 10 shifts the absorption spectrum characteristically; if this occurs, a presumption can be made that a barbiturate(s) is present. Measuring the difference in absorbance of the two spectra obtained at 260 nm enables a quantitative estimation of the barbiturate concentration. Should a qualitative identification be desired (and it should be) the solution just analyzed should be acidified and extracted with an organic solvent to separate the barbiturates. Evaporation of this solvent leaves a residue which can be analyzed by TLC (Procedure B) or by GC (Procedure C) to indicate which barbiturates are present. Actually, if a gas chromatograph is available, Procedure C is the method of choice because it provides a specific quantitative analysis of the biological specimen in a very simple way. The barbiturate is extracted into toluene and then concentrated upon reextraction into methanolic trimethylanilinium hydroxide, a reagent which derivatizes barbiturates upon injection of an aliquot into the gas chromatograph. The resulting chromatograph can be used to identify and quantitate the barbiturates present. An Alternate Type C Procedure is available for the direct analysis of a biological specimen – immunoassay. The principles and procedures of this method are discussed subsequently.

TYPE A PROCEDURE

James C. Valentour and Beverly Lorenzo

APPARATUS

1. Culture tubes with Teflon® lined screw-caps, 16 × 125 mm, (Kimax #45066A)
2. Test tubes, 15 × 100 mm
3. Filter paper (E & D 615, fast filtering), 9 cm
4. Centrifuge

REAGENTS

All chemicals should be analytical reagent grade.

1. Barbiturate stock solution, 50 mg/dl
   Dissolve 50.0 mg of phenobarbital in a small amount of dilute alkali, add slightly less than 100 ml of water, then acidify the solution with dilute acid and dilute to 100 ml.
2. Barbiturate reference solutions, 1.0 and 0.2 mg/dl
   Dilute 1.00-ml aliquots of the barbiturate stock solution to 50 and 250 ml, respectively, with water.
3. Phosphate buffer, pH 7.0
   Dissolve 1.2 g of sodium hydroxide in water,

add 15.5 g of potassium dihydrogen phosphate monohydrate, and dilute to one liter. Using a pH meter, adjust the buffer to pH 7.0 by adding dilute sodium hydroxide or potassium dihydrogen phosphate as required. Any other nonbarbiturate pH 7.0 buffer will suffice.

4. Dichloromethane
5. Mercuric chloride stock solution, 1.0 g/dl
   Dissolve 0.50 g of mercuric chloride in water, add three drops of concentrated nitric acid, and dilute to 50 ml.
6. Dilute mercuric chloride solution, 20 mg/dl
   Add 1.0 ml of the mercuric chloride stock solution to water containing 0.4 g of sodium bicarbonate and dilute to 50 ml. This solution is stable for 24 hr only.
7. Diphenylthiocarbazone (dithizone), 1 mg/dl
   Dissolve 10 mg of diphenylthiocarbazone in one liter of dichloromethane. Store the solution in a dark bottle at 4°C.

PROCEDURE

1. Pipet 5.0 ml of specimen (barbiturate reference solutions, blood, serum, plasma, urine, or stomach contents and an aqueous sample which serves as a reagent blank) into a screw-capped culture tube. Add 5.0 ml of pH 7.0 buffer and 5.0 ml of dichloromethane.
2. Cap the tubes and mix gently for 1 min. Centrifuge the tubes for 2 min; aspirate and discard the upper (aqueous) layer. To remove blood from the dichloromethane, filter the dichloromethane into a clean screw-capped culture tube.
3. Add 2.0 ml of the dilute mercuric chloride solution to each tube and mix gently for 1 min.
4. Centrifuge the tubes for 2 min; aspirate and discard all of the upper (aqueous) layer.
5. Add 10 ml of water to each tube and mix gently for 1 min.
6. Centrifuge the tubes for 2 min; aspirate and discard *all* of the upper (aqueous) layer. (Any entrained mercuric chloride could yield a false positive result.)
7. Filter the dichloromethane into clean test tubes and add 2.0 ml of the diphenylthiocarbazone solution.
8. Visually compare the color of the samples to those of the standards and reagent blank.

CALCULATION

The concentration of barbiturates present may be estimated by comparing the colors of the dichloromethane solutions of the samples to those of the standards, providing that diphenylthiocarbazone is present in excess. More diphenylthiocarbazone should be used to estimate barbiturate concentrations above 1 mg/dl. An orange color should result if the barbiturate concentration is 1.0 mg/dl or greater, a pale amber color if the barbiturate concentration is 0.2 mg/dl, and a blue color if the barbiturate concentration is lower than 0.2 mg/dl. Normal specimens of blood, urine, or stomach contents produce no color change in the diphenylthiocarbazone solution.

SENSITIVITY

The commonly encountered barbiturates (amobarbital, butabarbital, pentobarbital, secobarbital, and phenobarbital) have 0.2 mg/dl as a lower limit of detection by this method.

INTERPRETATION (see p. 7)

This test is semiquantitative at best. It may suffice when simplicity and time are compelling factors, but should always be confirmed by a more specific and quantitative method.

INTERFERING SUBSTANCES

The following substances also have been found to react with diphenylthiocarbazone to varying degrees: glutethimide, tolbutamide, chlorpropamide, diphenylhydantoin, and primadone. Extreme care must be exercised in performing this test. Incomplete separation or entrainment of the mercuric chloride in the chloroform extract may yield a false positive; hence, the need for a concomitantly analyzed aqueous sample and a confirmation of all positive results by some other analytical procedure.

REFERENCES*

Bjorling, C. O., Berggren, A., and Willman-Johnson, B., Determination of barbituric acid derivatives as mercury complexes, *J. Pharm. Pharmacol.*, 11, 297, 1959.

Curry, A. S., Rapid method for screening for barbiturates, *Br. Med. J.*, 2, 1040, 1973.

Helman, E. Z., Emergency screening of urine, plasma, or gastric contents for barbiturates, *Clin. Chem.*, 16, 797, 1970.

Lubran, M., A new color reaction for the detection and estimation of barbiturates in biological fluids, *Clin. Chim. Acta*, 6, 594, 1961.

Stevenson, W. G., Spectrophotometric determination of blood barbiturate, *Anal. Chem.*, 33, 1374, 1961.

Wallenius, G., Zaar, B., and Lausing, E., A rapid method for determination of barbiturates in serum or urine, *Scand. Lab. Invest.*, 15(Suppl. 69), 252, 1963.

Zaar, B. and Gronwall, A., A micro method for determination of barbiturates in serum as mercuric complexes, *Scand. Lab. Invest.*, 13, 225, 1961.

TYPE B PROCEDURE

Raymond Bath and Gerald Kananen

APPARATUS

1. Pasteur pipets
2. Bottles, glass-stoppered, 60 ml, or separatory funnels, 100 ml
3. Filter paper (E & D #615)
4. UV spectrophotometer, recording
5. Evaporating dishes, porcelain (Coors)
6. Thin-layer chromatography (TLC) equipment: (a) spotting pipets; (b) glass plates, coated with silica gel GF; (c) developing tanks; (d) spray bottles

REAGENTS

All chemicals should be analytical reagent grade.

1. Barbiturate stock solution, 50 mg/100 ml
   Dissolve 50.0 mg of a given barbiturate with water in a volumetric flask and dilute to 100 ml. If the free acid is used, add a trace of alkali to help dissolve the solid, add 50.0 ml of water, then acidify the solution and dilute it to 100 ml with water.
2. Barbiturate reference solution, 5.0 mg/100 ml
   Dilute 1.0 ml of the stock solution to 10.0 ml with water. Store all reference solutions in glass-stoppered bottles in a refrigerator. If enough acid is added to bring the pH to 4 or lower, these refrigerated solutions are stable for at least 3 months. If improperly stored in alkaline solutions, the long-acting barbiturates are the first to deteriorate. A basic solution of sodium phenobarbital deteriorates measurably after 4 days at room temperature.
3. Sodium dihydrogen phosphate, 2.25*M*
   Dissolve 310 g of the monohydrate salt in water and dilute to one liter. Store the solution in a polyethylene bottle.
4. Sodium hydroxide, 0.45*N*
   Dissolve 18 g of sodium hydroxide in water and dilute to one liter. Store the solution in a polyethylene bottle.
5. Alkaline buffer
   Add 0.5 ml of 2.25*M* sodium dihydrogen phosphate to 3.0 ml of 0.45*N* sodium hydroxide. The pH of this solution must be 10.3 ± 0.2. If it is not, suitably dilute either of the two components. The mixture's pH is critical within the stated limits. Once prepared, the component solutions are stable for at least 2 months if stored in polyethylene bottles.
6. Chloroform
   All chloroform should be obtained in glass containers. Extract an aliquot of each new lot with 0.45*N* sodium hydroxide. Compare the absorbance of this chloroform-saturated alkaline solution with that of 0.45*N* sodium hydroxide. There should be no significant absorption between 240 and 300 nm. If there is, wash the chloroform with dilute alkali, dilute acid, and water. Retest the washed chloroform prior to using it.
7. Sodium hydroxide, 0.1*N*
   Dissolve 4 g of sodium hydroxide in water and dilute to one liter.
8. Potassium dihydrogen phosphate, 0.1*M*
   Dissolve 13.6 g of potassium dihydrogen phosphate in water and dilute to one liter.
9. Phosphate buffer, pH 7.0
   Add 30.0 ml of 0.1*N* sodium hydroxide to 50.0 ml of 0.1*M* potassium dihydrogen phos-

*For an updated list of reference material, see References, p. 44.

phate and dilute the mixture to 100 ml with distilled water. Any other pH 7.0 buffer will suffice.

10. Hydrochloric acid, 6*N*
    Dilute 50.0 ml of concentrated hydrochloric acid to 100 ml with water.
11. Diisopropyl ether
12. Potassium permanganate, 100 mg/100 ml
    Dissolve 0.1 g of potassium permanganate in water and dilute to 100 ml.
13. Mercuric sulfate, 2 g/100 ml
    Suspend, with mixing, 5 g of mercuric oxide in 100 ml of water. Add, while stirring, 20.0 ml of concentrated sulfuric acid. Allow the mixture to cool, then dilute it to 250 ml with water.
14. Diphenylcarbazone (DPC), 10 mg/100 ml
    Dissolve 10.0 mg of diphenylcarbazone in 100 ml of chloroform. Store the solution in a dark bottle.

PROCEDURE, QUANTITATIVE

1. Pipet 3.0 ml of specimen (blood, serum, plasma, urine, or stomach content) into a 60-ml glass-stoppered bottle or 100-ml separatory funnel. Include a 3.0-ml sample of barbiturate reference solution and a 3.0-ml water sample for a reagent blank in each series of analyses.
2. Adjust the pH of all samples other than whole blood to 6.5.
3. Add 50.0 ml of chloroform to each sample and shake the container for 3 min.
4. Remove the aqueous phase from all samples except whole blood by aspiration and discard it. If whole blood was used, the chloroform layer may be carefully decanted. Filter each of the chloroform extracts obtained in Step 3 through E & D #615 filter paper.
5. Shake the chloroform filtrate of all samples other than whole blood with 5.0 ml of pH 7.0 phosphate buffer. Allow the layers to separate, then aspirate and discard the aqueous wash solution.
6. Place a 40.0-ml aliquot of each (washed) chloroform extract into a clean 60-ml glass-stoppered bottle.
7. Add 5.0 ml of 0.45*N* sodium hydroxide and

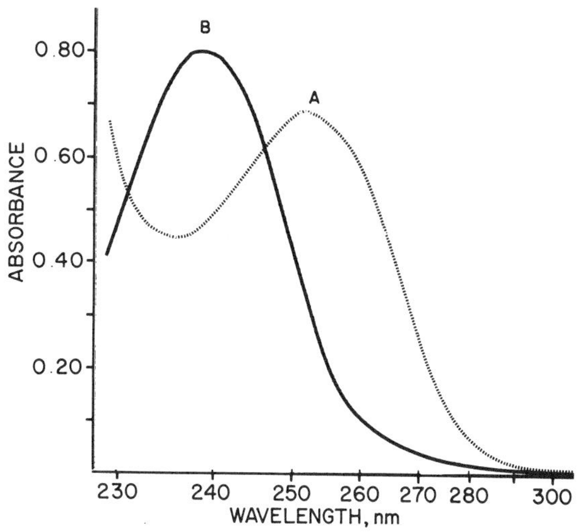

FIGURE 1. Absorption curves for barbiturates.

shake the mixture for 1 min. Add 10.0 ml of 0.45*N* sodium hydroxide to the extract of the reference solution.

8. Pipet the aqueous alkaline layer into a test tube and centrifuge it. The residual chloroform may be discarded or it can be reserved for determination of any neutral drugs it may contain.
9. Place 3.0 ml of the aqueous alkaline layer, which has a pH of 13, into a quartz cuvette and determine its UV absorbance (A_B) from 340 to 230 nm, using the extract of the water sample as the reference solution. If the absorption curve is similar to Curve A in Figure 1, proceed to Step 10 to confirm the presence of a 5,5-disubstituted barbituric acid. If a curve similar to Figure 2 is obtained, proceed as directed in Step 10 of the procedure for *N*-methylbarbituric acids.* If a curve similar to Figure 3 is obtained, proceed as directed in Step 7 of the procedure for thiopental.†
10. Add 0.5 ml of 2.25*M* sodium dihydrogen phosphate to each cuvette and mix well. Determine the UV absorbance of the solution, which now has a pH of 10.3 ± 0.2, from 340 to 230 nm (see Curve B, Figure 1).
11. If the UV absorption curve is atypical, acidify a known aliquot of the aqueous layer from Step 10 and extract it with 10.0 ml of chloroform. Aspirate the aqueous layer and discard it. Ex-

*See p. 248.
†See p. 374.

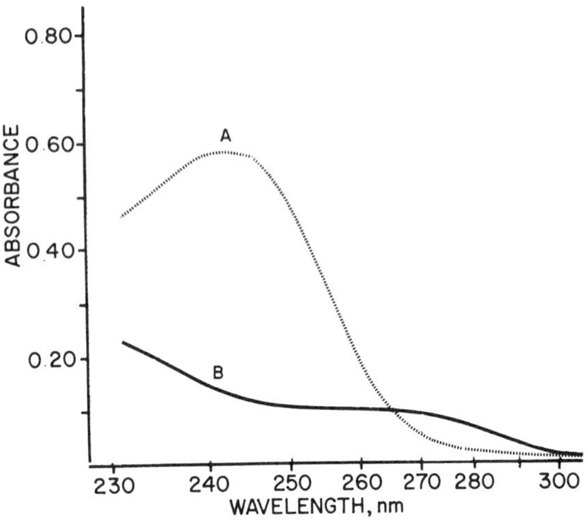

FIGURE 2. Absorption curves for *N*-methylbarbituric acids.

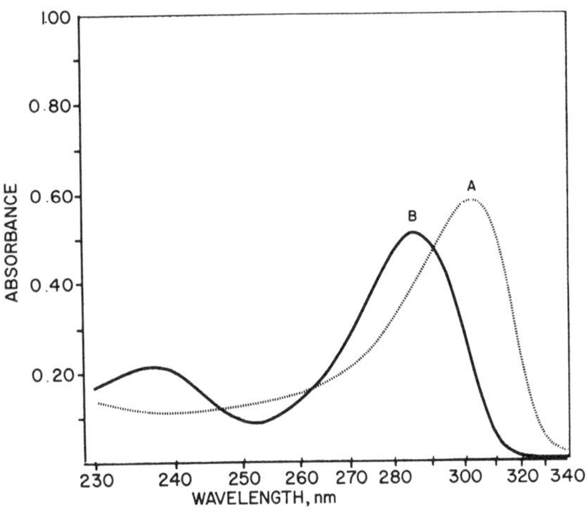

FIGURE 3. Absorption curves for thiopental.

tract an 8.0-ml aliquot of the organic layer with 4.0 ml of 0.45*N* sodium hydroxide and proceed as described in Step 8.

CALCULATION

1. Record the absorbance at 260 nm of the solution whose pH is 13 (A).
2. Record 7/6* of the absorbance at 260 nm of the solution whose pH is 10.3 ± 0.2(B).
3. Calculate the barbiturate concentration in the specimen as follows:

$$C_S = (A - B) \times \frac{5.0}{S^{b}\dagger}$$

If Step 11 was required, then (A − B) must be adjusted to compensate for the smaller aliquot used in this step.

ACCURACY AND PRECISION

The UV spectrophotometric data are easily reproducible to ± 5% of the true value if only one barbiturate is present, and its extinction is used to calculate the concentration. If the average extinction value for several common barbiturates is used, the result is ± 10% of the true value. If more than one barbiturate is present, the total concentration is within ± 10%, but the relative concentration of each must be determined by some other technique, preferably gas chromatography.

PROCEDURE, QUALITATIVE‡

1. Combine the aqueous alkaline layers from Steps 7 and 10 of the Quantitative Procedure in a 60-ml glass-stoppered bottle and acidify them with 6*N* hydrochloric acid.
2. Add 10.0 ml of chloroform and shake the mixture for 3 min.
3. Aspirate the aqueous layer. Filter the organic layer into an evaporating dish and evaporate it to dryness.

*The factor 7/6 is used to compensate for the addition of the 0.5 ml of buffer to the 3.0-ml sample.

†S is the comparable difference in absorbance that is obtained when 3.0 ml of a solution containing 5.0 mg of a barbiturate/100 ml is processed in a manner identical to that described above. If the identity of the barbiturate in the specimen is not known, S can be the average of the values obtained from analyzing the phenobarbital, secobarbital, pentobarbital, and amobarbital reference solutions. Typical S values for these barbiturates are 514, 463, 500, and 465, respectively, in a 1-cm cuvette at 260 nm.

‡A quick presumptive qualitative test may be made by extracting the pH 10.3 buffered solution (Step 10 above) with chloroform and then redetermining the UV absorption of the chloroform extracted buffer. Phenobarbital yields a spectrum which is relatively unchanged, secobarbital yields one which is significantly altered.

Table 1

R_f VALUES OF SEVERAL BARBITURATES AND DIPHENYLHYDANTOIN ON SILICA GEL G AFTER DEVELOPMENT IN DIISOPROPYL ETHER

		Sequential color reaction to sprays		
Compound	R_f Value	$KMnO_4$	$HgSO_4$	DPC
Amobarbital	0.78	–	Gray	Violet
Butabarbital	0.72	–	Gray	Violet
Diphenylhydantoin	0.35	–	Gray	Violet
Hexobarbital	0.62	Yellow	Gray	Violet
Pentobarbital	0.80	–	Gray	Violet
Phenobarbital	0.62	–	Gray	Violet
Secobarbital	0.87	Yellow	Gray	Violet

4. Dissolve the residue in 0.2 ml of chloroform and spot a portion on a TLC plate. Each plate must also contain spots of suitable reference barbiturates (or diphenylhydantoin).
5. Develop the plate in diisopropyl ether.
6. Allow the plate to air-dry.
7. Spray the plate sequentially with potassium permanganate, mercuric sulfate, and diphenylcarbazone. Note the results after each spraying. Typical R_f values and color reactions to the sprays are shown in Table 1.

INTERPRETATION (see p. 7)

Many investigators have studied the correlation between a patient's clinical condition and his blood barbiturate concentration. The reported data are summarized in Table 2. These data indicate that spontaneous recovery from phenobarbital intoxication occurs when the phenobarbital concentration is between 3.4 and 5.0 mg/100 ml of blood. Stage 2, defined as the patient's ability to respond to questioning, is the criterion used for describing recovery. In amobarbital intoxication, recovery was noted in the range from 1.5 to 2.0 mg/100 ml of blood. At amobarbital concentrations higher than 3.4 mg/100 ml of blood, which is the recovery level for phenobarbital intoxication, patients were always severely intoxicated. The recovery levels for pentobarbital and secobarbital range from 0.3 to 0.6 mg/100 ml of blood. Severe intoxication was noted when pentobarbital and secobarbital concentrations exceeded 1.5 mg/100 ml of blood. This emphasizes the need for qualitative as well as quantitative chemical analysis in all instances of barbiturate intoxication.

ACCURACY AND PRECISION

The UV spectrophotometric data are easily reproducible to ± 5% of the true value if only one barbiturate is present, and its extinction is used to calculate the concentration. If the average extinction value for several common barbiturates is used, the result is ± 10% of the true value. If more than one barbiturate is present, the total concentration is within ± 10%, but the relative concentration of each must be determined by some other technique, preferably gas chromatography.

INTERFERING SUBSTANCES

Several weakly acid drugs whose UV absorbances are significant at 260 nm can interfere, if present. Diphenylhydantoin (Dilantin®) is the most common. Megimide® and Ritalin®, "sulfa" drugs, and high concentrations of salicylic acid are also possible interferences. Except for Dilantin®, however, these drugs are seldom present concomitant with barbiturate poisonings.

Table 2

RELATION BETWEEN A PATIENT'S CLINICAL CONDITION AND THE BARBITURATE CONCENTRATION* IN HIS BLOOD

	Clinical stages†				
Barbiturate	**1**	**2**	**3**	**4**	**5**
Phenobarbital	1.0	3.4	5.5	8.0	15.0
Amobarbital	0.7	1.5	3.0	5.2	6.6
Pentobarbital	0.4	0.6	1.5	2.0	3.0
Secobarbital	0.3	0.5	1.0	1.5	2.0

* Concentration is expressed in mg/100 ml of blood. Each figure represents the concentration of barbiturate at which the average nontolerant patient enters into a given clinical stage. The figures given are averages from findings in at least four to six patients.

† The clinical conditions of the patients were grouped into five arbitrary categories on the basis of the following criteria

Stage 1: awake, competent, and mildly sedated.
Stage 2: sedated, reflexes present, prefers sleep, answers questions when roused, does not cerebrate.
Stage 3: comatose, reflexes present.
Stage 4: comatose areflexive.
Stage 5: comatose, circulatory and/or respiratory difficulty.

These stages do not have definite limits, but blend into each other as the patient progresses from stage to stage. The deep tendon reflexes were used as the criteria for presence or absence of reflexes. Corneal, pupillary, and abdominal responses are subject to more variability in relation to the levels of anesthesia. Gag and cough reflexes return at approximately the same time as the deep tendon reflexes; response to pain returns at a later time. The respiratory difficulty considered in Stage 5 is due to direct depression of the respiratory center in the medulla and should not be confused with the attendant respiratory difficulty due to pneumonia, which is always a possible complication in a heavily sedated individual.

REFERENCES*

Parker, K. D., et al., Blood and urine concentrations of subjects receiving barbiturates, meprobamate, glutethimide and diphenylhydantoin, *Clin. Toxicol.*, 3, 131, 1970.

Sunshine, I. and Maes, R., An evaluation of methods for the determination of barbiturates in biological materials, *Clin. Toxicol.*, 1, 281, 1968.

*For an updated list of reference material, see General References, p. 44.

TYPE C PROCEDURE

Gerald Kananen, Vijay Aggarwal, and Michael McGee

APPARATUS

1. Culture tubes with Teflon®-lined caps, 16 × 125 mm (Kimax #45066A)
2. Concentratubes®* (Concentratubes® are test tubes which hold about 20 ml and taper to a sharp tip which holds about 10 μl.)
3. Vortex mixer (Scientific Industries, Model #16-500J)
4. Syringe, 10 μl (Hamilton #701)
5. Syringe, 100 μl (Hamilton #710)
6. Integrator (Hewlett-Packard, Model 3373)
7. Recorder (Hewlett-Packard, Model 7127a)
8. Gas chromatograph, (Hewlett-Packard, Model 7621) dual FID equipped with a 6′ × 1/8″ i. d. stainless steel column containing 10% UCW-982 on Chromosorb W, HP, 80/100 mesh

Operating Conditions

Gas Flow Rates:
- air – 400 ml/min
- helium – 30 ml/min
- hydrogen – 30 ml/min

Temperatures:
- injection port – 260°C
- detector – 300°C
- oven – screening procedure, isothermal 230°C; quantitative procedure, programmed-initial temperature, 180°C; post injection delay, 10 min thereafter programmed at 20° C/min to 290°C, then hold at 290°C for 2 min

REAGENTS

All chemical should be analytical reagent grade.

1. Phosphoric acid, 0.2*M*
   Dilute 1.15 ml of 85% phosphoric acid to 100 ml with distilled water.
2. Concentrated trimethylanilinium hydroxide (TMAH)
   A mixture of 7.0 g of trimethylanilinium iodide (Aldrich Chemical #13, 914–9), 3.6 g of silver oxide, and 10 ml of methanol are placed in a screw-capped culture tube and shaken for 2 min. The mixture is then rotated on a mechanical rotator for 4 hr and then centrifuged. The supernatant is decanted and stored for subsequent use at 20°C. The molarity of the solution is 1.8 ± 0.2*M* and is stable for at least 4 weeks.
3. Aprobarbital stock solution, 5.0 mg/dl
   Dissolve 25.0 mg of aprobarbital in toluene and dilute to 500 ml.
4. Internal reference solution, 0.5 mg/dl
   Dilute 10 ml of the aprobarbital stock solution to 100 ml with toluene.
5. Barbiturate mixture stock solution, 50.0 mg/dl
   Transfer 27.3 mg of each of the sodium salts of amobarbital, pentobarbital, secobarbital, phenobarbital, and diphenylhydantoin to a 50-ml volumetric flask and add 40 ml of distilled water. Add enough 6*M* NaOH to dissolve the solids and dilute to volume with distilled water. At pH values where diphenylhydantoin is soluble, phenobarbital begins to decompose, so this solution should be used immediately.
6. Barbiturate reference solution, 2.0 mg/dl
   Dilute 4.0 ml of the barbiturate mixture stock solution to 100 ml with distilled water. When stored at 4°C, this reference solution is stable for at least 2 weeks.
7. Barbiturate serum reference solution, 2.0 mg/dl Dilute 4.0 ml of the barbiturate mixture
   Dilute 4.0 ml of the barbiturate mixture stock solution to 100 ml with serum. When for at least 2 weeks.
8. Glutethimide stock solution, 50.0 mg/dl
   Transfer 25.0 mg of glutethimide to a 50-ml volumetric flask. Add enough ethanol to just dissolve the powder. Dilute to volume with distilled water. The stock solution is stable for at least 4 weeks when stored at 4°C.
9. Glutethimide reference solution, 2.0 mg/dl

*Laboratory Research Co., P.O. Box 36509, Los Angeles, Cal. 90036.

Table 1

THE ABSOLUTE AND RELATIVE RETENTION TIMES OF SOME COMMONLY OCCURRING ACID DRUGS

	Screening Procedure		Quantitation Procedure		
Drug	RT (min)	RRT	RT (min)	RRT*	Response Factor†
Early phenobarbital‡	1.35	0.92	4.32	0.92	0.86
Aprobarbital	1.47	1.00	4.86	1.00	1.00
Butabarbital	1.67	1.14	5.25	1.12	0.80
Amobarbital	1.84	1.25	6.15	1.31	0.63
Pentobarbital	2.04	1.39	7.06	1.51	0.78
Secobarbital	2.29	1.56	7.89	1.68	0.69
Glutethimide	3.76	2.56	9.00	1.85	0.80
Phenobarbital	3.77	2.56	9.09	1.94	3.10
Primidone	5.55	3.29	14.09	2.80	4.50
Diphenylhydantoin	9.87	6.71	15.55	3.32	0.26

* Retention time relative to aprobarbital.
† Ratio of peak heights of 2.0 mg/dl of barbiturates to the aprobarbital internal standard.
‡ Product of phenobarbital decomposition (see Interfering Substances).

Dilute 4.0 ml of the glutethimide stock solution to 100 ml with distilled water. This solution is stable for at least 2 weeks when stored at 4°C.

PROCEDURE

1. To 2.0 ml of sample (blood, urine, or barbiturate reference solution) in a screw-capped culture tube, add 1.0 ml of 0.2*M* H_3PO_4 and 5.0 ml of the internal reference solution. Shake the tube for 2 min and then centrifuge for 5 min to separate the phases.
2. Transfer about 4 ml of the toluene phase to a Concentratube® using a Pasteur pipet. (A quantitative transfer is not necessary because an internal standard is in the toluene.)
3. Vortex the Concentratube® and while still vortexing slowly add 35 μl of the TMAH solution using a 100-μl syringe. Centrifuge the Concentratube® for 10 min to separate the TMAH from the toluene.
4. Set the chromatographic conditions described above for the screening procedure and slowly inject a 1-μl aliquot of the TMAH into the injection port over a 5-sec interval. This slow injection serves to reduce solvent tailing on many instruments.
5. If no peaks with retention times corresponding to any of the barbiturates, diphenylhydantoin, or glutethimide are observed, then none of these substances is present in the sample. A peak at the retention time corresponding to those listed in Table 1 indicates the presence of the substance in question.
6. If the presence of a drug is indicated by the screening procedure, inject 3 μl of the TMAH solution over a 10-sec interval into the injection port of a gas chromatograph set up with the conditions listed under Quantitative Procedure above (Figure 1).

CALCULATION

The concentration of barbiturate can be determined by using either peak height or peak area measurements and the following formula:

$$C_X = C_S \frac{P_X}{A_X} \times \frac{A_S}{P_S}$$

where

C_X = concentration of the drug in the sample;
C_S = concentration of the known drug in the barbiturate reference solution (2mg/dl);
P_X = peak height or peak area of the drug in the sample;
A_X = peak height or peak area of the aprobarbital internal standard peak in the sample;

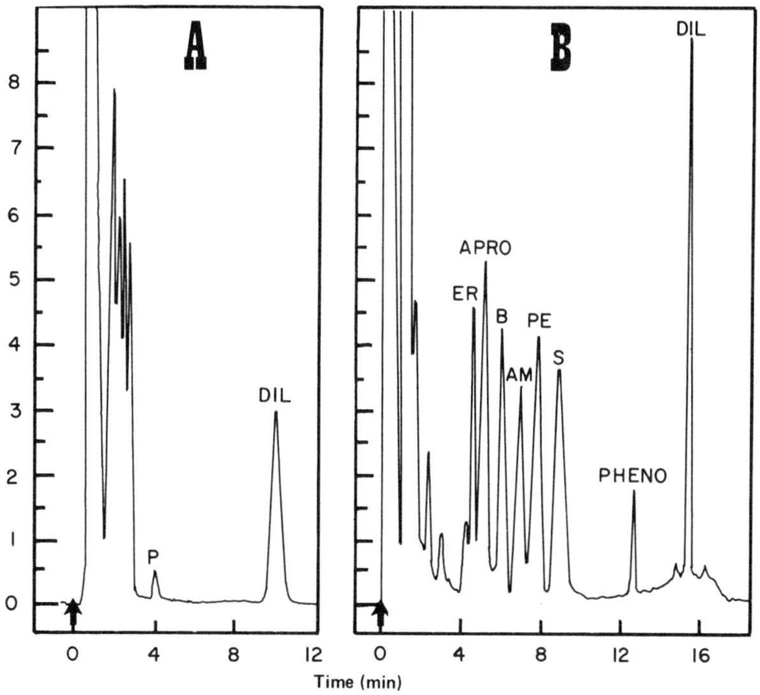

FIGURE 1. Chromatograms showing analyses using (A) the screening and (B) the quantitative procedure. ER = early phenobarbital; ARPO = aprobarbital; B = butabarbital; AM = amobarbital; PE = pentobarbital; S = secobarbital; PHENO = phenobarbital; and DIL = Dilantin®. (From Kananen, G., Osiewicz, R., and Sunshine, I., Barbiturate analysis – a current assessment, *J. Chromatogr. Sci.*, 10, 285, 1972. With permission.)

P_s = peak height or peak area of the known drug in the barbiturate reference solution;
A_s = peak height or peak area of the aprobarbital internal standard peak in the barbiturate reference solution.

INTERPRETATION (see p. 7)

Many investigators have studied the correlation between a patient's clinical condition and his blood barbiturate concentration. The reported data are summarized in Procedure B, Table 2. These data indicate that spontaneous recovery from phenobarbital intoxication occurs when the phenobarbital concentration is between 3.4 and 5.0 mg/100 ml of blood. Stage 2, defined as the patient's ability to respond to questioning, is the criterion used for describing recovery. In amobarbital intoxication, recovery was noted in the range from 1.5 to 2.0 mg/100 ml of blood. At amobarbital concentrations higher than 3.4 mg/100 ml of blood, which is the recovery level for phenobarbital intoxication, patients were always severely intoxicated. The recovery levels for phenobarbital and secobarbital range from 0.3 to 0.6 mg/100 ml of blood. This emphasized the need for qualitative as well as quantitative analysis in all instances of barbiturate intoxication. Analytical data obtained by this procedure are comparable to data obtained using double extraction procedures for gas chromatography or combined UV-TLC analysis.[1] The peak area ratios are linear functions of barbiturate concentration from 0.1 to 8 mg/dl. Minimum detectable amount is 0.1 mg/dl. The coefficient of variation for replicate analyses of 2.0 mg/dl reference solution is 2.0 to 3.0%.

INTERFERING SUBSTANCES

Osiewicz et al.[2] have shown that the peak areas of both phenobarbital and the phenobarbital decomposition product (*N*-methyl-α-phenylbutyramide) are linear with respect to concentration of phenobarbital. Glutethimide and several of its metabolites are extracted and derivatized by this procedure. The glutethimide peak (RRT 1.85) is poorly resolved from the phenobarbital peak (RRT 1.94). The absence of an early phenobarbital peak and the presence of several large peaks (due to glutethimide metabolites) between glutethimide (RRT 1.85) and diphenylhydantoin (RRT 3.3) is indicative of glutethimide. It is not possible to differentiate phenobarbital from mephobarbital since both drugs produce the same methylated derivatives. In addition, Aggarwal[3] has reported that sulfonylureas can be extracted by this procedure.

REFERENCES

1. **Kananen, G., Osiewicz, R., and Sunshine, I.,** Barbiturate analysis – a current assessment, *J. Chromatogr. Sci.,* 10, 285, 1972.
2. **Osiewicz, R., Aggarwal, V., Young, R., and Sunshine, I.,** The quantitative analysis of phenobarbital with trimethylanilinium hydroxide, *J. Chromatogr.,* 88, 157, 1974.
3. **Aggarwal, V. and Sunshine, I.,** Determination of sulfonylureas and metabolites by pyrolysis gas chromatography, *Clin. Chem.,* 20, 200, 1974.

GENERAL REFERENCES

Cleeland, R. et al., A simple, rapid, ^{125}I radioimmunoassay for the detection of barbiturates in hologreal fluids, *J. Forensic Sci.,* 20, 45, 1975.

Ehrnelo, M., Pharmacokinetics and distribution properties of phenobarbital in humans following oral and intravenous administration, *J. Pharm. Sci.,* 63, 1114, 1974.

Flynn, E. J. and Spector, S., Determination of barbiturate derivatives by radioimmunoassay, *J. Pharmacol. Exp. Ther.,* 181(3), 547, 1974.

Jatlow, P., Ultraviolet spectrophotometric analysis of barbiturates, *Am. J. Clin. Pathol.,* 59, 167, 1973.

MacGee, J., Rapid determination of diphenylhydantoin in blood plasma by GLC, *Anal. Chem.,* 42, 421, 1970.

Van Meter, J. C. and Gillen, H. W., A source of variation in the GC assay of phenobarbital treated with trimethylanilinium hydroxide, *Clin. Chem.,* 19, 359, 1973.

Watson, D. and Dillon, G., Use of the barbiturate-mercury reaction in clinical laboratory screening for barbiturate poisoning, *Am. J. Clin. Biochem.,* 10, 2, 1973.

ALTERNATIVE TYPE C PROCEDURE IMMUNOASSAY

Details for the EMIT procedure will be found on p. 401. Details for the RIA procedure will be found on p. 403.

BENZODIAZEPINES*

PRINCIPLE

Combining extractive information, thin-layer chromatographic R_f values and functional group sprays can lead to detection and tentative identification of different benzodiazepines. Additional UV spectrophotometric data may lead to identification of the specific bendiazepine.

TYPE A PROCEDURE

Paul R. Sedgwick

APPARATUS

1. Separatory funnels, 60, 120, and 250 ml
2. Filter paper (Whatman #1)
3. Beakers, 30, 100, and 250 ml
4. Pasteur pipets, disposable
5. Heating plate
6. UV spectrophotometer, scanning
7. Quartz cells, 1- and 5-cm pathlength, 3-ml volume
8. Centrifuge tubes, 12 and 40 ml
9. Measuring graduated cylinders, 15, 100, or 250 ml
10. Centrifuge
11. Thin-layer chromatography equipment: (a) micropipets (b) glass plates coated 0.25 mm thick with silica gel and a 254-nm fluorescent indicator; (c) developing tank; (d) UV light, 254 nm

REAGENTS

All chemicals should be analytical reagent grade.

1. Sodium hydroxide, 0.1*N*
   Add 4 g of sodium hydroxide to a one-liter volumetric flask and dilute to volume with water.
2. Potassium dihydrogen phosphate, 0.1*M*
   Add 13.6 g of potassium dihydrogen phosphate to a one-liter volumetric flask and dilute to volume with water.
3. Phosphate buffer, pH 7, 3*M*
   Add 30 ml of 0.1*N* sodium hydroxide and 50 ml of 0.1*M* potassium dihydrogen phosphate to a 100-ml volumetric flask and dilute to volume with water.
4. Diethyl ether
5. Chloroform
   Shake 10 parts of chloroform with 1 part of 0.45*N* sodium hydroxide. Remove the alkali and filter the chloroform through any fast filter paper to remove residual water.
6. Sulfuric acid, 0.2*N*
   Dilute 2.8 ml of sulfuric acid to 500 ml with water.
7. Sulfuric acid, 2*N*
   Dilute 28 ml of sulfuric acid to 500 ml with water.
8. Hydrochloric acid, 2*N*
   To 300 ml of water add 83.3 ml of concentrated (12*N*) hydrochloric acid and dilute the mixture to 500 ml.
9. Sodium hydroxide, 0.45*N*
   Dissolve 18 g of sodium hydroxide in water and dilute to one liter with water.
10. Sodium hydroxide, saturated
    Add 430 g of sodium hydroxide to 500 ml of water while stirring.
11. Ethanol
12. Acetone:benzene:chloroform mixture, 25:40:40
    Mix 25 ml of acetone, 40 ml of benzene, and 40 ml of chloroform.
13. Drug† spotting solutions, 1 mg/ml (for TLC only)
    Dissolve 10 mg of either the salt or the free drug in ethanol and dilute to 10 ml with ethanol.

*For quantitative procedures for chlordiazepoxide, see p. 75; for diazepam, see p. 119.

†Chlordiazepoxide HCl (Librium®), diazepam (Valium®), nitrazepam, medazepam (Nobrium®), flurazepam HCl (Dalmane®), and clonazepam may be obtained from Hoffman-LaRoche, Inc., Nutley, N.J.; chlorazepate dipotassium (Tranxene®) from Abbott Laboratories, North Chicago, Ill.; and oxazepam (Serax®) from Wyeth Labs., Philadelphia, Pa.

Table 1*

DISTRIBUTION OF BENZODIAZEPINES

	Ether (neutrals)	Hydrochloric acid (weaker bases)	Sulfuric acid (stronger bases)	Aqueous
Clorazepate	7	68	25	0
Chlordiazepoxide	1	15	84	0
Demoxepam			most	
Desmethylchlordiazepoxide-acid				
Oxazepam	39	60	1	0
Diazepam	5	85	10	0
Desoxydemoxepam		most		
Nitrazepam	0	90	10	0
Medazepam	1	13	86	0
Flurazepam	0	0	99	1
Clonazepam	69	31	0	0
Common interfering substances	caffeine fats	some caffeine methaqualone	nicotine putrescines quinine	

* The percentage of each drug which will be found in the several successive fractions used to extract benzodiazepines from the original pH 7 buffered sample. The solvent is diethyl ether.

14. Iodoplatinate spray, acidified
    Dissolve 9.0 g of reagent grade potassium iodide in 300 ml of water. Add 10 ml of 10% w/v chloroplatinic acid and 9 ml of hydrochloric acid. Mix well.

PROCEDURE

1. Add a 20-ml sample (whole blood, plasma, urine, or 10 g of liver homogenized with 10 ml of water) to 100 ml of diethyl ether in an appropriate separatory funnel. Add 5 ml of pH 7 phosphate buffer to urine samples. (Results may be obtained with as little as 5 ml of sample for high therapeutic levels, or even less sample in overdose cases.)
2. Shake vigorously for 3 min and centrifuge, if necessary, to break emulsions.
3. Discard the aqueous phase and filter the ether into a mixing cylinder through Whatman #1 paper.
4. Add 5 ml of 0.2*N* sulfuric acid and shake vigorously for 3 min to extract the more basic drugs (Table 1).
5. Withdraw the acid phase into a separatory funnel. Save the diethyl ether. Add 1 ml of saturated sodium hydroxide and 25 ml of chloroform to the acid extract. Shake vigorously and filter the chloroform through Whatman #1 paper into a beaker, and assist the initial evaporation with heat and air. Evaporate the last milliliter to dryness only at room temperature, with dry air or nitrogen, carefully, to avoid degrading or volatilizing the drugs.
6. Add 5 ml of 2*N* hydrochloric acid to the diethyl ether (Step 5) and extract the weaker bases by shaking the mixture. Withdraw the acid phase into a separatory funnel and again save the diethyl ether. Add 1 ml of saturated sodium hydroxide (be careful of splattering) and 25 ml of chloroform to the extract. Shake vigorously and filter the chloroform through Whatman #1 paper into a beaker. Evaporate as before.
7. Add 5 ml of 0.45*N* sodium hydroxide to the diethyl ether. Shake vigorously for 1 min. Withdraw and discard the aqueous phase. Filter and evaporate the diethyl ether (as described above for the chloroform extracts) to isolate the neutral drugs.
8. Add approximately 200 μl of chloroform to each beaker (Steps 5, 6, and 7) and triturate to reconstitute any drugs. Spot all three residues on the same thinlayer plate. Also, spot aliquots of the TLC reference solutions for each of the drugs suspected to be present. Place the spotted plate in a chromatographic tank

Table 2

THIN-LAYER CHROMATOGRAPHIC DATA*

Drug	$R_f \times 100$
Clorazepate	49
Chlordiazepoxide	20
Demoxepam†	36
Desmethylchlordiazepoxide†	08
Oxazepam	29
Diazepam	70
Desoxydemoxepam†	47
Nitrazepam	47
Medazepam	71
Flurazepam	08
Clonazepam	48

* Silica gel, 0.25-mm thick (thicker plates will require more acetone and vice versa), developed in acetone: benzene: chloroform, 25:40:40.
† Metabolites.

containing the acetone:benzene:chloroform solvent. The tank should be lined on one side with any suitable absorbent paper to speed the development.

9. When the plate is developed, dry it at room temperature or assist with a cool blower. Then view it under a 254-nm light source. Compare any spots obtained from the sample's extracts with those of the known drug reference solutions (Table 2).
10. If a strongly absorbing dark spot, corresponding with a benzodiazepine and/or a metabolite, is detected on the TLC plate, spray the plate with acidified iodoplatinate. A positive reaction is a purplish-brown spot. If both the parent drug and a recognized metabolite are observed from biological specimens, the probability of identification is increased. For confirmation of the drug, select a quantitative procedure (see Index) or treat the TLC plate as follows. (a) Scrape the suspected spot (all the silica gel) into a 12-ml centrifuge tube. (b) Add 1 ml of 0.45*N* sodium hydroxide and 10 ml of chloroform to the centrifuge tube containing the silica gel, and mix thoroughly with a disposable pipet. (c) Centrifuge the tube for 3 min at approximately 3,000 rpm. (d) Aspirate and discard the aqueous fraction, then filter the chloroform through Whatman #1 paper into a beaker. (e) Evaporate carefully as described before. (f) When dry, add 3 ml of 0.2*N* sulfuric acid and triturate, then determine the UV absorption spectrum of each fraction using a 5-cm pathlength quartz cell. Dilute as necessary to keep on scale (or transfer to a 1-cm cell). Compare the spectrum obtained with those of the reference solutions (Table 3). Further confirmatory data may be obtained by adding one or two drops of saturated sodium hydroxide to the solutions and comparing the shift in the UV absorption spectrum of the resulting basic solutions.
11. If no spots or only *very* weak spots are observed, a more sensitive test can be performed by soaking the plate until dripping wet with 2*N* sulfuric acid, letting the excess flow off with some drying (no more than 5 min) in a fume hood, and observing in a dark room or a viewing box with a 254-nm light source. A positive reaction for the benzodiazepines and metabolites is either a yellow-green or off-white fluorescent spot. A drug treated in this manner cannot be confirmed by UV scanning.

SENSITIVITY

Detection on the TLC plate is 1 to 2 μg; 3 μg total (3 ml in a 5 cm cell) will give a recognizable UV spectrum of any of the tested benzodiazepines.

Table 3

UV DATA FOR THE BENZODIAZEPINES*

Drug	Major peak, nm	Minor peak, nm
Chlorazepate†	238	284
Oxazepam†	237	286
Diazepam†	241	287
Flurazepam†	233	280
Chlordiazepoxide	246	305
Nitrazepam	280	
Clonazepam	275	
Medazepam‡	253	

* The UV absorption spectra of metabolites are similar to their respective parent compounds.
† Minor peak is 280 to 290 nm; major peak is <241 nm.
‡ Inflexion at 282 nm.

BISMUTH

PRINCIPLE

Bismuth salts, in the presence of a copper wire, will deposit on the copper (Procedure A). The bismuth thus isolated can be characterized by its reaction with quinine and potassium iodide (Procedure B).

TYPE A PROCEDURE

Sidney Kaye

REAGENTS

All chemicals should be analytical reagent grade.

1. Copper strip, 5 × 10 mm, or a spiral of #20 copper wire
2. Hydrochloric acid, concentrated
3. Hydrochloric acid, 1.2*N*
   Dilute 10.0 ml of concentrated hydrochloric acid to 100 ml with water.
4. Nitric acid, 8.2*N*
   Dilute concentrated nitric acid with an equal volume of water.
5. Bismuth stock solution, 1 mg/ml
   Dissolve 100 mg of metallic bismuth in 10.0 ml of 8.2*N* nitric acid, then dilute the solution to 100 ml with water. Store the solution in a Pyrex® bottle.
6. Bismuth reference solutions
   Dilute 10.0 ml of the bismuth stock solution to 100 ml with water. Quantities of 0.5, 1.0, and 1.5 ml of this solution correspond to 50, 100, and 150μg of bismuth, respectively.
7. Potassium cyanide, 10 g/dl
   Dissolve 10 g of potassium cyanide in water and dilute to 100 ml.

PROCEDURE

1. To an Erlenmeyer flask containing a copper strip or spiral, add 4.0 ml of concentrated hydrochloric acid and either a 20.0-ml aliquot of urine, vomitus, or stomach content or 10 g of macerated kidney diluted with 10.0 ml of water.
2. Heat this mixture gently, maintaining the original volume by adding 1.2*N* hydrochloric acid as required. If the mixture is heated gently, the need for additional hydrochloric acid is minimal.
3. After 45 min discard the digested sample. Retain the copper strip or spiral.
4. Wash the spiral with distilled water. Discard the wash water.
5. After repeated washings place the spiral on a piece of filter paper to remove any excess water.

INTERPRETATION (see p. 7)

A shiny black deposit indicates that 30 μg or more of bismuth may be present. On the basis of color comparison fairly reliable presumptive estimates may be made and reported in multiples of 50 μg as negative, small, moderate, or large amounts per unit of sample. The more sensitive quinine-potassium iodide reagent should be used to confirm and semiquantitate the bismuth.*

Bismuth may be a therapeutic ingredient in some gastrointestinal medicines and is fairly commonly used. Analytical findings must therefore be correlated with history, circumstances, symptoms, and clinical picture. Bismuth salts are not very toxic and may be tolerated in fair amounts.

ACCURACY AND PRECISION

The deposition of bismuth on copper is slow and

*See the semiquantitative procedure for bismuth on p. 49.

not complete (about 75%); however, it is useful as a rapid presumptive test.

INTERFERING SUBSTANCES

Arsenic, antimony, sulfur, selenium, and tellurium also produce dark deposits on copper. The arsenic deposit is a dull black; that of antimony, a shiny purple. Sulfur, selenium, and tellurium, if present in small amounts, do not deposit easily because the high acidity required for bismuth deposition will convert them to very volatile hydrides (H_2S, H_2Se, H_2Te). If their presence is suspected, place the copper into 1.0 ml of the potassium cyanide solution; dark deposits due to sulfide, selenium, or tellurium, and *also those due to arsenic,* will dissolve. If a dark residue still persists, it suggests the presence of bismuth or antimony. To rule out the latter, perform the semiquantitative bismuth determination.

REFERENCE*

Kaye, S. and Castillo, J. C., Rapid and specific method for the estimation of bismuth in urine, *Am. J. Clin. Pathol.,* 14, 81, 1944.

TYPE B PROCEDURE

Sidney Kaye

REAGENTS

All chemicals should be analytical reagent grade.

1. Copper strip, 5, × 10 mm, or a spiral of #20 copper wire
2. Hydrochloric acid, concentrated
3. Nitric acid, 3.3*N*
   Mix 1 vol of concentrated nitric acid with 4 vol of water.
4. Sodium sulfite, 5 g/dl
   Dissolve 5 g of sodium sulfite in water and dilute to 100 ml.
5. Quinine† -potassium iodide reagent
   Dissolve 1 g of quinine sulfate in 100 ml of distilled water containing 0.5 ml of concentrated nitric acid. After solution is complete, add 2 g of potassium iodide.
6. Bismuth stock solution, 1 mg/ml
   Dissolve 100 mg of metallic bismuth in 10.0 ml of 3.3*N* nitric acid, then dilute the solution to 100 ml with distilled water. Store the solution in a Pyrex® bottle.
7. Bismuth reference solution, 100 μg/ml
   Dilute 10.0 ml of the bismuth stock solution to 100 ml with water.

PROCEDURE

1. Prepare a bismuth deposit on copper as described in the presumptive test (Type A Procedure‡).
2. Remove and wash the copper strip or spiral.
3. Transfer the copper strip or spiral to a 1 × 10 cm test tube. Add 1.0 ml of the sodium sulfite solution.
4. Add 1.0 ml of 3.3*N* nitric acid. Shake the tube and allow the mixture to act on the copper. Agitate the contents frequently until the deposited bismuth is dissolved. If the deposit is not too heavy, a period of 5 min is usually sufficient.
5. In each of six small test tubes, similar to that used for the unknown, put 1.0 ml of the sodium sulfite solution and 1.0 ml of 3.3*N* nitric acid. Add, respectively, 0, 0.1, 0.2, 0.4, 0.7, and 1.0 ml of the bismuth reference solution. (These quantities correspond to 0, 10, 20, 40, 70, and 100 μg of bismuth.) Dilute the tube contents to 3.0 ml with distilled water.
6. Add 1.0 ml of distilled water and 1.0 ml of the quinine-potassium iodide reagent to each test

*For an updated list of reference material, see References, p. 50.
†Cinchanine may be used instead of quinine.
‡See p. 48.

solution (Step 4) and each of the reference solution (Step 5). Shake the tube, then remove the copper spiral with the aid of a wooden applicator.

7. Compare the suspension of quinine-bismuth-iodide with those obtained from a series of reference solutions processed simultaneously, as described in Step 5.

INTERPRETATION (see p. 7)

A shiny black deposit indicates that 30 μg or more of bismuth may be present. On the basis of color comparison fairly reliable presumptive estimates may be made and reported in multiples of 50 μg as negative, small, moderate, or large amounts per unit of sample. The more sensitive quinine-potassium iodide reagent should be used to confirm and semiquantitate the bismuth.

Bismuth may be a therapeutic ingredient in some gastrointestinal medicines and is fairly commonly used. Analytical findings must therefore be correlated with history, circumstances, symptoms, and clinical picture. Bismuth salts are not very toxic and may be tolerated in fair amounts.

ACCURACY, PRECISION, AND SENSITIVITY

Although the degree of darkening of the copper strip or spiral is a good indication of the amount of bismuth present in the urine, it was found that the quinine-bismuth-iodide reaction will detect deposits of bismuth not visible to the naked eye. The sensitivity of the presumptive test is approximately 30 μg. The sensitivity of the quinine-bismuth-iodide reaction, as described above, is faint for 10 μg and definite for 20 μg of bismuth. The suggested number of reference solutions is arbitrary. If greater accuracy is desired, a larger number of reference solutions with a narrower range may be used; however, the upper limit of sensitivity should be kept at 100 μg because, under the conditions of the test, differences in concentration of bismuth above this level are difficult to estimate. The best range for an accurate estimation is between 20 and 70 μg of bismuth. The total recovery of bismuth, as compared with directly analyzed reference solutions, is about 75%.

INTERFERING SUBSTANCES

By using copper for the isolation of bismuth, the interference of lead and/or iron is eliminated because these metals do not deposit on copper. None of the other metals that deposit on copper (mercury, arsenic, antimony, and silver) were found to give the double iodide reaction with the reagent under the conditions of this test. Experiments to determine the influence of these metals on the deposition of bismuth on copper indicate that the presence of 50 μg of either of these metals did not prevent the deposition of bismuth on the copper strip or spiral. The interference of copper is eliminated by the use of sodium sulfite.

REFERENCES

Bamford, F., *Poisons,* Blakiston, Philadelphia, 1940, 105.

Hall, R. J., Determination of bismuth in body tissues and fluids after administration of controlled doses, *J. Assoc. Off. Agric. Chem.,* 55, 639, 1972.

Kaye, S. and Castillo, J. C., Rapid and specific method for the estimation of bismuth in urine, *Am. J. Clin. Pathol.,* 14, 81, 1944.

Mahr, C., Colorimetric determination of bismuth, *Z. Anal. Chem.,* 94, 161, 1933.

Tompsett, S. L., Determination of bismuth in biologic material, *Analyst,* 63, 250, 1938.

BORATE

PRINCIPLE

Boric acid transforms yellow curcumin (tumeric, diferuloylmethane), through a loose intermediate addition product, into the red isomer rosocyanine. The rosocyanine turns blue when alkali is added. Addition of acid restores the red color (Procedure A). Should a quantitative analysis be required, the colored complex formed by boric acid with carminic acid is preferable (Procedure B).

TYPE A PROCEDURE

Fredric Rieders

APPARATUS

1. Spot plate, white porcelain (Coors No. 550, size 4/0)
2. Hot water bath

REAGENTS

All chemicals should be analytical reagent grade.

1. Boric acid, 50 mg/dl
   Dissolve 50.0 mg of boric acid in water and dilute to 100 ml with water.
2. Hydrochloric acid, 1.2*N*
   Add 10.0 ml of concentrated hydrochloric acid to distilled water, mix, then dilute to 100 ml. Store the solution in a glass-stoppered dropping bottle.
3. Curcuma tincture reagent
   Saturate 95% ethanol with curcumin by shaking with excess curcumin powder (Eastman 1179). Filter the solution through Whatman #1 filter paper. Store the reagent in a clear dropping bottle. The reagent is stable indefinitely.
4. Ammonium hydroxide, concentrated

SPECIMEN REQUIREMENTS

Urine

If the urine specimen is reasonably free of obvious mucus or heavy crystalline and amorphous solids, it may be used directly; if not, centrifuge the urine for 10 min at a speed between 3,500 and 5,000 rpm, then use the supernatant.

Gastric Content

Centrifuge the gastric content for 10 min at 5,000 rpm, then use the intermediate aqueous phase. If the gastric content is so thick that centrifugation does not yield a reasonably clear aqueous phase, mix 2.0 ml of gastric content with 2.0 ml of 1.2*N* hydrochloric acid. Centrifuge the mixture, then use the supernatant.

PROCEDURE

1. Into one well of a white porcelain spot plate place two drops of specimen (urine, gastric washings, clear aqueous centrifugate from gastric content, or other clear and essentially protein-free aqueous samples). Into a second well place two drops of water as a reagent blank. Into a third well place two drops of the boric acid solution for comparison.
2. To each well add, in succession, two drops of 1.2*N* hydrochloric acid and two drops of curcuma tincture reagent.
3. Place the spot plate on a hot water bath and observe the contents of each well. When the mixtures have completely dried, note any red

or red-brown coloration (rosocyanine formation).

4. Cool the spot plate, then moisten each residue with concentrated ammonium hydroxide and observe it for a color change, immediate or gradual, to blue, dark green, or greenish-black.

INTERPRETATION (see p. 7)

If the color changes described in the procedure occur as outlined, borate may be present in the sample. Positive results, although quite selective for boron, must be followed by quantification in blood or other tissues, since borates are ubiquitous and their presence in gastric contents and urine (e.g., from tooth powders) is not uncommon.

SENSITIVITY

1. 0.2/μg of boron in 2 drops of sample gives a positive reaction in both parts of the test.
2. 0.07/μg of boron in 2 drops of sample gives a positive (blue) reaction only in the second part of the test.

INTERFERING SUBSTANCES

1. Red-browns are also produced by ferric, molybdenum, titanium, niobium, tantalum, and zirconium compounds; however, the color is not changed to blue on addition of the ammonia.
2. The reaction is hindered by oxidants (peroxides, chromates, nitrites, and chlorate) as well as phosphoric acid and silicic acid.

TYPE B PROCEDURE

Fredric Rieders

APPARATUS

1. Photometer, photoelectric, with 1-cm cell and 600-nm filter

REAGENTS

All chemicals should be analytical reagent grade.

1. Ammonium sulfate, 4 g/dl
   Dissolve 4 g of ammonium sulfate in water and dilute to 100 ml.
2. Activated charcoal, Merck N.F.
3. Sulfuric acid, concentrated
4. Carminic acid reagent, 25 mg/dl
   Dissolve 125 mg of carminic acid (Eastman 1612) in 500 ml of concentrated sulfuric acid. This reagent is stable indefinitely if stored in a glass-stoppered glass bottle.
5. Boric acid stock solution, 29 mg/dl
   Dissolve 290 mg of orthoboric acid (H_3BO_3) in water and dilute to one liter with water.
6. Boric acid reference solutions
   Dilute 1.0, 2.0, and 4.0 ml of the boric acid stock solution to 10.0 ml with water to obtain solutions containing 29, 58, and 116 μg of boric acid, corresponding respectively to a boron content of 5, 10, and 20 μg/ml.

SPECIMEN REQUIREMENTS

Body fluids may be analyzed directly. Tissues must be minced before use.

PROCEDURE

1. Place 5.0 ml of the ammonium sulfate solution into a 15 ml centrifuge tube.
2. Add 1.0 ml of body fluid or 1.0 g of minced tissue and mix with a glass rod. Leave the glass rod in the tube.
3. Place the tube in boiling water for 15 min. Stir the tube contents gently at frequent intervals.
4. Remove the tube from the boiling water. Take out the glass rod and wash any adhering

residue into the tube, using a few milliliters of distilled water.

5. Centrifuge the tube and contents for 10 min at 3,500 rpm.
6. Decant the supernatant into a 10-ml volumetric flask.
7. Wash the precipitate with 1 to 2 ml of distilled water by suspending it therein with the aid of a glass rod, centrifuging as above, and decanting the supernatant into the 10-ml volumetric flask. Repeat this operation until the volumetric flask is filled to the 10-ml mark.
8. Add approximately 0.1 g of activated charcoal to the 10-ml flask and mix well. Continue to mix intermittently for 10 min, then allow the charcoal to settle for the next 5 min.
9. Decant the supernatant, then filter it through folded Whatman #42 filter paper.
10. Transfer 1.0* ml of the filtrate to a 100-ml beaker, then add, with constant agitation, 5.0 ml of concentrated sulfuric acid and 5.0 ml of the carminic acid reagent. Mix well. Process 1.0 ml of water (to be used as a reagent blank) and 1.0 ml of each reference solution in the same manner as the filtrate.
11. Transfer the mixture to the cuvette. Stopper the cuvette immediately. Allow the solution to stand for 10 min.
12. Determine the absorbance of the solution at 600 nm.

CALCULATION

Determine the borate concentration (mg/100 ml or mg/100 g) in the specimen by following formula:

$$C_x = 100 \times \frac{A_x}{A_R} \times C_R,$$

where

C_x = concentration of borate in the specimen;
A_x = absorbance of the specimen;
A_R = absorbance of the reference solution;
C_R = concentration of borate in the reference solution.

INTERPRETATION (see p. 7)

The normal blood borate content is less than 1.0 mg/100 ml. Toxic manifestations are usually associated with borate concentration in excess of 10.0 mg/100 ml of blood. Elevated blood borate concentrations associated with toxic manifestations are in most cases due to prolonged or chronic absorption of boric acid powders, ointments, or compresses placed on wounds or on large areas of denuded or damaged skin.

ACCURACY AND PRECISION

1. Recovery of added boron (in the form of boric acid) in the range from 10 to 30 μg/g of tissue is 98 ± 6%.
2. The average deviation of a single determination is 6.2%.

INTERFERING SUBSTANCES

Antimony (III), large amounts of iron (III), copper (II) and other colored ions, beryllium, and oxidizing acids interfere.

REFERENCES

Feigl, F., *Spot Tests,* Vol. 1, 4th ed., Elsevier, N. Y., 1954, 310.

Rieders, F. and Frere, F. J., Detection and estimation of toxicologically significant amounts of borate, chlorate, and oxalate in biologic material, *J. Forensic Sci.,* 8, 46, 1963.

*If the apparent boron content is greater than 20 μg/ml of filtrate (obtained in Step 9), take a smaller aliquot of the filtrate, dilute it to 1.0 ml, then process it as above.

BROMIDE

PRINCIPLE

Although bromide intoxication is seldom a problem because of the popularity of other tranquilizers, occasionally requests are received for the determination of a bromide. The simplest technique (Procedure A) depends on the formation of a colored complex gold salt. This is obtained by adding gold chloride to a protein-free sample of serum. The absorbance of this mixture is a function of its bromide content. A more elegant technique (Procedure B) depends on the oxidation of the bromide present in the protein-free filtrate by hypochlorous acid. This reacts with 2,4-dimethylphenol to produce a brominated compound which is easily detected by a gas chromatograph. Thus, the bromide content of the original sample may be measured.

TYPE A PROCEDURE

Irving Sunshine

APPARATUS

1. Photometer, photoelectric

REAGENTS

All chemicals should be analytical reagent grade.

1. Trichloroacetic acid, 10 g/100 ml
   Dissolve 10 g of trichloroacetic acid and 120 mg of sodium chloride in 100 ml of water.
2. Gold chloride, 500 mg/100 ml
   Dissolve 1 g of gold chloride in distilled water, then dilute to 200 ml. Store the solution in a glass-stoppered brown bottle.
3. Bromide stock solution, 300 mg/100 ml
   Dissolve 0.447 g of potassium bromide in water, then dilute to 100 ml.
4. Bromide reference solutions
   Transfer 5.0, 15.0, and 25.0 ml of the bromide stock solution to 50-ml volumetric flasks, then add distilled water to the calibration marks. The resulting solutions have bromide concentrations of 30.0, 90.0, and 150 mg/100 ml, respectively.

PROCEDURE

1. Place 2.0 ml of serum in a test tube. Slowly add 8.0 ml of the trichloroacetic acid solution and mix well. Process 2.0 ml of each bromide reference solution and 2.0 ml of water for a reagent blank in the same manner.
2. After about 15 min, centrifuge the tubes.
3. Filter the clear supernatant, protein-free solutions through Whatman #1 filter paper or its equivalent.
4. Place 4.0 ml of each filtrate into a cuvette and add 1.0 ml of the gold chloride solution.
5. Determine the absorbance of each mixture at 440 nm in a suitable photoelectric photometer, using the reagent blank as the reference solution.

CALCULATION

Compare the absorbance of the specimen with that of a suitably chosen reference solution processed in the same manner.

INTERPRETATION (see p. 7)

Serum bromide concentrations higher than 50 mg/100 ml are compatible with incipient toxicity. Many patients with this serum concentration appear confused. With bromide concentrations between 150 and 250 mg/100 ml of serum, uncoordination and emotional outbursts may be seen. Concentrations above 300 mg/100 ml may be fatal. Subsequent to removal of the patient from bromide therapy, the bromide is excreted along with chloride in essentially the same proportion in which they are present in plasma. Thus, serum bromide concentration decreases slowly and has a half-life of about 12 to 15 days unless special efforts are made to increase the bromide excretion rate by increasing chloride intake.

SENSITIVITY

15.0 mg/100 ml is detectable.

REFERENCE

Feigl, F., *Spot Tests,* Elsevier, Amsterdam, 1939, 163.

TYPE B PROCEDURE

G. Cimbura and J. Wells

APPARATUS

1. Centrifuge tubes, 15 ml
2. Vortex mixer (Vortex-Genie, Fisher Scientific Co.)
3. Centrifuge, clinical
4. Suitable microliter syringes
5. Gas chromatograph (Varian 1200, Varian Associates) equipped with a flame ionization detector and a 1 mV recorder, 6′ X ¼″ o.d. coiled aluminum column packed with 3% Poly-A103 on 80/100 mesh acid washed Gas Chrom Q (Applied Science Labs.)

   Operating Conditions

   Gas Flow Rate:
      nitrogen – 50 ml/min
   Temperature:
      column – 150°C

REAGENTS

All chemicals should be analytical reagent grade.

1. Bromide reference solution, 50 mg/100 ml
   Dissolve 64.34 mg of sodium bromide in water in a 100-ml volumetric flask and dilute to volume with water. Keep container well-closed.
2. Trichloroacetic acid, 20 g/100 ml
   Dissolve 20 g of trichloroacetic acid in water and dilute to 100 ml with water.
3. Sodium hypochlorite solution, 5% available chlorine B.D.H. Catalogue (1970–71) No. 7065. Store in refrigerator.
4. 2,4-Dimethylphenol(Eastman Koak)
   Dissolve 1 g in benzene and dilute to 100 ml with benzene.
5. Benzene, pesticide grade (Fisher Scientific Co.)

PROCEDURE

1. Pipet 0.5 ml of blood into each of two 15-ml centrifuge tubes (one of these will serve as a "blank"). Parallel each determination with one using the bromide reference solution.
2. Dilute the specimens with 0.5 ml of distilled water, and to each tube add 3 ml of the trichloroacetic acid solution. Agitate the mixtures on a Vortex mixer and centrifuge.
3. Transfer 3.0 ml aliquots of the protein-free solutions into two 15-ml centrifuge tubes.
4. a. Sample – Add 75 μl of the sodium hypochlorite solution, followed by 0.5 ml of the 2,4-dimethylphenol solution.
   b. "Blank" – Add 75 μl of the sodium hypochlorite solution, followed by 0.5 ml of benzene.
5. Stopper each tube tightly, agitate the mixtures on a Vortex mixer for about 2 min, and centrifuge.
6. Inject 2 μl of the upper benzene layers into the gas chromatograph.
7. If the bromide concentration is found to be greater than 100 mg/100 ml blood, it is necessary to dilute the blood with a suitable quantity of distilled water and repeat the experiment in order to insure a reliable result.

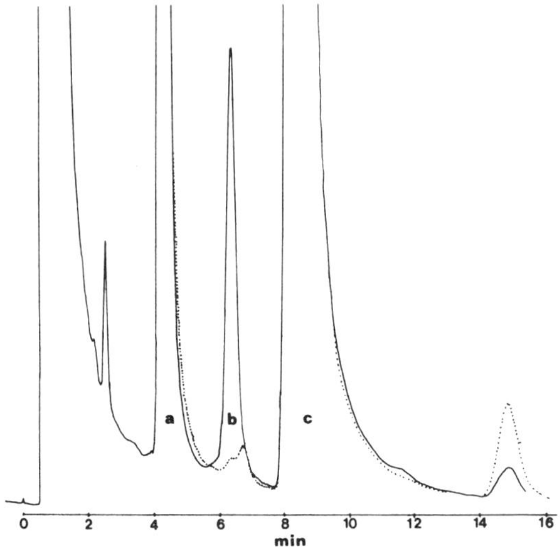

FIGURE 1. GC response (Poly-A103) to a blood sample treated as outlined under "Procedure" . . . . = Blank blood (no added bromide). = The same blood to which bromide has been added to give a bromide concentration of 25 mg/100 ml. Peak a product formed between the 2,4-dimethylphenol (Peak c) and hypochlorous acid. Peak b the bromination product, probably 6-bromophenol.

CALCULATION

To determine the concentration of bromide in the blood sample, compare the peak height of the bromo product (peak "b," Figure 1) with the height of the corresponding peak obtained by carrying the bromide reference solution through the "Procedure" for the sample.

INTERPRETATION (see p. 7)

Serum bromide concentrations higher than 50 mg/100 ml are compatible with incipient toxicity. Many patients with this serum concentration appear confused. With bromide concentrations between 150 and 250 mg/100 ml serum, uncoordination and emotional outbursts may be seen. Concentrations above 300 mg/100 ml may be fatal. Subsequent to removal of the patient from bromide therapy, the bromide is excreted along with chloride in essentially the same proportion in which they are present in plasma. Thus, serum bromide concentration decreases slowly and has a half-life of about 12 to 15 days unless special efforts are made to increase the bromide excretion rate by increasing chloride intake.

ACCURACY AND PRECISION

Duplicate analyses of five blood samples containing known concentrations of bromide in the 10 to 100 mg/100 ml range gave results within ±10% of the true values.

INTERFERING SUBSTANCES

The use of the "blank" in the procedure indicates the peaks other than the bromination product which may be found in the chromatogram.

REFERENCES

Wells, J. and Cimbura, G., The determination of elevated bromide levels in blood by gas chromatography, *J. Forensic Sci.,* 18(4), 437, 1973.

Wuth, O. J., Rational bromide pigment; New methods for its control, *JAMA,* 88, 2013, 1927.

CAFFEINE

PRINCIPLE

Caffeine is extracted from serum or urine with benzene, returned to an acid aqueous phase, and its absorbance is measured at 273 nm (Procedure B). After alkalinization of the aqueous phase, the caffeine is reextracted into chloroform. After evaporation to a residue, 50 μl of chloroform is added, and an aliquot of this solution is analyzed by gas chromatography, using a flame ionization detector (Procedure C).

TYPE B PROCEDURE

Joseph Routh

APPARATUS

1. Centrifuge tubes, glass-stoppered, 15 ml
2. Centrifuge
3. Mechanical shaker, horizontal
4. UV spectrophotometer

REAGENTS

All chemicals should be analytical reagent grade

1. NaCl
2. NaOH, 0.1*N*
   Dissolve 4g of sodium hydroxide in water and dilute to 100 ml with water.
3. Benzene
4. HCl, 6*N*
   Dilute 50 ml of concentrated hydrochloric acid to 100 ml with water.
5. Caffeine stock solution, 100 mg/dl
   Add 25 mg of caffeine alkaloid to a 25-ml volumetric flask and dilute to volume with water.
6. Caffeine, reference solutions, 1.0, 2.0, and 3.0 mg/dl
   Add 1.0 ml of caffeine stock solution to a 100-ml volumetric flask and dilute to volume with water. Repeat with 2.0 and 3.0 ml of caffeine stock solution.

PROCEDURE

1. Transfer 2.0 ml of sample (serum, urine, caffeine reference solutions, and water as a reagent blank) to a 15 ml glass-stoppered centrifuge tube. Add 1.5 g of NaCl, 0.5 ml of 0.1*N* NaOH, and 10 ml of benzene.
2. Stopper the tubes and mix the contents by inversion. Shake the tubes for 15 min on a horizontal mechanical shaker.
3. Centrifuge the tubes for 5 min and transfer an 8-ml aliquot of the benzene layer to another glass-stoppered centrifuge tube containing 4.0 ml of 6*N* HCl.
4. Shake the tubes for 5 min on the mechanical shaker and centrifuge the contents for 5 min.
5. Remove the benzene layer by careful aspiration and transfer a 3-ml aliquot of the aqueous layer to a 10-mm light path cuvette.
6. Determine the absorbance of the cuvette contents at 237 nm, using the solution obtained from the reagent blank in the reference cuvette.
7. Prepare a standard curve by plotting the absorbance of each reference solution against its concentration.

CALCULATION

Reagent blank, serum, and urine blank determinations should be carried out and used to correct the serum or urine values in the standard curve. In a random series of serum blanks on 39 specimens, the mean value was [0.024 A (SD ± 0.008)] 0.75 ± 0.25 μg/ml.

INTERPRETATION (see p. 7)

Caffeine is not found in normal serum or urine in

appreciable amounts. After the ingestion of a strong cup of coffee or two NoDoz® tablets (120 to 200 mg of caffeine), peak levels of 3 to 6 μg/ml in serum were reached in 60 to 90 min. Two to three hours after the ingestion, urine specimens contained from 2 to 6 μg/ml of caffeine.

ACCURACY AND PRECISION

Recovery values for the addition of caffeine to a series of serum specimens ranged from 95 to 106%.

INTERFERING SUBSTANCES

Metabolic products of caffeine and other interfering substances that may be present in urine are not extracted by benzene. The addition of 0.1*N* NaOH to the extraction mixture further reduces interference from these compounds, and extraction into 6*N* HCl eliminates most of the methylated xanthines from the final extract. The blank values in serum and urine may be due in part to small amounts of theobromine and theophylline that are not completely removed by the extraction process.

REFERENCES

Axelrod, J. and Reichenthal, J., The fate of caffeine in man and a method for its estimation in biological material, *J. Pharmacol. Exp. Ther.*, 107, 519, 1953.

Routh, J. I., Shane, N. A., Arredondo, E. G., and Paul, W. D., Determination of caffeine in serum and urine, *Clin. Chem.*, 15, 661, 1969.

TYPE C PROCEDURE

James C. Garriott and Susan Jones

APPARATUS

1. Screw-capped test tubes, 15 ml
2. Mechanical shaker
3. Centrifuge
4. Air source (compressed air tank)
5. Syringe, 10 μl (Hami... n Microliter #701)
6. Glass-stoppered centrifuge tubes, conical, 5 and 15 ml
7. Gas-liquid chromatograph equipped with a flame ionization detector, recorder, and coiled glass column, 6′ X 2 mm i.d., packed with 2.5% SE30 on 80 to 100 mesh Chromosorb G (AW/DMCS)

   Operating Conditions

   Gas Flow Rates:
   - nitrogen – 30 ml/min
   - hydrogen – 30 ml/min
   - air – 140 ml/min

   Temperatures:
   - column – 180°C
   - injection port – 200°C
   - detector – 300°C

REAGENTS

All chemicals should be analytical reagent grade.

1. Sodium chloride, solid
2. Benzene
3. Sodium hydroxide, 0.1*N*
   Dissolve 4.0 g of solid sodium hydroxide in water and dilute to one liter.
4. Hydrochloric acid, 5.0*N*
   Place 430 ml of concentrated (36%) hydrochloric acid in a volumetric flask, then dilute to one liter.
5. Caffeine stock solution, 100 mg/dl
   Add 25 mg of caffeine alkaloid to a 25 ml volumetric flask and dilute to volume with water.
6. Caffeine reference solutions, 1.0, 2.0, and 3.0 mg/dl
   Add 1.0 ml of caffeine stock solution to a 100-ml volumetric flask and dilute to volume with water. Repeat with 2.0 and 3.0 ml of caffeine stock solution.
7. Ammonium hydroxide, concentrated
8. Chloroform

9. Filter funnels and filter paper
10. Sodium sulfate, anhydrous, solid

PROCEDURE

1. To 2.0 ml of sample (blood, urine, tissue homogenate, or gastric contents) in a 15-ml test tube, add 1.5 g of sodium chloride, 0.5 ml of 0.1*N* sodium hydroxide, and 10.0 ml of benzene.
2. Add 2.0 ml of water and 2.0 ml of each caffeine reference solution to separate 15-ml tubes. Process each sample in the same manner as the specimen.
3. Extract each sample by shaking for 15 min on a mechanical shaker, then centrifuge for 5 min to separate the layers.
4. Transfer an 8-ml aliquot of the benzene layers from each tube to separate 15-ml tubes. Add 4.0 ml of 5*N* hydrochloric acid to each tube.
5. Extract each sample by shaking for 5 min on a mechanical shaker, then centrifuge for 5 min to effect separation of the layers.
6. Completely remove the benzene layer from each tube and discard. Remove the dissolved benzene in the aqueous phase by passing a stream of air through the solutions for 1 to 2 min using a fine-tipped glass tube or pipet attached to an air source.
7. Make each solution basic by adding concentrated ammonium hydroxide (approximately 2.0 ml) with mixing until an alkaline reaction is given with litmus paper.
8. Add 2.0 ml of chloroform to each tube and mix the solutions by shaking by hand for 3 min.
9. Remove and discard the upper aqueous layers. Transfer the chloroform to a 5-ml centrifuge tube by passing it through filter paper containing some sodium sulfate (about 300 mg) to remove any residual water. Rinse the filter paper with 2 ml of chloroform. Place the tube over a steam bath, and evaporate the solvent to dryness by directing a stream of air on the surface of the liquid. Dissolve the residue in 50 μl of chloroform and inject 3 μl into the gas chromatograph. Caffeine has an absolute retention time of 4.48 min under the conditions described.

CALCULATION

Calculate the caffeine concentration in the specimen by using the following formula:

$$C_S = C_R \times \frac{P_S}{P_R}$$

where

C_S = concentration of caffeine in the sample;
C_R = concentration of caffeine in the reference standard;
P_S = peak height of caffeine in the sample;
P_R = peak height of caffeine in the reference standard.

INTERPRETATION (see p. 7)

Caffeine is not found in normal serum or urine in appreciable amounts. After the ingestion of a strong cup of coffee or two NoDoz® tablets (120 to 200 mg of caffeine), peak levels of 3 to 6 μg/ml in serum were reached in 60 to 90 min (Table 1). Two to three hours after the ingestion, urine specimens contained from 2 to 6 μg/ml of caffeine. After a fatal overdose of caffeine in a 5-year-old girl a blood concentration of 15.8 mg/100 ml was found. Survival time was approximately 7 hr.

ACCURACY AND PRECISION

Extraction and recovery of caffeine from aqueous solutions is 100%. Recovery of caffeine from blood (0.40 mg/100 ml) is approximately 86%. As little as 0.10 mg/100 ml in blood can be detected.

INTERFERING SUBSTANCES

Although several drug substances have retention times similar to that of caffeine under these conditions, most would not be extracted by the procedure described. Lidocaine may be difficult to distinguish, if present.

Table 1

Subject	Taken	Caffeine, mg	Caffeine concentration (blood), mg/100 ml			
			½ Hr	1 Hr	2 Hr	3 Hr
No. 1 (R.N.) 160 lb	36 oz of Coca Cola®	150	0.13	0.13	0.05	0.05
No. 2 (F.S.) 115 lb	36 oz of Coca Cola®	150	0.20	0.22	0.21	0.17
No. 3 (S.J.) 130 lb	2 cups of coffee	302	0.54	0.47	0.43	0.41
No. 4 (J.D.) 200 lb	3 NoDoz® tablets	300	0.49 0.41(U)*	0.49 0.62(U)	0.41 0.53(U)	0.36 0.64(U)

* (U) = Urine

REFERENCES

Axelrod, J. and Reichenthal, J., The fate of caffeine in man and a method for its estimation in biological material, *J. Pharmacol. Exp. Ther.,* 107, 519, 1953.

DiMaio, V. J. M. and Garriott, J. C., Lethal caffeine poisoning in a child, *J. Forensic Sci.,* 3, 275, 1974.

Garriott, J. C., Caffeine concentrations in blood of subjects after consumption of coffee, Coca Cola or caffeine, *Forensic Sci. Gazette,* 5, 2, 1974.

Routh, J. I., Shane, N. A., Arredondo, G. G., and Paul, L. D., Determination of caffeine in serum and urine, *Clin. Chem.,* 45, 661, 1969.

CARBAMAZEPINE

PRINCIPLE

A single extraction is sufficient to remove carbamazepine from plasma. Interferences are eliminated by derivatization with dimethylformamide dimethylacetal. The resulting derivative is injected into a gas chromatograph, and the drug is quantitated by the internal standard technique.

TYPE C PROCEDURE

Robert J. Perchalski and B. J. Wilder

APPARATUS

1. Culture tubes with Teflon®-lined screw caps, 16 × 75 mm
2. Mechanical shaker
3. Conical reaction vials with Teflon®-lined screw caps, 5 ml*
4. Heating block or oil bath maintained at 100°C
5. Gas chromatograph (Varian Model 2100) with flame ionization detectors and 91.5 cm × 2 mm i.d. glass U-tube columns packed with 2.8% OV-210/3.2% OV-1 on 80/100 mesh Chromosorb W-HP (Packing preparation – Measure out 20 cc of 80/100 mesh Chromosorb W-HP and solution coat with 40 ml of chloroform containing 1.12 g of OV-210. Oven dry the packing at 80°C for 60 min. Weigh the packing into a large crystallizing dish and, using the slurry technique, coat with 3.2% OV-1. OV-101 may be substituted for OV-1.)

   Operating Conditions

   Gas Flow Rate:
      nitrogen (carrier gas) – 25 ml/min
   Temperatures:
      column – 215°C
      injection port – 250°C
      detector – 270°C

REAGENTS

All solvents and chemicals should be analytical reagent grade.

1. Carbamazepine stock solution, 50 mg/dl
   Dissolve 12.5 mg of recrystallized (isopropanol) carbamazepine in methanol and dilute to 25 ml with methanol.
2. Carbamazepine reference solutions, 0.25, 0.50, 0.75, 1.00, and 1.25 mg/dl
   To 1.00-ml aliquots of drug-free plasma in screw-capped culture tubes, add 5, 10, 15, 20, and 25 μl of carbamazepine stock solution.
3. Extracting solvent
   Benzene: ethyl acetate (4:1 by volume)
4. Derivatizing reagent
   Dimethylformamide dimethyl acetal,† redistilled and stored in a flask with a Teflon®-lined screw cap.‡ Store at 4°C and protect from light and moisture.
5. Carbon disulfide, redistilled
6. Dibenzo[*a*,*d*]-1,4-cycloheptadiene-5-carboxamide‡‡ internal standard solution, 20 mg/dl
   Dissolve 10 mg of cyheptamide in methanol and dilute to 50 ml with methanol. Store at 4°C.
7. Sodium phosphate buffer, 1*M*, pH 9.2

*Reacti-vial, Pierce Chemical Co., Rockford, Ill. 61105.
†Methyl-8, Pierce Chemical Co.
‡Reacti-flask, Pierce Chemical Co.
‡‡Cyheptamide, Ayerst Laboratories, N.Y., N.Y. 10017.

Dissolve 14.2 g of anhydrous dibasic sodium phosphate and 4.0 g of sodium hydroxide in water and dilute to 100 ml with water. Check the pH with a suitable pH meter.

PROCEDURE

1. Add 0.01 ml of the internal standard solution, 0.5 ml of the sodium phosphate buffer, and 3 ml of the extracting solvent to a 16 × 75-mm culture tube containing 1.00 ml of sample (plasma and each reference solution).
2. Shake the mixture mechanically for 10 min and centrifuge for 2 min.
3. Transfer the upper organic layer to a conical reaction vial and evaporate the extract to dryness at 55°C under a stream of nitrogen.
4. To the residue, add 0.030 ml of dimethylformamide dimethyl acetal, cap the vial, and place it in a 100°C oil bath for 10 min.
5. Allow the vial to cool and set it aside until just prior to injection.
6. Evaporate the excess reagent at room temperature using a stream of nitrogen and dissolve the residue in 25 μl of carbon disulfide.
7. Inject 1 μl into the gas chromatograph within 30 min after evaporation of the derivatizing reagent. Although the derivatives are stable for at least 17 hr in excess derivatizing reagent, the internal standard derivative begins to degrade after 30 min in CS_2.
8. Calculate the ratio of the peak height of carbamazepine to that of cyheptamide for each sample.
9. Prepare a standard curve of peak height ratio vs. concentration for the carbamazepine reference solutions.

CALCULATION

Determine the concentration of carbamazepine in the unknown sample by finding the peak height ratio (carbamazepine/cyheptamide) of the unknown on the standard curve prepared in Step 9.

INTERPRETATION (see p. 7)

The mean value of the plasma concentrations of carbamazepine in 59 epileptic patients receiving between 600 and 1200 mg/day of Tegretol® was 3.69 ± 1.58 μg/ml, ranging from a low of 1.09 to a high of 10.1 μg/ml. Meinardi[1] showed a good dose-response relationship up to 19 mg/kg/day and indicated that side effects, such as feelings of inhibition, dizziness, stomach cramps, headache, and disturbance of vision, occurred in 50% of all subjects at concentrations of 8.5 to 10 μg/ml.

SENSITIVITY AND PRECISION

The lower limit of detection of carbamazepine in plasma is 0.2 μg/ml. The standard curve is linear from the lower limit up to at least 15 μg/ml. Replicate determinations agree within 5%.

INTERFERING SUBSTANCES

Other anticonvulsants commonly prescribed with carbamazepine, including phenobarbital, primidone, diphenylhydantoin, and ethosuximide, do not interfere. The plastic serum separators which have recently come into wide use should be avoided during sample handling as interferences are introduced into the plasma. The small peak which elutes after cyheptamide in Figure 1A is produced by the extracting solvent and is constant, and therefore, noninterfering.

REFERENCE

1. **Meinardi, H.,** Carbamazepine in *Antiepileptic Drugs,* Woodbury, D. M., Penry, J. K., and Schmidt, R. P., Eds., Raven Press, N.Y., 1972, 487.

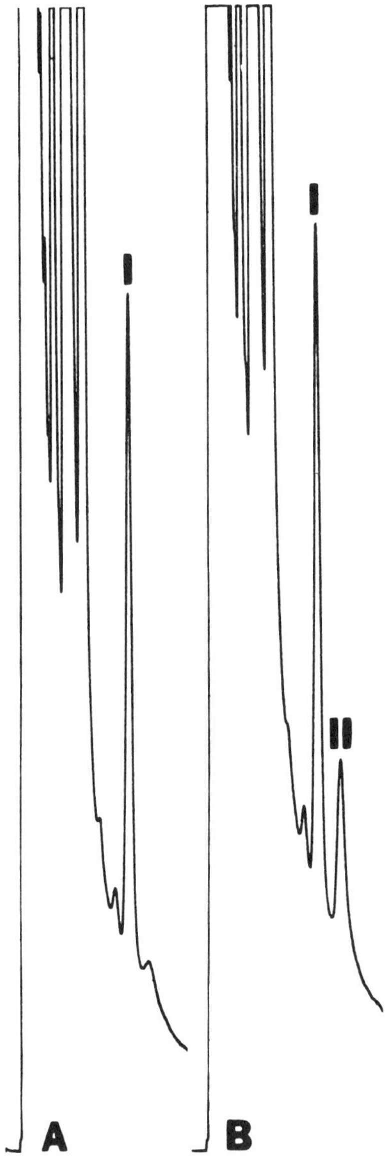

FIGURE 1. Chromatograms of extracts of a patient's plasma drawn just before (A) and 4 hr after (B) administration of 200 mg of Tegretol®, showing cyheptamide (I) and carbamazepine (II) with retention times of 5.65 and 6.90 min, respectively. The concentration of carbamazepine in B was 0.91 μg/ml. (From Perchalski, R. J. and Wilder, B. J., Rapid gas-liquid chromatographic determination of carbamazepine in plasma, *Clin. Chem.*, 20, 492, 1974. With permission.)

GENERAL REFERENCES

Faber, D. B. and Mann Intveld, W. A., A TLC method for determining carbamazepine in blood, *J. Chromatogr.*, 93, 1, 1974.

Frigerio, A., Finelli, R., Biandrati, P., Paserini, G., Morselli, P. L., and Garattini, S., Mass spectrometric characterization of carbamazepine-10,11-epoxide, a carbamazepine metabolite isolated from human urine, *J. Pharm. Sci.*, 61, 1144, 1972.

Kupferberg, H. J., GLC determination of carbamazepine in plasma, *J. Pharm. Sci.*, 61, 284, 1972.

Mashford, M. L., Ryan, P. L., and Thomson, W. A., Determination of carbamazepine in plasma, *J. Chromatogr.*, 89, 11, 1974.

Palmer, L., Bertilss, R. B., Collste, P., and Rawlins, M., Quantitative determination of carbamazepine in plasma by mass fragmentography, *Clin. Pharmacol. Ther.*, 14, 827, 1973.

Perchalski, R. J. and Wilder, B. J., Rapid gas-liquid chromatographic determination of carbamazepine in plasma, *Clin. Chem.*, 20, 492, 1974.

CARBON MONOXIDE

PRINCIPLE

Carbon monoxide determinations, seldom required in clinical toxicology, may be extremely important in forensic situations. This is particularly true in the investigation of a death associated with a fire. The presence or absence of carboxyhemoglobin has been used as an indication of whether the deceased was alive and died during the fire or whether the deceased was dead prior to the conflagration. This problem imposes a rigorous demand on the analyst for precision at concentrations at and below 10% carboxyhemoglobin.

Procedure A uses microdiffusion in a Conway cell. Adequate for high carboxyhemoglobin values, it does not permit a valid carboxyhemoglobin estimation below 10%. The technique depends on carbon monoxide being released from carboxyhemoglobin by free acid which is added to the blood sample. The carbon monoxide thus released diffuses in the Conway cell and reduces the palladium chloride in the center well to metallic palladium. A visual inspection indicates concentrations due to greater than 30% carboxyhemoglobin. The remaining unreacted palladium chloride in the center well can be ascertained by determining its absorbance at 278 nm. The absorbance difference between this result and an unreacted solution of palladium chloride can be used as a measure of the carbon monoxide evolved. The carboxyhemoglobin saturation can then be calculated if the hemoglobin content of the blood is determined. In Procedure B the percentage of carboxyhemoglobin in a suitably diluted specimen of whole blood is determined by simultaneous automated differential spectrophotometry at 548, 568, and 578 nm by means of a dedicated special purpose instrument (the Carboximeter) with an integral computational matrix and direct digital result presentation. The most reliable method is based on gas chromatography (Procedure C).

TYPE A PROCEDURE

Louis A. Williams

APPARATUS

1. Conway cells (Corning No. 3135)
2. UV spectrophotometer

REAGENTS

All chemicals should be analytical reagent grade.

1. Ucon® 2000 sealant (Union Carbide Corporation)
2. Hydrochloric acid, 0.1*N*
   Dilute 8.3 ml of concentrated hydrochloric acid to one liter with water.
3. Palladium chloride, 0.005*N*
   Dissolve 0.44 g of palladium chloride in 500 ml of 0.1*N* hydrochloric acid in a one-liter flask. Mix the solution, allow it to stand overnight, then dilute it to one liter with 0.1*N* hydrochloric acid. One ml of 0.005*N* palladium chloride is equivalent to 0.056 ml of carbon monoxide.
4. Sulfuric acid, 3.6*N*
   Dilute 10.0 ml of concentrated sulfuric acid to 100 ml with water.
5. Lead acetate-acetic acid solution
   Dilute 10.0 ml of glacial acetic acid to 100 ml with water. Saturate this solution with lead acetate.

PROCEDURE

1. On the lid of a Conway cell spread a thin layer of Ucon® in a circle comparable to the outer rim of the cell.
2. Pipet 3.0 ml of palladium chloride into the center well on the Conway cell.
3. Pipet 1.0 ml of 3.6*N* sulfuric acid into the outer well and place the cover over the cell, leaving an opening to permit addition of the blood specimen.

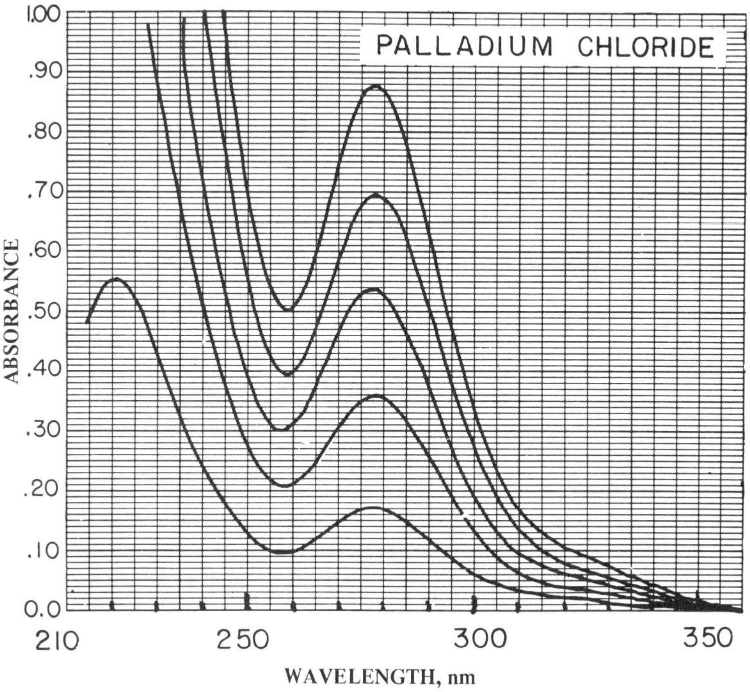

FIGURE 1. UV absorption spectra of various concentrations of palladium chloride. (Reproduced with permission of J. B. Lippincott Company, Philadelphia, from *Am. J. Clin. Pathol.*, 33, 334, 1960.)

4. Add 0.5 ml of blood, then slide the cover over the opening to seal the cell. Mix the contents of the outer well by gentle rotation, then allow the cell to stand for 2 hr at room temperature. *At this point, a semiquantitative estimate of carboxyhemoglobin can be made by observing the extent of the reduction that has occurred. The black film of metallic palladium that forms is a function of the amount of carbon monoxide released from the specimen. If a quantitative result is desired, proceed with Steps 5 to 8.*
5. Transfer the contents of the center well quantitatively to a 50-ml volumetric flask, rinsing three times with 3.0 ml of 0.1*N* hydrochloric acid.
6. Dilute the flask contents to 50.0 ml with 0.1*N* hydrochloric acid and mix well.
7. Using 0.1*N* hydrochloric acid as a reference solution, determine the absorbance of this solution in a 1-cm silica cuvette at 278 nm.
8. Using the same 0.1*N* hydrochloric acid reference solution, determine the absorbance of 3.0 ml of the 0.005*N* palladium chloride solution diluted to 50.0 ml with 0.1*N* hydrochloric acid using a 1-cm silica cuvette.

STANDARDIZATION AND CALCULATION

1. Dilute 0.5, 1.0, 1.5, 2.0, 2.5, and 3.0 ml of the 0.005*N* palladium chloride to 50.0 ml with 0.1*N* hydrochloric acid and mix well.
2. Using 1-cm silica cuvettes, determine the absorbance of the palladium chloride solutions against 0.1*N* hydrochloric acid at 278 nm (see Figure 1).
3. Plot the absorbances obtained as the ordinate against volumes of carbon monoxide/dl on the abscissa. The respective carbon monoxide values are as follows:

Volumes of palladium chloride, ml/50 ml	Volumes of carbon monoxide, ml/100 ml
3.0	0
2.5	5.6
2.0	11.2
1.5	16.8
1.0	22.4
0.5	28.0

4. Determine the carbon monoxide volumes from the reference curve. If the absorbance of the palladium chloride solution differs (at zero volume) from that shown on the curve, draw a new reference curve parallel to the old one, passing through the new zero point.
5. Perform a hemoglobin determination on an aliquot of the original specimen, then complete the calculation as follows:

$$\frac{\text{volumes of CO} \times 100}{\text{hemoglobin (g/100 ml)} \times 1.35} = \text{\% hemoglobin CO-saturated}$$

INTERPRETATION (see p. 7)

Hemoglobin has a 200-times greater affinity for carbon monoxide than for oxygen. For this reason oxygen can be replaced by carbon monoxide, producing a condition similar to anemia. The amount of hemoglobin saturation depends, for the most part, on the concentration of carbon monoxide in the atmosphere, the exposure time, the rate and depth of breathing, the absorption rate (which is related to temperature and humidity), and the hemoglobin concentration. Normal, healthy individuals may accumulate up to 10% carboxyhemoglobin from environmental causes such as cigarette smoking, working in an atmosphere polluted by gasoline engine exhaust fumes, or driving in an inadequately ventilated automobile with a faulty exhaust system. Major symptoms of carbon monoxide poisoning can be expected at blood saturation levels higher than 25%. This may be slightly lower in anemic or old persons. (In assessing a particular blood carbon monoxide saturation level, the age and health of the subject should be considered.) Lethal saturation levels range upwards from 50%, although they may be as low as 30% in old or diseased persons. Without treatment, death will certainly occur at saturation levels between 60 and 70%.

ACCURACY AND PRECISION

The coefficient of variation for this method is ± 5.2%.

INTERFERING SUBSTANCES

Sulfides can interfere if present in large quantities, as found in putrified blood. This interference, however, can be eliminated by substituting lead acetate-acetic acid solution for 3.6*N* sulfuric acid as the liberating solution.

REFERENCES

Frankel, S., Reitman, S., and Sonnenwirth, A. C., *Gradwohl's Clinical Laboratory Methods and Diagnosis,* C. V. Mosby, St. Louis, 1970, 303.

Williams, L. A., Linn, R. A., and Zak, B., Ultraviolet absorptiometry of palladium for determination of carbon monoxide hemoglobin, *Am. J. Clin. Pathol.,* 34, 334, 1960.

TYPE B PROCEDURE

A. Freireich, D. Landau, K. M. Dubowski, and N. C. Jain

APPARATUS

1. Centrifuge
2. Syringe, plastic, disposable, 2.5 ml, with a #19 needle, 1½ in. long
3. CO-Oximeter (Model 182)*
4. Swinny filter holder† (Cat. No. XX3001200), 13 mn

REAGENTS

All chemicals should be analytical reagent grade.

1. Co-Oximeter diluent solution* (120 g of Triton® X-100 per liter of water containing 1% Zephiran Chloride®)
2. Sodium hydrosulfite powder ($Na_2S_2O_4$)
3. CO-Oximeter zeroing solution*
   Dilute 10 ml of the diluent solution to 100 ml with water.
4. CO-Oximeter cleaning agent*
   Dilute 100 ml of Chlorox® to one liter with water.

SAMPLE PREPARATION

Fresh Blood

Only 0.4 ml of anticoagulated blood is required for the analysis. In actual practice, however, a 1 to 2-ml blood sample is convenient. The anticoagulant should be EDTA. Heparin can be used if the blood sample is fresh and is used immediately.

Old or Putrified Blood[‡1]

1. Centrifuge a 5-ml blood sample to separate the plasma from the red cells.
2. Aspirate and discard the supernatant plasma.
3. Add to the centrifuge tube a volume of CO-Oximeter zeroing solution equal to the volume of the red cells.
4. Shake the tube to hemolyze the cells. If clots are present, the entire mixture is thoroughly homogenized with a tissue grinder.
5. Add 10 mg of sodium hydrosulfite and mix well by shaking.
6. Centrifuge the tube. A film of fat may appear at the top of the tube contents.
7. Tilt the tube about 45° from a vertical position, then carefully insert the needle of a 2-ml syringe through the fat layer and remove 1 ml of the clear solution just below the fat layer. Discard the needle. The solution in the syringe is now ready for use in the CO-Oximeter.

PROCEDURE

1. Turn the instrument on. Allow 30 min warm-up for maximum stability.
2. With a syringe, introduce and pump zeroing solution through the instrument. Set Hb, HbO_2, and HbCO to zero.
3. Attach a Swinny filter filled loosely with glass wool to the syringe containing the blood sample. Introduce about 1 ml of the sample (fresh or the solution obtained from a

*Available from Instrumentation Laboratory, Inc., Lexington, Mass. 02173.
†Available from Millipore Corp., Bedford, Mass. 01730.
‡Specimens of blood from autopsy material often require a liberal interpretation of the term to qualify as "blood." In most instances the specimen is almost entirely a clot. In other instances the specimen may consist of about 5% or less of cells suspended in serum. When the specimen is not taken from the heart or from a major blood vessel, it is not unusual to have an admixture of the blood with pericardial or pleural fluid. Occasionally, one can distinguish globules of fats or oils or pieces of fatty tissue floating on the surface of the specimen.

putrefied sample in Step 7 of the sample preparation) and activate the pump.

4. Read value of Hb, HbO_2, and HbCO saturation directly displayed on the instrument 30 sec after the pump stops. This time interval allows the blood to equilibrate with the cuvette temperature.
5. Flush the instrument with zeroing solution to remove the blood from the system. Clean the system by two additional flush cycles using the zeroing solution, refilling the reservoir as required. After completion of the pump cycles, check zero readings for each channel. Failure to achieve zero settings to within ±0.2 of the zero values prior to analysis may indicate the presence of a blood clot in the cuvette and, hence, a questionable result.
6. Upon the completion of each set of measurements, introduce cleaning agent into the instrument and allow it to remain for 5 min or longer. Thereafter, flush the instrument and cuvette thoroughly with zeroing solution.

Note: When 100% CO saturated blood is processed through the method described above, the final 10 cc He/CO mixture in the syringe contains 0.094 cc carbon monoxide. Therefore, a 30 cc syringe containing 0.28 cc CO (i.e., $\frac{0.094}{10} \times 30$) diluted to 30 cc with helium is equivalent to the gas mixture resulting from 100% CO saturated blood analyzed by this method.

INTERPRETATION (see p. 7)

Normal Values

In normal nonsmoking subjects living in cities under conditions of minimal exposure to carbon monoxide, 0.25 to 2.1% HbCO saturations have been found; normal tobacco smokers were found to have HbCO saturations of 0.7 to 6.5%.[2,3] Occasionally, HbCO saturations as high as 12% were found in heavy cigarette smokers immediately after smoking.[4] Endogenous production of carbon from heme catabolism has been documented.[5]

Resume of Clinical Interpretations

Blood HbCO saturations below 5% are generally considered normal, and values below 10% may be compatible with normal environmental conditions for the subject. Concentrations below 10% HbCO saturation have in the past been generally considered as not detrimental to normal physical and mental performance, although Lilienthal[6] in laboratory studies found impairment of visual brightness at 4% HbCO saturation. Recent studies have demonstrated that low and commonly occurring HbCO concentrations may impair accurate estimation of time intervals, as well as performance of more complex psychomotor tasks.[5] Subjective symptoms (headache, nausea, mental confusion, restlessness, pallor, cold extremities, and a mild state of shock) have been observed in recumbent subjects at 15% HbCO saturation at a simulated altitude of 15,000 feet.[7] Some symptoms of acute carbon monoxide poisoning generally occur with approximately 20% HbCO and become severe at about 30% HbCO saturation.[8]

In fatal carbon monoxide poisoning, the HbCO saturation usually ranges from 60 to 80%, but death from the inhalation of carbon monoxide occasionally occurs with HbCO saturations below 60% and, in exceptional cases, the agonal saturation may be as low as 30 to 40%.[4,9]

ACCURACY AND PRECISION

Dubowski and Luke[10] found excellent correlation between carboxyhemoglobin values obtained on random post-mortem blood specimens directly with the Carboximeter® and by computation from gas-chromatographic analyses for carbon monoxide content plus photometric measurement of total hemoglobin content by a cyanmethemoglobin procedure. The main difference between the results obtained by gas chromatography and photometry and those obtained with the Carboximeter® was −0.35% HbCO in a series of 23 blood specimens ranging from 0 to 79% HbCO.

INTERFERING SUBSTANCES

It is extremely important that blood clots, protein, fat, or other interfering substances are not introduced into the flow cell of the CO-Oximeter. If any of these are present, erroneous results will be obtained. Old or putrified blood samples should, therefore, be treated as described above. The flow cell should also be free of air bubbles.

REFERENCES

1. **Freireich, A. W. and Landau, D.,** Determination of carbon monoxide in post-mortem clotted blood, *J. Forensic Sci.,* 16, 112, 1971.
2. **Gettler, A. O. and Mattice, M. R.,** The "normal" carbon monoxide content of the blood, *JAMA,* 100, 92, 1933.
3. **Trinder, P. and Harper, F. E.,** A colorimetric method for the determination of carboxyhemoglobin over a wide range of concentrations, *J. Clin. Pathol.,* 15, 82, 1962.
4. **Goldsmith, J. R. and Landsaw, S. A.,** Carbon monoxide and human health, *Science,* 162, 1352, 1968.
5. **Dubowski, K. M.,** Unpublished observations.
6. **Lilienthal, J. L., Jr.,** Carbon monoxide, *Pharmacol. Rev.,* 2, 324, 1950.
7. **Allen, T. H. and Allard, R. W.,** Fundamental parameters influencing the accumulation and elimination of carbon monoxide in adult human beings, Report No. 261, U.S. Army Medical Research and Nutrition Laboratory, Denver, 1961.
8. **Rowan, T. and Coleman, F. C.,** Carbon monoxide poisoning, *J. Forensic Sci.,* 7, 103, 1962.
9. **Gettler, A. O. and Freimuth, H. C.,** The carbon monoxide content of the blood under various conditions, *Am. J. Clin. Pathol.,* 11, 603, 1940.
10. **Dubowski, K. M. and Luke, J. L.,** Measurement of carboxyhemoglobin and carbon monoxide in blood, *Ann. Clin. Lab. Sci.,* 3, 53, 1973.

TYPE C PROCEDURE

Bryan S. Finkle

APPARATUS

1. Serological pipet, 5 ml
2. Measuring cylinder, ground-glass-stoppered, 25 ml
3. Glass syringes, fitted with Luer locks, 30 ml
4. Hypodermic needles (B-D), # 20
5. Hypodermic needle, plugged, #20, for use as a syringe stopper
6. Mechanical shaker, wrist-action (Burrell)
7. Glass syringe, fitted with a Luer lock two-way valve, 100 ml
8. Gas chromatograph (Beckman GC-2), fitted with a microthermal-conductivity detector (Carle 100), and a stainless-steel column, 4 X 1/8″ o.d., packed with 42/60-mesh 5A Linde molecular sieve

Operating Conditions

Gas Inlet Pressure:
helium (carrier gas) – 14 lbs
Temperatures:
oven – 40°C
injection port – Beckman gas-sampling valve, fitted with a 1-ml sample loop
Detector current: 25 mA, dc
Attenuation: X 5

REAGENTS

All chemicals should be analytical reagent grade.

1. Igepal® detergent, 250 μl/dl
   Dissolve 250 μl of the detergent in water and dilute to 100 ml.
2. Mineral oil, light viscosity
3. Carbon monoxide gas, lecture bottle
4. Helium
5. Potassium ferricyanide, 5 g/dl
   Dissolve 5 g of potassium ferricyanide in water and dilute to 100 ml.

PROCEDURE

1. Pipet 1.5 ml of whole blood* into a 25-ml ground-glass-stoppered measuring cylinder and dilute it to the 18-ml mark with the Igepal® detergent. Mix gently. Allow the blood to hemolyze by letting the mixture stand 1 min.
2. Draw 8.0 ml of the hemolyzed, diluted blood into a 30-ml glass syringe that has been lightly lubricated with mineral oil and fitted with a #20 B-D hypodermic needle.
3. Draw the remainder (approximately 10 ml) of the blood into a second similar syringe. Expel

*On removal from an exposure, a patient will lose a significant amount of carboxyhemoglobin just by breathing air; hence, any assessment of a living person's exposure requires that a blood sample be taken as soon as possible, preferably at the time and site of the exposure.

excess air. Keep the syringe stoppered with a plugged #20 hypodermic needle at all times except when introducing or expelling gases or liquids.

4. Saturate the blood in the second syringe with carbon monoxide in the following manner: (a) Introduce approximately 10 ml of carbon monoxide gas from a lecture bottle into the syringe. Shake the syringe for 10 min: (b) Expel all excess gas, then shake the blood with three separate 10-ml volumes of air for 2 min each.
5. Shake the blood in both syringes with 10-ml volumes of helium for 2 min, then expel the gas. A 100-ml helium reservoir in a glass syringe fitted with a Luer lock two-way valve provides a ready supply of gas and simple means of transfer to the sample syringes. The reservoir can be supplied from the injection port of the gas chromatograph.
6. Adjust the volume of blood in each syringe to 5.0 ml, then draw in 5.0 ml of potassium ferricyanide reagent.
7. Add 11 ml of helium to each syringe.
8. Adjust the volumes to 20.0 ml, allowing excess helium to escape. Stopper the syringes, agitate them for 20 min on the mechanical shaker, then allow the solutions to settle.
9. Inject about 8 ml of each gas mixture into the gas chromatograph.
10 Measure the carbon monoxide peak heights for the unknown and the 100%-saturated blood sample aliquots.

CALCULATION

Calculate the present carbon monoxide saturation of the blood specimen by direct proportion as follows:

$$\%\text{ carbon monoxide saturation of blood sample} = \frac{U}{S} \times 100,$$

S = CO peak height of the sample aliquot saturated to 100%;
U = CO peak height of the unknown sample aliquot.

INTERPRETATION (see p. 7)

Normal Values

In normal nonsmoking subjects living in cities under conditions of minimal exposure to carbon monoxide, 0.25 to 2.1% HbCO saturations have been found; normal tobacco smokers were found to have HbCO saturations of 0.7 to 6.5%.[1,2] Occasionally, HbCO saturations as high as 12% were found in heavy cigarette smokers immediately after smoking.[3] Endogenous production of carbon from heme catabolism has been documented.[4]

Resume of Clinical Interpretations

Blood HbCO saturations below 5% are generally considered normal, and values below 10% may be compatible with normal environmental conditions for the subject. Concentrations below 10% HbCO saturation have in the past been generally considered as not detrimental to normal physical and mental performance, although Lilienthal[5] in laboratory studies found impairment of visual brightness at 4% HbCO saturation. Recent studies have demonstrated that low and commonly occurring HbCO concentrations may impair accurate estimation of time intervals, as well as performance of more complex psychomotor tasks.[4] Subjective symptoms (headache, nausea, mental confusion, restlessness, pallor, cold extremities, and a mild state of shock) have been observed in recumbent subjects at 15% HbCO saturation at a simulated altitude of 15,000 feet.[6] Some symptoms of acute carbon monoxide poisoning generally occur with approximately 20% HbCO and become severe at about 30% HbCO saturation.[7]

In fatal carbon monoxide poisoning, the HbCO saturation usually ranges from 60 to 80%, but death from the inhalation of carbon monoxide occasionally occurs with HbCO saturations below 60% and, in exceptional cases, the agonal saturation may be as low as 30 to 40%.[3,8]

ACCURACY AND PRECISION

Dubowski and Luke[9] found excellent correlation between carboxyhemoglobin values obtained on random post-mortem blood specimens directly with the Carboximeter® and by computation from gas-chromatographic analyses for carbon monoxide content plus photometric measurement of total hemoglobin content by a cyanno-methemoglobin procedure. The main difference between the results obtained by gas chromatography and photometry and those obtained with the Carboximeter® was −0.35% HbCO in a series of 23 blood specimens ranging from 0 to 79% HbCO.

REFERENCES

1. **Gettler, A. O. and Mattice, M. R.,** The "normal" carbon monoxide content of the blood, *JAMA*, 100, 92, 1933.
2. **Trinder, P. and Harper, F. E.,** A colorimetric method for the determination of carboxyhemoglobin over a wide range of concentrations, *J. Clin. Pathol.*, 15, 82, 1962.
3. **Goldsmith, J. R. and Landsaw, S. A.,** Carbon monoxide and human health, *Science*, 162, 1352, 1968.
4. **Dubowski, K. M.,** Unpublished observations.
5. **Lilienthal, J. L., Jr.,** Carbon monoxide, *Pharmacol. Rev.*, 2, 324, 1950.
6. **Allen, T. H. and Allard, R. W.,** Fundamental parameters influencing the accumulation and elimination of carbon monoxide in adult human beings, Report No. 261, U.S. Army Medical Research and Nutrition Laboratory, Denver, 1961.
7. **Rowan, T. and Coleman, F. C.,** Carbon monoxide poisoning, *J. Forensic Sci.*, 7, 103, 1962.
8. **Gettler, A. O. and Freimuth, H. C.,** The carbon monoxide content of the blood under various conditions, *Am. J. Clin. Pathol.*, 11, 603, 1940.
9. **Dubowski, K. M. and Luke, J. L.,** Measurement of carboxyhemoglobin and carbon monoxide in blood, *Ann. Clin. Lab. Sci.*, 3, 53, 1973.

GENERAL REFERENCES

Curry, A., *Poison Detection in Human Organs*, 2nd ed., Charles C Thomas, Springfield, Ill., 1969, 43.

Dubowski, K. M. and Luke, J. L., Measurement of carboxyhemoglobin and carbon monoxide in blood, *Ann. Clin. Lab. Sci.*, 3(1), 53, 1973.

Maehly, A. C., Quantitative determination of carbon monoxide, in *Methods of Forensic Science*, Vol. 1, Lundquist, F., Ed., Interscience, N.Y., 1962, 539.

CHLORAL HYDRATE AND TRICHLOROETHANOL

PRINCIPLE

Chloral hydrate and its major metabolite, trichloroethanol, are halogenated hydrocarbons and are, thus, detectable in low concentrations by electron-capture gas chromatography. Advantage of this extreme sensitivity is taken to inject small amounts of biological specimens, including blood, tissue homogenate, and urine, directly into a 15% FFAP* (free fatty acid phase) gas-chromatographic column. Chlorobutanol is used as an internal standard.

Following ingestion, chloral hydrate is immediately metabolized into trichloroethanol. The reduction to trichloroethanol is very rapid and takes place even in vitro when a standard solution of chloral hydrate is prepared in blood. This enzymatic action necessitates making aqueous standard solutions of chloral hydrate. In case of chloral ingestion, only the trichloroethanol will be found in body fluids. Gastric contents may contain some unchanged drug.

TYPE B PROCEDURE

Naresh C. Jain

APPARATUS

1. Blender (Waring)
2. Centrifuge (International Size 2)
3. Gas chromatograph (Aerograph Hy-Fi Model 600-D), equipped with an electron-capture detector, a 1 mV recorder (Leeds and Northrup Speedomax H), a spiral stainless steel column, 5′ X 1/8″ o.d., packed with 15% FFAP (free fatty acid phase) on 60 to 80 mesh acid-washed Chromosorb W (A coil of stainless steel wire gauze in the injection chamber serves as a filter for solids in the biological material.)

   Operating Conditions

   Gas Flow Rates:
   nitrogen (carrier gas) – 8 ml/min

   Temperatures:
   column – 105°C for separating a mixture of chloral hydrate and trichloroethanol, 120°C for trichloroethanol alone
   injection port – 165°C
   detector – 180°C

REAGENTS

All chemicals should be analytical reagent grade.

1. Potassium carbonate, saturated aqueous solution
2. Chloral hydrate stock solution, 100 mg/mg/dl
   Dissolve 100 mg of chloral hydrate in water and dilute to 100 ml with water.
3. Chloral hydrate reference solutions
   Respectively, dilute 0.125, 0.250, 0.500, 0.75, and 1.00 ml of the chloral hydrate stock solution to 100 ml with water.
4. Trichloroethanol stock solution, 150 mg/dl
   Dilute 1.0 ml of trichloroethanol to one liter with water.
5. Trichloroethanol reference solutions
   Respectively, dilute 0.125, 0.250, 0.500, 0.75, and 1.00 ml of the trichloroethanol stock solution to 100 ml with water.
6. Chlorobutanol stock solution, 100 mg/dl
   Dissolve 100 mg of chlorobutanol (Baker) in 100 ml of a 1:1 mixture of ethanol and water.
7. Chlorobutanol internal standard solution
   Dilute 0.500 ml of the chlorobutanol stock

*Chloral hydrate is very rapidly metabolized to trichloroethanol. If ingestion of chloral hydrate is suspected, unmetabolized chloral hydrate will most likely not be found, but trichloroethanol will be present.

solution to 100 ml with a 1:1 mixture of ethanol and water.

8. Perchloric acid, 0.5*N*
   Dilute 10.0 ml of 70% perchloric acid to 140 ml with water.

SPECIMEN REQUIREMENTS

Fluids

Whole blood, urine, and stomach content can be analyzed directly.

Tissues

1. Homogenize a 20-g aliquot of tissue in the covered glass container of a Waring blender to which 80.0 ml of 0.5*N* perchloric acid has been previously added. Adjust the final volume to 100 ml with water.
2. Centrifuge the homogenate in a stoppered glass bottle for 30 min at 3,000 rpm.
3. Place a 10.0-ml aliquot of the supernatant in a glass-stoppered centrifuge tube. Slowly add the saturated potassium carbonate solution until the pH is between 5 and 6. Chilling of the supernatant prior to this step helps reduce the effervescence caused by the liberation of carbon dioxide. Note the final volume (F_x).
4. Centrifuge the mixture for 10 min at 1,500 rpm.

PROCEDURE

1. Examine the gas chromatograph to be sure that the operating conditions stated above are met. Inject 1 μl of the reference solutions. At a column temperature of 105°C, chloral hydrate, trichloroethanol, and chlorobutanol have retention times of 1.3, 5.6, and 10.1 min, respectively; at a column temperature of 120°C, the retention times for trichloroethanol and chlorobutanol are 2.8 min and 4.7 min, respectively.
2. Dilute 1.0 ml of specimen (whole blood, urine, stomach content, or the solution obtained from tissue homogenate) with 1.0 ml of the internal control solution of chlorobutanol. Process 1.0 ml of each reference solution in the same manner as the specimen.
3. Inject a 1-μl aliquot of each solution into the gas chromatograph.
4. Quantitate chloral hydrate or trichloroethanol in the specimen by comparison of the average peak area ratio (compound/internal standard) with the average peak area ratio of the reference solutions.

CALCULATION

Calculate the drug concentration in the biological specimen preparation as follows: in blood or urine,

$$C_x = C_S \times \frac{H_x}{R_x} \times \frac{R_S}{H_S},$$

in tissue,

$$C_x = C_S \times \frac{H_x}{R_x} \times \frac{R_S}{H_S} \times \frac{F_x}{2},$$

where

C_x = concentration of the specimen mixture;
C_S = concentration of the substance to be assayed in the reference mixture;
H_S = peak area of the substance to be assayed in the reference mixture;
H_x = peak area of the specimen mixture at the retention time of the substance to be assayed;
R_S = peak area of the internal control in the reference mixture;
R_x = peak area of the internal control in the specimen mixture;
F_x = final volume of the solution obtained from tissue homogenate.

INTERPRETATION (see p. 7)

Chloral hydrate is immediately metabolized. Shortly after oral ingestion only trichloroethanol can be found in blood. In man, after an oral dose of 1 g of chloral hydrate, the highest blood concentrations of trichloroethanol, ranging from 0.8 to 1.2 mg/dl, are reached between 30 and 60 min after ingestion. The rate of disappearance is slow; after 6 hr, the blood concentrations of trichloroethanol range from 0.3 to 0.6 mg/dl.

ACCURACY AND PRECISION

The response of the electron-capture detector to either chloral hydrate or trichloroethanol is linear in the concentration range from 0.00125 to 0.005 mg/ml. Specimens of biological materials whose concentrations of these substances exceed 0.005 mg/ml must, therefore, be diluted with distilled water. Recovery values for chloral hydrate and trichloroethanol from tissue homogenate range from 98 to 100%.

INTERFERING SUBSTANCES

No substances were found to interfere. Chloral hydrate and trichloroethanol may be determined simultaneously and do not interfere with each other.

PRECAUTIONS

Reference solutions of chloral hydrate should only be made in water. Blood should not be used, because chloral hydrate will be enzymatically metabolized to trichloroethanol. Aqueous solutions of chloral hydrate are stable if stored in a refrigerator.

REFERENCES

Breimer, D. D., Katelaars, H. C. J., and VanRossum, J. M., Gas chromatographic determination of chloral hydrate, trichloroethanol and trichloroacetic acid in blood and in urine employing head-space analysis, *J. Chromatogr.,* 88, 55, 1974.

Friedman, P. J. and Cooper, J. R., Determination of chloral hydrate, trichloracetic acid and trichloroethanol, *Anal. Chem.,* 30, 1674, 1958.

Garrett, E. R. and Lambert, H. J., Gas-chromatographic analysis of trichloroethanol, chloral hydrate, trichloroacetic acid and trichloroethanol glucuronide, *J. Pharm. Sci.,* 55, 812, 1966.

Jain, N. C., et al., A rapid gas-chromatographic method for the determination of chloral hydrate and trichloroethanol in blood and other biological materials, *J. Forensic Sci.,* 12, 497, 1967.

Kaplan, H. L., Forney, R. B., Hughes, F. W., and Jain, N. C., Chloral hydrate and alcohol metabolism in human subjects, *J. Forensic Sci.,* 12, 295, 1967.

Marshall, E. K., Jr. and Owens, A. H., Jr., Absorption, excretion and metabolic fate of chloral hydrate and trichloroethanol, *Bull. Johns Hopkins Hosp.,* 95, 1, 1954.

Moss, M. S. and Kenyon, M. W., The detection of trichlorosedatives in urine, *Analyst,* 89, 802, 1964.

CHLORDIAZEPOXIDE (LIBRIUM®)

PRINCIPLE

Chlordiazepoxide is extracted into an organic solvent from the biological fluid. In Procedure A the extract is evaporated to dryness, hydrolyzed, diazotized, and coupled to an aromatic amine, forming a purple solution which can be used for quantitation. In Procedure B this organic extract is reextracted into dilute acid, and the UV absorption spectrum of this solution is used to quantitate the drug. In Procedure C the extract is analyzed by gas chromatography, using an electron-capture detector.

TYPE A PROCEDURE

Gerald Kananen

APPARATUS

1. Bottles, ground-glass-stoppered, 60 ml, or separatory funnels
2. Filter paper (E & D) #615)
3. Photometer, photoelectric

REAGENTS

All chemicals should be analytical reagent grade.

1. Chlordiazepoxide stock solution, 100 mg/dl
   Dissolve 100 mg of chlordiazepoxide in water and dilute to 100 ml with water.
2. Chlordiazepoxide reference solution, 1 mg/dl
   Dilute 1.0 ml of the chlordiazepoxide stock solution to 100 ml with water. This solution is stable for at least 1 week if stored at 4°C.
3. Potassium carbonate, anhydrous
4. Ether, anhydrous
5. Sodium sulfate, anhydrous
6. Hydrochloric acid, 6*N*
   Mix equal volumes of concentrated hydrochloric acid and water.
7. Sodium nitrite, 1 g/l
   Dissolve 0.1 g of sodium nitrite in water and dilute to 100 ml with water.
8. Ammonium sulfamate, 500 mg/dl
   Dissolve 0.5 g of ammonium sulfamate in water and dilute to 100 ml with water.
9. *N*-1-Naphthylethylenediamine hydrochloride, 100 mg/dl
   Dissolve 100 mg of *N*-1-naphthylethylenediamine hydrochloride in water and dilute to 100 ml with water.

PROCEDURE

1. Pipet a 5.0-ml aliquot of specimen (whole blood, serum, or urine) into a 60-ml ground-glass-stoppered bottle or separatory funnel. Process 5.0 ml of reference solution and 5.0 ml of water for a reagent blank in the same manner.
2. Add 0.5 g of anhydrous potassium carbonate to each sample and dissolve it by swirling.
3. Add 30 ml of ether to each bottle and shake for about 1 min. Let the bottles stand for 5 to 10 min to allow the phases to separate.
4. Remove and discard the aqueous layers. Wash each ether layer twice, using a 5.0-ml aliquot of water each time. Discard the wash water.
5. Filter the ether through E & D #615 filter paper containing about 5 g of anhydrous sodium sulfate in its apex. Place 20 ml of each filtrate in a clear bottle or separatory funnel.
6. Add 5.0 ml of 6*N* hydrochloric acid to each sample and shake for 1 min. Allow the phases to separate, then remove the ether layers by aspiration and discard them.
7. Transfer a 4.0-ml aliquot of each acid extract to a test tube. Heat the tubes for 30 min in a boiling water bath. Shake the tubes several times during the first minute to permit rapid and even evaporation of any dissolved ether present.

8. Allow the solutions to cool, then dilute each to 5.0 ml with 6*N* hydrochloric acid.
9. Add 0.5 ml of the sodium nitrite solution and mix gently. Wait 3 min.
10. Add 0.5 ml of the ammonium sulfamate solution and mix gently. Wait 10 min.
11. Add 0.5 ml of the *N*-1-naphthylethylenediamine hydrochloride solution. Wait 1 hr.
12. Determine the absorbance of each solution at 550 nm using the extract from the reagent blank as the reference solution. The absorbance is stable for 16 hr.

CALCULATION

The absorbance of chlordiazepoxide is a linear function of concentration over a range from 0.1 to 1.0 mg/dl.

1. Compare the absorbance of the solution obtained from the specimen with the absorbance of the solution obtained from the reference sample.
2. Calculate the chlordiazepoxide concentration in the specimen by the following formula:

$$C_S = C_R \times \frac{A_S}{A_R},$$

where

C_S = concentration of the specimen;
C_R = concentration of the reference solution;
A_S = absorbance of the reference solution at 550 nm;
A_R = absorbance of the specimen at 550 nm.

INTERPRETATION (see p. 7)

Blood concentration is at a maximum between 2 and 4 hr after oral ingestion. Following therapeutic doses, the maximum concentration is 0.2 to 0.3 mg/100 ml.

ACCURACY AND PRECISION

With reasonable care, duplicate determinations will agree within ±5% of their mean value.

INTERFERING SUBSTANCES

Any substance containing a diazotizable amino group on a basic compound can interfere. The most common of these are the "sulfa" drugs.

REFERENCES

Pribilla, O., Chlordiazepoxide, *Arzneim-Forsch,* 14, 723, 1969.

Randall, L. O., Pharmacology of chlordiazepoxide, *Dis. Nerv. Syst.,* Suppl. 22, 7, 1961.

Roche Laboratories Products Reference Manual, Roche Laboratories, Nutley, N. J., 1970.

Smyth, D. and Pennington, G. W., The detection and excretion of chlordiazepoxide in human plasma and urine, *Arch. Int. Pharmacodyn. Ther.,* 145, 154, 1963.

TYPE B PROCEDURE

Clifford B. Walberg

APPARATUS

1. Centrifuge tubes, glass-stoppered, 50 and 15 ml
2. Centrifuge
3. Filter paper (Whatman #31), 11.0 cm
4. Separatory funnels, 60 ml with polyethylene (Kimax 28160 TS 13) stoppers
5. Volumetric pipet, 4 ml
6. UV spectrophotometer

REAGENTS

All chemicals should be analytical reagent grade.

1. Chlordiazepoxide stock solution, 100 mg/dl
   Add 28.04 mg of chlordiazepoxide (Librium®) hydrochloride* to a 25-ml volumetric flask and dilute to volume with distilled water. Store in a brown glass bottle at 4°C.
2. Chlordiazepoxide reference solution, 2 mg/dl
   Transfer 2.0 ml of the chlordiazepoxide stock solution to a 100-ml volumetric flask and dilute it to volume with pooled drug-free serum.
3. Phosphate buffer, 3*M* (approx. pH 3.6)
   Dissolve 42.4 g of sodium phosphate monohydrate, $HaH_2PO_4 \cdot H_2O$, in water and dilute to 100 ml with water.
4. Sodium hydroxide, 0.45*N*
   Dissolve 18 g of sodium hydroxide in water and dilute to one liter. Store the solution in a polyethylene bottle.
5. Chloroform (spectroquality, MCB #CX1050 or its equivalent
   If reagent grade chloroform is used, it must be washed with dilute alkali, dilute acid, and water until all artifacts are removed.
6. Sulfuric acid, 0.5*N*
   Dilute 7.0 ml of concentrated sulfuric acid to 500 ml with distilled water.

PROCEDURE

1. Transfer 2.0 ml of specimen (serum, urine, or stomach content) to a 50-ml glass-stoppered centrifuge tube. Transfer 2.0 ml of chlordiazepoxide reference solution to a second centrifuge tube.
2. Add 0.1 ml of 3*M* phosphate buffer.
3. Add 20 ml of chloroform. (The volume is not critical.) Stopper the tubes and shake them for 5 min. Allow the layers to separate. Centrifuge briefly to hasten the separation.
4. Aspirate as much of each (aqueous) top layer as possible without removing any of the chloroform layer. Decant each chloroform layer through Whatman #31 filter paper into a 60-ml separatory funnel. (Make sure that the chloroform saturates the filter paper first; if any residual aqueous phase touches the paper first, filtration will be prolonged.)
5. Add 4.0 ml of 0.45*N* sodium hydroxide to each filtrate.
6. Shake the chloroform-sodium hydroxide mixture for 2 to 3 min. Allow the layers to separate.
7. Drain each chloroform layer through Whatman #31 filter paper into a clean separatory funnel. Discard the sodium hydroxide.
8. Add 4.0 ml of 0.5*N* sulfuric acid to the chloroform, shake, then allow the layers to separate.
9. Drain each chloroform layer through Whatman #31 filter paper into a 15-ml centrifuge tube. Save these fractions for determinations of "neutral" drugs,† should they be required.
10. Drain each acid layer into a tube, then centrifuge it briefly.
11. Transfer at least 3 ml of each acid fraction to a silica cuvette.
12. Determine the UV absorption spectrum of each acid fraction from 320 to 220 nm, using 0.5*N* sulfuric acid as the reference solution. It is not necessary to extract the reference solution with chloroform.

CALCULATION

Determine the chlordiazepoxide concentration (mg/100 ml) in the sample C_S by the following formula:

$$C_S = \frac{(A_{245} - A_{290})\ \text{sample}}{(A_{245} - A_{290})\ \text{reference}} \times 2$$

Note: The wavelengths given are the second maximum (245 nm) and the first minimum (290 nm) when interpreting the UV absorption curve from 320 nm to the lower wavelengths (see Figure 1). Use the actual absorbance at maximum and minimum in these areas if the curve does not correspond exactly to the wavelengths given. Chlordiazepoxide concentrations lower than 0.3 mg/100 ml may be difficult to determine with this procedure. If this is the case, another procedure may be preferable.

*Available from Roche Laboratories, Nutley, N.J.
†See Diazepam (Valium®), p. 119.

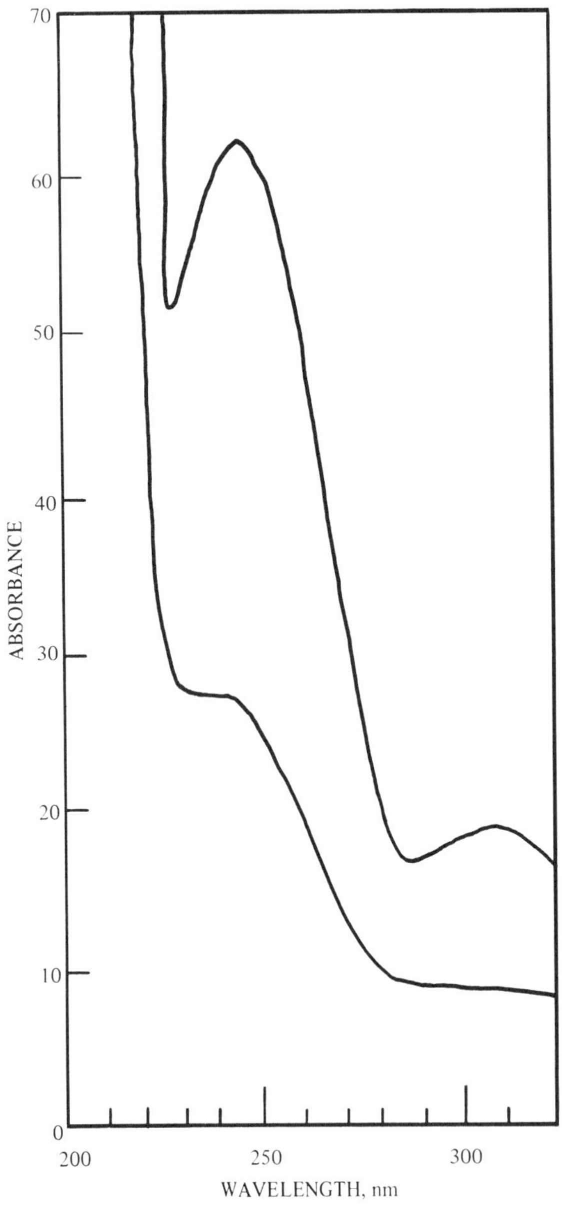

FIGURE 1. UV absorbance of chlordiazepoxide from 320 to 220 nm.

Sample Calculation

$(A_{245} - A_{290})$ sample = 0.253–0.072

$(A_{245} - A_{290})$ reference = 0.603–0.153

$$\frac{(0.253 - 0.072)}{(0.603 - 0.153)} \times 2 = 0.80 \text{ mg/100 ml}$$

INTERPRETATION (see p. 7)

Peak blood concentrations occur several hours after oral administration of Librium®. Blood concentrations following therapeutic doses of 5 to 10 mg three times a day are in the range 0.1 to 0.5 μg/ml. A single dose of 50 mg may produce blood concentration of 1.0 μg/ml in an average 150-lb individual. After the drug is discontinued, plasma concentrations decline slowly over several days. Librium® excretion in urine is slow, approximately 12% in 4 days; 1 to 2% is excreted in unchanged form and 3 to 6% appears as a conjugate. Blood concentrations in excess of 1.0 μg/ml indicate overdose, 10 to 20 μg/ml induce coma, and greater than 20 μg/ml endanger life, particularly if taken along with alcohol.

The effect of Librium® is enhanced in combination with drugs that have additive or supra-additive effects, such as alcohol, barbiturates, phenothiazines, MAO inhibitors, and imipramine-like compounds. Physical dependence may occur in patients receiving large daily doses.

ACCURACY AND PRECISION

Twenty-nine individual analyses of the same sample gave a mean average of 0.435 mg/100 ml with a standard deviation of 0.023 mg.

INTERFERING SUBSTANCES

Other benzodiazepines or their metabolites may interfere.

REFERENCES

Goodman, L. S. and Gilman, A., *The Pharmacological Basis of Therapeutics,* Macmillan, N. Y., 1964, 187.
Randall, L. O., Pharmacology of chlordiazepoxide (Librium), *Dis. Nerv. Syst.,* Suppl. 22, 7, 1961.
Roche Laboratories Product Reference Manual, Roche Laboratories, Nutley, N. J., 1970, 74.

TYPE C PROCEDURE

James Valentour

APPARATUS

1. Test tubes with screw-cap Teflon® liners, 16 × 125 mm
2. Multipurpose rotator
3. Integrator (Hewlett-Packard 3373B or Perkin-Elmer PEP-1)
4. Centrifuge
5. Gas chromatograph (Hewlett-Packard 5713) equipped with a pulsed linearized ^{63}Ni electron-capture detector with a 5′ × 1/4″ o.d. glass column, packed with 5% OV-7 on 80 to 100 mesh Chromosorb WHP. (A 2′ × 1/4″ o.d. glass column, packed with 3% OV-17 on 80 to 100 mesh Chromosorb WHP is also acceptable.)

Operating Conditions

Gas Flow Rate:
argon-methane (95:5) – 60 ml/min
Temperatures:
column – 285°C
no injection port heater
detector – 300°C

Attenuation: × 64

REAGENTS

All chemicals should be analytical reagent grade.

1. Extraction solvent, toluene-hexane-isoamyl alcohol, 78:20:2 by volume
2. Buffer, pH 9.2
   Add concentrated ammonium hydroxide to a saturated ammonium chloride solution until pH 9.2 is attained. (Other comparable buffers are suitable.)
3. Chlordiazepoxide stock solution, 50 mg/dl
   Dissolve 50 mg of chlordiazepoxide or 56 mg of chlordiazepoxide hydrochloride in water, and dilute to 100 ml.
4. Chlordiazepoxide reference solutions, 1.0, 0.50, 0.25, 0.10 mg/dl
   Add 10.0, 5.00, 2.50, and 1.00 ml of the stock solution to each of four volumetric flasks, and dilute each to 500 ml with water.
5. Flurazepam stock solution, 50 mg/dl
   Dissolve 50 mg of flurazepam in water, and dilute to 100 ml.
6. Flurazepam internal standard solution, 0.25 mg/dl
   Add 2.5 ml of the stock solution to a 500-ml volumetric flask, and dilute to 500 ml with water.

PROCEDURE

1. Place 2.00 ml of each of the sample specimens and the reference solutions in a screw-capped extraction tube.
2. To each tube add 1.00 ml of the flurazepam

internal standard solution, 2.0 ml of the pH 9.2 buffer, and 2.0 ml of the extraction solvent.
3. Rotate the capped tubes for 20 min at approximately 8 rpm.
4. Centrifuge the tubes for 5 min at approximately 2,000 rpm.
5. Inject 3 ml of the upper (organic) layer into the gas chromatograph at the stated operating conditions. The retention time of chlordiazepoxide is approximately 7 min.
6. Determine the ratio of the peak area due to chlordiazepoxide to that due to flurazepam (R).

CALCULATION

Calculate the chlordiazepoxide concentration in the specimen by the following formula:

$$C_p = \frac{R_p}{R} \times C$$

where

C_p = chlordiazepoxide concentration in the specimen peak;
R_p = ratio of the peak area (or height) of chlordiazepoxide in the specimen to the peak area (or height) of flurazepam;
R = ratio of the peak area (or height) of chlordiazepoxide in the standard(s) to the peak area (or height) of flurazepam;
C = chlordiazepoxide concentration of a suitable standard.

INTERPRETATION (see p. 7)

Listed below are relative retention times of some of the common benzodiazepines and benzodiazepine metabolites detected by this procedure:

	RRT on 5% OV-7	RRT on 3% OV-17
Oxazepam	.44	.42
Diazepam	.53	.55
N-des-Alkylflurazepam	.65	.67
N-des-Methyldiazepam	.76	.79
Demoxepam	.78	.88
3-Hydroxydiazepam	0.94	1.10
Flurazepam	1.00	1.00
Chlordiazepoxide	1.47	1.93
N-des-Methylchlordiazepoxide	1.58	0.75

Therapeutic administration of chlordiazepoxide reportedly produced peak plasma concentrations of 0.8 to 2 μg/ml. The concentrations of unmetabolized chlordiazepoxide, diazepam, and flurazepam in urine are reportedly quite low and fall below minimum detectable levels by this method under most circumstances.

SENSITIVITY

The minimum detectable concentration of chlordiazepoxide by this procedure is approximately 0.3 μg/ml. The range of linear response exceeds 5 μg/ml.

INTERFERING SUBSTANCES

The benzodiazepines listed above respond to electron-capture detection at low concentrations, but are distinguishable from chlordiazepoxide. By varying the reference solutions and, if necessary, the selection of the internal standard, others in this list may be quantitatively determined in biological fluids, provided that their concentrations are greater than about 0.1 to 0.3 μg/ml. Therapeutic concentrations of some of these substances, however, may lie below this concentration range.

REFERENCES

deSilva, J. A. F. and Puglisi, C. V., Determination of medazepam (Nobrium), diazepam (Valium) and their major biotransformation products in blood and urine by electron capture gas-liquid chromatography, *Anal. Chem.*, 42, 1725, 1970.

Garatini, S., Mussini, E., and Randall, L. O., *The Benzodiazepines*, Raven Press, New York, 1973.

Zingales, I., Determination of chlordiazepoxide plasma concentrations by electron capture gas-liquid chromatography, *J. Chromatogr.*, 61, 237, 1971.

Zingales, I., Diazepam metabolism during chronic medication, unbound fraction in plasma, erythrocytes and urine, *J. Chromatogr.*, 75, 55, 1973.

CHLORINATED HYDROCARBON PESTICIDES

PRINCIPLE

The pesticide is extracted from the sample with hexane. An aliquot of the concentrated hexane extract is then analyzed by gas chromatography, using an electron capture detector.

TYPE B PROCEDURE

Robert A. Maes

APPARATUS

1. Centrifuge tubes, conical, ground-glass-stoppered, 15 ml
2. Mixer (Vortex-Genie, Model K-550-G)
3. Centrifuge
4. Pipets, disposable, glass, 9″ long, fitted with rubber bulbs
5. Concentrator tubes, graduated, with 19/22 standard taper joints (Kontes No. K-570050), 25 ml
6. Evaporative concentrator assembly, small-scale, equipped with micro Synder columns, concentrator tubes, and springs (Kontes No. K-569250)
7. Glass beads, plain, 3 mm
   Wash the beads with *n*-hexane before use.
8. Syringes (Hamilton), 10 μl
9. Gas chromatograph (Varian Aerograph Model 1400), equipped with a nickel electron-capture detector, a 1 mV recorder (Varian Aerograph Model 20) with attached Disc integrator, and a glass column, 6′ × 1/8″ o.d., packed either with 3% OV-1 or with 10% DC-200 on Gas Chrom Q, 80 to 100 mesh, equipped with a Pyrex® injector insert proximal to the injection port, and silanized *in situ* with bistrimethylsilylacetamide

   Operating Conditions

   Gas Flow Rates:
   nitrogen (carrier gas) – 70 ml/min on 3% OV-1, 100 ml/min on 10% DC-200

   Temperatures:
   column – 180°C on 3% OV-1, 200°C on 10% DC-200
   injection port – 200°C on 3% OV-1, 210°C on 10% DC-200
   detector – 210°C on 3% OV-1, 230°C on 10% DC-200

Condition the column for 24 hr at 220°C.

REAGENTS

All chemicals should be analytical reagent grade.

1. *n*-Hexane, Mallinckrodt Nanograde
2. Chlorinated hydrocarbon stock solutions, 1 μg/ml
   Using *n*-hexane as the solvent, prepare stock solutions from any or all of the following compounds: aldrin; α-BHC; *p,p*′-DDD, *p,p*′-DDE; *o,p*′-DDT; *p,p*′-DDT; dieldrin; heptachlor; heptachlorepoxide; lindane.
3. Chlorinated hydrocarbon reference solutions
   Using *n*-hexane as the diluent, dilute each of the stock solutions as needed to obtain the following concentrations: aldrin, 0.01 to 0.05 μg/ml; α-BHC, 0.01 to 0.05 μg/ml; *p,p*′-DDD, 0.02 to 0.10 μg/ml; *p,p*′-DDE, 0.02 to 0.10 μg/ml; *o,p*′-DDT, 0.02 to 0.10 μg/ml; *p,p*′-DDT, 0.1 to 0.5 μg/ml; diedrin, 0.01 to 0.05 μg/ml; heptachlor, 0.01 to 0.05 μg/ml; heptachlorepoxide, 0.10 to 0.25 μg/ml; lindane, 0.01 to 0.05 μg/ml.

PROCEDURE

1. Place 2.0 ml of specimen (whole blood, serum, or plasma) into a 15-ml conical centrifuge tube. Prepare a series of reference solutions in the same manner. Add 6.0 ml of *n*-hexane to each tube, stopper, and mix the contents of each tube for about 1 min on a Vortex mixer.
2. Centrifuge the tubes for 5 min at 2,000 rpm or until separation is achieved.
3. Carefully transfer each upper *n*-hexane layer to a 25-ml evaporative concentrator tube, using disposable pipets fitted with rubber bulbs.
4. Repeat the extraction twice, using 6.0 ml of *n*-hexane each time (centrifuge if necessary). Combine the three extracts obtained from each sample in a concentrator tube.
5. Add a glass bead to each concentrator tube. Fit each tube with a modified micro Snyder column and concentrate the pooled *n*-hexane extracts to 500 μl on a steam bath. Avoid residue losses by rinsing the sides of the Snyder columns and concentrator tubes with *n*-hexane and by taking care that temperatures are not higher than 40°C and that evaporation does not proceed to dryness.
6. Inject 5 μl of each *n*-hexane extract into the gas chromatograph to determine the final dilution, making sure that the operating conditions stated above are met. The final volume of each *n*-hexane extract can be adjusted by concentrating it with a gentle stream of clean, dry nitrogen or by diluting it with *n*-hexane to a level consistent with the concentration of residues present in the sample.

CALCULATION

Determine the concentration of chlorinated hydrocarbon in the specimen by the following formula:

$$C_x = \frac{C_s \times P_x}{4 \times P_s},$$

where

C_x = concentration of chlorinated hydrocarbon in the specimen;
C_s = concentration of the chlorinated hydrocarbon in the reference solution;
P_x = peak area obtained from the specimen;
P_s = peak area obtained from the reference solution.

INTERPRETATION (see p. 7)

The interpretation of the results obtained depends on the pesticide involved. In the blood of unexposed persons, normal dieldrin concentrations range from 0.0001 to 0.0004 mg/100 ml, and *p,p'*-DDE or *p,p'*-DDT concentrations range from 0.001 to 0.004 mg/100 ml. Exposed asymptomatic workers have dieldrin concentrations ranging from 0.003 to 0.005 mg/100 ml blood. Toxic effects due to dieldrin are observed at blood concentrations of 0.02 mg/100 ml and fatalities at blood concentrations above 0.2 mg/100 ml.*

ACCURACY AND PRECISION

Using the procedure described above, recovery of various chlorinated hydrocarbons added to blood ranges from 85 to 94%. Because of the change in the standing current of the electron-capture detector after prolonged use, reference samples must be analyzed with each injection.

INTERFERING SUBSTANCES

No significant gas-chromatographic response is observed from normal blood constituents that might be extracted.

REFERENCES

Dale, W. E., Curley, A., and Cueto, C., Hexane-extractable chlorinated insecticides in human blood, *Life Sci.,* 5, 47, 1966.

Narayanaswami, K., Moitra, B., Kotangle, R. S., and Bami, H. L., Thin-layer chromatography in the detection of poisoning by pesticides, *J. Chromatogr.,* 95, 181, 1974.

*Additional data can be found in the *Handbook of Analytical Toxicology,* Chemical Rubber Co., Cleveland, Ohio, 1969, 566.

CHLOROQUINE

PRINCIPLE

An alkalinized specimen is extracted into chloroform and this extract is reextracted into acid. The UV absorption spectrum of the acid solution is used to identify and quantitate the chloroquine.

TYPE C PROCEDURE

Leo Kazyak

APPARATUS

1. pH Paper (Hydrion)
2. Graduated tubes or cylinders
3. Cuvettes, quartz or fused silica
4. Spectrophotometer, preferably ratio-recording, with linear-absorbance slide wire and expanded 0 to 0.1 absorbance range.

REAGENTS

All chemicals should be analytical reagent grade.

1. Potassium hydroxide, saturated aqueous solution
2. Chloroquine stock solution, 10 mg/100 ml
   Dissolve 16 mg of chloroquine diphosphate ($C_{18}H_{26}ClN_3 \cdot 2H_3PO_4$) in 100 ml of water.
3. Chloroquine reference solution
   Dilute 1.0 ml of the chloroquine stock solution to 100 ml with water. The resulting solution contains 1.0 μg chloroquine base/ml. The absorbance of this solution at 343 nm should be 0.06 ± 0.001 with 1-cm light path cuvettes.
4. Chloroform
5. Hydrochloric acid, 0.1*N*
   Dilute 8.25 ml of concentrated hydrochloric acid to one liter with water.

PROCEDURE

1. Add a drop of saturated potassium hydroxide solution to 3 ml of each sample (blood, plasma, red cells or urine specimen, reference solution, and water for a reagent blank). Test the specimen for alkalinity with Hydrion pH paper. Add more potassium hydroxide, if necessary.
2. Extract each sample with 30 ml of chloroform. Shake the extraction vessel for 5 min. Allow the solvent and aqueous phases to separate completely.
3. Carefully transfer 20.0 ml of each solvent phase to a clean glass-stoppered graduated tube or cylinder. Do not use anhydrous sodium sulfate or pass the solvent through filter paper to remove traces of aqueous phase, because some of the chloroquine will also be removed and significantly reduce the recovery.
4. Reextract the solvent with 3.0 ml of 0.1*N* hydrochloric acid. Shake the tube or cylinder for at least 3 min to insure complete recovery of the chloroquine from the solvent.
5. When the aqueous acidic phase has separated and cleared, aspirate it and transfer it to a clean quartz or fused silica cuvette.
6. Determine the absorbance of the acidic phase in a spectrophotometer that has an expanded 0.0 to 0.1 absorbance range, i.e., expandable

to full recorder scale for added sensitivity. Use the acidic phase obtained by processing the water sample as a reference solution.

CALCULATION

1. If the absorbance difference between 380 and 370 nm is greater than 0.002 on the expanded scale or 0.01 on a normal scale, the following base line correction must be made:

$$B = A_2 - 2.7\,(A_1 - A_2)$$
$$A_3' = A_3 - B$$

where

A_1 = absorbance at 380 nm;
A_2 = absorbance at 370 nm;
A_3 = absorbance at 343 nm;
A_3' = corrected absorbance at 343 nm.

2. When absorbance at 343 nm has been corrected, or if no correction is necessary, determine the chloroquine concentration (μg/ml) in the specimen of the following formula:

$$\frac{A_3'}{A_R} \times C_R \times \frac{V}{V_a} \times \frac{H}{S} = C_S,$$

where

A_R = absorbance of the chloroquine reference solution;
C_R = chloroquine concentration of the reference solution;
V = initial volume of the solvent;
V_a = volume of the solvent aliquot;
H = volume of 0.1*N* hydrochoric acid used;
S = volume of the specimen;
C_S = chloroquine concentration of the specimen.

3. The absorbance has a linear relationship to chloroquine concentrations from 0.3 to 1.3 μg/ml on the expanded 0.0 to 0.1 scale or from 3.0 to 13 μg on a normal 0.0 to 1.0 scale.

INTERPRETATION (see p. 7)

Therapeutic concentrations of chloroquine range from 0.01 to 0.10 mg/100 ml in blood cells and plasma. Concentrations as high as 0.35 mg/100 ml have been detected in blood cells without causing fatality; values above 0.4 mg/100 ml are compatible with fatality. However, there have been instances of increased chloroquine concentration in post-mortem blood in contradistinction to ante-mortem blood chloroquine concentrations that were in the therapeutic range. Cases of confirmed fatal chloroquine overdoses manifest blood concentrations of 1.0 mg/100 ml or higher. Following therapeutic use, urine chloroquine concentrations range from 1.0 to 10.0 mg/100 ml.

ACCURACY AND PRECISION

The spectrum of chloroquine (Figure 1) is specific for chloroquine and its analogues, e.g., Plaquenil® (hydroxychloroquine) and the monethyl metabolite of chloroquine. Recovery of chloroquine is about 90 ± 2%.

INTERFERING SUBSTANCES

Quinine will interfere with the analysis because it absorbs UV energy in the region of 343 nm and is present in concentrations 10 to 50 times that of the chloroquine. If the red cells can be separated from the plasma in blood specimen, chloroquine can frequently be determined in the presence of quinine by differential spectrophotometry in the region of 340 to 370 nm. Primaquine will also interfere with the determination of chloroquine; however, it is not recovered unchanged from biological specimens, and in specimens other than stomach content, where it remains intact, interference from primaquine is unlikely.

REFERENCE

Schulman, S. G. and Young, J. F., A modified fluorimetric determination of chloroquine in biological samples, *Anal. Chim. Acta,* 70, 229, 1974.

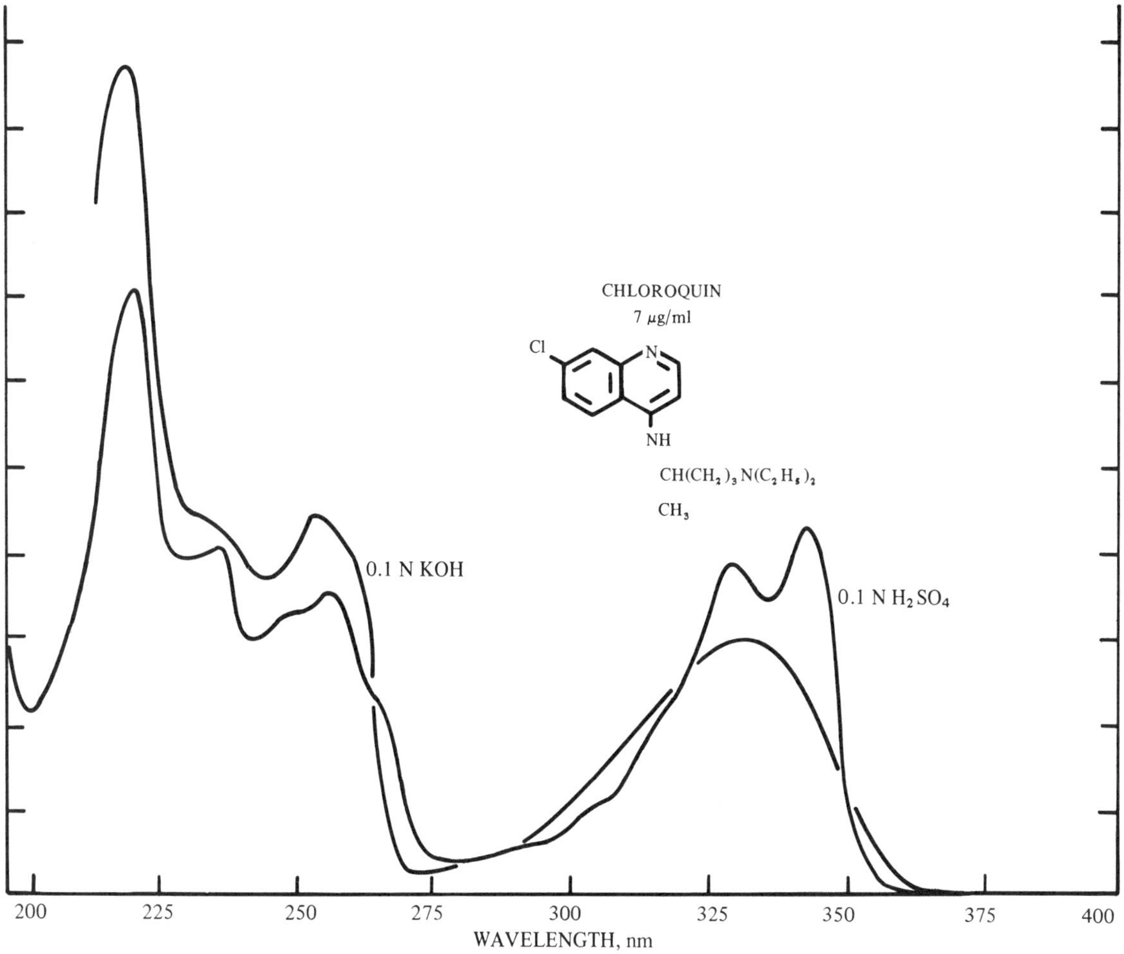

FIGURE 1. UV spectrum of chloroquine. (Reproduced with permission of the U.S. Army.)

CHOLINESTERASE

USE AND INTERPRETATION OF CHOLINESTERASE MEASUREMENTS

Charles R. Crane, Donald C. Sanders, and John K. Abbott

Two basic types of cholinesterase activity are found in the tissues of all animals. True cholinesterase, found in erythrocytes and nerve tissues, exhibits a substrate preference for acetylcholine. (Acetylcholine serves as a neurotransmitter at parasympathetic nerve terminals, in sympathetic ganglia, at somatic motor end plates, and within the central nervous system.) Pseudocholinesterase, found principally in plasma, preferentially hydrolyzes butyrylcholine, but will hydrolyze acetylcholine at a lesser rate. Although the total physiological role of plasma pseudocholinesterase is not well-defined, the enzyme is known to function in the hydrolysis of biologically active esters in the blood. Quantitative determination of blood cholinesterase activity as a clinical procedure is of significance in a variety of situations.

The localized and short-acting properties of succinylcholine muscle relaxants are primarily due to their rapid hydrolysis by plasma cholinesterase. Individuals with lowered levels of cholinesterase activity are poor candidates for these drugs because severe and prolonged apnea and paralysis may ensue. For this reason, a preliminary cholinesterase assay is sometimes performed on the serum of a patient scheduled for these drugs; a low serum activity is a definite contraindication unless supportive measures are taken. In 3 to 5% of the population a persistently low enzyme level is the result of a defective cholinesterase molecule, which is genetically controlled. Individuals whose serum activity is low because they possess this defective gene can be identified by measurement of their cholinesterase activity in the presence and absence of dibucaine.

Pseudocholinesterase activity has been used as a test of liver function. The synthesis of the enzyme by the parenchymal cells of the liver is associated with serum albumin synthesis; therefore, liver dysfunction may be reflected in abnormal levels of both these proteins in blood plasma. Decreased plasma or serum cholinesterase activity has been found in decompensated cardiac function with congestion of the liver, in cancer of the liver, and in any liver disease that affects the parenchymal cells, such as cirrhosis, hepatitis, or cholangitis.

A third use for clinical cholinesterase determinations, and one of increasing importance, is in the diagnosis of suspected cases of organophosphate poisoning. Essentially all of the organophosphate and carbamate pesticides are potent cholinesterase inhibitors, and most of them inhibit both types of the enzyme. The activity of the plasma enzyme is usually, but not invariably, inhibited more rapidly than that of the true cholinesterase of the erythrocyte. Characteristically, it also recovers more rapidly due to synthesis of new enzymes by the liver, while the recovery of erythrocyte activity is governed by the relatively slow production of new cells. Since the range of "normal" cholinesterase activity is quite broad, it is desirable that persons working with cholinesterase inhibitors have a preexposure assay performed to establish their individual normal enzyme levels. The initial determination should be followed by periodic assays during the working season, so that changes can be detected before exposure reaches a serious level. Activity must drop below 80% of the preexposure value (a 20% inhibition) before it becomes significant as an indicator of exposure.

Though diagnostically less specific than in the above cases, the pseudocholinesterase level has been shown to decrease in the case of duodenal ulcer, pancreatitis, cancer of the lung or pancreas, malnutrition, cachexia, myocardial infarction, acute and chronic infections, toxemia of pregnancy, dermatomyositis, and various forms of anemia, such as pernicious, hemorrhagic, hemolytic, or sprue. Certain drugs and chemicals also have been shown to decrease the activity of pseudocholinesterase. These include, among many others, physostigmine (eserine), prostigmine, and neostigmine; carbamates; sulfonates, and sulfates; fluorides, oxalates, and citrates; oximes and quaternary ammonium compounds; phenothiazines (chlorpromazine, imipramine, etc.); LSD-25; atropine, hyoscyamine, and scopolamine; benactyzine; some antibiotics (streptomycin and chloramphenicol); estrogenic and cortisone-like hormones; and exogenous serum albumin due to transfusions, injections, or other methods of administration.

The measurement of whole blood cholinesterase finds its greatest usefulness in the analysis of hemolyzed samples. When hemolysis is present in an ante-mortem blood specimen, calculation of activity may be made on a volume basis and compared to the normal range of values. In the interpretation of these values, it can be assumed that the erythrocyte enzyme contributes most of the measured activity when acetylcholine is used as the substrate. The analysis of post-mortem specimens presents special problems. Since the separation of cellular and plasma components in blood begins when circulation ceases, the relative amounts of erythrocytes and plasma in post-mortem blood may be quite different from those in circulating ante-mortem blood. When extensive hemolysis is present in post-mortem specimens, it is not valid to relate the whole blood activity to either volume or hematocrit, but activity can be expressed as units per gram of hemoglobin. For the purpose of relating such a value to the normal range of the method employed, a nominal hemoglobin value of 15 g may be assumed; however, such values should be interpreted cautiously and with regard for the assumptions therein.

REFERENCES

Kalow, W. and Genest, K., A method for the detection of atypical forms of human serum cholinesterase. Determination of dibucaine numbers, *Can. J. Biochem. Physiol.,* 35, 339, 1957.

Richterich, R., *Clinical Chemistry, Theory and Practice,* Academic Press, N. Y., 1969, 441.

PRINCIPLE

In Procedure A application of a serum aliquot to a test paper impregnated with a choline ester substrate and a pH indicator causes a color change due to the enzymatic release of the acid moiety from the substrate. Cholinesterase activity is inversely proportional to the time interval required for the color of the test paper to match that of a control paper. Procedure B is based on the color change of phenol red in a buffered enzyme-substrate-indicator solution produced by the enzymatic release of acetic acid from acetylcholine. Enzyme activity is proportional to the ratio of final to initial absorbance after a 30-min incubation period. In Alternate Procedure B a choline ester substrate is hydrolyzed in a buffer-substrate-enzyme solution and the change in pH over a 1-hr period is measured directly using an expanded scale pH meter. Activity is proportional to the change in pH corrected for nonenzymatic hydrolysis. The pH-Stat procedure (C) measures the rate of base addition required to hold an enzyme-substrate mixture at a constant pH under controlled temperature conditions. Enzyme activity, expressed in micromoles of substrate hydrolyzed per minute per volume of enzyme, is identical to the micromoles of base per minute required to hold the pH of the incubation mixture constant.

TYPE A PROCEDURE

Charles R. Crane, Donald C. Sanders, and John K. Abbott

APPARATUS

1. Tweezers, fine tipped
2. Paper punch, ¼ in. diameter
3. Microscope slides, precleaned glass, 1 × 3 in.
4. Micropipets, calibrated to deliver 7 μl
5. Stopwatch

REAGENTS

All chemicals should be analytical reagent grade.

1. Acholest™ test paper kit* – (a) test papers (Bottle #1); (b) control papers (Bottle #2)

PROCEDURE

Preparation of Test Papers

1. Wash the tweezers and paper punch thoroughly. Rinse them first with distilled water, then with alchohol. Allow them to dry.
2. Being careful not to touch the paper with the fingers, punch ¼ in. discs from the test and control papers. Return the discs to their respective containers.

Cholinesterase Assay

1. Using a separate clean slide for each specimen to be assayed, place six 7.0-μl drops of serum or plasma, evenly spaced, along a microscope slide. Record the ambient temperature.
2. Using the tweezers, place three discs of test paper and three discs of control paper flat onto the drops. Start the stopwatch.
3. Cover the discs with a second slide, pressing gently to assure complete saturation of the paper discs with the specimen.
4. Record the time required for the test discs to match the color of the control discs.

CALCULATION†

1. Determine the average time required by the three replicate test discs.
2. Temperature adjustments must be made when groups of Acholest values are to be compared. From 15 to 30°C, color-matching time *decreases* with an *increase* in temperature at the rate of 4%/°C, but is nonlinear beyond this range. Thus, a matching time of 20 min measured at 21°C is equivalent to a matching time of 16.8 min at 25°C (i.e., 4°C × 4%/°C =

*Available from E. Fougera & Co., Inc., Hicksville, N.Y. 11802.

†For conversion of Acholest units to units of other methods, see p. 100.

16%; 16% of 20 min = 3.2 min; 20 min − 3.2 min = 16.8 min).

INTERPRETATION* (see p. 7)

The time required for the color of the test disc to match the color of the control disc reflects the cholinesterase activity of the specimen. Interpret the test results according to the table below, which shows the results obtained at room temperature (25°C) and is supplied with the Acholest™ kit.

Minutes to color match	Cholinesterase activity
<5	Increased
7–18	Normal
20–35	Decreased
35–150	Strongly decreased

Experiments with 277 males have established a mean value and normal range by the pH-Stat method.† Conversion of these values to Acholest units (minutes) yields the following data: mean value = 5 min (at 25°C); normal range = 2 to 13 min (95% confidence limits).

ACCURACY AND PRECISION

Braid[1] has reported a standard deviation of ± 8% of the population mean (coefficient of variation), with no single value differing by more than 13% from the population mean.

INTERFERING SUBSTANCES

1. Matching time is best observed against a dark background illuminated by either daylight or tungsten lighting. Fluorescent lighting is unsatisfactory.
2. Any trace of hemolysis in the plasma or serum specimen must be avoided. If plasma is used, the anticoagulant of choice is heparin. Citrate, oxalate, and particularly fluoride must be avoided.
3. Some detergents inhibit cholinesterase activity in plasma and serum. All glassware, including the microscope slides, should therefore be thoroughly rinsed before using.

REFERENCE

1. **Braid, P. E. and Nix, M. S.,** Modification of a test paper procedure for determination of human serum cholinesterase activity, *Arch. Environ. Health,* 17, 986, 1968.

GENERAL REFERENCE

Fleisher, J. H., Woodson, G. S., and Simet, L., A visual method for estimating blood cholinesterase activity, *Arch. Ind. Health,* 14, 510, 1956.

TYPE B PROCEDURE

Charles R. Crane, Donald C. Sanders, and John K. Abbott

APPARATUS

1. Test tubes
2. Constant-temperature bath, 25°C ± 1°C
3. Spectrophotometer, visible-range, or photoelectric colorimeter

REAGENTS

All chemicals should be analytical reagent grade.

1. Sodium hydroxide, 0.01*N*
   Dissolve 4 g of sodium hydroxide in one liter

*For assessment of the test results, see p. 86.
†See Type C Procedure, p. 96.

of water. Dilute 10 ml of this solution to 100 ml.

2. Phenol red, 100 mg/dl
   Grind 100 mg of phenol red with 28.0 ml of 0.01*N* sodium hydroxide in a mortar until completely dissolved. Dilute the solution to 100 ml with distilled water.
3. Buffer-indicator mixture, pH 8.00, 0.05*M*
   Dissolve 6.65 g of anhydrous dibasic sodium phosphate (Na_2HPO_4) and 0.43 g of anhydrous monobasic potassium phosphate (KH_2PO_4) in distilled water. Add 10 ml of the phenol red solution, then dilute to one liter, mixing thoroughly. The pH of this mixture should be 8.0 ± 0.1; if not, adjust it to this range by adding either hydrochloric acid or sodium hydroxide. Stored in a tightly stoppered Pyrex® or alkali-resistant bottle, this mixture is stable for at least 3 months; however, it should be checked periodically to see whether its absorbance at 540 nm or its pH has changed.
4. Acetylcholine perchlorate* substrate solution, 0.663*M*
   Dissolve 4.074 g of dried acetylcholine perchlorate in distilled water and dilute to 25 ml. Stored at 4°C, this substrate solution is stable for 1 month.

SPECIMEN PREPARATION

Either serum or plasma may be used. If plasma is used, the anticoagulant of choice is heparin; the use of fluoride, citrate, or oxalate as anticoagulants or preservatives is not recommended. Each serum or plasma sample should be assayed in duplicate. If the available volume of serum or plasma is limited, the method can be adapted by reducing all aliquots proportionately. The lower limit of the final assay volume is obviously fixed by the sample-size requirements of the available photometer.

PROCEDURE

Assay

1. For each unknown to be assayed, set up two test tubes. (Matched colorimeter tubes or cuvettes may be used, if desired, to avoid transfer of the solutions for the absorbance measurement.) Into each tube pipet 5.0 ml of the buffer-indicator mixture and 0.5 ml of serum or plasma. Mix the contents of each tube by inversion.
2. Prepare a set of duplicate control tubes for each series of unknowns by pipeting 5.0 ml of the buffer-indicator mixture and 0.5 ml of distilled water into each of two tubes. Mix the contents of each tube by inversion.
3. To establish temperature equilibrium, place the tubes for 10 min in a 25°C water bath.
4. Using distilled water as the reference solution, zero the photometer at 540 nm.
5. After 10 min, remove the first tube from the bath. Add 0.5 ml of the substrate solution. Quickly mix the contents of the tube by several gentle inversions, then measure and record the absorbance (A_1) at 540 nm. Note the exact time of the absorbance reading, or start an interval timer or a stopwatch. Replace the tube in the constant-temperature bath immediately after making the absorbance measurement.
6. Repeat this process at timed intervals for the duplicate specimen and the control samples.
7. After an interval of slightly less than 30 min following the first absorbance measurement, remove the first tube from the water bath, allowing just enough time to wipe it dry and place it in the photometer. Record its absorbance (A_2) at precisely 30 min after reading its initial absorbance (A_1).
8. Repeat this process for each remaining tube, timing the second absorbance readings at the same intervals as the first, so that for each sample the time between the addition of the substrate and the reading of A_2 is exactly 30 min.

Preparation of a Standard Curve

If more than one unknown is to be assayed, aliquots of each plasma or serum specimen can be pooled for use in the standard curve.

1. Prepare a standard stock solution of 0.15*N* acetic acid by diluting 8.62 ml of glacial acetic acid (17.4*M*) to one liter with distilled, CO_2-

*The perchlorate is preferred over the bromide, iodide, or chloride because it is less hygroscopic. It should be dried over Drierite® in a vacuum desiccator and stored therein until required for use.

free water. Check the solution against a primary standard.

2. Prepare eight standardized solutions of acetic acid with concentrations of 0.01, 0.03, 0.05, 0.07, 0.09, 0.11, 0.13, and 0.15*N* by making accurate dilutions of the stock solution with distilled CO_2-free water. These solutions correspond respectively to 10, 30, 50, 70, 90, 110, 130, and 150 units of cholinesterase activity per milliliter plasma or serum.
3. Pipet 5.0 ml of the buffer-indicator mixture into each of nine test tubes.
4. Add 0.5 ml of (pooled) plasma or serum to each tube.
5. To eight of the tubes add 0.5 ml of acetic acid solution, using a different concentration in each tube. To the ninth tube add 0.5 ml of water instead of acetic acid; this represents 0 cholinesterase units. Mix the contents of each tube by gentle inversion.
6. Measure the absorbance of each reference solution at 540 nm, using distilled water to zero the instrument. The time at which this measurement is made is not critical because the color is quite stable. The reference solutions may be prepared and their absorbances measured either before or after the specimens are assayed.
7. Calculate the ratio of the absorbance of each acetic acid standard (A_{10}, A_{30}, etc.) to the absorbance of the tube containing no acetic acid (A_0).
8. Plot these ratios ($\frac{A_{10}}{A_0}$, $\frac{A_{30}}{A_0}$, etc.) on the log axis of semi-log paper against the corresponding cholinesterase units on the linear axis $\frac{A_{10}}{A_0}$ *vs* 10, $\frac{A_{30}}{A_0}$ *vs* 30, etc.). This constitutes the standard curve.

Note: In Caraway's method[1] the standard curve was composed of 15 points. The authors of this modification have found nine points to be adequate and have on occasion, when pressed for time, used only five. The points chosen should be evenly spaced between 0 and 0.15*N*. In laboratories where this test is infrequently performed, a standard curve constructed from pooled serum or plasma may be used for subsequent assays, provided that the reagent solutions have not changed. It is advisable to check at least one point on the standard curve (near the normal values) to determine if any major change has occurred. Whenever new reagents are prepared, a new standard curve must be established.

CALCULATION*

1. Calculate the ratio of the absorbance at 30 min (A_2) to the initial absorbance (A_1) for each specimen.
2. Determine the number of cholinesterase units in each specimen by comparison with the standard curve.
3. Determine the cholinesterase activity for the control tubes in the same manner, then calculate the average.
4. Subtract the average control value from that obtained for each specimen. The control value corrects for nonenzymatic hydrolysis of the substrate.
5. The activity units are expressed as μmoles of acetylcholine hydrolyzed by the enzyme in 1 ml of plasma or serum under the conditions specified (μmoles/ml/30 min).

Sample Calculation

Specimen: $A_1 = 1.037; A_2 = 0.589; \frac{A_2}{A_1} = \frac{0.589}{1.037} = 0.568$
ChE units (from the standard curve) = 97

Control: $A_1 = 0.925; A_2 = 0.906; \frac{A_2}{A_1} = \frac{0.906}{0.925} = 0.979$
ChE units (from the standard curve) = 2

Activity: 97 − 2 = 95 units

INTERPRETATION† (see p. 7)

The original publication of the Caraway method[1] quotes a normal range of 55 to 100 units. Subsequently, measurements on 277 blood specimens from male subjects gave a normal range of 45 to 113 units (95% confidence limits) for plasma values, with a mean of 79 units.

ACCURACY AND PRECISION

The precision of this method yields a coefficient of variation (standard deviation/mean) of 1 to 2% for replicate analyses of the same sample.

*For conversion of Caraway units to units of other methods, see p. 99.
†For assessment of the test results, see p. 86.

INTERFERING SUBSTANCES

Since this is a photometric method, any turbidity or extraneous color contributes equally to the A_1 and to the A_2 readings, which results in an increased $\frac{A_2}{A_1}$ ratio and a decrease in apparent ChE activity.

Hemolytic serum or plasma is not suitable for the assay. According to Caraway, lipemic or icteric specimens can be analyzed by the following procedure. After the second absorbance measurement of specimen (A_2, at 30 min), add 1 drop of 6*N* hydrochloric acid to the tube, then measure the absorbance again (A_3). In the same manner make a third absorbance measurement (A'_3) on a sample of normal serum or plasma. Subtract A'_3 from A_3. Adjust the ratio $\frac{A_2}{A_1}$ for the specimen by subtracting the absorbance increment ($A_3 - A'_3$) from each of the original absorbances (A_1 and A_2). Determine the number of ChE units corresponding to the adjusted ratio by comparison with the standard curve, then proceed with the calculation.

REFERENCE

1. **Caraway, W. T.**, Photometric determination of serum cholinesterase activity, *Am. J. Clin. Pathol.*, 26, 945, 1956.

ALTERNATE TYPE B PROCEDURE

Charles R. Crane, Donald C. Sanders, and John K. Abbott

APPARATUS

1. Vacutainer® tubes, heparinized (Becton, Dickinson & Co.), or heparinized syringes
2. Sahli pipets, 20 μl
3. Test tubes, 12 ml
4. Magnetic stirrer and Teflon®-covered stirring bars
5. Constant-temperature bath, 25°C ± 0.5°C
6. pH Meter, sensitive to ± 0.01 pH unit, preferably with a combination electrode that will fit in 12-ml test tubes
7. Clinical centrifuge
8. Capillary tubes, heparinized
9. Hematocrit centrifuge

REAGENTS

All chemicals should be analytical reagent grade.

1. Saponin solution
   Dissolve 10.0 mg of saponin in 100 ml of distilled water. Prepare this solution fresh each day it is to be used.
2. Buffer stock solution
   Dissolve 4.124 g of sodium barbital, 0.545 g of potassium phosphate, monobasic (KH_2PO_4), and 44.730 g of potassium chloride in distilled water and dilute to 200 ml. (Dehydrate the phosphate and barbital salts for 2 hr at 110°C and store them in a disiccator prior to weighing.) Store the solution in a polyethylene bottle.
3. Hydrochloric acid, 0.1*N*
   Dilute 8.6 ml of concentrated hydrochloric acid to one liter with water.
4. Buffer solution for whole blood or plasma
   Dilute 6.4 ml of buffer stock solution with 75.0 ml of distilled water. Adjust the pH to 8.00 with 0.1*N* hydrochloric acid, then dilute the solution to 100 ml.
5. Substrate solution for whole blood or plasma
   Dissolve 0.405 g of acetylcholine perchlorate* in 10.0 ml of distilled water. (Dry the acetylcholine perchlorate overnight in a vacuum desiccator over Drierite® prior to weighing.) This solution is stable for 4 weeks if stored in a refrigerator.
6. Buffer solution for red cells
   Dilute 20.0 ml of the buffer stock solution with 75.0 ml of distilled water. Adjust the pH to 8.10 with 0.1*N* hydrochloric acid, then dilute the solution to 100 ml.
7. Substrate solution for red cells
   Dissolve 0.270 g of acetylcholine perchlorate in 10.0 ml of distilled water. (Dry acetylcholine perchlorate overnight in a vacuum

*Available from K & K Laboratories, Plainview, N.Y. 11803.

desiccator over Drierite® prior to weighing.) This solution is stable for 4 weeks if stored in a refrigerator.

PROCEDURE

Whole Blood

1. Collect a blood specimen in a heparinized Vacutainer® tube or in a heparinized syringe. Rock the specimen gently to promote even distribution of red cells.
2. Using a Sahli pipet, withdraw a 20.0-μl aliquot for each replicate analysis desired. Duplicate samples are recommended. Wipe the pipet tip, then expel each aliquot into a 12-ml test tube containing 1.0 ml of the saponin solution. Rinse the pipet three times by drawing the saponin-whole blood mixture into the pipet and expelling it into the tube. Swirl the tube gently to mix the cells and promote rapid hemolysis.
3. Add 1.0 ml of the appropriate buffer solution to the hemolysate and mix. For rapid and efficient mixing, place a small Teflon®-covered magnetic stirring bar in each test tube. Place each tube in a small test tube rack, then mount the rack over the magnetic stirrer with the pH electrode support mounted over the rack.
4. For each group of specimens to be assayed, prepare two control tubes, each containing 1.0 ml of the saponin solution and 1.0 ml of the appropriate buffer solution. Mix the contents of each control tube.
5. Place both the test and the control tubes for 10 min in a 25°C constant-temperature bath. Stirring may be continued if the bath can be mounted on the magnetic stirrer (see Step 8).
6. Measure and record the pH to the nearest 0.01 unit for each replicate specimen and each control tube (pH_1).
7. Add 0.2 ml of the appropriate substrate solution to each test and control tube, mix, then return the tubes to the water bath. Time and record the intervals at which the addition to each tube is made.
8. After exactly 1 hr measure and record the pH of each test and control sample again (pH_2). Measurements of pH may be made while the magnetic stirrer is in operation, provided that the initial buffer calibration of the pH meter is also made with the stirrer operating.

Plasma

1. Collect a blood specimen in a heparinized Vacutainer® tube or in a heparinized syringe. Separate cells and plasma by centrifugation. Alternatively, blood may be collected directly in a heparinized capillary tube from a free-flowing deep finger puncture, allowing one tube per replicate analysis. Duplicate samples are recommended. Draw the blood to within ½ in. of the end, then seal the end with the flame of a microburner, taking care not to heat the blood. Allow the tube to cool, then centrifuge it in a standard hematocrit centrifuge for 4 min.
2. Using a Sahli pipet, withdraw a 20.0-μl aliquot of plasma for each replicate analysis desired. Duplicate samples are recommended. Wipe the pipet tip, then expel each aliquot into a 12-ml test tube containing 1.0 ml of distilled water. Rinse the pipet three times by drawing the water-plasma mixture into the pipet and expelling it into the tube. Swirl the tube gently to mix the contents. If the alternate method of specimen collection was used, score the capillary tube a few millimeters above the plasma-cell interface. Break the tube where scored, then place a Sahli pipet squarely against the opening. Allow the pipet to fill to the 20-μl mark by capillary action. Wipe the pipet tip, expel the plasma, and rinse as described above.
3. Add 1.0 ml of the appropriate buffer solution to the diluted plasma specimen and mix.
4. For each group of specimens to be assayed, prepare two control tubes each containing 1.0 ml of distilled water and 1.0 ml of the appropriate buffer solution. Mix the contents of each control tube.
5. Place both the test and the control tubes for 10 min in a 25°C constant-temperature bath.
6. Measure and record the pH to the nearest 0.01 unit for each replicate specimen and each control tube (pH_1).
7. Add 0.2 ml of the appropriate substrate solution to each test and control tube, mix, then return the tubes to the water bath. Time and record the intervals at which the addition to each tube is made.

8. After exactly 1 hr, measure and record the pH of each test and control sample again (pH_2).

Red Cells

1. Collect a blood specimen in a heparinized Vacutainer® tube or in a heparinized syringe. Mix by gentle inversion to dissolve and distribute the heparin. Fill capillary tubes with this well-mixed blood to within ½ in. of the ends, allowing one tube for each replicate analysis. Duplicate samples are recommended. Alternatively, blood may be collected directly in heparinized capillary tubes, one for each replicate analysis, from a free-flowing deep finger puncture. Seal the filled capillary tubes on one end in the flame of a microburner, taking care not to heat the blood. Allow the tubes to cool, then centrifuge them in a standard hematocrit centrifuge for 4 min.
2. Score each capillary tube a few millimeters below the plasma cell interface. Break the tube where scored, then place the tip of a 20-μl Sahli pipet squarely against the opening of the capillary tube. Invert the assembly so that the tip of the pipet points upward, then gently draw the cells into the pipet to the 20-μl mark. Wipe the pipet tip, then expel the cells into a 12-ml test tube containing 1.0 ml of the saponin solution. Rinse the pipet three times by drawing the saponin red-cell mixture into the pipet and expelling it into the tube. Swirl the tube gently to mix the cells and promote rapid hemolysis.
3. Add 1.0 ml of the appropriate buffer solution to the hemolysate.
4. For each group of specimens to be assayed, prepare two control tubes, each containing 1.0 ml of the saponin solution and 1.0 ml of the appropriate buffer solution. Mix the contents of each control tube.
5. Place both the test and the control tubes for 10 min in a 25°C constant-temperature bath.
6. Measure and record the pH to the nearest 0.01 unit for each replicate specimen and each control tube.
7. Add 0.2 ml of the appropriate substrate solution to each test and control tube, mix, then return the tubes to the water bath. Time and record the intervals at which the addition to each tube is made.
8. After exactly 1 hr, measure and record the pH of each test and control sample again (pH_2).

CALCULATION*

The ΔpH units of the Michel method are calculated by the following equation:

$$\Delta \text{ pH units/hr} = \Delta \text{ pH(specimen)} - \Delta \text{ pH(control)}$$

To calculate the activity, proceed as follows:

1. Subtract the final pH (pH_2) of each *control* tube from its initial pH (pH_1) to obtain the value ΔpH(control). Thus,

$$\Delta \text{ pH(control)} = pH_1 - pH_2$$

2. Subtract the final pH (pH_2) of each *specimen* tube from its initial pH (pH_1) to obtain the value ΔpH(specimen). Thus,

$$\Delta \text{ pH(specimen)} = pH_1 - pH_2$$

3. Subtract ΔpH(control) from ΔpH(specimen) to correct for nonenzymatic hydrolysis in the pH measurement of the specimen. The corrected value represents the change in pH per hour due to enzyme activity and is the figure reported to the physician.

Sample Calculation

Control #1	pH_1 = 8.00; pH_2 = 7.93
Control #2	pH_1 = 8.00; pH_2 = 7.93
Specimen #1	pH_1 = 7.94; pH_2 = 7.04
Specimen #2	pH_1 = 7.94; pH_2 = 7.08
ΔpH (control)	8.00 – 7.93 = 0.07 for #1
	8.00 – 7.93 = 0.07 for #2
	Average = 0.07 ΔpH units/hr
ΔpH(specimen)	7.94 – 7.04 = 0.90 for #1
	7.94 – 7.08 = 0.86 for #2
	Average = 0.88 ΔpH units/hr
Corrected value	ΔpH units/hr = 0.88 – 0.07 = 0.81

*For conversion of Michel units to units of other methods, see p. 99.

INTERPRETATION* (see p. 7)

Whole Blood

The normal range of activity (95% confidence limits) for whole blood cholinesterase, as reported by Grainger et al.[1] is between 1.06 and 1.59 ΔpH units/hr, with a population mean of 1.33.

Plasma

The normal range of activity (95% confidence limits) for plasma is between 0.49 and 1.24 ΔpH units/hr, with a population mean of 0.86, as established by the authors from tests on a group of 277 male subjects.

Red Cells

The normal range of activity (95% confidence limits) for red blood cells, as reported by Wolfsie and Winter,[2] is between 0.68 and 1.04 ΔpH units/hr, with a population mean of 0.86.

ACCURACY AND PRECISION

Whole Blood

The analysis of 12 replicate samples taken from constantly stirred whole blood provided the following precision statistics: mean, 1.134 ΔpH units/hr; standard deviation, 0.013 ΔpH units/hr; coefficient of variation, 1.15%.

Plasma

The analysis of 12 replicate samples from the same plasma specimen provided the following precision statistics: mean, 0.689 ΔpH units/hr; standard deviation, 0.010 ΔpH units/hr; coefficient of variation; 1.45%.

*For assessment of the test results, see p. 86.

Red Cells

The analysis of 12 replicate samples taken from constantly stirred heparinized whole blood provided the following precision statistics: mean, 0.845 ΔpH units/hr; standard deviation, 0.0089 ΔpH units/hr; coefficient of variation, 1.06%.

INTERFERING SUBSTANCES

Heparin is the anticoagulant of choice; fluoride, citrate, and oxalate should be avoided. Since pseudocholinesterase is inhibited by many detergents and a portion of the whole blood activity is contributed by the plasma enzymes, all glassware should be thoroughly rinsed before use. Values obtained from plasma showing visible hemolysis should be interpreted with caution. Since erythrocytes normally contain relatively large amounts of acetylcholinesterase, even slight hemolysis may release enough of the enzyme into the plasma to mask the effects of inhibition of the plasma enzyme.

REFERENCES

1. **Grainger, M. M., Groff, W. A., and Ellin, R. I.,** Blood cholinesterase values, *Arch. Environ. Health,* 16, 821, 1968.
2. **Wolfsie, J. H. and Winter, G. D.,** Statistical analysis of normal human red blood cell and plasma cholinesterase activity values, *A.M.A. Arch. Ind. Hyg. Occup. Med.,* 6, 43, 1952.

GENERAL REFERENCES

Larson, E. F., *Microelectrometric Method for Blood Cholinesterase Determinations,* California State Department of Public Health, Division of Laboratories, Sacramento, 1957.

Michel, H. O., An electrometric method for the determination of red blood cell and plasma cholinesterase activity, *J. Lab. Clin. Med.,* 34, 1564, 1949.

TYPE C PROCEDURE

Charles R. Crane, Donald C. Sanders, and John K. Abbott

APPARATUS

1. Vacutainer® tubes (B-D), or syringes, heparinized
2. Pasteur pipets
3. Volumetric flasks, 10 ml
4. Clinical centrifuge
5. Centrifuge tubes, conical, 12 ml
6. Hematocrit centrifuge
7. pH-Stat, equipped with thermostat-controlled reaction vessel and constant-temperature circulating water bath

REAGENTS

All chemicals should be analytical reagent grade.

1. Hemolyzing agent, 20 mg/dl
   Add 20 ml of Triton® X-100* to 80 ml of distilled water, mix thoroughly, then store the solution at room temperature.
2. Ringer's salts solution
   Dissolve 9 g of sodium chloride, 0.3 g of potassium chloride, 0.25 g of calcium chloride, and 0.2 g of sodium bicarbonate in distilled water and dilute to one liter.
3. Titrant, 0.005*N*
   Dissolve 200 mg of sodium hydroxide in CO_2-free distilled water. Dilute this solution to one liter, using CO_2-free distilled water. Store the solution in full, tightly capped bottles. Protect titrant stored in the reservoir of the pH-Stat from CO_2 absorption by placing a drying tube filled with Mallcosorb® (Mallinckrodt®), 30 to 50 mesh, over the air inlet. Standardize this solution daily before use by titration with potassium hydrogen phthalate (primary standard grade).
4. Substrate for whole blood and red cells, 0.102*M*
   Dry acetylcholine perchlorate† overnight in a vacuum desiccator over Drierite® and store it therein until required for use. Dissolve 250 mg of the salt in distilled water, then dilute to 10.0 ml. If stored at 4°C, the solution is stable for 1 month.
5. Substrate for plasma, 0.163*M*
   Dry butyrylcholine iodide‡ overnight in a vacuum desiccator over Drierite® and store it therein until required for use. Dissolve 490 mg of the salt in distilled water, then dilute to 10.0 ml. If stored at 4°C, this solution is stable for 2 weeks.

SPECIMEN PREPARATION

Collect blood specimens in heparinized Vacutainer® tubes or in heparinized syringes.

Whole Blood

Add 0.1 ml of the Triton® X-100 solution to a 10-ml volumetric flask. Pipet 2.0 ml of whole blood into the flask, then mix by swirling. Allow the mixture to stand for 3 to 5 min or until hemolysis is complete, then dilute it to volume with Ringer's salts solution.

Plasma

Centrifuge approximately 3.0 ml of whole blood until cells and plasma are separated. Carefully withdraw a 1.0-ml aliquot of the plasma fraction, transfer it to a 10-ml volumetric flask, then dilute it to volume with Ringer's salts solution.

Red Blood Cells

Pipet exactly 2.0 ml of whole blood into a 12-ml conical centrifuge tube. Separate cells and plasma by centrifugation. Using a Pasteur pipet, withdraw the plasma, being careful not to remove any red cells. Fill the tube almost to the top with Ringer's salts solution (approximately 10 vol), cover it with

*Available from Rohm and Haas, Philadelphia, Pa. 19116.
†Available from K & K Laboratories, Plainview, N.Y. 11803.
‡Available from Mann Research Laboratories, N.Y., N.Y. 10018.

Parafilm®, then mix the contents gently but thoroughly by inversion. Centrifuge the tube again, then remove the Ringer's salts solution with a Pasteur pipet and discard it. Repeat the washing with Ringer's salts solution. After removal of the second wash solution, add 0.1 ml of the Triton® X-100 solution to the packed red cells and mix by swirling. Allow the cells to hemolyze for 3 to 5 min, then transfer the hemolysate quantitatively to a 10-ml volumetric flask. Using Ringer's salts solution, rinse the centrifuge tube and add the washings to the volumetric flask. Dilute the flask contents to volume with Ringer's salts solution.

PROCEDURE

1. Add 1.0 ml of the enzyme solution (diluted plasma, or the hemolysate of whole blood or red cells) to the pH-Stat reaction vessel, turn on the magnetic stirrer of the unit, and allow the reaction vessel to come to a temperature equilibrium at 25°C.
2. Adjust the pH of the enzyme solution to 8.10 by gradual addition of the dilute sodium hydroxide, using a Pasteur pipet or a small syringe.
3. With the pH-Stat unit adjusted to maintain a constant pH of 8.10, add the appropriate substrate (100 μl of the acetylcholine perchlorate solution for the hemolysates of whole blood and red blood cells, or 0.50 ml of the butyrylcholine iodide solution for the diluted plasma). Turn on the unit's chart drive and titrator.
4. Allow the reaction to continue for a minimum of 3 min or until a titrant volume of 0.5 ml has been added.*

CALCULATION†

1. Measure a 3-min interval on the recorder trace during which the slope was constant, disregarding any nonlinear "overshoot" at the beginning of the titration.
2. Determine the number of recorder chart scale divisions, representing titrant volume, which were traversed during the 3-min interval.
3. Divide the number of scale divisions by 3 to obtain the reaction rate in scale divisions per minute.
4. Calculate the activity per milliliter of undiluted specimen as micromoles of substrate hydrolyzed per minute, using the following formula:

$$\text{activity} = 1{,}000 \times S \times T \times N \times D,$$

where

S = scale divisions per minute;
T = milliliters of titrant per scale division;
N = normality of base;
D = dilution factor.‡

Sample Calculations

Assume the following conditions: normality of base = 0.00512 (calculated prior to assay); milliliters of titrant (base) per scale division = 0.025 (this constant will vary with the burette and instrument selected). After the assay, a linear 3-min section of the recorder trace traverses 21.5 scale divisions. The activity is calculated as follows:

$$\text{scale divisions/min} = 21.5/3 = 7.17 \text{ scale divisions/min} \quad (1)$$

$$\text{activity} = (1{,}000) \times (7.17) \times (0.025) \times (0.00512) \times (10) = 9.18\ \mu\text{mol/min/ml plasma} \quad (2)$$

*These limits are based on obtaining a precision of 1% in reading the recorder chart trace. Select a chart speed that will allow a 3-min trace to be read with a precision of at least 1%, e.g., 2 cm/min or faster. If the recorder chart is divided into 100 divisions (full-scale), then the minimum volume of titrant delivered to allow 1% precision in its measurement would be about 20% full-scale travel of the pen. With the use of a 2.5-ml automatic burette, full-scale pen travel represents 2.5 ml of titrant, and 20% of full-scale pen travel represents 0.5 ml of titrant. Both of these limits (3 min in time and 20% of full-scale pen travel) represent minima and should be exceeded in the assay to insure 1% precision in these measurements.

†For conversion of pH-Stat units to units of other methods, see p. 100.

‡The dilution factor for a 1-in-5 dilution of whole blood is 5; for a 1-in-10 dilution of plasma, the dilution factor is 10. The dilution factor for red blood cells is Hct, where Hct is the fractional hematocrit value of the whole blood. Correction of assay values to a hypothetical 50% hematocrit, thereby effectively providing assay values for 1.0 ml of packed red cells under the standard conditions of the hematocrit centrifugation, generally proves more satisfactory than attempting to sample washed and packed red cells directly.

If the same titration values had been obtained from whole blood, the only factor that would change would be the dilution factor. Thus,

$$\text{activity} = (1{,}000) \times (7.17) \times (0.025) \times (0.00512) \times (5) = 4.59\ \mu\text{mol/min/ml whole blood} \quad (3)$$

With the same titration values for a red cell hemolysate prepared from whole blood with a hematocrit of 0.45, the dilution factor would be calculated as follows:

$$\text{dilution factor} = \frac{5}{\text{Hematocrit}} = \frac{5}{0.45} = 11.11 \quad (4)$$

Thus,

$$\text{activity} = (1{,}000) \times (7.17) \times (0.025) \times (0.00512) \times (11.11) = 10.20\ \mu\text{mol/min/ml red cells} \quad (5)$$

When multiple assays are performed on one type of specimen, e.g., plasma, calculation may be simplified by multiplying the last four factors in the activity equation to form a new factor, K, by which each (scale division/min) unit is multiplied to obtain the activity.

Thus,

$$K_{(\text{plasma})} = (0.025) \times (0.00512) \times (1{,}000) \times (10) = 1.28000 \quad (6)$$

Then, for (scale division/min) obtained in Equation 1,

$$\text{activity} = (K_{\text{plasma}}) \times (\text{scale divisions/min}) = (1.28000) \times (7.17) = 9.18\ \mu\text{mol/min/ml plasma} \quad (7)$$

INTERPRETATION* (see p. 7)

The mean and normal range of values given in the table below were determined on a population of 277 male subjects.

	Plasma	Whole blood	Red blood cells
Number of subjects	277	243	241
Mean	7.70	4.51	8.28
Standard deviation	1.61	0.58	1.12
Range (mean ±2 standard deviations)	4.48–10.93	3.35–5.67	6.04–10.52

ACCURACY AND PRECISION

The sequential analysis of 24 aliquots taken from constantly stirred heparinized whole blood or plasma provided the following precision statistics:

	Plasma	Whole blood	Red blood cells
Number of aliquots	24	24	24
Mean	8.22	4.47	10.05
Standard deviation	0.14	0.15	0.40
Coefficient of variation, %	1.70	3.35	3.98

Storage Stability

If adequately heparinized, whole blood hemolysates, prepared as described, maintain at least 90% of their original cholinesterase activity for up to 6 days when stored at room temperature. When refrigerated or frozen, they retain the 90% activity level for up to 50 days.

Hemolysates of red blood cells exhibit a rapid loss of cholinesterase activity at room temperature, dropping to about 90% of their initial activity in the first 12 hr and less than 60% within 3 days. Refrigeration maintains the activity at the 90% level for about 3 days; freezing extends storage time up to 50 days.

Plasma, either whole or diluted 1:10 with Ringer's salts solution, maintains the 90% activity level for

*For assessment of the test results, see p. 86.

about 6 days at room temperature and up to 50 days when refrigerated or frozen.

A stringy, gelatinous precipitate occasionally appears in frozen whole blood and red cell hemolysates upon subsequent thawing, making the pipeting of homogeneous samples difficult; therefore, unless long-term storage of specimens is necessary, freezing should be avoided. No problems were encountered in assaying frozen plasma specimens.

No experimental data are available on the effect of storage at ambient temperatures above 25°C; therefore, specimens taken elsewhere and mailed to the laboratory should be kept cold during transit.

INTERFERING SUBSTANCES

Oxalate, citrate, and particularly fluoride should not be used as anticoagulants or preservatives in blood collected for cholinesterase analysis. The plasma enzyme is inhibited by most detergents, including the Triton® X-100 used to hemolyze cells for erythrocyte and whole blood analysis. All glassware should therefore be carefully rinsed with distilled water. The effects of mild hemolysis in plasma are minimized by the selection of butyrylcholine as a substrate, because the hydrolysis rate of this substrate by the erythrocyte enzyme is less than 5% of its hydrolysis rate by the plasma enzyme. An occasional elevated value within replicate erythrocyte samples is apparently due to an aggregation of red cell membranes after hemolysis. Careful mixing just prior to sampling will usually prevent this error. Unlike colorimetric methods, the pH-Stat procedure is unaffected by color or turbidity in the specimen; icteric or lipemic plasma may be used.

REFERENCES

Crane, C. R., Sanders, D. C., and Abbott, J. K., Studies on the Storage Stability of Human Blood Cholinesterases, I, Report No. AM 70-4, Federal Aviation Administration, Office of Aviation Medicine, Civil Aeromedical Institute, Oklahoma City, 1970.

Nabb, D. P. and Whitfield, F., Determination of cholinesterase by an automated pH-Stat method, *Arch. Environ. Health,* 15, 147, 1967.

CONVERSION OF PLASMA CHOLINESTERASE ACTIVITY UNITS

Charles R. Crane, Donald C. Sanders, and John K. Abbott

Since the range of normal values for serum and plasma cholinesterase is quite broad, most clinical interpretations should consider an elevation or depression of activity on the basis of the individual's baseline or preexposure value. Any change from the baseline activity is easily noted if both values are expressed in the same units; however, the units of activity obtained by the various commonly used cholinesterase methods are neither identical nor heretofore readily interconvertible. By use of the following conversion (regression) equations, activity units obtained by one method may be readily transformed to the corresponding units of any other. To provide a broad gradient of enzyme activity, these equations were prepared by performing simultaneous assays by each method on aliquots of plasma samples containing mixtures of fresh and heat-denatured plasma in varying proportions. Consequently, these conversion relationships are valid for activity levels from near zero to the upper limits of activity found in normal human plasma. Correlation coefficients are included for each conversion equation.

1. To convert pH-Stat units to Michel units (ΔpH): Michel units = 0.117 × (pH-Stat units) − 0.039; correlation coefficient = 0.986.
2. To convert pH-Stat units to Caraway units (ChE): Caraway units = 10.67 × (pH-Stat units) − 3.15; correlation coefficient = 0.989.

3. To convert pH-Stat units to Acholest units (T at 25°C): Acholest units = $\frac{81.4}{(\text{pH-Stat units})} - 5.19$; correlation coefficient = 0.991.
4. To convert Michel units (ΔpH) to pH-Stat units: pH-Stat units = 8.32 × (Michel units) + 0.41; correlation coefficient = 0.986.
5. To convert Caraway units (ChE) to pH-Stat units: pH-Stat units = 0.092 × (Caraway units) + 0.366; correlation coefficient = 0.989.
6. To convert Acholest units (T at 25°C) to pH-Stat units: pH-Stat units = $\frac{44.9}{T} + 0.827$, where T = minutes required to match color by the Acholest method at 25°C; correlation coefficient = 0.991.

Example:

To convert a Michel plasma value of 0.47 ΔpH units to its equivalent value in pH-Stat units, use Equation 4. By substituting 0.47 ΔpH units in Equation 4,

$$\text{pH-Stat units} = (8.32 \times 0.47) + 0.41 = 4.32.$$

Michel, Caraway, and Acholest units can be converted from one to another by first converting them to pH-Stat units. Note that the conversion equation for Acholest units applies only to data at 25°C; to convert Acholest units obtained at any other temperature, the temperature correction factor described in that method (Type A Procedure)* must be applied prior to use of the regression equation.

Interconversion data for the pH-Stat method as applicable to the Sigma† and Boehringer‡ commercial-kit methods have been published;[1] the use of these additional data would permit interconversion of activity units among any of six methods.

REFERENCE

1. **Crane, C. R., Sanders, D. C., and Abbott, J. K.,** A Comparison of Three Serum Cholinesterase Methods, Rep. No. 70-13, Federal Aviation Administration, Office of Aviation Medicine, Civil Aeromedical Institute, Oklahoma, 1970.

CHOLINESTERASE AND PSEUDOCHOLINESTERASE (DIBUCAINE NUMBER)

PRINCIPLE

Persons exposed to organophosphate pesticides may develop symptoms due to the inhibition of cholinesterase activity by these compounds. In these persons, cholinesterase activity can serve as a measure of exposure and hazard.

Benzoylcholine is hydrolyzed by the enzyme cholinesterase to form benzoic acid. Benzoylcholine exhibits much greater absorbance in the UV range than does benzoic acid. Thus, the decrease in absorbance at 240 nm after incubation of a sample with benzoylcholine can be used as a direct measurement of enzyme activity. This substrate may be used to indicate exposure to pesticide cholinesterase inhibitors. The addition of dibucaine to the substrate readily distinguishes the typical (normal) from the atypical (succinylcholine sensitive) cholinesterase by differential inhibition. Dibucaine inhibits the normal enzyme while the atypical enzyme is less subject to its inhibitory effect.

*See p. 88.

†Kit 420-CC. Sigma Chemical Co., 3500 Dekalb Street, St. Louis, Missouri 63118.

‡Kit TC-Ce, Cat. No 15948 TCAB Boehinger-Mannheim Corp., 219 East 44th Street, N.Y., N.Y. 10017.

TYPE B PROCEDURE

Clifford B. Walberg

APPARATUS

1. Recording UV spectrophotometer
2. Volumetric pipet, 3 ml

REAGENTS

All chemicals should be analytical reagent grade.

1. Sorensen phosphate buffer, pH 7.4, $M/15$
2. Benzoylcholine chloride solution, $1 \times 10^{-3} M$
   Dissolve 24.4 mg of benzoylcholine in the Sorensen buffer and dilute to 100 ml with the buffer. Divide into 2.5-ml aliquots, freeze, and store at $-10°C$. Frozen, the reagent is stable for at least 6 to 12 months.
3. Dibucaine solution, $4 \times 10^{4} M$
   Dissolve 15.2-mg dibucaine (nupercaine hydrochloride) in the Sorensen buffer and dilute to 100 ml with the buffer. Divide into 1.5-ml aliquots, freeze, and store at $-10°C$. Frozen, the reagent is stable for at least 6 to 12 months.
4. Substrate solution
   Mix two parts of the benzoylcholine chloride solution with 38 parts of the buffer. Prepare fresh daily.
5. Inhibition solution
   Mix two parts of the benzoylcholine chloride solution, one part of the dibucaine solution, and 37 parts of the buffer. Prepare fresh daily.

PROCEDURE

If the serum cholinesterase level after exposure to organophosphate pesticides is desired, perform Method A only (temperature 25°C). To determine the dibucaine number (sensitivity to succinylcholine), perform Methods A and B in sequence and without delay to avoid variation due to ambient temperature.

Note: Adjust the spectrophotometer to zero at 240 nm using the appropriate blank (substrate for Method A, inhibition solution for Method B). The spectrophotometer must be ready for immediate use after mixing the serum with the reaction solution.

A. Serum Cholinesterase (Organophosphate Poisoning)

1. Transfer 3.0 ml of substrate solution into a cuvette.
2. Add 0.02 ml of serum.
3. Mix well and place in the spectrophotometer immediately. Use a solution of the substrate as the reference solution.
4. Measure the absorbance each minute for 5 min.
5. Determine the rate of change of absorbance per minute. Use only the linear decrease for calculations (see Figures 1 and 2).

B. Dibucaine Number (Succinylcholine Sensitivity)

1. Transfer 3.0 ml of inhibition solution into a cuvette.
2. Add 0.02 ml serum.
3. Mix well and place in the spectrophotometer immediately. Use the inhibition solution as the reference solution.
4. Measure the absorbance each minute for 5 min.
5. Determine the rate of change of absorbance per minute. Use only the linear decrease for calculations (see Figures 3 and 4).

CALCULATIONS

Calculate the International Units (I.U.) for Procedure A to determine organophosphate pesticide poisoning, and for Procedure A and B to determine the Dibucaine Number (D.N.).

$$\text{I.U. } (\mu\text{mol/min/liter}) = \frac{\Delta\ \text{A/min}}{6{,}600 \times 1} \times 10^{6} \times \frac{3.02}{0.02}$$

$$\text{I.U.} = \Delta\ \text{A/min} \times 22{,}880$$

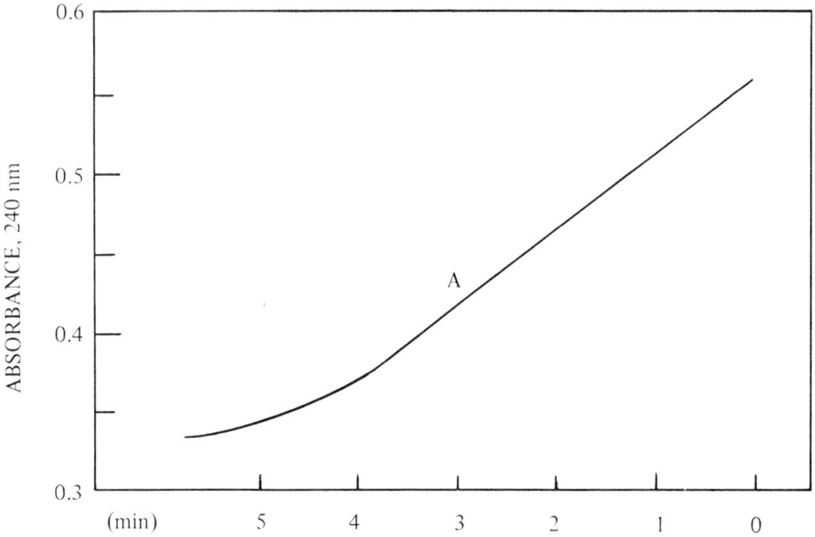

Calculations

Substrate solution (A):

A_0 min = 0.562

A_3 min = 0.410

ΔA = 0.152

$\Delta A/\text{min} = \frac{0.152}{3} = 0.051$

$0.051 \times 22880 = 1167$ I.U.

A = Substrate solution

FIGURE 1. Normal cholinesterase activity.

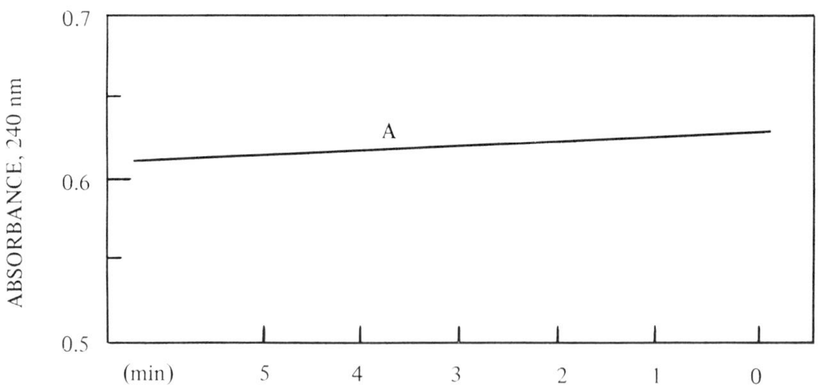

Calculations

Substrate solution (A):

A_0 min = 0.632

A_5 min = 0.617

ΔA = 0.015

$\Delta A/\text{min} = \frac{0.015}{5} = 0.003$

$0.003 \times 22880 = 69$ I.U.

A = Substrate solution

FIGURE 2. Example of patient exposed to parathion (low cholinesterase activity).

Note: The molar absorptivity is 6,600 and refers to the difference between the absorbance of benzoylcholine chloride and benzoic acid at 240 nm. The molar absorptivity and the factor may be verified for each laboratory.[1]

$$\text{D.N.} = 100 - 100\,\frac{I_B}{I_A}$$

where

I_B = I.U. test-inhibition solution (B);
I_A = I.U. test-substrate solution (A);

NOTES

1. A "normal" serum should be analyzed in the same manner and used as a control.

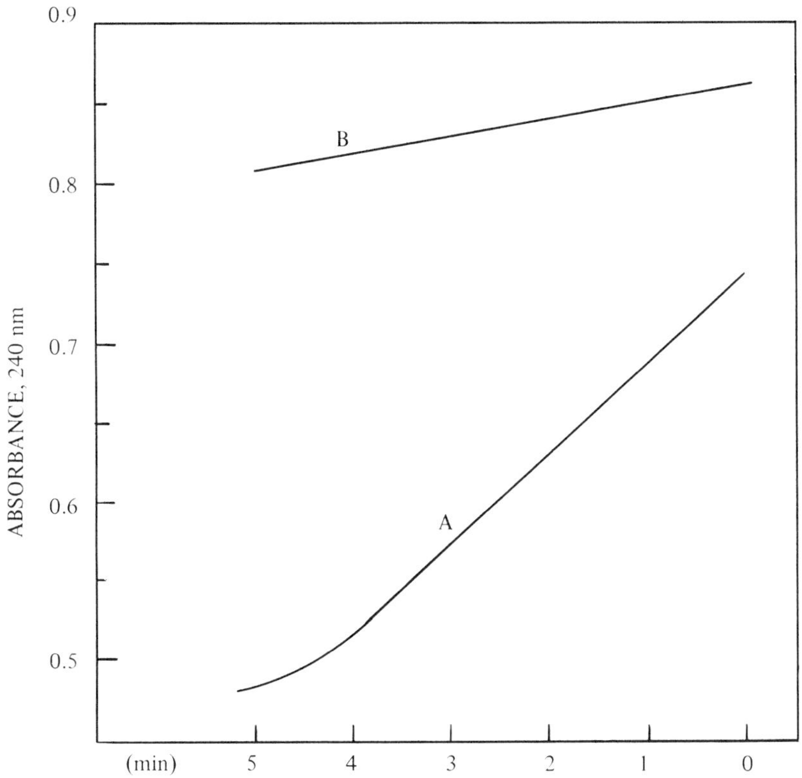

A = Substrate solution only
B = Inhibition solution

Inhibition solution (B):

A_0 min = 0.860

A_3 min = 0.833

ΔA = 0.027

$\Delta A/\text{min} = \frac{0.027}{3} = 0.009$

$0.009 \times 22880 = 206$ I.U.

Substrate solution (A):

A_0 min = 0.750

A_3 min = 0.576

ΔA = 0.174

$\Delta A/\text{min} = \frac{0.174}{3} = 0.058$

$0.058 \times 22880 = 1327$ I.U.

Dibucaine Number (D.N.):

$\text{D.N.} = 100 - (100 \times \frac{206}{1327})$

$\text{D.N.} = 100 - 16$

$\text{D.N.} = 84$

FIGURE 3. Example of patient with normal dibucaine number (normal cholinesterase and normal inhibition).

2. Normal levels for serum cholinesterase are given for assays performed at 25°C. The usual precautions for enzyme determinations should be observed.
3. The reaction is fast. The rate of change of absorbance is usually linear for 5 min or less.

INTERPRETATION (see p. 7)

Total Activity

Normal serum cholinesterase activity ranges from 559 to 1,483 I.U. This activity is decreased on exposure to organophosphate pesticides, in some organic disease states, and in those individuals having the genotype for atypical cholinesterase.

Dibucaine Number

The percent inhibition of cholinesterase activity produced by the local anesthetic dibucaine may be used to identify the genotype of the individual. The percent inhibition converted to a whole number is the Dibucaine Number (D.N.) and it is independent of the enzyme activity even when organic disease has reduced the activity to low levels.

Normal cholinesterase (homozygous)	D.N. = approximately 80
Heterozygous	D.N. = approximately 60
Atypical (homozygous)	D.N. = approximately 20

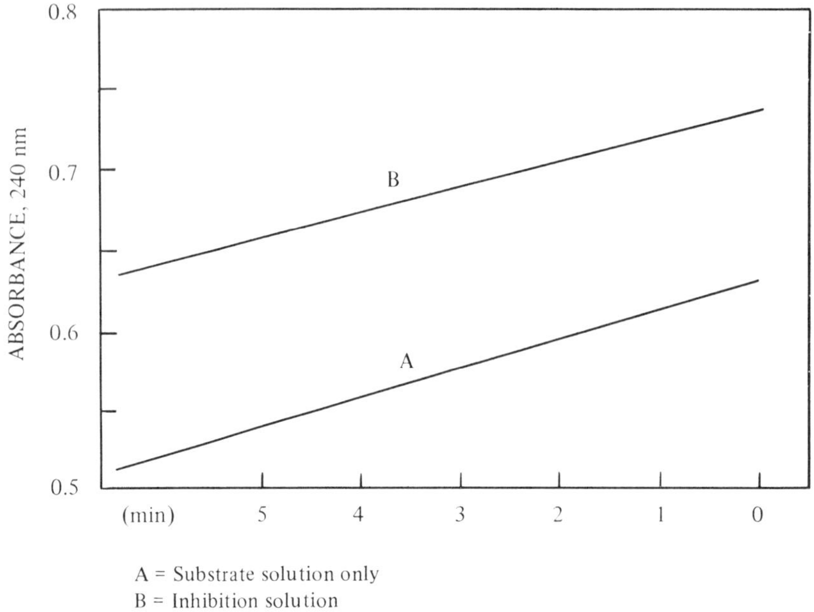

Inhibition solution (B):

$A_0 \text{ min} = 0.740$

$A_5 \text{ min} = 0.660$

$\Delta A = 0.080$

$\Delta A/\text{min} = \frac{0.080}{5} = 0.016$

$0.016 \times 22880 = 366$ I.U.

Substrate solution (A):

$A_0 \text{ min} = 0.630$

$A_5 \text{ min} = 0.530$

$\Delta A = 0.100$

$\Delta A/\text{min} = \frac{0.100}{5} = 0.020$

$0.020 \times 22880 = 458$ I.U.

Dibucaine Number (D.N.):

$\text{D.N.} = 100 - (100 \times \frac{366}{458})$

$\text{D.N.} = 100 - 80$

$\text{D.N.} = 20$

FIGURE 4. Example of patient with prolonged effect of succinylcholine (low dibucaine number).

Patients having the atypical genotype are extremely sensitive to succinylcholine and may suffer from paralysis and prolonged apnea when this muscle relaxant is administered.

ACCURACY AND PRECISION

The precision of this method yields a coefficient of variation of 6% for replicate analyses of the same sample.

REFERENCE

1. **Kalow, W., Genest, K., and Staron, N.,** Kinetic studies on the hydrolysis of benzoylcholine by human serum cholinesterase, *Can. J. Biochem. Physiol.*, 34, 637, 1956.

GENERAL REFERENCES

Kalow, W. and Genest, K., A method for the detection of atypical forms of human serum cholinesterase. Determination of dibucaine numbers, *Can. J. Biochem. Physiol.*, 35, 339, 1957.

Richterich, R., *Clinical Chemistry, Theory and Practice*, Academic Press, N.Y., 1969, 441.

COPPER

PRINCIPLE

In Procedure B protein-free filtrates of sera are exposed to several reagents which react with the cations in question to produce colored solutions whose absorbances are used to measure the cation concentrations. (This procedure is also applicable to iron and zinc.) When exposed to a suitable ligand, such as bathocuproine sulfonate, copper salts form a characteristic colored complex whose absorbance can be used to measure the copper concentrations. If serum copper concentrations are required, this reaction can be applied to a protein-free filtrate of the serum with high specificity and adequate sensitivity. A more elegant technique requires the extraction of a suitable copper complex into methyl isobutyl ketone (Procedure C). This extract can then be aspirated into an atomic absorption spectrometer, and its copper content thus may be determined.

TYPE B PROCEDURE

Bennie Zak

APPARATUS

1. Automatic pipets and diluters
2. Centrifuge
3. Spectrophotometer, visible-range (Coleman II, Bausch and Lomb Spectronic 70 or 100, Turner 330 or 350, Gilford 300N, Beckman DBG, Hitachi 124, or any other comparable spectrophotometer)

REAGENTS

All chemicals should be analytical reagent grade and as free of trace metals as possible.

1. Trichloroacetic acid (TCA) stock solution, 100 g/dl
   Dissolve 100g of iron-free trichloroacetic acid* in metal-free distilled water in a glass-stoppered graduate to a volume of 100 ml. The accuracy of this measurement is not critical.
2. Trichloroacetic acid-ascorbic acid (TCA-AA) solution
   Pipet 20 ml of TCA stock solution into a 100-ml volumetric flask containing 50 to 60 ml of metal-free water. Add 1 g of ascorbic acid, then dilute to the mark with water.
3. Metal stock solutions
   For each metal, dilute three different concentrations of commercial atomic absorption standards so that each contains 50 μg/ml of solution.
4. Copper reference solutions
   Prepare reference solutions with concentrations ranging from 0 to 300 μg/100 ml by pipeting 0.0, 1.0, 2.0, and 3.0 ml of the copper stock solution into 100-ml volumetric flasks containing 50 ml of the TCA-AA solution. Dilute the solution in each flask to the mark with metal-free water. These filtrate-like solutions contain 0, 50, 100, and 150 μg of copper/100 ml, respectively, and they correspond to 0, 100, 200, and 300 μg/100 ml. In everyday practice, only the 100 μg/100 ml reference solution need be prepared.
5. Iron reference solutions
   Prepare iron reference solutions in the same manner as copper reference solutions, using aliquots of the iron stock solutions instead of copper.
6. Zinc reference solutions
   Prepare zinc reference solutions in the same manner as copper or iron reference solutions, using aliquots of the zinc stock solutions instead of copper or iron.
7. Ammonium acetate, 50 g/100 ml
   Dissolve 500 g of ammonium acetate in water and dilute to one liter.
8. Bathocuproine sulfonate (BCS) solution, 30 mg/100 ml

*Available from G. F. Smith Chemical Co., Columbus, Ohio.

Dissolve 30.0 mg of bathocuproine sulfonate in the ammonium acetate solution. Dilute this solution to 100 ml with ammonium acetate solution.

9. Bathophenanthroline sulfonate (BPS) solution, 30 mg/100 ml
   Dissolve 30.0 mg of bathophenanthroline sulfonate in the ammonium acetate solution. Dilute this solution to 100 ml with ammonium acetate solution.
10. Bathophenanthroline sulfonate (BPS) solution, 10 mg/ml
    Dissolve 100 mg of bathophenanthroline sulfonate in 10.0 ml of metal-free water. This solution is used only when copper and iron are to be determined sequentially.
11. Zincon®, 35 mg/100 ml
    Dissolve 35.0 mg of Zincon® in 2.0 ml of Brij 35® solution (Atlas Chemical Industries, Inc.) and dilute to 100 ml with metal-free water.
12. Chloral hydrate, 60 g/100 ml
    Dissolve 6 g of chloral hydrate in metal-free water. Dilute this solution to 10.0 ml with metal-free water.
13. Sodium hydroxide solution, 4*N*
    Dissolve 160 g of sodium hydroxide in metal-free water and dilute to one liter.
14. Borate buffer solution
    Weigh 4.5 g of sodium borate decahydrate into a 50-ml flask containing about 15 ml of metal-free water. Add 75 mg of sodium cyanide and 20 ml of the sodium hydroxide solution. When the solids are dissolved, dilute the solution to 50 ml with metal-free water. Pipet 1.0 ml of the buffer into 4.0 ml of the 0.0 μg/100 ml reference solution, then measure the pH. This should be between 8.5 and 9.5. If the pH is below 8.5, prepare the solution again, using 22 ml of the sodium hydroxide solution. Test the buffer solution again to see if the appropriate pH value is acheived.

PROCEDURE[1]

The preparation of the filtrate from the specimen and reference solutions is identical for any or all of the determinations of the three metals. The volume relationships will be described for a Coleman II spectrophotometer. If another spectrophotometer is used, the suggested volumes may have to be modified in proportion.

Determination of Copper or Iron

1. Pipet 3.0 ml of serum into 3.0 ml of TCA-AA solution. Mix well. Allow the mixture to stand for a few minutes, then centrifuge it for 10 min at 3,000 rpm.
2. Pipet a 4.0-ml aliquot of the filtrate into a 19 *N* 105-mm cuvette.
3. If copper is to be determined, add 0.5 ml of the BCS solution to the filtrate.
4. Measure the absorbance at 484 nm against a reference sample prepared by substituting 4.0 ml of the 0.0 μg/100 ml reference solution for the filtrate. Elevate the cuvette in its carrier by a suitable support, because the minimum volume for the cuvette in this carrier is ordinarily 5.5 ml.
5. If iron is to be determined, use the identical process, but substitute the 30 mg/100 ml BPS solution for the BCS reagent. Measure the absorbance at 534 nm against a reference sample prepared by substituting 4.0 ml of the 0.0 μg/100 ml reference solution for the filtrate.

Determination of Zinc

1. Prepare a filtrate in the same manner as for the copper or iron determination.
2. Pipet 1.0 ml of borate buffer into 4.0 ml of the filtrate. Process a reagent blank prepared with the 0.0 μg/100 ml reference solution in the same manner as the specimen for use as a reference sample.
3. Pipet 0.1 ml of Zincon® reagent into the filtrate and mix well.
4. Set the instrument for 0 absorbance at 630 nm, then add 0.1 ml of the chloral hydrate solution to the cuvette and mix.
5. Read the increased absorbance of this solution at 630 nm. Note that both readings are made in the same cuvette and that the principle of self-blanking after demasking the zinc complex is used. Although the color is stable for more than 10 min, the nature of the procedure dictates that the operator read the generated absorbance immediately and then proceed to demask the zinc complex in the filtrate of the

next sample. The use of an automatic pipet simplifies all reagent additions and is recommended.

Sequential Determination of Copper and Iron

1. Pipet 0.5 ml of BCS solution into 4.0 ml of filtrate, then determine the absorbance of the solution at 484 nm (A_1) and at 534 nm (A_2). The absorbance at 484 nm is used to determine the copper, while the absorbance at 534 nm serves as a reference value for the subsequent determination of iron. Use a 4.0-ml sample of the 0.0 μg/100 ml reference solution, processed in the same manner, as a reagent blank.
2. Pipet 40 μl of the 10 mg/ml BPS solution into both the specimen and the reagent blank and then read the additional absorbance at 534 nm (A_3). Subtract A_2 from A_3 to obtain the absorbance of the specimen due to iron.

Determination of Copper, Iron, and Zinc from the Same Filtrate

1. Pipet 2.0 ml of the filtrate into a cuvette. Treat this with half the volumes of the reagents used for the sequential determination of copper and iron, proceeding in the same manner.
2. Pipet 2.0 ml of the filtrate into a second cuvette. Treat this with half the volumes of the reagents used for the determination of zinc, proceeding in the same manner.

CALCULATION

Copper and Iron

Read the absorbances of the reference solutions against the reagent blank at 484 nm for copper and at 534 nm for iron. Plot the three absorbances against the concentrations from which they were obtained. The absorbances are stable for several hours and usually yield a straight line.

Zinc

Determine the absorbance changes for the reagent blank and reference solutions. Subtract the value obtained from the reagent blank from that obtained from the reference solutions. A plot of the resultant absorbances against concentrations yields a straight line from 0.0 to 300 μg/ml. The determination of the absorbance difference from each demasked reference solution should be made individually rather than by batch processing, since the color is not as stable as the colors for copper and iron.

INTERPRETATION (see p. 7)

The procedures described above permit determination of copper and iron by sequential reaction on a single aliquot, or of all three metals by the use of two aliquots of the same filtrate. Usually only one elevated metal concentration is encountered in a toxic circumstance; therefore, the directions for the determination of any of the metals on a single aliquot are probably the most important. For situations where either copper or iron may be elevated, the sequential procedure is presented so that both metals can be determined on a single aliquot. The zinc determination must be performed on a second aliquot.

In the normal range one would encounter 60 to 150 μg/100 ml for iron,[2] 80 to 160 μg/100 ml for copper,[3] and 76 to 132 μg/100 ml for zinc.[4] In a known pathological circumstance where a constituent-elevating disease is encountered, any of the three metals could be elevated above these ranges; this factor would have to be considered in deciding whether part of the elevated metal concentration was exogenous in origin.

The ligands described were selected on the basis of their specificity, selectivity, and the relative ease of determination with common laboratory equipment. For the determination of either copper or iron only two chemical steps are involved; for the determination of both copper and iron only three steps are needed. The determination of zinc involves only four chemical steps. In practice the process is easily simplified with the use of automatic diluters, while the reaction is simplified by the principle of internal self-blanking.[5]

There are more sensitive reagents for iron, such as 2,4-di-[pyridyl-(2)-4-(p-methaxyphenyl)]-pyridine sulfonate with a molar absorptivity of 26,900,[6] 3-(2-pyridyl)-5,6-diphenyl-1,2,4-triazine sulfonate with a molar absorptivity of 27,900,[7,8] and 2,6-bis-(4-phenyl-2-pyridyl)-4-phenyl pyridine with a molar absorptivity of 30,200.[9,10] For copper there are the condensation products of oxalylhydrazide and acetaldehyde which have a molar absorptivity of 22,000,[11] N,N,N^1 N^1-tetraethylthiuram disulfide with a molar absorptivity of 33,000,[12] or its pyridine analogue, bis-(1-piperidyl-thiocarbonyl) disulfide with a molar absorptivity of 37,500.[13] For zinc there is dithizone[14] or the much more sensitive 1-(2-pyridylazo)-2-napthal with a molar absorptivity of 52,800.[15] The latter compound is used in a modification of the Zincon® procedure described here and makes use of the same differential demasking phenomenon.[1,5] In toxic conditions, however, one expects to find elevated values, and all the procedures described have proven to be adequately sensitive in cases of normal or low concentrations.[1,16,17] In addition, copper and iron both produce colors in the same reaction medium when they are determined sequentially. The substitution of the more sensitive ligands for the three metal ions is easily possible at the discretion of the user.

ACCURACY AND PRECISION

Bathophenanthroline sulfonate and bathocuproine sulfonate are ideally suited for quantitative analysis because they are virtually specific for iron and copper, respectively. They react instantaneously at pH 4 to 5, and they have reliable molar absorptivities and strong binding constants, which ensure that the colored complexes formed are reproducible even when they are formed in each other's presence. For sequential color formation of copper and iron in the same aliquot, the order of reactions is chosen so that the color for copper forms first. The copper spectrum gives virtually no interference at 534 nm, whereas, if the order of the reactions were reversed, the ferrous BPS spectrum would present the problem of a huge value for the reagent blank in the subsequent copper determination. Less than a 3% error is expected in serum determinations in the normal ranges for copper and iron, and the accuracy is markedly increased if higher concentrations are present.

Although there are interferences in the zinc reaction, the procedural characteristics used for serum obviate interference by the use of differential demasking, during which zinc is selectively released for individual reaction. The accuracy for serum zinc in the normal range, using this procedure, is between 3 and 5%. The accuracy is increased if the concentration becomes abnormally high.

INTERFERING SUBSTANCES

In zinc determination, copper and iron are the main interferences; however, a differential demasking technique is used, in which copper, iron, and zinc are first complexed as cyanides in the presence of the color reagent Zincon®. At this point in the procedure neither of the three metals can react with the Zincon® and the sample is now its own blank. With the addition of chloral hydrate, the excess cyanide is rapidly destroyed. The zinc ions are liberated from the weakest of the three complexes, and the reaction with the ligand takes place. Liberation of cyanide from the copper and iron complexes does not occur under the selected condition, because the addition of ascorbic acid for reduction of copper and iron to lower valence states ensures stability of their cyanide complexes. If any other interfering color reactions occur in serum filtrates that are unrelated to the cyanide complexation and demasking steps, they presumably become a part of the sample blank. In that case, they are read before the addition of chloral hydrate and are not affected by the demasking processes.[1]

The bathophenanthroline sulfonate, used for the determination of iron, and the bathocuproine sulfonate, used for the determination of copper, are very selective under the reaction conditions described. No known interfering color reactions for either metal ligand occur in TCA filtrates of serum. In addition, when the ferrous BPS reaction is carried out in the presence of cuprous BCS, no interaction of any kind occurs to enhance or inhibit the color complexes of either metal. Zinc may react with the ligands of the other two metals, but the complex formed is colorless. As long as a reasonable excess of both ligands is present, no problems are encountered. Besides, Cu(I) reacting with BCS and Fe(II) reacting with BPS have very strong binding constants. This aids in the avoidance of interference from other potentially competing metals.

REFERENCES

1. **Watkins, R., Weiner, L. M., and Zak, B.,** Determination of copper, iron and zinc from a single small sample, *Microchem. J.,* 16, 14, 1971.
2. **Boutwell, J. H.,** *Clinical Chemistry, Laboratory Manual and Methods,* Lea and Febiger, Philadelphia, 1961, 204.
3. **Weissman, N. and Pileggi, V. J.,** Inorganic ions, in *Clinical Chemistry, Principles and Technics,* Henry, R. J., Cannon, D. C., and Winkelman, J. W., Eds., Harper and Row, N.Y., 1974, chap. 19.
4. **Prasad, A. S., Oberleas, D., and Halsted, J. A.,** Determination of zinc in biological fluids by atomic-absorption spectrophotometry in normal and cirrhotic subjects, *J. Lab. Clin. Med.,* 66, 508, 1965.
5. **Williams, L. A., Cohen, J. S., and Zak, B.,** Study of a differential demasking technique for serum zinc, *Clin. Chem.,* 8, 502, 1962.
6. **Schmidt, R., Weis, W., Klingmüller, V., und Standinger, Hj.,** Eine Methode der automatischen Bestimmung des Gesamteisen in Blutserum und Urin mit 2,6-de-[pyridyl-(2)]-4-[p-methoxyphenyl]-pyridine and seiner Sulfosaüre, *Z. Klin. Chem. Klin. Biochem.,* 6, 39, 1967.
7. **Stookey, L. L.,** Ferrozine, a new spectrophotometric reagent for iron, *Anal. Chem.,* 42, 779, 1970.
8. **Manasterski, A., Weiner, L. M., and Zak, B.,** Spectrophotometric study of the reaction of 3-(2-pyridyl)-5,6-bis (4-phenylsulfonic Acid)-1,2,-4-triazine with iron and copper, *Microchem. J.,* 16, 245, 1971.
9. **Zak, B., Baginski, E. S., Epstein, E., and Weiner, L. M.,** Comparison of sensitivity and specificity of iron chromogens: Measurement of serum iron with a new aqueous color reagent, *Ann. Clin. Lab. Sci.,* 1, 14, 1971.
10. **Zak, B., Baginski, E. S., Epstein, E., and Weiner, L. M.,** Determination of serum iron with a new color reagent, *Clin. Toxicol.,* 4, 621, 1971.
11. **Nilsson, G.,** A new color reaction on copper and certain carbonyl compounds, *Acta Chem. Scand.,* 4, 205, 1950.
12. **Watkins, R. and Zak, B.,** Sensitive microreacting ligand for serum copper, *Microchem. J.,* 16, 304, 1971.
13. **Carter, P. F.,** Submicrogram serum copper quantification by spectrophotometry with bis (1-piperidylthiocarbonyl) disulfide, *Clin. Chim. Acta,* 39, 497, 1972.
14. **Sandell, E. B.,** *Colorimetric Determination of Traces of Metals,* 3rd ed., Interscience, 1959, chap. 49.
15. **Carter, P. F.,** Spectrophotometric submicrogram serum Zinc assay: An application for the routine service laboratory, *Clin. Chim. Acta,* 52, 277, 1974.
16. **Landers, J. W. and Zak, B.,** Determination of copper and iron in a single small sample, *Am. J. Clin. Pathol.,* 29, 590, 1958.
17. **Zak, B.,** Simple procedure for the single sample determination of copper and iron, *Clin. Chim. Acta,* 3, 328, 1958.

TYPE C PROCEDURE

F. William Sunderman, Jr.

APPARATUS

1. Centrifuge tubes, glass-stoppered, 12 and 50 ml
2. Mixer (Vortex)
3. Centrifuge
4. Erlenmeyer flasks, 125 ml
5. Beads (Pyrex®)
6. Hot plate, electric
7. pH Meter, equipped with probe-type electrode
8. Tissue homogenizer, Teflon®-glass, motor-driven
9. Spectrometer, atomic absorption (Perkin-Elmer Model 303), fitted with a copper hollow-cathode lamp and a "high-solids" Lundegardh burner

REAGENTS

All chemicals used should be analytical reagent grade. Use distilled demineralized water to prepare all solutions.

1. Copper stock solution, 100 μg/ml
   Dissolve 0.03928 g of copper sulfate pentahydrate in water and dilute to 100 ml.
2. Copper reference solutions
   Dilute 0.25, 0.5, 1.0, 2.0, and 3.0 ml of the copper stock solution to 100 ml with water.
3. Hydrochloric acid, 1.4*N*
   Dilute 58.0 ml of concentrated hydrochloric acid to 500 ml with water.
4. Trichloroacetic acid, 20 g/100 ml

Dissolve 20 g of trichloroacetic acid in water and dilute to 100 ml with water.

5. Nitric acid, concentrated, 15.4*N*
6. Sulfuric acid, concentrated, 36*N*
7. Perchloric acid, 70%
8. Sodium acetate, 5 g/dl
   Dissolve 5 g of sodium acetate in water and dilute to 100 ml with water.
9. Ammonium hydroxide, concentrated, 15*N*
10. Ammonium hydroxide, 0.5*N*
    Dilute 5.0 ml of concentrated ammonium hydroxide to 150 ml with water.
11. Ammonium pyrrolidine dithiocarbamate, 5 g/dl
    Dissolve 5 g of ammonium pyrrolidine dithiocarbamate in water and dilute to 100 ml with water.
12. Methylisobutylketone, redistilled

PROCEDURE

Specimen Preparation

Serum

1. Transfer each of the following to 12-ml glass-stoppered centrifuge tubes: 2.0 ml of serum, 2.0 ml of water (to serve as a reagent blank), and 2.0 ml of each copper reference solution.
2. Add 2.0 ml of 1.4*N* hydrochloric acid to each tube and mix, using a Vortex mixer. Allow the tubes to stand for 30 min at room temperature.
3. Add 2.0 ml of the trichloroacetic acid solution and mix again. Allow the tubes to stand for 30 min at room temperature.
4. Centrifuge the tube containing the serum for 10 min at 2,000 rpm, then transfer the protein-free supernatant to a clean tube. The samples (reagent blank, reference, and serum) are now ready for measurement by atomic absorption.

Urine

1. Transfer each of the following to 125-ml Erlenmeyer flasks: 50.0 ml of urine, 50.0 ml of water (to serve as a reagent blank, and 1.0 ml of each copper reference solution. Add 50.0 ml of water to each reference sample.
2. Add to each flask 6.0 ml of nitric acid, 3.0 ml of sulfuric acid, and 3 Pyrex® beads. Heat the flasks on an electric hot plate in a fume hood until the urine sample is charred to a dark brown color and the sample volumes are reduced to approximately 4 ml.
3. After the flasks have cooled to room temperature, add 2.0 ml of nitric acid and 1.5 ml of perchloric acid. Heat the flasks on the hot plate until dense white fumes appear.
4. Add 10.0 ml of sodium acetate solution to each flask.
5. Measure the pH of the samples, using a probe-type pH electrode. Add concentrated ammonium hydroxide until the contents of the flasks reach a pH of approximately 4.
6. Cool the contents of the flasks to room temperature, then add 0.5*N* ammonium hydroxide to adjust the pH to 5.5.
7. Decant the contents of the flasks into 50-ml glass-stoppered centrifuge tubes together with 3 small washings of water.
8. Add 1.0 ml of ammonium pyrrolidine dithiocarbamate solution to each tube and mix.
9. Add 6.0 ml of methylisobutylketone to each tube and mix, using a Vortex mixer.
10. Centrifuge the tubes for 5 min at 2,000 rpm, then transfer the supernatant methylisobutylketone extracts to 12-ml glass-stoppered centrifuge tubes. The extracts are now ready for measurement by atomic absorption.

Fecal and Tissue Samples

1. Homogenize aliquots of feces and tissues (0.5 g wet weight) in 10.0 ml of water, using a motor-driven Teflon®glass tissue homogenizer.
2. Transfer the homogenates to 125-ml Erlenmeyer flasks together with four 10.0-ml washings of distilled water. Into additional flasks transfer 50.0 ml of water (to serve as a reagent blank) and 1.0 ml of each copper reference solution. Add 50.0 ml of water to each reference sample.
3. Digest the samples with nitric, sulfuric, and perchloric acids and extract the copper into methylisobutylketone as described under the preparation of urine samples.

Adjustment of the Atomic-Absorption Spectrometer

1. Adjust the atomic absorption spectrometer to the following operating conditions:
   Lamp Current: 15 mA
   Absorption Wavelength: 3247 nm
   Entrance Slit: 4 μ
   Scale Expansion: 10 X
   Meter Response: position 4
   Air Pressure: 25 lb
   Air Flow: 10-m units
   Acetylene Pressure: 10 psi
   Acetylene Flow: 6.5-m units
   Sample Aspiration Rate: 3 ml/min

2. Set the potentiometer knob at 0% absorption. While water is aspirated into the burner, set the null meter at the null point by means of the background adjustment knob.
3. Verify the stability of the burner and of the optical and electronic systems by monitoring the null meter for several minutes while water is continuously aspirated into the burner.

Atomic Absorption Measurements

1. Aspirate the extracts obtained from the reagent blank, reference samples, and specimen into the flame.
2. Determine the percent absorption (%A) of the samples by adjusting the null meter to the null point, using the potentiometer knob.

CALCULATION

1. Convert the measurements of percent absorption (%A) into absorbance (A) units by the equation:

$$\text{Absorbance (A)} = 2 - \log_{10} (100 - \%A)$$

2. Determine the amount of copper in the specimen by comparing its absorbance with that of a suitable reference sample. For determinations on a large number of specimens, a standard curve may be prepared by plotting the absorbances of the reference solutions against their respective copper concentrations.

INTERPRETATION (see p. 7)

The normal values for copper are as follows:[1,4]

Serum (N = 58): mean = 119 μg/100 ml, S.D. ± 18.8;
range 70–165 μg/100 ml
Urine (N = 21: mean = 1.68 μg/100 ml, S.D. ± 0.70;
range = 0.61 – 3.03 μg/100 ml
mean = 18.4 μg/day, S.D. ± 8.4;
range = 7.5 – 33.8 μg/day
Sweat (N = 330: mean = 55 Mg/100 ml, S.D. ± 35
range = 3.0 – 146
Sweat (N = 150): mean = 14.8 Mg/100 ml S.D. ± 61;
range = 59 – 228

According to Morell et al.,[2] the normal mean concentration of hepatic copper is 31.5 ± 6.8 μg/g (dry weight). Sternlieb[3] considers 100 μg of copper/g (dry weight) the upper normal limit for hepatic copper. Untreated patients with hepatolenticular degeneration usually have more than 250 μg of copper/g of dry liver.

ACCURACY AND PRECISION

The coefficients of variation for replicate analyses of copper in serum and urine are 1.4 and 4.6%, respectively.[1] Measurements of the recovery of copper added to serum, urine, feces, and liver average 101, 96, 94, and 94% respectively.[1] Measurements of copper in serum, urine, and tissues by the atomic absorption technique do not differ significantly ($p > 0.05$) from measurements by the spectrophotometric technique of Morell et al.[2]

INTERFERING SUBSTANCES

Despite thorough search, no other element interferes with the determination of copper in biological materials by atomic absorption spectrometry.[1]

REFERENCES

1. **Sunderman, F. W., Jr. and Roszel, N. O.,** Measurements of copper in biological materials by atomic-absorption spectrometry, *Am. J. Clin. Pathol.,* 48, 286, 1967.
2. **Morell, A. G., Windsor, J., Sternlieb, I., and**

Scheinberg, I. H., Spectrophotometric determination of microgram quantities of copper in biological materials, in *Laboratory Diagnosis of Liver Disease,* Sunderman, F. W. and Sunderman, F. W., Jr., Eds., Warren H. Green, Inc., St. Louis, 1968, 196.

3. **Sternlieb, I.,** Laboratory diagnosis of hepatolenticular degeneration, in *Laboratory Diagnosis of Liver Disease,* Sunderman, F. W. and Sunderman, F. W., Jr., Eds., Warren H. Green Inc., St. Louis, 1968, 189.
4. **Hohnadel, D. C., Sunderman, F. W., Jr., Nechay, M. W., and McNeely, M. D.,** Atomic absorption spectrometry of nickel, copper, zinc, and lead in sweat collected from healthy subjects during sauna bathing, *Clin. Chem.,* 19, 1288, 1973.

GENERAL REFERENCE

Yee, H. Y. and Goodwin, J. F., Simultaneous determination of copper and iron in a single aliquot of serum, *Clin. Chem.,* 20, 189, 1974.

CYANIDE

PRINCIPLE

Cyanide may be liberated from biological fluids by acidification. The evolved hydrogen cyanide is absorbed in alkali and the sodium cyanide thus formed is qualitatively and/or quantitatively determined by measuring the absorbance of chromophores formed by interaction of the cyanide ion with suitable reagents (Procedures A and B). Procedure C presents a sensitive gas-chromatographic method for the determination of cyanide in biological specimens, based on its conversion to cyanogen chloride using chloramine-T. The cyanogen chloride thus formed is extracted with hexane and injected into a gas chromatograph equipped with an electron-capture detector for its quantitation.

TYPE A PROCEDURE

Fredric Rieders

REAGENTS

All chemicals should be analytical reagent grade.

1. Methyl Cellosolve® (2-methoxyethanol, Eastman 2381)
2. *p*-Nitrobenzaldehyde, 0.05*M*
   Dissolve 0.755 g of *p*-nitrobenzaldehyde (Eastman 2408) in 100 ml of methyl Cellosolve®. Store the reagent in a ground-glass-stoppered amber bottle. Prepare fresh at least every 6 months.
3. *o*-Dinitrobenzene, 0.05*M*
   Dissolve 0.840 g of *o*-dinitrobenzene (Aldrich 12, 663-2) in 100 ml of methyl Cellosolve®. Store the reagent in a ground-glass-stoppered amber bottle. Prepare fresh at least every 6 months.
4. Sodium hydroxide, 0.05*N*
   Dissolve 2 g of sodium hydroxide pellets in 100 ml of distilled water. Store the reagent in a polyethylene-stoppered borosilicate bottle. Keep exposure to room air at a minimum. Prepare fresh every 2 weeks.
5. Cyanide stock solution, 100 mg of CN^-/100 ml
   Dissolve 0.250 g of potassium cyanide in about 50 ml of distilled water. Add 20 ml of 0.5*N* sodium hydroxide. Dilute the mixture to 100 ml with distilled water. Store the solution in a screw-capped polyethylene container. Prepare fresh at least every 3 months.
6. Cyanide reference solution, 0.05 mg of CN^-/100 ml
   Dilute 0.5 ml of the cyanide stock solution to one liter with distilled water. Prepare fresh just prior to use.

PROCEDURE[1,2]

1. To a clean, dry 10 × 75 mm borosilicate test tube, add successively 0.5 ml of 0.05*M* *p*-nitrobenzaldehyde in methyl Cellosolve®, 0.1 ml of specimen (whole blood, plasma, serum, cerebrospinal fluid, urine, bile, gastric content, or solid tissue fluidized prior to the analysis by homogenizing 1 part tissue with 2 parts water), and 0.5 mg of 0.005*M* *o*-dinitrobenzene in methyl Cellosolve®. Add the same reagents to two other tubes, one containing a 0.1-ml aliquot of the reference solution and the other 0.1 ml of water.
2. Agitate each mixture for 30 sec by flicking the container with either a finger or a vibrator.
3. Centrifuge the tubes for 3 min at 3,000 rpm.
4. Transfer 0.5 ml of each supernatant to a clean, dry 10 × 75 mm test tube. Add 0.05 ml of 0.5*N* sodium hydroxide. Mix by shaking.
5. Observe the samples for about 1 min for development of a violet color, then place the tubes in the dark for 15 min and observe them again.

INTERPRETATION (see p. 7)

The development of a violet color within the first minute of observation indicates the presence of a potentially acutely toxic concentration of cyanide. The origin of such cyanide concentrations may be from cyanide salts and complexes, hydrocyanic acid inhalation[3] (e.g., from combustion fumes of plastics), or from biotransformation of nitriles or thiocyanates. Blood stored at 5°C can develop significant concentrations of cyanide within 24 hr, especially if it is contaminated with pyocyaneous organisms.[4]

ACCURACY AND PRECISION

The minimum concentration that can be detected by this procedure is approximately 0.03 mg of cyanide ion/100 ml of blood. In symptomatic cyanide intoxications, concentrations are usually well in excess of 0.07 mg of cyanide/100 ml of blood.

INTERFERING SUBSTANCES

Up to 0.5*M* F^-, Br^-, Cl^-, $BO_3^=$, SCN^-, OCN^-, $CO_3^=$, $SO_4^=$, $SO_3^=$, $PO_4^=$, NO_3^-, citrate, tartrate, and acetate do not interfere. Nitrite and sulfide at 0.5*M* concentrations result in rapid browning of the solution; below 0.1*M*, this is not the case.

REFERENCES

1. **Rieders, F. and Garcia, C. A.,** A rapid specific, sensitive screening test for cyanide in biologic materials, *Acta Pharmacol. Toxicol. Scand.*, in press.
2. **Guilbault, G. G. and Kramer, D. N.,** Ultra sensitive, specific method for cyanide using *p*-nitrobenzaldehyde and *o*-dinitrobenzene, *Anal. Chem.*, 38, 834, 1966.
3. **Wetherell, H. R.,** The occurrence of cyanide in the blood of fire victims, *J. Forensic Sci.*, 11, 167, 1966.
4. **Sunshine, I. and Finkle, B.,** The necessity for tissue studies in fatal cyanide poisonings, *Int. Arch. Arbeitsmed.*, 20, 588, 1964.

TYPE B PROCEDURE

Fredric Rieders

APPARATUS

1. Conway microdiffusion dishes, porcelain, with glass cover (A. H. Thomas Co., Cat. No. 4472-F), 68-mm diameter
2. Spectrophotometer or photoelectric colorimeter
3. Interval timer

REAGENTS

All chemicals should be analytical reagent grade.

1. Silicone lubricant (Dow Corning Silicone A)
2. Sodium hydroxide, 0.1*N*
   Dissolve 4 g of sodium hydroxide pellets in distilled water and dilute to one liter with water. Store the reagent in a polyethylene-stoppered borosilicate bottle. Keep exposure to room air at a minimum. Prepare fresh every 2 weeks.
3. Cyanide stock solution, 100 mg of CN^-/100 ml
   Dissolve 0.250 g of potassium cyanide in about 50 ml with distilled water. Add 2.0 ml of 0.5*N* sodium hydroxide. Dilute the mixture to 100 ml with distilled water. Store the solution in a screw-capped polyethylene container. Prepare fresh at least every 3 months.
4. Cyanide internal control solution, 10 μg of CN^-/ml (high)
   Dilute 1.0 ml of the cyanide stock solution to 100 ml with distilled water. Prepare fresh just prior to use.
5. Cyanide internal control solution, 2 μg of CN^-/ml (low)
   Dilute 2.0 ml of the cyanide stock solution to one liter with distilled water. Prepare fresh just before use.
6. Sulfuric acid, 3.6*N*
   Dilute 10 ml of concentrated sulfuric acid to 100 ml with water.
7. Sodium phosphate, monobasic, 1*M* (13.8 g/100 ml)
   Dissolve 13.8 g of $NaH_2PO_4 \cdot H_2O$ in water and dilute to 100 ml with water.
8. Chloramine-T, 0.25 g/100 ml

Dissolve 0.25 g of chloramine-T in water and dilute to 100 ml with water. Store at 4°C.

9. Color reagent
   Put 3.0 g of barbituric acid, 15 ml of pyridine, and 3.0 ml of 12*N* HCl in a 25-ml volumetric flask. Mix until dissolved. Dilute to volume with H_2O, and filter. Must be prepared fresh each day.

PROCEDURE

Simultaneously analyze all samples (blood, urine, water as a reagent blank, and both control reference solutions).

1. Lightly coat the rim of each Conway cell with the silicone lubricant. To the inner compartment of each Conway cell add 0.5 ml of 0.1*N* NaOH (absorbing solution).
2. To the outer compartment of each Conway cell add 0.5 ml of 3*N* sulfuric acid (liberating solution).
3. Place the glass covers on each Conway cell so that there is an opening to the outer chamber through which addition of samples and controls may be made to the outer compartment.
4. To the outer chamber add, without mixing, 0.5 ml of sample.
5. Seal the cells by sliding the cover over the exposed outer chamber and gently tip and rotate cells to mix the contents, being careful not to mix the contents of the outer and inner chambers.
6. Allow the samples to diffuse for 2 hr at room temperature. (Diffusion time can be decreased by increasing temperature.)
7. After 2 hr transfer 0.10 ml of the contents of the inner chamber of each cell to a 5-ml labeled test tube.
8. To each tube add 1 ml of 1*M* NaH_2PO_4 and 0.5 ml of chloramine-T solution.
9. Mix and let stand for 2 to 3 min.
10. Add 1.5 ml of the color reagent, mix, and let stand for 10 min. The development of a red color indicates cyanide ions are present.
11. Determine the absorbance of each solution at 580 nm, placing the solution obtained by processing the water in the reference cuvette.

CALCULATION

Calculate the cyanide concentration:

$$C_X = A_X \times \frac{10}{A_H}$$

where

C_X = cyanide concentration of the specimen;
A_X = absorbance of the specimen;
A_H = absorbance of the high internal control solution at 580 nm (if the absorbance of low internal control solution is used, use 2.0 instead of 10).

INTERPRETATION (see p. 7)

Normal cyanide content of fresh blood, as determined by the above method, is less than 10 μg of CN^-/100 ml. Following the ingestion of ionizable cyanides, signs of acute toxicity are associated with blood concentrations above 50 μg of CN^-/100 ml. Acute fatalities usually contain more than 100 μg of CN^-/100 ml. Tissue cyanide concentrations, with the possible exception of spleen, are often slightly lower than that of blood, while cyanide in the urine is often below several micrograms per milliliter. Inhalation of hydrocyanic acid results in signs and symptoms of acute toxicity at blood concentrations at or above 20 μg of CN^-/100 ml. Blood concentrations in fatal cases may be below 100 μg of CN^-/100 ml. In clinical poisonings by ionizable cyanides in which the patient has survived the acute episode, the cyanide concentration in the blood declines rapidly due to detoxication. Following the absorption of such cyanogens as aliphatic nitriles, nitrile glucosides, or large doses of thiocyanate, prolonged elevated cyanide concentrations in the blood are associated with varying degrees of toxic signs.

REFERENCES

Feldstein, M. and Klendshoj, N. D., The determination of volatile substances by microdiffusion analysis, *J. Forensic Sci.*, 2(1), 30, 1957.

Guatelli, M. A., The toxicity of cyanides, in *Methods of Forensic Science*, Curry, A., Ed., Interscience, N.Y., 1964, 322.

Sunshine, I. and Finkle, B., The necessity for tissue studies in fatal cyanide poisonings, *Int. Arch. Arbeitsmed.*, 20, 588, 1964.

Wawschinek, O., Paletta, H., and Beyer, W., Identification of cyanide in biological material, *Arch. Toxikol.*, 23, 52, 1968.

TYPE C PROCEDURE

James C. Valentour

APPARATUS

1. Microdiffusion cells (Scientific Products, Cat. #D1815-1)
2. Screw-capped culture tubes, 13 × 100 mm (Scientific Products, Cat. #T1346-1)
3. Ice bath
4. Gas chromatograph (Hewlett-Packard Model 5713) equipped with a ^{63}Ni pulsed linearized electron-capture detector, a 6′ × ¼″ o.d. stainless steel column, packed with 7% Halcomid M-18 on Anakrom ABS, 90 to 110 mesh, and a suitable 1 mV recorder

   Operating Conditions

   Gas Flow Rate:
      5% methane in argon (carrier gas) – 35 ml/min
   Temperatures:
      oven – 55°C
      detector – 200°C

REAGENTS

All chemicals should be analytical reagent grade unless stated otherwise.

1. Cyanide stock solution, 100 mg of cyanide ion/dl
   Dissolve 250 mg of potassium cyanide in distilled water, add a trace of alkali, and dilute to 100 ml with distilled water.
2. Cyanide ion reference solutions, 10.0, 1.00, and 0.100 mg/dl
   Dilute 10.0, 1.00, and 0.10 ml of the stock solution to 100 ml, respectively, with water.
3. Sodium hydroxide, 0.1*N*
   Dissolve 4 g of sodium hydroxide in water and dilute to one liter.
4. Sodium dihydrogen phosphate, 1*M*
   Dissolve 138 g of sodium dihydrogen phosphate monohydrate in water and dilute to one liter.
5. Chloramine-T solution, 250 mg/100 ml
   Dissolve 250 mg chloramine-T (sodium *p*-toluene sulfonchloramide) in water and dilute to 100 ml. When kept at 4°C this solution is stable for at least 2 weeks.
6. Sulfuric acid, 3.6*N*
   Cautiously add 100 ml of concentrated sulfuric acid to water and dilute to one liter.
7. Acidified microdiffusion cell sealant
   Add several drops of 3.6*N* sulfuric acid to several grams Ucon® 2000 sealant, (Union Carbide) and mix thoroughly.
8. *n*-Hexane, spectrograde

PROCEDURE

1. Soak all glassware to be used in 3.6*N* sulfuric acid for ½ hr or more, rinse with water, and dry.
2. To each outer reservoir of a series of microdiffusion cells, add 3.0 ml of the samples (cyanide reference solutions, blood, urine, or other specimens to be analyzed).
3. To each inner reservoir of the microdiffusion cells, add 3.0 ml of 0.1*N* sodium hydroxide.
4. Spread the acidified sealant on each microdiffusion cell cover in a ring equal in diameter to that of the outer rim of the Conway cell.
5. Add 1.0 ml of 3.6*N* sulfuric acid to each outer reservoir of the microdiffusion cells, cover, and seal each cell immediately after the addition of the acid by placing a sealant ringed lid over the cell.
6. After allowing the microdiffusion cells to stand overnight, remove the cell covers and transfer 1.00 ml of sodium hydroxide from each inner reservoir to a screw-capped culture tube. Place the culture tubes in an ice bath.
7. To one tube add 2.00 ml of *n*-hexane, 2.0 ml of 1.0*M* sodium dihydrogen phosphate, and 1.0 ml of chloramine-T solution. Cap the tube, shake the mixture briefly, and replace it in the ice bath. After approximately 5 min, shake the tube thoroughly and again replace it in the ice bath.
8. After the hexane (top) layer has separated, inject 1 to 3 μl into the gas chromatograph (Figure 1).
9. Process the sodium hydroxide solution from

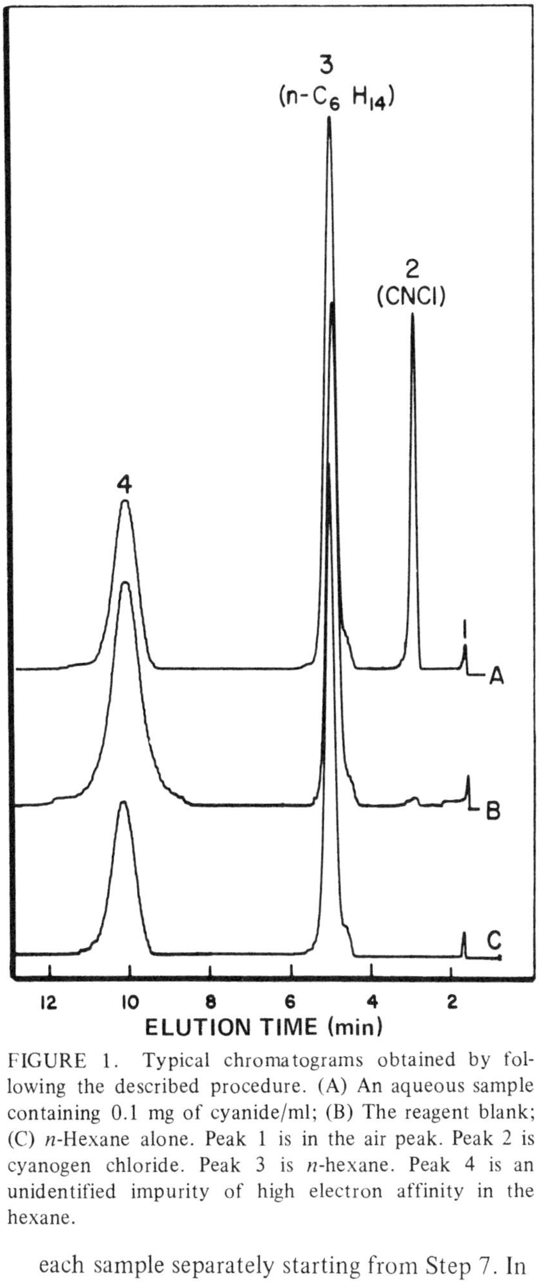

FIGURE 1. Typical chromatograms obtained by following the described procedure. (A) An aqueous sample containing 0.1 mg of cyanide/ml; (B) The reagent blank; (C) *n*-Hexane alone. Peak 1 is in the air peak. Peak 2 is cyanogen chloride. Peak 3 is *n*-hexane. Peak 4 is an unidentified impurity of high electron affinity in the hexane.

each sample separately starting from Step 7. In order to minimize loss of the volatile product, cyanogen chloride, begin Step 7 for each subsequent sample after injecting an aliquot of the preceding sample.

CALCULATION

1. Measure the peak heights or peak areas of cyanogen chloride and *n*-hexane.
2. Calculate the response ratios:

$$\frac{\text{cyanogen chloride response}}{\text{n-hexane response}} = R$$

3. Calculate the concentrations of cyanide in the specimens by following formula:

$$C_S = \frac{R_S}{R_r} \times C_r,$$

where

C_r = concentration of cyanide ion in the reference solution;
C_S = concentration of cyanide ion in the specimen;
R_s = response ratio of the specimen;
R_r = response ratio of the reference solution.

INTERPRETATION (see p. 7)

Normal cyanide content of fresh blood, as determined by the above method, is less than 10 μg of CN^-/100 ml. Following the ingestion of ionizable cyanides, signs of acute toxicity are associated with blood concentrations above 50 μg of CN^-/100 ml. Acute fatalities usually contain more than 100 μg of CN^-/100 ml. Tissue cyanide concentrations, with the possible exception of spleen, are often slightly lower than that of blood, while cyanide in the urine is often below several micrograms per milliliter. Inhalation of hydrocyanic acid results in signs and symptoms of acute toxicity at blood concentrations at or above 20 μg of CN^-/100 ml. Blood concentrations in fatal cases may be below 100 μg of CN^-/100 ml. In clinical poisonings by ionizable cyanides in which the patient has survived the acute episode, the cyanide concentration in the blood declines rapidly due to detoxication. Following the absorption of such cyanogens as aliphatic nitriles, nitrile glucosides, or large doses of thiocyanate, prolonged elevated cyanide concentrations in the blood are associated with varying degrees of toxic signs.

PRECISION

The relationship between cyanide concentration and response ratios (cyanogen chloride vs *n*-hexane) is linear between 0.025 μg/ml (minimal detectable amount) and 100 μg/ml. The coefficient of variation for replicate analyses is 2.5%.

INTERFERING SUBSTANCES

Thiocyanate yields a peak coincident to that resulting from cyanide. When taken through the entire procedure, the thiocyanate response is 2 to 3% of that from an equal concentration of cyanide.

REFERENCES

Scoggins, N. W., UV determination of cyanide ion, *Anal. Chem.*, 4(7), 1294, 1974.

Valentour, J. C., Aggarwal, V., and Sunshine, I., Sensitive gas chromatographic determination of cyanide, *Anal. Chem.*, 46, 924, 1974.

DIAZEPAM (VALIUM®)

PRINCIPLE

Diazepam is extracted from serum into chloroform at approximately pH 6.5. The chloroform is evaporated and the dry residue is dissolved in *n*-hexane. Diazepam is extracted from the hexane with hydrochloric acid. The acid solution of diazepam has absorption maxima at 285 and 240 nm and a minimum at 265 nm. Quantitation is made by relating the absorbance difference of the sample between 240 and 265 nm to that of a serum pool containing a known amount of diazepam assayed simultaneously (Procedure B). After using *n*-butyl chloride to extract the diazepam from the biological specimen, it is reextracted into acid. The acid is made alkaline, and the diazepam is extracted into 75 μl of chloroform. An aliquot of this is analyzed by gas chromatography (Procedure C).

TYPE B PROCEDURE

Clifford B. Walberg

APPARATUS

1. Centrifuge tubes, ground-glass-stoppered, 50 and 15 ml
2. Centrifuge
3. Filter paper, Whatman # 31, 11.0 cm
4. Funnel, glass, 65 mm top diameter
5. Separatory funnels, 60 ml with linear high density polyethylene stoppers (Kimax #28160, TS 13)
6. Volumetric pipet, 4 ml
7. Heating block, 56°C
8. UV spectrophotometer, scanning, and companion recorder

REAGENTS

All chemicals should be analytical reagent grade.

1. Hydrochloric acid, 2*N* (approx)
   Dilute 16.7 ml of concentrated hydrochloric acid to 100 ml with water.
2. Diazepam stock solution, 40 mg/100 ml
   Transfer 10 mg of diazepam (Valium®) to a 25-ml volumetric flask containing just enough 2*N* hydrochloric acid to cover the bottom of the flask, then dilute to volume with distilled water. Store at 4°C.
3. Diazepam reference solution, 2 mg/100 ml
   Transfer 5.0 ml of the diazepam stock solution to a 100-ml volumetric flask and dilute it to volume with pooled drug-free serum.
4. Phosphate solution, 3*M* (approx pH 3.6)
   Transfer 42.4 g of sodium dihydrogen phosphate, $NaH_2PO_4 \cdot H_2O$, to a 100-ml volumetric flask. Dilute to volume with distilled water.
5. Sodium hydroxide, 0.45*N*
   Dissolve 18 g of sodium hydroxide in water and dilute to one liter. Store the solution in a polyethylene bottle.
6. Chloroform, spectroquality MCB #CX1050 or its equivalent
   If reagent grade chloroform is used, it must be washed with dilute alkali, dilute acid, and water until all artifacts are removed.
7. Sulfuric acid, 0.5*N*
   Dilute 7.0 ml of concentrated sulfuric acid to 500 ml with distilled water.
8. *n*-Hexane, spectroquality

PROCEDURE

1. Transfer 2.0 ml of serum to a 50-ml glass-stoppered centrifuge tube. Transfer 2.0 ml of diazepam reference solution to a second centrifuge tube.
2. Add 0.1 ml of 3*M* phosphate solution.
3. Add 2 ml of spectroquality chloroform (the volume is not critical). Stopper the tubes and shake them on a mechanical shaker for 5 min.

Allow the layers to separate. (Centrifuge briefly to hasten the separation.)

4. Aspirate as much of each (aqueous) top layer as possible without removing any of the chloroform layer. Decant each chloroform layer through Whatman # 31 filter paper into a 60-ml separatory funnel. (Make sure that the chloroform saturates the filter paper first; if any residual aqueous phase touches the paper first, filtration will be prolonged.)
5. Add 4.0 ml of 0.45*N* sodium hydroxide to each filtrate.
6. Shake the chloroform-sodium hydroxide mixture for 3 to 4 min. Allow the layers to separate.
7. Drain the chloroform layer through Whatman #31 filter paper into a 15-ml graduate centrifuge tube with glass stopper. The sodium hydroxide fraction may be saved for a barbiturate determination if required. If the presence of Librium® is suspected, the chloroform fraction should be extracted with 4.0 ml of 0.5*N* sulfuric acid. Save the acid solution for the analysis of Librium®.
8. Evaporate each chloroform filtrate (Step 7) to dryness in a 56°C heating block.
9. Dissolve each residue in 5.0 ml of *n*-hexane. The addition of *n*-hexane prior to extraction with hydrochloric acid (Step 10) prevents turbidity, which occurs if the residue is dissolved directly in acid. The turbidity may be due to lipids, which are insoluble in acid.
10. Add 4.0 ml of 2*N* hydrochloric acid to each of the *N*-hexane solutions. Stopper the tubes, shake them for less than 30 sec, then centrifuge briefly to hasten separation.
11. Remove the hexane layers by aspiration. Transfer at least 3 ml of each aqueous fraction to a silica cuvette.
12. Determine the absorbances of the aqueous fractions from 320 to 220 nm (Figure 1). Use 2*N* hydrochloric acid as the reference solution. (It is not necessary to extract this hydrochloric acid with hexane.)

CALCULATION

Determine the diazepam concentration (mg/100 ml) in the sample (C_S) by the following formula:

$$C_S = \frac{(A_{240\,nm} - A_{265\,nm})\ \text{sample}}{(A_{240\,nm} - A_{265\,nm})\ \text{reference}} \times 2$$

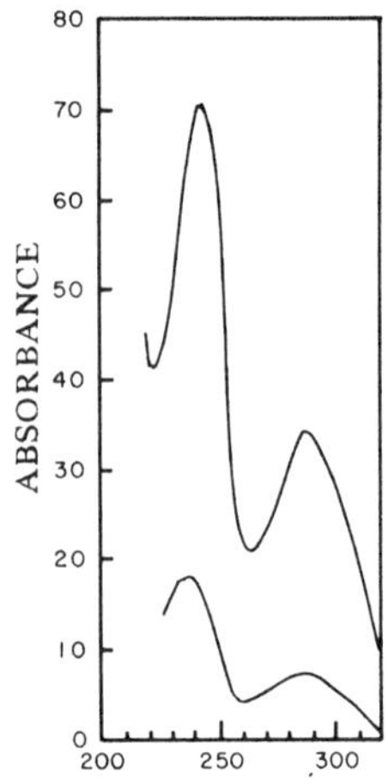

FIGURE 1. UV absorbance of diazepam from 320 to 220 nm.

Typical Calculation

$$\frac{0.189 - 0.035}{0.700 - 0.207} \times 2 =$$

0.6 mg/100 ml

$(A_{240\,m} - A_{265\,m})$ reference = 0.700 − 0.207

$(A_{240\,nm} - A_{265\,nm})$ sample = 0.189 × 0.035

Note: The wavelengths given are the maximum at 240 nm and the minimum at 265 nm. Diazepam concentration lower than 0.3 mg/100 ml may be difficult to determine with this procedure. Should such low concentrations be expected, another procedure may be preferable.

INTERPRETATION (see p. 7)

Blood concentrations of up to 0.20 mg/100 ml may be expected following a maximum therapeutic dosage of 40 mg of diazepam/day. The usual finding, however, is 0.02 to 0.05 mg/100 ml after single dosages of 5 or 10 mg. Peak concentrations are obtained within 1 hr of oral administration and the half-life is 2 to 3 hr. It is excreted exclusively in metabolized form, predominantly as oxazepam glucuronide. Serax® (oxazepam) is a metabolic product of Valium®. No measurable amounts of intact Valium® are excreted in urine. Serum concentrations of 1 mg/100 ml are compatible with coma.

INTERFERING SUBSTANCES

Other bendiazepines or their metabolites may interfere. Extraction of Dalmane® or Serax® added to serum produces similar curves with this method, but the absorbance difference between 240 and 265 nm is less than that of Valium®. At a drug concentration of 2 mg/100 ml serum, the absorbance difference for Dalmane® is approximately 0.220 and that for Serax® is approximately 0.315.

REFERENCES*

deSilva, J. A. F. and Puglisi, C. V., Determination of medazepam (Nobrium), diazepam (Valium) and their major biotransformation products in blood and urine by electron-capture gas-liquid chromatography, *Anal. Chem.*, 42, 1725, 1970.

Roche Laboratories Product Reference Manual, Roche Laboratories, Nutley, N.J., 1970, 177.

TYPE C PROCEDURE

James C. Garriatt

APPARATUS

1. Centrifuge tubes, glass-stoppered with conical tips, 15 and 5 ml
2. Centrifuge
3. Pasteur pipets
4. Syringes, 100 μl (Hamilton Microliter #710), 10 μl, (Hamilton Microliter #701)
5. Vortex mixer
6. A gas-liquid chromatograph equipped with a flame ionization detector, linear temperature programmer, recorder and 2 coiled glass columns, 6′ × 2 mm i.d., one packed with 3% OV-1 on 80 to 100 mesh Chromosorb W, A/W DMCS, the other packed with 3% OV-17 on 80 to 100 mesh Chromosorb W, A/W DMSC

Operating Conditions

Gas Flow Rates:
- nitrogen (carrier gas) – 30 ml/min
- hydrogen – 30 ml/min
- air – 240 ml/min

Temperatures:
- column – programmed at 8°C/min from 190 to 270°C; initial temperature held for 2 min and final temperature held for 8 min
- injection part – 200°C
- detector – 300°C

REAGENTS

All chemicals should be analytical reagent grade,

1. *n*-Butyl chloride [Eastman (Cat. #52) 1-chlorobutane]
   Redistill before using.
2. Concentrated ammonium hydroxide
3. Hydrochloric acid, 1.0*N*
   Dilute 8.0 ml of concentrated hydrochloric acid to 100 ml with water.
4. Chloroform (Matheson Coleman Bell), reagent grade
5. Diazepam (Hoffmann-LaRoche, Inc.)
6. Diazepam stock solution, 1 mg/ml
   Transfer 25 mg of diazepam to a 25-ml volumetric flask and dilute to volume with absolute ethanol. Place the solution in a screw-top test tube and store away from light. Ethanol solutions have been found to be more stable than those in weak hydrochloric acid and were stable at room temperature for 3 months.

PROCEDURE

1. Transfer 5 ml of sample (whole blood, serum, plasma, or tissue homogenate) to a 15-ml glass-stoppered centrifuge tube. Transfer 5 μl of diazepam stock solution to a second centrifuge tube, using a 10-μl syringe, and add 5 ml water. (Extraction from blood and aqueous solutions has been shown to be equally complete.) Additional standards equivalent to therapeutic concentrations of 0.02 mg/100 ml and 0.05 mg/100 ml can be prepared by adding 1.0 and 2.5 μl of the reference solution to 5 ml of water.
2. To each tube add 0.1 ml of concentrated ammonium hydroxide.
3. To each tube add 5 ml of *n*-butyl chloride. Stopper the tubes and extract by gentle inversion for 3 to 5 min. Centrifuge at 2,000 rpm for 3 min to achieve separation of phases.
4. With a Pasteur pipet, remove the entire upper *n*-butyl chloride layer from each tube and place it into clean 15-ml centrifuge tubes.

*For an updated list of reference material, see References, p. 123.

5. Repeat Steps 3 and 4 with 5-ml aliquots of *n*-butyl chloride and add these extracts to their respective counterparts from the first extractions.
6. To each of the combined *n*-butyl chloride extracts, add 5 ml of 1.0*N* hydrochloric acid. Stopper the tubes and mix by inversion or on the vortex mixer. Centrifuge for 3 min to achieve separation of the aqueous and organic phases.
7. Aspirate and discard the top *n*-butyl chloride layers.
8. Pass clean air through the hydrochloric acid solution in each tube for 1 min to remove any remaining *n*-butyl chloride. (Failure to remove all of the *n*-butyl chloride will introduce error as a result of increase in the apparent volume of chloroform in the final extract.)
9. With a volumetric pipet, transfer 4.0 ml of the 1.0*N* hydrochloric acid in each tube to 5-ml conical centrifuge tubes.
10. To each tube add 0.8 ml of concentrated ammonium hydroxide and mix by inversion.
11. Using a 100-μl syringe, add 75 μl of chloroform to each tube and mix with a vortex mixer.
12. Centrifuge at 2,000 rpm for 5 min and, with a Pasteur pipet or vacuum aspirator, remove all but about 0.1 ml of the upper aqueous layer from the chloroform in the tip of each of the centrifuge tubes. (A small volume of aqueous fluid over the chloroform prevents evaporation.)
13. Inject 4 μl of the chloroform extract sequentially into the gas chromatograph with a 10-μl syringe. On the OV-1 column, diazepam has a retention time of 9.4 min and the demethylated metabolite a retention time of 10.2 min.
14. Measure the peak heights of diazepam.

CALCULATION

The peak height is directly proportional to the concentration of the drug in blood or serum over the range from 0 to 1.0 mg/100 ml. Use the following formula:

$$C_S = C_R \times \frac{P_S}{P_R},$$

where

C_S = concentration of diazepam in sample;
C_R = concentration of diazepam in reference standard;
P_S = peak height of diazepam (sample);
P_R = peak height of diazepam (reference standard).

INTERPRETATION (see p. 7)

Blood concentrations of up to 0.20 mg/100 ml may be expected following a maximum therapeutic dosage of 40 mg of diazepam/day. The usual finding, however, is 0.02 to 0.05 mg/100 ml after single dosages of 5 or 10 mg. Peak concentrations are obtained within 1 hr of oral administration and the half-life is 2 to 3 hr. It is excreted exclusively in a metabolized form, predominantly as oxazepam glucuronide. Serax®, oxazepam, is a metabolic product of Valium®. No measurable amounts of intact Valium® are excreted in urine. Serum concentrations of 1 mg/100 ml are compatible with coma.

PRECISION AND SENSITIVITY

Peak height is proportional to concentration over the range from 0 to 1.0 mg/ 100 ml. Mean recovery of diazepam added to blood (or to aqueous solution) over this range is 66% ± 8%. In 11 duplicate analyses of concentrations of reference standard corresponding to blood concentrations of 0.05 to 0.30 mg/100 ml, the variability of the peak heights did not exceed ± 6.1%. The average variability was 2%. Samples with diazepam concentrations of 0.02 to 0.05 mg/100 ml give peaks easily matched with those of extracted diazepam standards prepared by using as little as 1.0 or 2.5 μl of the reference solution in 5 ml water. Thus, blood concentrations associated with therapeutic dosage can be detected as well as concentrations resulting from overdose. The detection limit is approximately 0.01 mg/100 ml.

INTERFERING SUBSTANCES

This procedure extracts many other drugs with basic properties, some of which may have reten-

Table 1

RETENTION TIMES OF SOME DRUGS ENCOUNTERED WITH *n*-BUTYL CHLORIDE EXTRACTION

	3% OV-1 Column (min)	3% OV-17 Column (min)
Methadone metabolite	5.3	8.2
Propoxyphene metabolite	6.3	–
Methadone	6.6	9.4
Methaqualone	6.6	11.0
Propoxyphene	7.0	9.8
Oxazepam	8.4	12.9
Propoxyphene metabolites	8.8	12.9
(doublet)	9.0	
Methaqualone metabolite	9.0	14.6
Diazepam	9.4	14.5
Demethyldiazepam (Roche #2180)	10.2	16.5
Propoxyphene metabolite	10.4	15.6
Flurazepam	12.3	19.9

tion times similar to those of diazepam and its demethylated metabolite (Table 1). On the OV-1 column, for example, diazepam is not separated from metabolites of propoxyphene. On the OV-17 column, however, the retention times are sufficiently different to allow positive identification and quantitation of diazepam. The use of two GC columns is recommended in order to establish a higher probability of identification.

REFERENCES

deSilva, J. A., Koechlin, B. A., and Bader, G., Blood level distribution patterns of diazepam and its major metabolite in man, *J. Pharmacol. Sci.,* 85, 692, 1966.

Foerster, E. and Mason, M. F., Preliminary studies on the use of *n*-butyl chloride as an extract in a drug screening procedure, *J. Forensic Sci.,* 19, 155, 1974.

Greaves, M. S., Quantitative determination of medazepam, diazepam, and nitrazepam in whole blood by TLD GC, *Clin. Chem.,* 20, 141, 1974.

Hellestad, L., et al., Diazepam metabolism in man, *Clin. Pharmacol. Ther.,* 15, 479, 1974.

Kaplan, S. A., Jack, M. L., Alexander, K., and Weinfeld, R. E., Pharmacokinetic profile of diazepam in man following single intravenous and oral and chronic oral administrations, *J. Pharm. Sci.,* 62, 1789, 1973.

Zingales, I. A., Diazepam metabolism during chronic medication; unbound fraction in plasma, erythrocytes, and urine, *J. Chromatogr.,* 75, 55, 1973.

DIGITOXIN

PRINCIPLE

Digitoxin, a cardiac glycoside, is measured by radioimmunoassay. In this method the glycoside present in the patient's serum competes with a fixed amount of radioactive derivative of the drug for binding sites on an exact amount of antiserum. Subsequently, any of the drug remaining unbound by the antibody (both the endogenous and the radioactive) is adsorbed on charcoal and can be separated from the bound form by centrifugation. The bound glycoside, which remains in the supernatant, is then counted in a scintillation spectrometer. Calculations are made with reference to a calibration curve made from appropriate standards.

TYPE A PROCEDURE

Louis A. Williams and Joseph S. Annino

APPARATUS

1. Plastic test tubes, 12 × 75 mm
2. Ice bath
3. Centrifuge
4. Liquid scintillation radiation counter
5. Vials for liquid scintillation counter

REAGENTS*

All chemicals should be analytical reagent grade.

1. Stock standard, 1 mg/ml
   Dissolve 25 mg of digitoxin in 95% ethanol and dilute to 25 ml with 95% ethanol; if necessary, warm to effect solution. Stable indefinitely if stored in tightly sealed containers at −20°C.
2. Intermediate standard, 10 μg/ml
   Dilute 1 ml of digitoxin stock standard to 100 ml with 95% ethanol. Stable for 6 months if stored at −20°C.
3. Dilute standard, 50 μg/l (S_6)
   Dilute 100 μl of intermediate standard to 20 ml with bovine serum.
4. Working standards
   Make dilutions of the dilute standard with bovine serum according to the following table (stable for 1 week if stored at 4°C):

Working standard	Dilute standard (ml)	Bovine serum (ml)	Concentration (μg/l)
S5	9	6	3
S4	6	9	1.5
S3	4.5	10.5	1.5
S2	3	12	1.0
S1	1.5	13.5	0.5
S1	0	15	0

5. Barbital buffer, pH 7.4
   Dissolve 2.94 g of sodium barbital, 1.94 g of sodium chloride in 1,900 ml of deionized sodium chloride in 1900 ml of deionized water. Check pH and adjust to 7.4 ± 0.05 with 0.1*N* hydrochloric acid or 0.1*N* sodium hydroxide. Dilute to 2,000 ml with deionized water and store at 4°C. Stable for 1 month.
6. Tritiated digitoxin
   Dilute ^{3}H-digitoxin[†] to 100 ng/ml with 95% ethanol. Store at 4°C.
7. Dextran-coated charcoal
   Dissolve 1.0 g of dextran-70 in 200 ml of barbital buffer. Suspend 10 g of Norit® A charcoal in 200 ml of barbital buffer. Mix these 2 solutions together, stir for 5 min, then store at 4°C. Stable for 1 month.
8. Antiserum
   Add 10 mg of bovine albumin (Fraction V) to a vial of digitoxin antiserum,[‡] followed by 30 ml of barbital buffer; swirl until dissolved. If stored at 4°C, it is stable for 1 month.
9. Stannous chloride solution, 40 g/l

*Although suppliers are indicated for certain materials, other sources may be suitable.

†New England Nuclear, Boston, Mass.

‡Wien Laboratories, Succasunna, N.J.

Dissolve 8 g of stannous chloride dihydrate ($SnCl_2 \cdot 2H_2O$) in a small amount of 1*N* hydrochloric acid and dilute to 200 ml with the 1*N* hydrochloric acid.

10. Counting solution
To 3,000 ml of toluene add 125 ml of Liquifluor®,* cap, and mix well. Add 600 ml of Scintisol-GP,† cap, and mix well. Store in a dark bottle.
11. Bovine serum

PROCEDURE

Perform duplicate analyses on all samples. Sera showing visible hemolysis or bilirubin require quench correction. Because of the possibility of changes with the time of contact with the charcoal, no more than 40 samples should be analyzed at one time.

1. To 12 × 75 mm plastic tubes, add 0.2 ml of sample (test sera and each of the working standards). For samples requiring quench correction (QC), measure 0.2 ml of serum and 0.8 ml of buffer directly into counting vials.
2. Add 0.2 ml of bovine serum and 0.8 ml of buffer directly into two counting vials for total count (TC).
3. To all tubes (including QC and TC vials) add 50 μl of ^{3}H-digitoxin solution, mix each tube well, and allow them to stand 5 min. Place QC and TC vials aside until step 9.
4. To all tubes add 300 μl of digitoxin antiserum (Reagent 7). Mix well and allow to stand for 15 min.
5. Place all tubes in an ice bath for 5 min.
6. Resuspend the cold dextran-coated charcoal suspension by use of a magnetic stirrer.
7. Using an automatic pipettor with a plastic tip, add 0.5 ml of the mixed charcoal suspension to all tubes. Mix each tube well.
8. Centrifuge for 10 min at full speed.
9. While centrifugation is taking place, add 0.2 ml of stannous chloride solution to counting vials, including QC and TC.
10. After centrifugation, *immediately* decant each supernatant solution into properly labeled counting vials and mix well.
11. Add 15 ml of the counting solution to each vial, including the QC and TC vials.
12. Cap, mix well, and allow to stand for 10 min in the dark.
13. Count the radiation in a liquid scintillation counter set at 1% error and a 5 min maximum counting time.

CALCULATION

1. Plot the count rate of the working standards (ordinate) against their respective concentrations in μg/l (abscissa) on semilog graph paper.
2. Determine the concentrations of the test sera from their count rate readings using the standard curve.
3. For samples requiring quench corrections, correct the counts as follows before calculating:

$$\frac{\text{cpm of TC}}{\text{cpm of QC}} \times \text{cpm of test} = \text{corrected sample cpm}$$

Note: Calculate percent binding as follows:

$$\frac{\text{SO}}{\text{TC}} \times 100 = \%\ \text{binding}$$

where

SO = the counts per minute for the zero working standard
TC = the total counts per minute.

The percent binding may vary with different lots of antiserum, but a level of at least 40% should be obtained for adequate sensitivity. This may require experimental adjustment of the antiserum dilution.

INTERPRETATION (see p. 7)

Digitoxin is a cardiotonic secondary glycoside derived from the leaves of several suitable species of digitalis. Since it does not occur naturally in the

*New England Nuclear, Boston, Mass.
†Isolab, Inc., Akron, Ohio

body, its concentration (measured in serum or plasma) is used to confirm toxicity or as a guide in the establishment of therapeutic levels. As with most drugs, there is some overlap of the toxic level with the optimal range for therapy. The generally accepted therapeutic range for digitoxin in serum is 14 to 30 μg/l (ng/ml). Concentrations above 30 μg/l (ng/ml) are considered potentially toxic.

A certain amount of cross-reactivity is displayed by the antibodies currently available for use in tests. Some manufacturers, in fact, use the same antibody for both digitoxin and digoxin. The therapeutic range for digitoxin is approximately ten times that of the optimal concentration of digoxin; therefore, it is possible to obtain positive results using the digoxin method when the drug in the sample is, in fact, digitoxin. Since the names of the drugs are so similar, it is extremely important that the physician and the nursing staff clearly and accurately identify the drug that the patient is receiving in order that the appropriate methodology can be used.

REFERENCES

Beller, G. A., Smith, T. W., Abelman, W. H., Haber, E., and Hood, W. B., Jr., Digitalis intoxication: Clinical correlations with serum levels, *N. Engl. J. Med.*, 284, 989, 1971.

Bentley, J. D., Burnett, G. H., and Conklin, R. L., et al., Clinical application of serum digitoxin levels – a simplified plasma determination, *Circulation*, 41, 67, 1970.

Butler, V. P., Jr., Digoxin: Immunologic approaches to measurement and reversal of toxicity, *N. Engl. J. Med.*, 283, 1150, 1970.

Cerceo, E. and Elloso, C. A., Factors affecting the radioimmunoassay of digoxin, *Clin. Chem.*, 18, 539, 1972.

Hayes, A. H., Jr., Pharmacodynamic and pharmacokinetic measurements in cardiovascular-renal drugs, *Clin. Pharmacol. Ther.*, 16, 201, 1974.

Park, H. M., et al., Clinical evaluation of radioimmunoassay digoxin, *J. Nucl. Med.*, 14, 531, 1973.

Smith, T. W., Radioimmunoassay for serum digitoxin concentration: Methodology and clinical experience, *J. Pharmacol. Exp. Ther.*, 175, 352, 1970.

Smith, T. W., Butler, V. P., and Haber, E., Determination of therapeutic and toxic serum digoxin concentrations by radioimmunoassay, *N. Engl. J. Med.*, 281, 1212, 1969.

DIGOXIN

PRINCIPLE

Digoxin, a cardiac glycoside, is measured by radioimmunoassay. In this method the glycoside present in the patient's serum competes with a fixed amount of a radioactive derivative of the drug for binding sites on an exact amount of antiserum. Subsequently, any of the drug remaining unbound by the antibody (both the endogenous and the radioactive) is adsorbed on charcoal and can be separated from the bound form by centrifugation. The latter, which remains in the supernatant, is then counted in a scintillation spectrometer. Calculations are made with reference to a calibration curve made from appropriate standards.

TYPE A PROCEDURE

Louis A. Williams and Joseph S. Annino

APPARATUS

1. Plastic test tubes, 12 X 75 mm
2. Centrifuge
3. Liquid scintillation radiation counter
4. Vials for liquid scintillation counter

REAGENTS*

All chemicals should be analytical reagent grade.

1. Stock standard, 1 mg/ml
   Dissolve 25 mg of digoxin in 95% ethanol and dilute to 25 ml; if necessary, warm to effect solution. Stable indefinitely if stored at −20°C.
2. Intermediate standard, 1 μg/ml
   Dilute 0.1 ml of stock standard to 100 ml with 95% ethanol. If stored at −20°C, the solution is stable for 6 months.
3. Dilute standard, 5 μg/l
   Dilute 250 μl of intermediate standard to 50 ml with bovine serum.
4. Working standards
   Make dilutions of the dilute standard with bovine serum according to Table 1 (if stored at 4°C, solutions are stable for 1 week).

Table 1

Working standard	Dilute standard (ml)	Bovine serum (ml)	Concentration (μg/l)
S5	3	2	30
S4	2	3	20
S3	1.5	3.5	15
S2	1	4	10
S1	0.5	4.5	5
S0	0	5	0

5. Buffer, pH 7.4
   Dissolve 8.77 g of sodium chloride, 1.74 g of monobasic potassium phosphate, and 1 g of sodium azide in approximately 950 ml of water. Adjust pH to 7.4 ± 0.05 with 0.1*N* hydrochloric acid or 0.1*N* sodium hydroxide, then dilute with water to one liter. Store at 4°C.
6. Tritiated digoxin
   Dilute the tritiated digoxin (general tag)† with 50% ethanol so that 50 μl will contain 0.8 ng (16 ng/ml). Store at 4°C.
7. Dilute antiserum
   Upon receipt, aliquot 1 ml of the digoxin antiserum‡ into screw-capped tubes. Store the aliquots at −20°C. Thaw 1 ml of antiserum and dilute to 40 ml with buffer. When stored at 4°C the diluted solution is stable 1 week.
8. Charcoal suspension
   Suspend 5 g of charcoal (Norit® A) in 500 ml of pH 7.4 buffer. Using a magnetic stirrer, mix for 10 min. Store at 4°C.

*Although suppliers are indicated for certain materials, other sources may be suitable.

†New England Nuclear, Boston, Mass.

‡Antibodies, Inc., Davis, California.

9. Stannous chloride, 40 g/l
   Dissolve 8 g of stannous chloride dihydrate ($SnCl_2 \cdot 2H_2O$) in 1*N* hydrochloric acid and dilute to 200 ml with the 1*N* hydrochloric acid.
10. Counting solution
    To 3,000 ml of toluene add 125 ml of Liquifluor®,* cap, and mix well. Add 600 ml of Scintisol-GP,† cap, and mix well. Store in a dark bottle.

PROCEDURE

Perform duplicate analyses on all samples. Sera showing visible hemolysis or bilirubin require quench correction. Because of the possibility of changes with the time of contact with the charcoal, no more than 40 samples should be analyzed at one time.

1. To each of two 12 X 75 mm plastic tubes, add 0.5 ml of sera to be assayed and each of the working standards. For samples requiring quench correction (QC), add 0.5 ml of serum and 0.8 ml of buffer directly into counting vials.
2. Add 0.5 ml of bovine serum and 0.6 ml of buffer directly into each of two counting vials for total count (TC).
3. To all tubes (including QC and TC vials), add 50 μl of tritiated digoxin, mixing each tube well after addition. Put QC and TC vials aside until Step 9.
4. Add 100 μl of dilute antiserum to all tubes. Mix each tube after addition.
5. Let stand 15 min at room temperature.
6. Resuspend the charcoal by mixing with a magnetic stirrer and continue the mixing until all additions have been made. Using an automatic pipettor with a plastic tip, add 0.5 ml of the charcoal suspension to each tube. Mix each tube.
7. Let stand 15 min at room temperature.
8. Centrifuge all tubes simultaneously at full speed for 5 min.
9. While centrifugation is taking place add 0.2 ml of stannous chloride solution to the properly labeled counting vials, including QC and TC.
10. After centrifugation, *immediately* decant the supernatant into the counting vials and mix.
11. Add 12 ml of the counting solution to all vials. Cap and mix well. Add counting solution to the QC and TC vials as well.
12. Allow to stand 10 min in the dark.
13. Determine the count rate for each vial using a liquid scintillation counter set at 3% error using a maximum counting time of 5 min.

*New England Nuclear, Boston, Mass.
†Isolab, Inc., Akron, Ohio.

CALCULATION

1. Plot the count rate of the working standards (ordinate) against their respective concentrations in μg/l (abscissa) on semi-log graph paper.
2. Determine the concentrations of the test sera from their count rates using the standard curve.
3. For samples requiring quench corrections, correct the counts as follows before calculating:

$$\frac{C_T}{C_Q} \times C_R = C_{cor}$$

C_T = count rate of TC;
C_Q = count rate of QC;
C_R = count rate of test;
C_{cor} = corrected sample count rate.

Note: Calculate % binding as follows:

$$\frac{S_O}{Tc} \times 100 = \%\ \text{binding}$$

where

S_o = the counts per minute for the zero working standard;
TC = the total counts per minute.

The binding may vary with different lots of antiserum but a level of at least 40% should be obtained for adequate sensitivity. This may require experimental adjustment of the antiserum dilutions.

INTERPRETATION (see p. 7)

Digoxin is a cardiotonic, secondary glycoside derived from the leaves of several suitable species of digitalis. It is available under such trade names as Lanoxin® or Davoxin®. Since it does not occur naturally in the body, its concentration (measured in serum or plasma) is used to confirm toxicity or as a guide in the establishment of therapeutic levels. As with most drugs, there is some overlap of the toxic level with the optimal range for therapy. The therapeutic range usually specified for digoxin is 0.9 to 2.0 μg/l (ng/ml). Concentrations above 2.0 μg/l (ng/ml) should be considered potentially toxic.

A certain amount of cross-reactivity is displayed by the antibodies currently available for use in tests. Some manufacturers, in fact, use the same antibody for both digoxin and digitoxin. The therapeutic range for digitoxin is approximately 10 times that of the optimal concentration of digoxin, and therefore, it is possible to obtain positive results using the digoxin method when the drug in the sample is, in fact, digitoxin. Since the names of the drugs are so similar, it is extremely important that the physician and the nursing staff clearly and accurately identify the drug that the patient is receiving in order that the appropriate methodology can be used.

REFERENCES

Beller, G. A., Smith, T. W., Abelman, W. H., Haber, E., and Hood, W. B., Jr., Digitalis intoxication: Clinical correlations with serum levels, *N. Engl. J. Med.,* 284, 989, 1971.

Bentley, J. D., Burnett, G. H., Conklin, R. L., et al., Clinical application of serum digitoxin levels – a simplified plasma determination, *Circulation,* 41, 67, 1970.

Butler, V. P., Jr., Digoxin: Immunologic approaches to measurement and reversal of toxicity, *N. Engl. J. Med.,* 283, 1150, 1970.

Cerceo, E. and Elloso, C. A., Factors affecting the radioimmunoassay of digoxin, *Clin. Chem.,* 18, 539, 1972.

Goldman, R. H., The use of serum digoxin levels in clinical practice, *JAMA,* 229(3), 331, 1974.

Hayes, A. J., Jr., Pharmacodynamic and pharmacokinetic measurements in cardiovascular-renal drugs, *Clin. Pharmacol. Ther.,* 16, 201, 1974.

Karjalainen, J., Ojala, K., and Reissell, P., Tissue concentrations of digoxin in autopsy material, *Acta Pharmacol. Toxicol.,* 34, 385, 1974.

Park, H. M., et al., Clinical evaluation of radioimmunoassay digoxin, *J. Nucl. Med.,* 14, 531, 1973.

Smith, T. W., Radioimmunoassay for serum digitoxin concentration: Methodology and clinical experience, *J. Pharmacol. Exp. Ther.,* 175, 382, 1970.

Smith, T. W., Butler, V. P., and Haber, E., Determination of therapeutic and toxic serum digoxin concentrations by radioimmunoassay, *N. Engl. J. Med.,* 281, 1212, 1969.

DIPHENHYDRAMINE*

PRINCIPLE

Diphenhydramine is extracted into an organic solvent from an alkaline solution of the sample. It is purified by reextraction into acid which is then alkalinized and reextracted with a solvent. An aliquot of this solvent is then gas chromatographed.

TYPE B PROCEDURE

T. J. Siek

APPARATUS

1. Separatory funnels, 125 ml
2. Microliter syringe, 5 or 10 μl capacity
3. Gas chromatograph (Perkin-Elmer, Model 900), with dual column oven, dual electrometers, flame ionization detectors, 1 mV recorder, temperature programming, and two glass columns, 8′ × 2 mm i.d. and 8′ × 4 mm o.d.; Column A packed with 10% OV-1 on 80 to 100 mesh Gas Chrom Q† and Column B packed with 3% OV-17 on 100 to 120 mesh Gas Chrom Q

   Operating Conditions

   Gas Flow Rates:
   - helium (carrier gas) – 27 ml/min
   - air – approximately 400 ml/min
   - hydrogen – approximately 30 ml/min

   Temperatures:
   - oven – 240°C
   - injection port – 280°C
   - detector (manifold on Perkin-Elmer 900) – 280°C

REAGENTS

All chemicals should be analytical reagent grade unless otherwise specified.

1. Chloroform, reagent grade, further purified by distillation in a large scale all glass distillation assembly or washed with aqueous base, aqueous acid, and water prior to use
   Add about 1% absolute ethanol after distillation or washing to serve as a preservative.
2. Sulfuric acid, 1*N*
   Add 28 ml of concentrated sulfuric acid to water (caution) and dilute with water to one liter.
3. Sodium hydroxide, 1*N* and 10*N*
   For 1*N* dissolve 40 g of sodium hydroxide in water and dilute to one liter; 10*N* requires 400 g of sodium hydroxide/liter of solution.
4. Folded filter paper, S & S number 588, 12.5 cm
5. Internal standard solution, 100 μg/ml
   Dissolve 10 mg of *n*-eicosane (normal C_{20} hydrocarbon) in hexane or chloroform and dilute to 100 ml with the same solvent.
6. Diphenhydramine, 100 μg/ml
   Dissolve 11.4 mg of diphenhydramine hydrochloride in water, add a few milliliters of 1*N* sodium hydroxide, and extract quantitatively with purified chloroform. Dilute the extract to 100 ml with purified chloroform.

PROCEDURE

1. To respective 125-ml separatory funnels, add 5 ml of each specimen to be analyzed (blood or urine), 2 ml of 10*N* sodium hydroxide, and 60 ml of chloroform.

*If dimenhydrinate (Dramamine®) is suspected to be the offending agent, then one should analyze the sample for diphenhydramine and 8-chlorotheophylline, the other component of Dramamine®. This may be done by using the procedure described for theophylline (see p. 369).

†Applied Science Laboratories, Inc., State College, Pennsylvania.

2. Extract gently but thoroughly for several minutes; do not shake the funnel vigorously.
3. Place about 6 g of anhydrous sodium sulfate on a folded filter paper. Prior to filtering the chloroform extract, rinse this filter with reagent chloroform (discarding the rinse). Then filter the extract and save the filtrate. Rinse the filter with small quantities of chloroform and add this wash solution to the original filtrate.
4. Evaporate the filtrate to 10 ml on a steam bath in a fume hood, using a stream of air or nitrogen.
5. Extract the chloroform with 10 ml of 1*N* sulfuric acid.
6. To the aqueous extract add 1.5 ml of 10*N* sodium hydroxide to bring the pH of the solution to greater then 10. Cool and extract this solution twice with 5 ml of chloroform, each time, and filter the chloroform extracts, as in Step 3, through anhydrous sodium sulfate.
7. To the pooled filtrates add 1 ml of internal standard and reduce the volume to about 1 ml.
8. With the gas chromatograph fully warmed-up and stable, check the retention times of diphenhydramine and *n*-eicosane on the two columns. With a clean syringe inject 1 to 3 μl of extract (approximately 50 μl total volume) onto each column. Attenuate the signal so that a large *n*-eicosane peak is traced. If diphenhydramine is shown to be present by retention times on both columns, measure peak areas of *n*-eicosane and diphenhydramine on one of the columns. On OV-1 diphenhydramine has a retention time of 4.24 min, and *n*-eicosane, 5.58 min. On OV-17, diphenhydramine and *n*eicosane retention times are 2.04 and 1.44 min, respectively.

n-eicosane retention times are 2.04 and 1.44

CALCULATION

$$C_D = E\frac{A_D}{A_E} \times \frac{100}{R} \times \frac{100}{U_S} \times F \times \frac{1\text{ mg}}{1000\ \mu g}$$

where

C_D = mg% diphenhydramine in the specimen
E = micrograms *n*-eicosane added to the extract
A_D = area of diphenhydramine peak in specimen extract
A_E = area of *n*-eicosane peak in specimen extract
R = percent recovery of diphenhydramine (90%)
F = 1.43, a factor which corrects for the difference in response of the flame detector to *n*-eicosane and diphenhydramine
V_S = volume of specimen extracted

Following the procedure above, the calculation reduces to:

$$C_D = \frac{16}{V_S}\frac{A_D}{A_E}$$

when $V_s = 5$ then $C_D = 3.2\frac{A_D}{A_E}$

INTERPRETATION (see p. 7)

Therapeutic diphenhydramine concentrations in blood are less than 0.1 mg%.

ACCURACY AND PRECISION

Following this procedure, the results obtained should be within 10% of the true concentration. The least precise part of the analysis is the steps preceding chromatography.

INTERFERING SUBSTANCES

No basic drug has been found which gives retention times on the two columns matching diphenhydramine.

REFERENCE

Bilzer, W. and Gundert-Remy, V., Determination of nanogram quantities of diphenhydramine and or phenadrine in human plasma using gas-liquid chromatography, *Eur. J. Clin. Pharmacol.*, 6, 268, 1973.

DIPHENYLHYDANTOIN (DILANTIN®)

PRINCIPLE

Serum is acidified, extracted into ethylene dichloride, and then back-extracted into 1.0*N* NaOH. Refluxing the NaOH with potassium permanganate, 8*N* NaOH, and *n*-heptane hydrolyzes and oxidizes the diphenylhydantoin to benzophenone, which is selectively extracted into the heptane. The concentration of benzophenone and thus that of the diphenylhydantoin is determined spectrophotometrically (Procedure B). Barbiturates do not interfere, as they are converted to nonultraviolet absorbing compounds by the oxidative process.[1] In Procedure C the diphenylhydantoin is extracted from the sample with toluene and reextracted into a dilute solution of trimethylanilinium hydroxide (TMAH) prepared in ethylene glycol. The extracted barbiturates and diphenylhydantoin in this reagent are stable for at least 24 hr. Thus, many samples can be extracted simultaneously and analyzed sequentially. This is particularly valuable if an automated GC procedure is used. Phenobarbital forms only one derivative, *N,N'*-dimethylphenobarbital, and weak acids, such as glutethimide and primidone, are not coextracted. An Alternate Type C Procedure is available for the direct analysis of a biological specimen – immunoassay. The principles and procedures of this method are discussed subsequently.

TYPE B PROCEDURE

Bradford R. Hepler and Jack E. Wallace

APPARATUS

1. Separatory funnels, 250 ml
2. Round-bottom flasks, 250 ml
3. Reflux condensers
4. Graduated cylinders, glass-stoppered, 50 ml
5. Heating mantles for 250-ml round-bottom flasks
6. Magnetic stirrers and Teflon® stirring bars
7. Rheostat, capable of delivering 60 V
8. UV recording spectrophotometer
9. Filter paper (Whatman #541)
10. Long-stemmed glass funnels
11. Centrifuge tubes, 15 ml
12. Centrifuge

REAGENTS

All chemicals used should be analytical reagent grade.

1. Ethylene dichloride, spectrograde
2. *n*-Heptane, spectrograde
3. HCl, 1.0*N*
   To a one-liter graduated cylinder, add approximately 800 ml of deionized water. Add 83 ml of concentrated HCl and mix. Dilute to one liter with deionized water and mix well.
4. NaOH, 1.0*N*
   Dissolve 40 g of sodium hydroxide in deionized water and dilute to one liter with deionized water.
5. NaOH, 8.0*N*
   Dissolve 160 g of NaOH in 400 ml of deionized water contained in a 500-ml volumetric flask. Mix and cool under running tap water, releasing the pressure occasionally. Dilute to volume with deionized water and mix well.
6. Potassium permanganate, solid
7. Stock Dilantin® standard, 100 mg/dl
   The sodium salt of 5,5-diphenylhydantoin (Sigma Chemical Co.) is dried overnight in a desiccator containing magnesium perchlorate. Weigh 108.7 mg of the sodium salt, and quantitatively transfer it to a 100-ml volumetric flask. Add approximately 50 ml of deionized water and 5 drops of 1.0*N* NaOH, mix well, and dilute to volume with deionized water. Store 5.0-ml aliquots of the stock standard in plastic bottles at 0°C.
8. Working serum standard, 2 mg/dl
   Pipet 500 μl of stock standard into a 25-ml

volumetric flask. Dilute to volume with serum. Mix well. Pipet 3.0-ml aliquots into plastic tubes, cap, and store at 0°C.

9. Quality control
   This can be either purchased or prepared by pooling specimens obtained from patients who have taken Dilantin®. As components of the pool are collected, they should be stored at 0°C. When 50 ml has been collected, it may be thawed, mixed, and filtered; 3.0-ml aliquots should then be stored in capped plastic tubes.

PROCEDURE

1. Add 2 ml of sample (patient serums, working serum standard, quality control serum, and water as a reagent blank) to separately marked 250-ml separatory funnels.
2. Add 1.0 ml of 1*N* HCl to the contents of each funnel.
3. Add 40.0 ml of ethylene dichloride to each funnel, stopper, and shake vigorously for 1 min.
4. Allow the layers to separate. Filter the ethylene dichloride through the Whatman #541 filter paper into a 50-ml glass-stoppered cylinder, and discard all solvent in excess of 30 ml.
5. Add 5.0 ml of 1*N* NaOH to each cylinder.
6. Stopper and shake each cylinder vigorously for 3 min.
7. Allow the layers to separate. Using one disposable pipet for each sample, remove as much of the NaOH layer as possible to appropriately labeled 15-ml centrifuge tubes.
8. Centrifuge the 1.0*N* NaOH solutions at 3,000 rpm for 5 min.
9. Pipet 4.0 ml of each 1*N* NaOH solution into appropriately labeled 250-ml round-bottom flasks. Be certain that none of the NaOH adheres to any of the ground glass joints of the flasks.
10. To each of the round-bottom flasks, add 0.2 g of potassium permanganate. Be certain that none of the potassium permanganate adheres to any of the ground glass joints.
11. Through a long-stemmed glass funnel placed in the mouth of each flask, add 20 ml of 8.0*N* NaOH. The funnel prevents any of the NaOH from adhering to the ground glass joint. Should any NaOH collect on the joint of the flask, wipe the joint clean with a tissue. If any does adhere to the joint, the condenser and flask may freeze together during the reflux step.
12. Add 5.0 ml of *n*-heptane to each flask.
13. Add a 1-in. magnetic stirring bar to each flask. Join the flask to a reflux condenser, place the heating mantles around the flasks, and carefully place each apparatus on a magnetic stirrer.
14. Adjust the rheostat to 60 V for each heating mantle, and allow the refluxing to begin.
15. Reflux the mixtures for 30 min. Periodically check to insure that water is flowing through the condensers, that the stirrers are stirring, and that all seals are tight between the round-bottom flasks and condensers.
16. After 30 min, turn off the heat, remove the heating mantles, and allow the flasks to cool for 10 min.
17. Add approximately 100 ml of deionized water through the open end of the reflux condenser, and remove the cooled flasks from their respective condensers.
18. Add additional water to the flasks to permit the *n*-heptane layer to float to the neck of each flask so that it may be removed easily.
19. Remove 3.0 ml of the *n*-heptane layer from each flask into appropriately labeled tubes.
20. Determine the UV absorption spectrum of each solution using the prepared water reagent blank as the reference solution.
21. Record the absorbance at 247 nm, the peak absorbance of the prepared benzophenone derivative (Figure 1).

CALCULATION

$$\frac{A_u}{A_s} \times C_s = C_u$$

where

A_u = the absorbance of the sample at 247 nm
A_s = the absorbance of the standard at 247 nm
C_s = the concentration of the standard
C_u = the concentration of the sample

INTERPRETATION (see p. 7)

Vincent[2] states that 1.0 to 2.0 mg/dl of blood is the range for therapeutic control of seizures, with

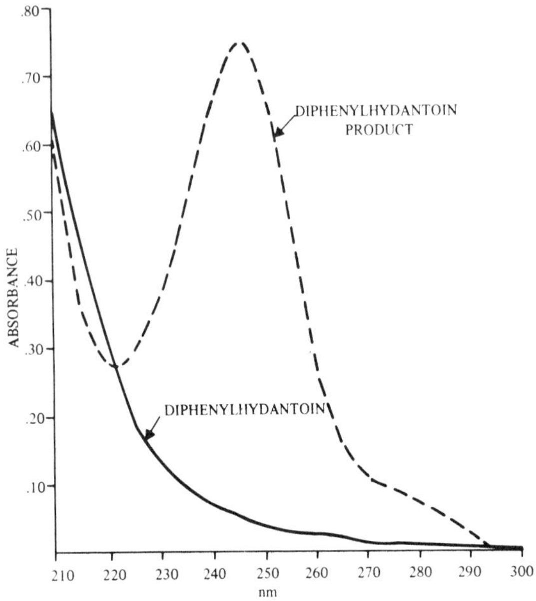

FIGURE 1. UV absorption spectrum of diphenylhydantoin and its oxidation product, both at 10 μg/ml in water and *n*-heptane, respectively.

minimal side effects. Less than 1.0 mg/dl may be considered therapeutically unsatisfactory. Weissman[3] states that although the usual range of a therapeutically beneficial diphenylhydantoin concentration is between 1.0 to 2.0 mg/dl, in some patients this may reach 5.0 mg/dl. Wallace[4] states that the therapeutic range for serum diphenylhydantoin levels is 0.8 to 1.5 mg/dl, with a toxic-comatose range in the area of 8 to 10 mg/dl.

PRECISION

On a 2.0 mg/dl concentration of diphenylhydantoin, the coefficient of variation is 4.5%.

INTERFERING SUBSTANCES

Barbiturates do not interfere. Hydantoins containing less than two phenyl groups bonded at any one carbon atom also do not interfere.

REFERENCES*

1. **Wallace, J. E.,** Simultaneous spectrophotometric determination of diphenylhydantoin and phenobarbitol in biological specimens, *Clin. Chem.*, 15, 323, 1969.
2. **Vincent, T. S.,** Importance of Dilantin blood levels in managing epilepsy, Tex. Med., 69, 67, 1973.
3. **Weissman, N.,** *Laboratory Aids in Toxicological Problems,* Copyright Bio-Science Lab., Van Nuys, Calif., 1973, 10.
4. **Wallace, J. E. and Ladd, S. L.,** Determination of drugs in biologic specimens, *Ind. Med.*, 39, 23, 1970.

GENERAL REFERENCES

Kutt, H., Pharmacodynamic and pharmacokinetic measurements of antiepileptic drugs, *Clin. Pharmacol. Ther.*, 16, 243, 1974.

Wallace, J. E., Farquhar, J. K., Hamilton, H. E., and Everhart, B. A., Comments on the determination of diphenylhydantoin, *Clin. Chem.*, 20, 515, 1974.

TYPE C PROCEDURE

Robert Osiewicz and James Valentour

APPARATUS

1. Culture tubes with Teflon®-lined caps, 16 × 125 ml (Kimax #45066A)
2. Concentratubes®† (Concentratubes® are test tubes which hold about 20 ml and taper to a sharp tip which holds about 10 μl)
3. Vortex mixer (Scientific Industries, Model #16-500J)
4. Syringe, 100 μl (Hamilton #710), 10 μl (Hamilton #701)
5. Integrator (Hewlett-Packard Model 3373B)
6. Recorder (Hewlett-Packard Model 7127A)
7. Gas Chromatograph (Hewlett-Packard Model 7621), dual FID equipped with 6′ × 1/8″ i.d. stainless steel column containing 10% UCW-982 on Chromosorb W, HP, 80 to 100 mesh

Operating Conditions

Gas Flow Rates:
helium or nitrogen – 30 ml/min

*For an updated list of reference material, see General References, p. 136.

†Available from Laboratory Research Co., P.O. Box 36509, Los Angeles, Cal. 90036.

hydrogen – 30 ml/min
air – 400 ml/min
Temperatures:
injection port – 260°C
detector – 300°C
oven – injection temperature 180°C, post injection delay 10 min, thereafter programmed at 20°C/min to 290°C, then hold at 290°C for 2 min

REAGENTS

All chemicals should be analytical reagent grade.

1. Phosphoric acid, 0.2*M*
   Dilute 1.15 ml of 85% phosphoric acid to 100 ml with distilled water.
2. Concentrated trimethylanilinium hydroxide (TMAH)
   A mixture of 7.0 g of trimethylphenylammonium iodide (Eastman #4423), 3.6 g of silver oxide, and 10 ml of methanol are placed in a screw-capped culture tube and rotated for 4 to 6 hr. The mixture is then centrifuged and the liquid phase decanted and stored for subsequent use. When stored at 20°C, it is stable for 1 month. The solution should be 1.8 ± 0.2*M*.
3. Dilute trimethylanilinium hydroxide (TMAH)
   Dilute 1 ml of the concentrated TMAH solution to 10 ml with ethylene glycol. When stored at 20°C, it is stable for 1 month
4. Aprobarbital stock solution, 5.0 mg/dl
   Dissolve 25.0 mg of aprobarbital in toluene and dilute to 500 ml with toluene.
5. Internal reference solution, 0.5 mg/dl
   Dilute 10 ml of stock solution to 100 ml with toluene.
6. Diphenylhydantoin-phenobarbital stock solutions, 50 mg/dl
   Transfer 27.5 mg each of the sodium salts of phenobarbital and diphenylhydantoin to a 25-ml volumetric flask, and dilute to volume with distilled water.
7. Diphenylhydantoin-phenobarbital aqueous reference solution, 2 mg/dl
   Dilute 4 ml of the barbiturate stock solution to 100 ml with distilled water.
8. Diphenylhydantoin-phenobarbital serum reference solution, 2 mg/dl
   Dilute 4 ml of the barbiturate stock solution to 100 ml with serum.

PROCEDURE

1. To 2 ml of sample (blood, urine, or barbiturate reference solution) in a screw-capped culture tube, add 1.0 ml of 0.2*M* H_3PO_4 and 5.0 ml of the internal reference solution. Shake the tubes for 2 min and then centrifuge then for 5 min to separate the phases.
2. Transfer about 4 ml of the toluene layer to a Concentratube® using a Pasteur pipette. (A quantitative transfer is not necessary because an internal standard is in the toluene.)
3. Vortex each Concentratube® and while still vortexing, add 20 µl of the diluted TMAH using a 100-µl Hamilton syringe. Centrifuge the Concentratube® for 10 min at 2,000 rpm.
4. Inject 3 µl of the TMAH into the injection port over a 5 to 10 sec interval, using the chromatographic conditions listed above for the quantitative procedure.
5. Calculate the barbiturate and diphenylhydantoin peak heights (or area) and that of aprobarbital Table 1.

CALCULATION

The calculation can be performed by using either peak height or peak area measurements and the following formula:

$$C_X = C_s \times \frac{P_X}{A_X} \times \frac{A_S}{P_s}$$

where

C_X = concentration of the drug in the sample;
P_X = peak height or peak area of the drug in the sample;
A_X = peak height or peak area of the aprobarbital internal standard peak in the extract of the sample solution;
C_s = concentration of the known drug in the standard solution (2 mg/dl);
P_s = peak height or peak area of the known drug in the standard solution;
A_s = peak height or peak area of the aprobarbital internal standard in the extract of the standard solution.

Table 1
THE ABSOLUTE AND RELATIVE RETENTION TIMES OF SOME ORGANIC ACID DRUGS

Drug	RRT*	RT(min)	Response factor†
Aprobarbital	1.00	4.86	1.00
Butabarbital	1.12	5.25	1.19
Amobarbital	1.31	6.15	1.03
Pentobarbital	1.51	7.06	0.98
Secobarbital	1.68	7.89	0.93
Phenobarbital	1.94	9.09	1.12
Diphenylhydantoin	3.32	15.55	1.07

* Retention time relative to a probarbital.
† Ratio of peak heights of 2.0 mg/dl of barbiturates to 2.5 mg/dl aprobarbital, internal standard.

INTERPRETATION (see p. 7)

Vincent[1] states that 1.0 to 2.0 mg/dl of blood is the range for therapeutic control of seizures, with minimal side effects. Less than 1.0 mg/dl may be considered therapeutically unsatisfactory. Weissman[2] states that although the usual range of a therapeutically beneficial diphenylhydantoin concentration is between 1.0 to 2.0 mg/dl, in some patients this may reach 5.0 mg/dl. Wallace[3] states that the therapeutic range for serum diphenylhydantoin levels is 0.8 to 1.5 mg/dl, with a toxic-comatase range in the area of 8 to 10 mg/dl.

PRECISION

One plasma sample, prepared to contain 2.5 mg/dl of phenobarbital, diphenylhydantoin, and three other barbiturates, was analyzed 50 times by this procedure. The standard deviations ranged from 0.20 to 0.33.

INTERFERING SUBSTANCES

It is not possible to differentiate phenobarbital from meprobarbital since both drugs produce the same methylated derivatives.

REFERENCES

1. **Vincent, T. S.**, Importance of Dilantin blood levels in managing epilepsy, *Tex. Med.*, 69, 67, 1973.
2. **Weissman, N.**, *Laboratory Aids in Toxicological Problems,* Copyright Bio-Science Lab., Van Nuys, Cal., 1973, 10.
3. **Wallace, J. E. and Ladd, S. L.**, Determination of drugs in biologic specimens, *Ind. Med.*, 39, 23, 1970.

GENERAL REFERENCES

Aggarwal, V. and Sunshine, I., Determination of sulfonylureas and metabolites by pyrolysis gas chromatography, *Clin. Chem.*, 20, 200, 1974.

Atkinson, A. J. and Shaw, J. M., Pharmacokinetic study of a patient with diphenylhydantoin toxicity, *Clin. Pharmacol. Ther.*, 14, 521, 1973.

Dill, W. A. and Glazko, A. J., Fluorimetric assay of diphenylhydantoin in plasma or whole blood, *Clin. Chem.*, 18, 675, 1972.

Kananen, G., Osiewicz, R., and Sunshine, I., Barbiturate analysis – a current assessment, *J. Chromatogr. Sci.*, 10, 284, 1972.

MacGee, J., Rapid determination of diphenylhydantoin in blood plasma by GLC, *Anal. Chem.*, 42, 421, 1970.

Osiewicz, R., Aggarwal, V., Young, R. M., and Sunshine, I., The qualitative analysis of phenobarbital with trimethylanilinium hydroxide, *J. Chromatogr.*, 88, 157, 1974.

Saitoh, Y., Improved micro determination for diphenylhydantoin in blood by UV spectrophotometry, *J. Pharm. Sci.*, 62, 206, 1973.

Van Meter, J. C. and Gillen, H. W., A source of variation in the GC assay of phenobarbital treated with trimethylanilinium hydroxide, *Clin. Chem.*, 19, 359, 1973.

Wilder, B. J., Serrano, E. E., and Ramsay, R. E., Plasma diphenylhydantoin levels after loading and maintenance doses, *Clin. Pharmacol. Ther.*, 14, 797, 1973.

ALTERNATE TYPE C PROCEDURE IMMUNOASSAY

Details for the EMIT procedure will be found on p. 401. Details for the RIA procedure will be found on p. 403.

DIQUAT

PRINCIPLE

When urine containing diquat is treated with sodium dithionite, a characteristic color forms (Procedure A). This reaction can be the basis for a quantitative determination (Procedure B) if the diquat is separated from the urine. This separation is performed by column chromatography using ammonium chloride to elute the adsorbed diquat.

TYPE A PROCEDURE

D. J. Berry and J. Grove

REAGENTS

All chemicals should be analytical reagent grade.

1. Sodium hydroxide, 1*N*
   Dissolve 40 g of sodium hydroxide in water and dilute to one liter.
2. Sodium dithionite, 1 g/100 ml
   Immediately prior to use, dissolve 1 g of sodium dithionite in 100 ml of 1*N* sodium hydroxide This reagent should be discarded after 2 hr.

PROCEDURE

1. Pipet 10 ml of urine into a 15-ml glass-stoppered test tube.
2. Add 2 ml of dithionite reagent, stopper, and invert tube twice (do not shake).
3. Observe color. The formation of an apple-green color due to the diquat-free radical is indicative of diquat ingestion.

INTERPRETATION (see p. 7)

This reaction is an "early warning" test and is influenced by urine volume and the time after ingestion. Confirmation should be sought using Procedure B if a positive result is obtained.

INTERFERING SUBSTANCES

Urine pigments can cause difficulty in detecting very low concentrations of diquat.

TYPE B PROCEDURE

D. J. Berry and J. Grove

APPARATUS

1. Burette, 25 ml
2. Reflux condenser and flask
3. Buchner funnel
4. Filter paper (Whatman #5)
5. Beaker, 2 liter
6. pH test paper (Universal)
7. Separatory funnel
8. Test tubes, glass-stoppered, 15 ml
9. UV spectrophotometer

REAGENTS

All chemicals should be analytical reagent grade.

1. Sulfuric acid, concentrated
2. Sodium hydroxide, 10*N*
   Dissolve 40 g of sodium hydroxide in water and dilute to 100 ml.
3. EDTA, calcium salt, 5 g/100 ml
   Dissolve 5 g of the salt in water and dilute to 100 ml.

4. Sodium chloride, saturated aqueous solution
5. Cation-exchange resin column (Permutit Zeo-Karb® 225, 52 to 100 mesh, 8% DVB, sodium from 0.9 to 1.1 WR)
   Wash 3.5 g of resin with water into a 25-ml burette in which a glass wool pad has been placed near the stopcock. Pass through the column, at a rate of 5 ml/min, first 20 ml of saturated sodium chloride solution and then 50 ml of water. The column is now ready for use. Use a new column for each test.
6. Ammonium chloride, 2.5 g/100 ml
   Dissolve 25 g of ammonium chloride in water and dilute to one liter.
7. Ammonium chloride, saturated aqueous solution
8. Sodium hydroxide, 0.3*N*
   Dissolve 1.2 g of sodium hydroxide in water and dilute to 100 ml.
9. Reducing agent
   Dissolve 0.2 g of sodium dithionite and 0.2 g of sodium metabisulfite in 100 ml of 0.3*N* sodium hydroxide. Prepare this reagent just prior to use; it must be used within 1 hr of its preparation. (Solid sodium dithionite should be stored in a desiccator.)
10. Diquat stock solution, 250 μg/ml
    Dissolve 0.1229 g of diquat dibromide monohydrate in 250 ml of saturated ammonium chloride solution.
11. Diquat reference solutions: Solution A, 10 μg/ml – Dilute 10.0 ml of the diquat stock solution to 250 ml with saturated ammonium chloride solution. Solution B, 1.5 μg/ml – Dilute 15.0 ml of Solution A to 100 ml with saturated ammonium chloride solution. Solution C, 1 μg/ml – Dilute 10.0 ml of Solution A to 100 ml with saturated ammonium chloride solution. Solution D, 0.5 μg/ml – Dilute 5.0 ml of Solution A to 100 ml with saturated ammonium chloride solution. Solution E, 0.25 μg/ml – Dilute 2.5 ml of Solution A to 100 ml with saturated ammonium chloride solution. These solutions are stable under normal laboratory conditions, provided they are not exposed to sunlight.

PROCEDURE

1. Add enough concentrated sulfuric acid to the whole specimen so that the solution is 2*N*. Boil this solution under reflux for 1 hr, with occasional swirling of the flask to prevent local overheating. Allow the contents to cool to room temperature.
2. Filter the contents of the flask through a Buchner funnel containing Whatman #5 filter paper.
3. Wash the filter paper with water.
4. Transfer the filtrate to a 2-liter beaker and dilute the solution to 0.5*N* with water.
5. Adjust the solution to a pH between 8 and 9 by careful addition of 10*N* sodium hydroxide, using a strip of Universal test paper as the indicator.
6. Add 50 ml of the EDTA solution and mix. The pH of the solution should now be between 6 and 7.
7. Refilter the solution, using vacuum. Transfer the filtrate to a separatory funnel.
8. Allow the filtrate to percolate through the prepared resin column at a flow rate of 5 to 10 ml/min.
9. Wash the column with 150 ml of 2.5% ammonium chloride at a flow rate of 3 to 4 ml/min.
10. Elute the diquat by passing saturated ammonium chloride solution through the resin column at a rate of 1 ml/min. Collect 50 ml of the effluent in a 50-ml volumetric flask and mix.
11. Pipet 10.0 ml of the effluent into a 15-ml glass-stoppered test tube, then add 2.0 ml of reducing reagent and mix by inverting twice.
12. Within 5 min of adding the reducing reagent, measure the absorbances of the solution at 375, 379, 383, and 385 nm in a 4-cm glass cell, using as reference solution a mixture containing 10.0 ml of saturated ammonium chloride solution and 2.0 ml of reducing reagent. Designate these as E_{375}, E_{379}, E_{383}, and E_{385}, respectively. If the absorbance of the solution is too high, use a smaller aliquot of the effluent and dilute it with saturated ammonium chloride to 10 ml; correct for this dilution in the final calculation.
13. With each series of analyses, measure concomitantly the absorbances at 379 nm of 10-ml aliquots of reference Solutions B, C, D, and E after adding 2 ml of reducing reagent to each solution.

CALCULATION

1. Correct the absorbance at 379 nm (E_{379}) of the sample solution for irrelevant absorption by means of Equations 1 and 2. Designate the corrected absorbances as E_{379} (corrected 1) and E_{379} (corrected 2), respectively.

$$E_{379}\text{ (corrected 1)} = 3.79\,E_{379} - 2.28E_{375} - 1.52E_{385} \quad (1)$$

$$E_{379}\text{ (corrected 2)} = 2.49\,(2\,E_{379} - E_{375} - E_{383}) \quad (2)$$

2. Determine the average of E_{379} (corrected 1) and E_{379} (corrected 2). Designate this as E_{379} (mean corrected). Using E_{379} (mean corrected), calculate the amount of diquat present by comparison with E_{379} of the reference solutions.

INTERPRETATION (see p. 7)

Information regarding diquat excretion is lacking. A case reported by Oreopoulas and McEvoy[1] showed diquat in the urine 11 days after ingestion.

ACCURACY AND PRECISION

Solutions of diquat obey Beer's law. The recovery of diquat added to urine is 90 to 100%.

INTERFERING SUBSTANCES

Background absorption has been eliminated by using the equations based on the method of Morton and Stubbs.[2] Blank urines carried through this procedure do not give any measurable absorbance.

REFERENCES

1. **Oreopoulas, D. G. and McEvoy, J.**, Diquat poisoning, *Postgrad. Med. J.*, 45, 635, 1969.
2. **Morton, R. A. and Stubbs, A. L.**, Photoelectric spectrometry applied to the analysis of mixtures and Vitamin A oils, *Analyst*, 71, 348, 1946.

GENERAL REFERENCE

Calderbank, A. C., Morgan, C. B., and Yuen, S. H., Determination of diquat residues in potato tubers, *Analyst*, 86, 569, 1961.

DIURETICS

PRINCIPLE

The diuretics can be extracted from acid media with ethyl acetate. They can be selectively reextracted from this solution with weak and strong alkali. Thus separated, these extracts can be acidified and reextracted with ethyl acetate. These ethyl acetate extracts can be concentrated and aliquots chromatographed. The drugs can then be visualized by their UV absorption and by the characteristic colored complex they form with sodium, 1,2-naphthoquinone-4-sulfonate.

TYPE B PROCEDURE

Robert A. Maes

APPARATUS

1. Thin-layer chromatography (TLC) equipment: (a) spotting pipets; (b) glass plates, coated with silica gel F_{254}; (c) developing tanks; (d) spray bottles
2. UV lamp, 254 nm radiation
3. Separatory funnels, 250 ml
4. Evaporator reduced pressure, rotary (Büchi)
5. Beakers, 100 ml

REAGENTS

All chemicals should be analytical reagent grade.

1. Lead acetate, 10 g/dl
   Dissolve 10 g of lead acetate in water and dilute to 100 ml with water.
2. Hydrochloric acid, concentrated (35%)
3. Hydrochloric acid, 1*N*
   Dilute 86.0 ml of concentrated (35%) hydrochloric acid to one liter with water.
4. Ethyl acetate, Mallinckrodt Nanograde®
5. Sodium bicarbonate, freshly prepared saturated aqueous solution
6. Sodium hydroxide, 0.25*N*
   Dissolve 9.9 g of sodium hydroxide in water and dilute to one liter with water.
7. Anhydrous sodium sulfate
8. Diuretic reference solutions
   Stock solutions of 1 mg/ml in acetone were made of the following diuretics: chlorexolone, quinethazone, acetazolamide, chlorthalidone, epithiazide, bendroflumethiazide, cyclopenthiazide, and trichlormethiazide.
9. TLC developing solvents
   (a) Solvent #1 – Mix 40.0 ml of *n*-hexane with 40.0 ml of acetone and 20.0 ml of diethylamine; (b) Solvent #2 – Mix 80.0 ml of chloroform with 15.0 ml of methanol and 5.0 ml of diethylamine. Prepare the developing solvents just prior to use. Line the developing tank with filter paper.
10. Spray reagents
   (a) Sodium hydroxide, 1*N*; (b) A saturated solution of sodium 1,2-naphthoquinone-4-sulfonate in a mixture of ethanol-water (1:1). Spray (a) followed by (b).

PROCEDURE

1. To 30 ml of urine add 5 ml of the lead acetate solution and then adjust the pH of the mixture to pH 2 to 3 with 1.0*N* HCl.
2. Filter the mixture through glass wool.
3. Extract the filtrate with 60 ml of ethyl acetate by shaking in a separatory funnel for 5 min.
4. Discard the aqueous layer.
5. Wash the ethyl acetate extract twice with 25 ml of a freshly prepared saturated sodium bicarbonate solution. Save the wash solutions.

6. Wash the ethyl acetate twice with 10 ml of 0.25*N* sodium hydroxide. Save the wash solutions.
7. Using concentrated hydrochloric acid, acidify both the pooled bicarbonate as well as the sodium hydroxide washings (Steps 5 and 6, respectively).
8. Extract each pooled acidified washing with 30 ml of ethyl acetate. Separate the ethyl acetate layers. Discard the aqueous phases.
9. Dry each ethyl acetate extract with anhydrous sodium sulfate.
10. Evaporate each dried extract in a rotary evaporator at 20°C.
11. Dissolve each residue in 0.2 ml of acetone and spot each solution on a thin-layer chromatographic silica gel F_{254} plate.
12. Spot about 10 μl of the diuretic reference solutions on the same plate and chromatograph in saturated chromatotanks using developing Solvent 1 at room temperature. Allow the solvent front to rise 15 cm.
13. Remove the plate from the developing tank and dry it at 100°C.
14. Place the plate under the UV lamp and locate the spots. The diuretics appear as violet spots on exposure to UV light.
15. If positive, run a second plate in saturated chromatotanks using developing Solvent 2 at room temperature. Allow the solvent front to rise 15 cm.
16. Repeat as indicated in Steps 13 and 14.
17. Spray the plate with the sodium hydroxide spray followed by the NQS reagent and allow it to air-dry. Within 15 min after spraying with the NQS reagent, the drugs appear as stable pale orange spots which become more pronounced after storing in the dark for 1 or 2 days. R_f values of the different compounds are listed in Table 1. Most of the listed diuretics are extracted into the sodium hydroxide fraction, but chlorexolone and chlorthalidone are in the bicarbonate fraction.

Table 1

R_f VALUES (× 100) OF COMMON DIURETICS

Diuretic	Solvent system #1	Solvent system #2
Chlorexolone	61	91
Quinethazone	32	49
Acetazolamide	2	22
Chlorthalidone	55	58
Epithiazide	24	46
Bendroflumethiazine	46	75
Cyclopenthiazide	70	76
Trichlormethiazide	7	40

INTERPRETATION (see p. 7)

The method provides a qualitative and semiquantitative analysis of the different diuretics. Ethyl acetate extractions were made at two different pH levels because of the differing pKa values of the diuretics. Because the low concentrations of these drugs in blood make detection difficult, urine is the specimen of choice. After an oral intake of 4 mg of epithiazide or trichlormethiazide, the drug easily can be found within 6 hr after ingestion.

SENSITIVITY

The detection limit is 2 to 5 μg.

INTERFERING SUBSTANCES

No significant spots are observed from the analysis of drug-free urine.

REFERENCE

Maes, R., Gijbels, M., and Laruelle, L., Detection of some diuretics in biological fluids, *J. Chromatogr.*, 53, 408, 1970.

DOXEPIN

PRINCIPLE

Doxepin can be extracted from an alkaline solution into an organic solvent. Aliquots of this extract can be used for gas chromatography or thin-layer chromatography. Reextraction of the remainder of the extract into acid yields a solution whose UV absorption spectrum is characteristic and useful for confirmation of the chromatographic data.

TYPE C PROCEDURE

Philip C. Reynolds

APPARATUS

1. Extraction tubes with Teflon®-lined screw caps, 20 × 125 mm
2. Mechanical shaker
3. Centrifuge tubes, 12 ml
4. Thin-layer chromatography (TLC) equipment (Brinkmann Instruments): (a) micropipets; (b) glass plates, coated with silica gel G; (c) developing tanks; (d) spray bottles
5. Extraction tubes with Teflon®-lined screw caps, 13 × 100 mm
6. Mixer (Vortex)
7. UV spectrophotometer (Perkin Elmer Model 402)
8. Gas chromatograph (Perkin Elmer Model 900), equipped with dual flame ionization detectors, two 1 mV recorders, and two glass columns, 6′ × 1/4″ o.d. × 1/8″ i.d., packed respectively with 3% S.E. 30 ultraphase and 3% OV-17 on Chromosorb W (HP), 80/100 mesh*

   Operating Conditions

   Gas Flow Rates:
   air, nitrogen, and hydrogen – optimal for maximum response per manufacturer's instructions

   Temperatures:
   column – 240°C
   injection port – 240°C
   detector – 290°C
   manifold – 290°C

*Pierce Chemical Co., Rockford, Ill.

REAGENTS

All chemicals should be analytical reagent grade.

1. Doxepin stock solution, 1 mg/ml
   Dissolve 28.26 mg of doxepin hydrochloride in water and dilute to 25 ml.
2. Doxepin reference solutions, 0.5, 1.0, and 2.0 mg/100 ml
   Dilute 0.5, 1.0, and 2.0 ml of the doxepin stock solution to 100 ml respectively.
3. Hydrochloric acid, 6*N*
   Dilute concentrated hydrochloric acid with an equal volume of water.
4. Chloroform
   It is mandatory that each lot of solvent be carried through the entire procedure to assure the absence of excessive UV background or extraneous gas-chromatographic peaks.
5. Sodium hydroxide, 4*N*
   Dissolve 160 g of sodium hydroxide in water and dilute to one liter.
6. Glass wool
7. Sodium sulfate, anhydrous
8. Codeine phosphate internal standard control solution, 1 mg/ml
   Dissolve 25 mg of codeine phosphate in methanol. Dilute this solution to 25 ml with methanol.
9. TLC developing solutions
   Solution A, methanol-ammonium hydroxide, 100:1.5; Solution B, ethanol-dioxane-benzene-ammonium hydroxide, 6:40:50:5
10. Platinum chloride, 10 g/100 ml

Dissolve 10 g of platinum chloride in water and dilute to 100 ml with water.

11. Iodoplatinate reagent
    Dissolve 10 g of potassium iodide in 240 ml of water. Add 10.0 ml of the platinum chloride solution, then dilute the mixture to 500 ml with water.
12. Sodium sulfite
13. Ammonium hydroxide, concentrated
14. Ethyl ether
15. Hydrochloric acid, 0.5*N*
    Dilute 4.0 ml of concentrated hydrochloric acid to 100 ml with water.

SPECIMEN PREPARATION

Urine

1. To 5.0 ml of urine add 0.2 ml of 6*N* hydrochloric acid and 10.0 ml of chloroform. Shake the mixture for 5 min on a mechanical shaker. Process 5.0 ml of water for a reagent blank and 5.0 ml of each doxepin reference solution concomitantly and in the same manner.
2. Centrifuge the samples for 5 min. Transfer the supernatants to clean tubes and discard the solvent layers.
3. Add 0.5 ml of 4*N* sodium hydroxide and 10.0 ml of chloroform to each sample. Shake the mixtures for 5 min on a mechanical shaker.
4. Centrifuge the samples, then aspirate and discard the supernatants. Use the chloroform extracts for the analysis.

Blood or Tissue

1. To 5.0 ml of blood or tissue slurry add enough 4*N* sodium hydroxide to bring the pH to 9.5. Add 10.0 ml of chloroform, then shake the mixture for 5 min on a mechanical shaker. Process 5.0 ml of water for a reagent blank and 5.0 ml of each doxepin reference solution concomitantly and in the same manner.
2. Centrifuge the samples for 5 min. Aspirate and discard as much of the supernatant aqueous layers as possible, leaving only the solvent and firmly packed proteinogenous layers.
3. Separate the chloroform extracts by filtering them through small pledgets of glass wool and anhydrous sodium sulfate. Avoid the use of filter paper. Use the filtrates for the analysis.

PROCEDURE

1. Transfer 8.0 ml of the solvent phase obtained from each sample (unknown, reagent blank, and reference solutions) to a 12-ml centrifuge tube.
2. Add 50 μl of the codeine phosphate internal standard control solution to each extract and mix well.
3. Evaporate the solvent to about 50 μl in a 50°C water bath with the aid of a gentle air stream.
4. Inject 1 to 3 μl of the concentrated mixture into each column of the gas chromatograph. The retention times of doxepin relative to codeine are approximately 0.64 for the S.E. 30 column and 0.69 for the OV-17 column.
5. Record the retention distance of each peak (measured in millimeters) from the solvent front. At a recorder speed of ¾″/min the unknown should agree within ±1 mm when compared to those obtained from the injected reference solutions.

Confirmation

6. Spot equal volumes of the final extracts obtained from the specimen and from the reference solutions 2.0 mm from the base of each of two TLC plates.
7. Place one plate in developing solution A and the other in developing solution B.
8. Allow the developing solutions to rise about 140 mm from the point of application.
9. Remove the plates from the tank. Place them in a fume hood to dry for at least 1 hr.
10. Spray each plate lightly with iodoplatinate reagent. Doxepin will have an R_f value of about 0.51 in System A and about 0.95 in System B. At least one metabolite will be found in overdose cases. This metabolite is iodoplatinate-positive and trails doxepin in both systems.
11. For final confirmation, scrape the reactive spots from the TLC plates and transfer the scrapings to 13 × 100 mm screw-capped tubes.
12. Add 0.5 ml of water, a few milligrams of sodium sulfite, and 2 drops of concentrated ammonium hydroxide to the scrapings.
13. Add about 5 ml of ethyl ether to each tube, then mix the contents for 20 sec, using a Vortex mixer.
14. Centrifuge the tubes for 3 min. Transfer the

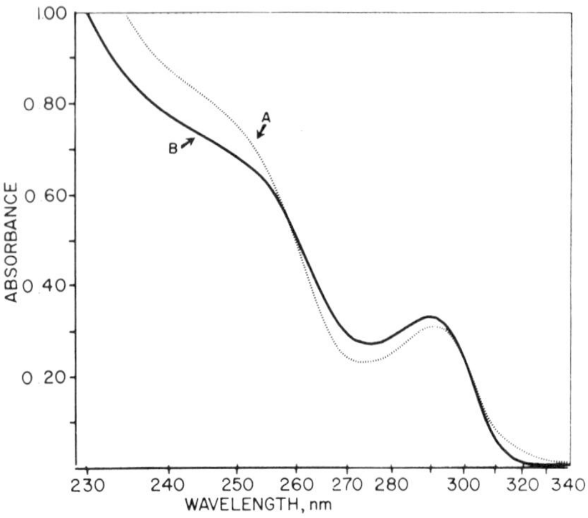

FIGURE 1. UV spectrum for doxepin. A = 25 μg/ml (in 0.5*N* HCl); B = 25 μg/ml (in 0.5*N* NaOH).

supernatant ether layers to another set of tubes.

15. Add 1.1 ml of 0.5*N* hydrochloric acid to the ether, then mix the tube contents for 20 sec, using a Vortex mixer.
16. Scan each hydrochloric acid layer in the spectrophotometer from 220 to 350 nm. Doxepin has a characteristic curve with a maximum at 294 nm and shoulder at 235 to 245 nm (Figure 1).

CALCULATION

Compare the peak height ratio of the unknown relative to codeine with the ratio of a suitable doxepin reference solution relative to codeine. The gas-chromatographic response of these ratios is linear for concentrations from 0 to 3 mg/100 ml original solution.

INTERPRETATION (see p. 7)

In one case, a concentration of 1 mg doxepin/100 ml blood was judged consistent with death. No other information is available at this time.

ACCURACY AND PRECISION

This method is capable of detecting doxepin concentrations of 0.2 mg/100 ml blood, with a coefficient of variation of 7%. More precise results at low concentrations can be obtained by using a smaller amount (15 to 25 μg) of internal control.

INTERFERING SUBSTANCES

Any basic organic drug is potentially interfering. However, if the GLC, TLC, and UV criteria are met, the drug is easily identified and quantitated.

REFERENCES

Cochin, J. and Daly, W. J., Rapid identification of analgesic drugs in urine with TLC, *Experientia*, 18, 294, 1962.

Sunshine, I., Use of TLC in the diagnosis of poisoning, *Am. J. Clin. Pathol.*, 40, 576, 1963.

ETHANOL

PRINCIPLE

Ethanol determinations are usually based on its volatility and/or its redox potential. Both these properties are utilized in Procedure A. A Conway microdiffusion cell, with potassium dichromate in the center well and the sample in the outer well, suffice. If ethanol is present, it will diffuse out of the sample and react with the dichromate. The extent of this reduction can be used qualitatively, semiquantitatively, or quantitatively to indicate the probable ethanol content of the sample. Although nonspecific, this procedure is very adequate for many applications, if all its limitations are understood.

Some laboratories prefer to use a more elegant distillation procedure to separate the ethanol from a biological matrix. A very simple direct distillation unit is described in Procedure B. The distillate is tested with dichromate. If a positive reaction ensues and the specificity of the procedure is in question, then specific tests for other volatile reducing substances, such as methanol or isopropanol, are indicated. One distillation method that attempts to minimize the problem of interference has been described by Kozelka and Hine.[1] This procedure requires special glass apparatus not usually available in many laboratories, and hence was not included in this volume. It should be considered by those who may have the opportunity to do more than an occasional ethanol determination by distillation.

Many of the problems of precision, accuracy, and specificity are resolved by the gas-chromatographic procedure (C). Valuable as this procedure is, it is impractical unless one column in a gas chromatograph is always available for this determination. Few substances other than the "volatiles" can be sought on this column, and it is impractical to insert and remove a column if infrequent analyses are required. Hence, despite the advantages of the gas-chromatographic procedure, unless a laboratory has a significant daily demand for ethanol determinations, a distillation method may be more desirable. Those laboratories that have a daily demand for many ethanol determinations may be predisposed to an automated head space analyzer. This unit, not described below, has the advantage of speed, specificity, and accuracy, and is very desirable for laboratories with a large daily work load.

TYPE A PROCEDURE

Arthur J. McBay

APPARATUS

1. Modified Conway microdiffusion dish

REAGENTS

All chemicals should be analytical reagent grade.

1. Potassium dichromate
   Dissolve 1.0 g of potassium dichromate in 500 ml of water. Add 0.1 g of silver nitrate to the solution. Carefully add 500 ml of concentrated sulfuric acid. This mixture is stable for at least 1 year if protected from direct sunlight and atmospheric water vapor. For use, the reagent is conveniently dispensed from a 1-oz dropping bottle of amber glass.

PROCEDURE

1. Cover the bottom of the middle ring of the dish with blood or urine by pouring directly from the specimen container.
2. Add a few drops of potassium dichromate to the center well from a dropping bottle.
3. Place the cover on the dish and allow it to stand at room temperature.

INTERPRETATION (see p. 7)

The reagent will change color in 15 min to 1 hr if ethanol or another volatile reducing substance is present. The color change is from yellow to green to blue. A discernible change has been observed in less than 1 hr when 1.0 ml of blood containing 200 μg of either methanol, ethanol, or isopropanol was allowed to react with about 0.3 ml of dichromate reagent. In 2 hr the reagent turns blue. This method is not specific for ethanol.

REFERENCE

1. **Kozelka, F. L. and Hine, C. H.,** Method for the determination of ethyl alcohol for medicolegal purposes, *Ind. Eng. Anal. Ed.*, 13, 905, 1941.

TYPE B PROCEDURE

Irving Sunshine

APPARATUS

1. Direct distillation apparatus[1] (Scientific Glass Apparatus Co., Inc., Cat. No. JD-1390) or any similar all glass distillation apparatus
2. Volumetric flasks, 10 ml
3. Test tubes
4. Spectrophotometer or photoelectric photometer

REAGENTS

All chemicals should be analytical reagent grade.

1. Ethanol reference solutions
   Add absolute ethanol to blood that has been previously checked to insure that volatile reducing substances are not present. The ethanol concentrations of the reference solutions should range from 0 to 320 mg/100 ml of blood in gradations of 40 mg/100 ml.
2. Sulfuric acid, 1*N*
   Cautiously add 28 ml of concentrated sulfuric acid to 100 ml of water. After cooling the solution to room temperature, dilute it to one liter with water.
3. Sodium tungstate, 112 g/liter
   Dissolve 112 g of sodium tungstate in water and dilute to one liter.
4. Sulfuric acid, 18*N*
   Dilute 500 ml of concentrated sulfuric acid to one liter with water.
5. Potassium dichromate
   Dissolve 1.0500 g of potassium dichromate in one liter of 18*N* sulfuric acid. This reagent is stable for at least 1 year if protected from direct sunlight and atmospheric water vapor.

PROCEDURE

1. To each of a series of distillation flasks add successively 20 ml of water, 2.0 ml of sample (blood or urine specimen, duplicates of each reference solution, and water for a reagent blank), 5.0 ml of 1*N* sulfuric acid, and 5.0 ml of the sodium tungstate solution. Mix the contents of each flask by swirling. Allow the protein in the mixtures to precipitate.
2. After the protein precipitation is complete, start the distillation.
3. During an 8- to 10-min distillation period collect 8 to 9 ml of each distillate in a 10-ml volumetric flask. Dilute the contents of each flask to 10.0 ml with water and mix.
4. Add 1.0 ml of each distillate to a series of test tubes containing 3.0 ml of the potassium dichromate solution. Mix the contents of each tube.
5. Place the tubes in a boiling water bath. Be sure that the level of the boiling water is higher than the volume of liquid in the test tubes.
6. After 15 min remove the tubes from the water bath and allow them to cool to room temperature.
7. Determine the absorbance of each solution at 450 or 350 nm. Use the solution obtained by processing the water samples as the reference solution.

CALCULATION

1. Measure the absorbance of the final dichromate solution of each reference sample at 450 or 350 nm against the reagent blank.
2. Plot the absorbances of the reference solutions against their ethanol concentrations on rectilinear graph paper. A straight line will result.
3. Determine the ethanol concentration of the specimen by comparing its absorbance with those of the reference solutions.

INTERPRETATION (see p. 7)

No significant quantities of ethanol are present in biological specimens obtained from living subjects who have abstained from intake of ethanol. Table 1 gives the estimated blood-ethanol concentrations one might expect in a healthy person following absorption of various amounts of ingested ethanol. The principal effect of ethanol of significance for the diagnosis of acute alcoholic intoxication is its action as a central nervous system (CNS) depressant. While the CNS-depressant action of ethanol is on a continuum ranging from no discernible effect at very low blood-alcohol concentrations (e.g., 10 mg/dl) to ultimate severe respiratory depression and death at very high blood-alcohol concentrations (e.g., 500 mg/dl), it is convenient to describe these effects in terms of separate, though overlapping, stages of acute alcoholic influence. Table 2 shows a simple classification of acute alcoholic influence stages, together with typical effects, at various blood-alcohol concentrations. Ethanol concentrations in blood (and other biological liquids such as cerebrospinal fluid, urine, etc.) are commonly expressed in milligrams of ethanol per 100 ml of the specimen (mg/dl) for clinical applications.

Special statutory provisions in all states and federal jurisdictions govern the interpretation of concentrations of ethanol in blood with respect to the presumption of fitness to operate a motor vehicle. The following provisions of the Uniform Vehicle Code are widely followed:

Upon the trial of any civil or criminal action or proceeding arising out of acts alleged to have been commited by any person while driving or in actual physical control of a vehicle while under the influence or intoxicating liquor, the amount of alcohol in the person's blood, urine, breath, or other bodily substance shall give rise to the following presumptions:

1. If there was at that time 0.05 percent or less by weight of alcohol in the person's blood, it shall be presumed that the person was not under the influence of intoxicating liquor.

2. If there was at that time in excess of 0.05 percent but less than 0.10 percent by weight of alcohol in

Table 1

APPROXIMATE ETHANOL CONCENTRATIONS (mg/100 ml) IN BLOOD

Body weight, lb	Total number of drinks* 1	2	3	4	5	6	7	8	9	10
100	38	75	113	150	188	225	263	300	338	375
120	31	63	94	125	156	188	219	250	281	313
140	27	54	80	107	134	161	188	214	241	268
150	25	51	75	101	126	151	176	201	226	251
160	23	47	70	94	117	141	164	188	211	234
180	21	42	63	83	104	125	146	167	188	208
200	19	38	56	75	94	113	131	150	169	188
220	17	34	51	68	85	102	119	136	153	170
240	16	31	47	63	78	94	109	125	141	156

* If these drinks were not taken within 1 hr, deduct one drink from the total number of drinks for each hour that elapsed between the first and the last drink. A drink is defined as 1 oz of 100-proof "hard liquor" (whiskey, vodka, gin, etc.), 12 oz of 4% beer, or 3 oz of fortified wine.

Table 2

MAJOR EFFECTS OF ACUTE ALCOHOLIC INFLUENCE

Ethanol concentration in blood	Stage of alcoholic influence	Typical effects
10–50 mg/dl	Euphoria	Euphoria, decreased inhibitions, diminished attention and judgment
50–100 mg/dl	Excitement	Sedation, impaired muscular coordination, decreased sensitory response
150–300 mg/dl	Confusion	Disorientation, disturbances of sensation, impaired balance, slurred speech
250–400 mg/dl	Stupor	Markedly decreased response to stimuli, marked muscular incoordination, incontinence of urine and feces, sleep or stupor
400–500 mg/dl	Coma	Complete unconsciousness, depressed reflexes, subnormal temperature, respiratory and circulatory collapse, death

the person's blood, such fact shall not give rise to any presumption that the person was or was not under the influence of intoxicating liquor, but such fact may be considered with other competent evidence in determining whether the person was under the influence of intoxicating liquor.

3. If there was at that time 0.10 percent or more by weight of alcohol in the person's blood, it shall be presumed that the person was under the influence of intoxicating liquor.

4. Percent by weight of alcohol in the blood shall be based upon grams of alcohol per 100 cubic centimeters of blood.

These interpretation standards have been endorsed by the National Safety Council's Committee on Alcohol and Drugs and the House of Delegates of the American Medical Association.

ACCURACY AND PRECISION

"Blank" blood and urine solutions give "apparent" ethanol concentrations of less than 1 mg/100 ml. The recovery of ethanol is 99.7%. The precision of the method was determined by analyses performed by different laboratories on aliquots of the same samples; the results had a mean deviation of 2.7% of the actual ethanol present.

INTERFERING SUBSTANCES

Acetone and chlorinated hydrocarbons do not interfere. Methanol, paraldehyde, isopropanol, and formaldehyde will interfere. Their presence or absence must be determined by additional tests on other aliquots of the distillate.

REFERENCE

1. **Dubowski, K. and Shupe, L.,** Improved semimicro distillation apparatus, *Am. J. Clin. Pathol.*, 22, 709, 1952.

GENERAL REFERENCE

Dubowski, K., Tests for alcohol, in *Alcohol and the Impaired Driver*, Committee on Medicolegal Problems, Ed., American Medical Association, Chicago, Ill., 1968, 61.

TYPE C PROCEDURE

Kurt M. Dubowski

APPARATUS

1. Septum vials, 15 mm, screw-capped with butyl rubber stoppers
2. Water bath (e.g., Lauda-Brinkmann Model K-4) with ± 0.01 to 0.05°C regulation.
3. Tuberculin syringe, plastic, 1 ml with a 25-gauge 1½-in. needle
4. Chaney adaptor
5. Gas chromatograph, equipped with a flame ionization detector (e.g., Varian Model 1860), a stainless steel (or glass) column, 6′ × 1/8″ i.d., packed with Porapak S (80 to 100 mesh), and a suitable potentiometer recorder (1 mV full-scale sensitivity and 250-mm chart width). An electronic or recorder-coupled mechanical integrator is very desirable. If liquid samples are to be injected, the injection port is fitted with a removable glass liner. Operating conditions and electrometer settings of the chromatograph should be adjusted so that injection of 2 μl of 200 mg/dl of ethanol produces a full-scale recorder response with a retention time of approximately 2 min. A recorder chart speed of 5 mm/min is used if peak heights are employed for quantitation; higher chart speeds can be used if peak areas are measured. (Other column packings may be used for the analysis of volatile substances. Table 1 provides reference data relative to these other materials.)

   Operating Conditions

   (Typical operating conditions are shown for a Varian Model 1860-3 gas chromatograph.)

   Gases:

	Inlet pressure	Flow rate
helium or nitrogen (carrier gas)	55 psig	45 ml/min
hydrogen	20 psig	45 ml/min
air	15 psig	330 ml/min

   Temperatures:

   column – 165°C
   injection port – 175°C
   detector – 225°C

REAGENTS

All chemicals should be analytical reagent grade.

1. Mixed volatiles reference solutions
   Using absolute ethanol and chromatographically pure absolute acetone, isopropanol, and methanol, prepare the following low concentration and high concentration solutions.

Mixed Volatiles Reference Solution

	Low concentration	High concentration
Acetone	50 mg/dl	100 mg/dl
Ethanol	100 mg/dl	200 mg/dl
Isopropanol	50 mg/dl	100 mg/dl
Methanol	50 mg/dl	100 mg/dl

   In sealed glass containers at 4°C, these reference solutions are stable for at least 6 months.
2. Diluent internal standard solution
   Dissolve 12 g of Triton® X-100 in water, add 1.80 g(= 2.2 g/ml at 20°C) of acetonitrile, and dilute to one liter.

PROCEDURE

Head Space Analysis Procedure

1. Into a 15-ml screw-capped septum vial with a butyl rubber septum stopper, place 1.0 g of sodium chloride and 1 ml of well-mixed whole blood (or other liquid sample). Close the vial and mix well by rotation and lateral shaking (swirling).
2. Prepare vials (following the same procedure)

Table 1

ABSOLUTE RETENTION TIMES FOR ETHANOL USING THE DESCRIBED GAS-CHROMATOGRAPHIC CONDITIONS

Packing	Temperature, °C	Absolute retention time for ethanol (min)
1. 0.5% Carbowax K-600 and 3.8% Hallcomid 18 on Teflon® 6 HC 40 to 60 mesh	100	0.24
2. 0.5% Carbowax K-600 and 3.8% Hallcomid 18 on Teflon® 6 HC 40 to 60 mesh	50	1.8
3. 0.4% Carbowax 1500 on Carbopak A	80	1.47
4. Porapak Q, 80 to 100 mesh	155	1.60
5. Chromosorb 102, 100 to 120 mesh	155	2.16
6. 15% Carbowax 1500 on Celite 525, 80 to 100 mesh	80	2.58
7. Porapak S, 80 to 100 mesh	155	2.51
8. 30% Carbowax 20*M** on Chromosorb W, AW, 60 to 80 mesh	130	2.12

* 6′ × ¼″ o.d. column, rather than the 6′ × 1/8″ size used for the other supports.

containing 1 ml of low concentration and 1 ml of high concentration mixed volatiles reference solution, respectively. For specimens of limited volume, the same procedure is followed with 0.2 g of sodium chloride and 0.1 ml of specimen.

3. Place all vials into a water bath maintained at 38 ± 0.05°C and allow the vials (immersed to just below the screw caps) to equilibrate for 45 min.
4. Using a plastic 1-ml tuberculin syringe fitted with a volume-limiting Chaney adaptor and a 25-guage 1½-in. needle preheated to 38°C, withdraw a fixed volume (approximately 0.25 ml) of the head space vapor (after repeated pumping to obtain an equilibrated sample aliquot) and immediately inject it into the gas chromatograph. (For gas chromatographs equipped with a heated gas-sampling valve and a 0.25-ml sample loop, a larger head space sample can be withdrawn from a septum vial and transferred to the gas-sampling valve.) Thoroughly purge the syringe and needle by rapid repetitive intake and expulsion of room air.
5. Record each chromatogram for 5 min.
6. It is convenient and advisable to sample and chromatograph the head space vapors in the following sequence: low concentration reference solution, unknown specimen(s), and high concentration reference solution. The reference solutions (or at least one reference solution) should be analyzed completely in parallel with every unknown specimen (or repeated with every ten unknown specimens). The same syringe is used for all unknown and reference specimens.
7. For analyses of critical importance, repeat Steps 4, 5, and 6 after allowing the vials to equilibrate for at least 20 min after the prior head space vapor withdrawal.
8. Identify ethanol in the unknown specimen, if present, by its retention time in comparison with the reference solutions. For the system described, the volatile substances appear in the following order: methanol, ethanol, acetone,

Table 2

TYPICAL RELATIVE RETENTION TIMES* OF VOLATILE SUBSTANCES

(On Porapak S Column)

Compound	Relative retention time*
Acetone	1.44
Acetonitrile	1.23
Ethanol	1.00
Isopropanol	1.80
Methanol	0.48

* Retention times relative to that of ethanol, whose absolute retention time for this analytical system is 2.0 min.

and isopropanol. Typical retention times are shown in Table 2.

9. If ethanol is present in the unknown specimen, its concentration in the original blood (or other) specimen is determined with the following formula:

$$\frac{P_A}{P_R} \times C_R = C_A$$

where

P_A = peak area of ethanol of unknown specimen;
P_R = peak area of ethanol of reference specimen;
C_R = reference concentration of ethanol;*
C_A = ethanol concentration of unknown (mg/dl).

Direct Injection Procedure

1. With a fully quantitative technique, add exactly equal volumes of the well-mixed whole blood (or other liquid sample) and the diluent internal standard solution to a suitable container, and mix thoroughly. (Glass-stoppered microcentrifuge tubes are convenient for this purpose; use of a high precision manual or mechanical sampler/diluter is helpful when many specimens are to be analyzed.)
2. Mix exactly equal volumes of low concentration and high concentration mixed volatiles reference solution, respectively, and diluent internal standard solution.
3. Centrifuge all mixtures briefly in closed containers, if necessary, to obtain a perfectly clear mixture free of debris, blood cell ghosts, etc.
4. Using a suitable gas-chromatographic syringe, inject 2 μl of each unknown and reference specimen, prepared as per Step 1 or 2 above, into the gas chromatograph. Immediately after each injection separate the syringe plunger and barrel, and thoroughly clean and dry them.
5. Record each chromatogram for 5 min.
6. It is convenient and advisable to sample and chromatograph low concentration reference solution, unknown specimen(s), and high concentration reference solution, in that sequence. The reference solutions (or at least one reference solution) should be analyzed completely in parallel with every unknown specimen (or repeated with every 10 unknown specimens). Different syringes can be used to inject the several specimens.
7. For analyses of critical importance, repeat Steps 4, 5, and 6.
8. Identify ethanol in the unknown specimen, if present, by its retention time in comparison with the simultaneously analyzed reference solutions. For the system described, the volatile substances appear in the following order: methanol, ethanol, acetonitrile, acetone, and isopropanol. Typical retention times are shown in Table 2.
9. If ethanol is present in the unknown specimen, its concentration in the original blood (or other specimen) is determined with the following formula:

$$\frac{S_E/S_R}{K_E/K_R} \times C_R = C_E$$

where

S_E = peak area of ethanol in unknown sample and diluent internal standard mixture;
S_R = peak area of acetonitrile in unknown sample and diluent internal standard mixture;
K_E = peak area of ethanol in reference sample and diluent internal standard mixture;
K_R = peak area of acetonitrile in reference

*Low concentration is 100 mg/dl; high concentration is 200 mg/dl.

Table 3

APPROXIMATE ETHANOL CONCENTRATIONS (mg/100 ml) IN BLOOD

Body weight, lb	Total number of drinks* 1	2	3	4	5	6	7	8	9	10
100	38	75	113	150	188	225	263	300	338	375
120	31	63	94	125	156	188	219	250	281	313
140	27	54	80	107	134	161	188	214	241	268
150	25	51	75	101	126	151	176	201	226	251
160	23	47	70	94	117	141	164	188	211	234
180	21	42	63	83	104	125	146	167	188	208
200	19	38	56	75	94	113	131	150	169	188
220	17	34	51	68	85	102	119	136	153	170
240	16	31	47	63	78	94	109	125	141	156

* If these drinks were not taken within 1 hr, deduct one drink from the total number of drinks for each hour that elapsed between the first and the last drink. A drink is defined as 1 oz of 100-proof "hard liquor" (whiskey, vodka, gin, etc.), 12 oz of 4% beer, or 3 oz of fortified wine.

sample and diluent internal standard mixture;

C_R = reference sample concentration of ethanol;

C_E = ethanol concentration of unknown (mg/dl).

INTERPRETATION (see p. 7)

No significant quantities of ethanol are present in biological specimens obtained from living subjects who have abstained from intake of ethanol. Table 3 gives the estimated blood ethanol concentrations one might expect in a healthy person following absorption of various amounts of ingested ethanol. The principal effect of ethanol of significance for the diagnosis of acute alcoholic intoxication is its action as a central nervous system (CNS) depressant. While the CNS-depressant action of ethanol is on a continuum ranging from no discernible effect at very low blood-alcohol concentrations (e.g., 10 mg/dl) to ultimate severe respiratory depression and death at very high blood-alcohol concentrations (e.g., 500 mg/dl), it is convenient to describe these effects in terms of separate, though overlapping, stages of acute alcoholic influence. Table 4 shows a simple classification of acute alcoholic influence stages, together with typical effects, at various blood-alcohol concentrations. Ethanol concentrations in blood (and other biological liquids such as cerebrospinal fluid, urine, etc.) are commonly expressed in milligrams of ethanol per 100 ml of the specimen (mg/dl) for clinical applications.

Special statutory provisions in all states and federal jurisdictions govern the interpretation of concentrations of ethanol in blood with respect to the presumption of fitness to operate a motor vehicle. The following provisions of the Uniform Vehicle Code are widely followed:

Upon the trial of any civil or criminal action or proceeding arising out of acts alleged to have been committed by any person while driving or in actual physical control of a vehicle while under the influence of intoxicating liquor, the amount of alcohol in the person's blood at the time alleged as shown by chemical analysis of the person's blood, urine, breath, or other bodily substance shall give rise to the following presumptions:

1. If there was at that time 0.05 percent or less by weight of alcohol in the person's blood, it shall be presumed that the person was not under the influence of intoxicating liquor.

2. If there was at that time in excess of 0.05 percent but less than 0.10 percent by weight of alcohol in the person's blood, such fact shall not give rise to any presumption that the person was or was not under the influence of intoxicating liquor, but such fact may be

Table 4

MAJOR EFFECTS OF ACUTE ALCOHOLIC INFLUENCE

Ethanol concentration in blood	Stage of alcoholic influence	Typical effects
10–50 mg/dl	Euphoria	Euphoria, decreased inhibitions, diminished attention and judgment
50–100 mg/dl	Excitement	Sedation, impaired muscular coordination, decreased sensitory response
150–300 mg/dl	Confusion	Disorientation, disturbances of sensation, impaired balance, slurred speech
250–400 mg/dl	Stupor	Markedly decreased response to stimuli, marked muscular incoordination, incontinence of urine and feces, sleep or stupor
400–500 mg/dl	Coma	Complete unconsciousness, depressed reflexes, subnormal temperature, respiratory and circulatory collapse, death

considered with other competent evidence in determining whether the person was under the influence of intoxicating liquor.

3. If there was at that time 0.10 percent or more by weight of alcohol in the person's blood, it shall be presumed that the person was under the influence of intoxicating liquor.

4. Percent by weight of alcohol in the blood shall be based upon grams of alcohol per 100 cubic centimeters of blood.

These interpretation standards have been endorsed by the National Safety Council's Committee on Alcohol and Drugs and the House of Delegates of the American Medical Association.

ACCURACY AND PRECISION

When peak area measurements are used to calculate sample ethanol concentrations, the standard deviation and coefficient of variation (= relative standard deviation) of replicate analyses for the procedures described above are as follows for specimens with a mean ethanol concentration of 100 mg/dl:

	Head space analysis	Direct injection
Standard deviation	± 2.80 mg/dl	2.8%
Coefficient of variation	± 2.18 mg/dl	2.2%

When peak height measurements are used to calculate sample ethanol concentrations, the standard deviation and coefficent of variation of replicate analyses are somewhat greater than listed above, unless the procedure is fully optimized with respect to sample size, peak slope, chart speed, and other gas-chromatographic analysis conditions.

Accuracy of the procedures is highly satisfactory for identification of ethanol and its quantitation in biological liquids, as judged by performance in the analysis of proficiency tests and other "blind" specimens; analysis results are always within ± 10 mg/dl of the target values.

INTERFERING SUBSTANCES

Commonly occurring volatile substances are shown in Table 2. These compounds can be readily separated from each other and identified by their relative retention time according to the procedures outlined. In critically important analyses, it is good and recommended practice to confirm the tentative identifications based on a single set of gas-chromatographic conditions by additional methods, which can include reanalysis of the prepared sample by gas-chromatographic means with a different column and other conditions. If an internal standard with a retention time different than that of acetonitrile is desired, *n*-propanol, *tert*-butanol, and dioxane, among others, are suitable compounds.

REFERENCES

Baker, R. N., et al., Toxic volatiles in alcoholic coma, *Bull. Los Angeles County Neurol. Soc.*, 33, 140, 1968.

Wallace, J. E. and Dahl, E. V., Rapid vapor phase method for determining ethanol in blood and urine by gas chromatography, *Am. J. Clin. Pathol.*, 46, 152, 1966.

ETHCHLORVYNOL

PRINCIPLE

Ethchlorvynol reacts with diphenylamine to form a pink color. The absorbance can be used for qualitative identification and quantitative measurement of the ethchlorvynol concentration in urine or protein-free filtrates of blood (Procedures A and B). Ethyl acetate will extract ethchlorvynol from biological fluids, and aliquots of the extract can be analyzed by gas chromatography (Procedure C).

TYPE A PROCEDURE

Bryan S. Finkle and Raymond Bath

APPARATUS

1. Centrifuge tubes, 10 ml
2. Mixer (Vortex)
3. Centrifuge

REAGENTS

All chemicals should be analytical reagent grade.

1. Trichloroacetic acid, 10.0 g/100 ml
   Dissolve 10.0 g of trichloroacetic acid and 1.0 g of sodium chloride in water and dilute to 100 ml.
2. Ethchlorvynol stock solution, 10 mg/100 ml
   Dissolve 10.0 mg of ethchlorvynol in approximately 50.0 ml of ethanol and dilute to 100 ml with water.
3. Ethchlorvynol reference solutions
   Dilute appropriate volumes of the stock solution to obtain solutions containing 0.05 to 0.5 mg of ethchlorvynol/100 ml.
4. Color reagent
   Dissolve 1.0 g of diphenylamine in 50.0 ml of concentrated sulfuric acid. Carefully add this solution, while stirring, to a mixture of 50.0 ml of water and 50.0 ml of glacial acetic acid.
5. Control reagent
   Carefully add 50.0 ml of concentrated sulfuric acid, while stirring, to a mixture of 50.0 ml of water and 50.0 ml of glacial acetic acid.

PROCEDURE

1. To 2.0 ml of serum or plasma add 8.0 ml of the trichloroacetic acid solution, mix in a Vortex mixer, then centrifuge.
2. Add 3.0 ml of color reagent to a 2.0 ml aliquot of the supernatant from Step 1 (or 2.0-ml of urine or centrifuged gastric content), 2.0 ml of each reference solution, and 2.0 ml of the control reagent.
3. If ethchlorvynol is present, a stable red color will develop, slowly at first, but with increasing intensity up to 2 hr. The red color is partially extractable into chloroform.

INTERPRETATION (see p. 7)

No meaningful interpretation related to the subject's behavior or condition can be made from Procedure A. A positive result simply indicates that the subject ingested ethchlorvynol, in which case this test should be followed by a quantitative procedure for ethchlorvynol.* A positive result with the control reagent indicates that a phenothiazine may be present.

ACCURACY AND PRECISION

This procedure will detect 0.01 mg of ethchlorvynol/100 ml of specimen.

*See pp. 156 and 157.

Note: It is extremely important to smell the gastric content. Ethchlorvynol has a very characteristic pungent odor even at a very low concentration.

INTERFERING SUBSTANCES

The test using the control reagent is necessary to rule out interference from phenothiazines and related drugs.

REFERENCES*

Andryauskas, S., Matusiak, W., and Dal Cortivo, L. A., Ethchlorvynol in toxicological analysis, *Int. Microfilm J. Legal Med.*, *2*, Card 4, 1967.

Frings, C. S. and Cohen, P. S., Rapid colorimetric method for the quantitative determination of ethchlorvynol (placidyl) in serum and urine, *Am. J. Clin. Pathol.*, 54, 833, 1970.

TYPE B PROCEDURE

Bryan S. Finkle and Raymond Bath

APPARATUS

1. Centrifuge tubes, 10 ml
2. Mixer (Vortex)
3. Centrifuge
4. Serological pipets, 5 ml
5. Spectrophotometer

REAGENTS

All chemicals should be analytical reagent grade.

1. Trichloroacetic acid, 10 g/100 ml
   Dissolve 10.0 g of trichloroacetic acid and 1.0 g of sodium chloride in water and dilute to 100 ml.
2. Ethchlorvynol stock solution, 10 mg/100 ml
   Dissolve 10.0 mg of ethchlorvynol in approximately 50.0 ml of ethanol and dilute to 100 ml with water.
3. Ethchlorvynol reference solutions
   Dilute appropriate volumes of the stock solution to obtain solutions containing 0.05 to 0.5 mg of ethchlorvynol/100 ml.
4. Color reagent
   Dissolve 1.0 g of diphenylamine in 50.0 ml of concentrated sulfuric acid. Carefully add this solution, while stirring, to a mixture of 50.0 ml of water and 50.0 ml of glacial acetic acid.
5. Control reagent
   Carefully add 50.0 ml of concentrated sulfuric acid, while stirring, to a mixture of 50.0 ml of water and 50.0 ml of glacial acetic acid.

PROCEDURE

1. To 2.0 ml of blood add 8.0 ml of the trichloroacetic acid solution, mix in a Vortex mixer, then centrifuge.
2. Into duplicate sets of clean test tubes place 2.0-ml aliquots of the clear supernatant from Step 1, or 2.0 ml of urine or centrifuged gastric content, and 2.0 ml of each reference solution.
3. Add 3.0 ml of the color reagent to one set of tubes and 3.0 ml of the control reagent to the other. The latter will serve as reagent blanks for the corresponding sample solutions.
4. Mix each solution in a Vortex mixer.
5. After 2 hr measure the absorbance of each sample solution at 510 nm, using the corresponding reagent blank as reference. The color is stable for 8 hr.

CALCULATION

1. The relationship between the absorbance and the concentration of ethchlorvynol is linear from 0.02 to 0.2 mg/100 ml and is valid when intensely colored unknowns are diluted with color reagent. Determine the ethchlorvynol concentration in the specimen by comparing

*For an updated list of reference material, see References, p. 159.

its absorbance with that of a suitably chosen reference solution.

2. Calculate the ethchlorvynol concentration in the specimen by using the following formula:*

$$C_S = \frac{A_S}{A_R} \times C_R,$$

where

C_S = concentration of the specimen;
A_S = absorbance of the specimen;
A_R = absorbance of the reference solution;
C_R = concentration of the reference solution.

INTERPRETATION (see p. 7)

Following oral ingestion of 200 mg of ethchlorvynol, the highest concentration in blood occurred within 1 to 2 hr and ranged up to 0.15 mg/100 ml. After 1 hr blood concentrations ranged from 0.06 mg to 0.15 mg/100 ml. The half-life of ethchlorvynol is estimated to be 1 hr.

Blood concentrations following continuous therapeutic dosages rarely exceed 1.0 to 2.0 mg/100 ml. Blood concentrations higher than 5.0 mg/100 ml will almost certainly result in coma and can, without medical aid, cause death.

Fatal blood and liver concentrations vary greatly. When only ethchlorvynol is involved, blood concentrations are usually higher than 6.0 mg/100 ml; however, in conjunction with relatively small amounts of ethanol (0.05 to 0.15%), ethchlorvynol concentrations as low as 2.5 mg/100 ml can prove fatal. The complete circumstances of a fatality (particularly the victim's health before death and the time interval between ingestion and death) must be considered when judging the significance of blood and tissue concentrations. Following long coma, post-mortem blood concentrations are often lower than ante-mortem concentrations.

ACCURACY AND PRECISION

Recovery of ethchlorvynol from blood and urine is 85 to 95%. The sensitivity of the color reaction is approximately 0.01 mg/100 ml. The coefficient of variation at 1.3 mg/100 ml is 3%.

INTERFERING SUBSTANCES

Concentrations of formaldehyde, acetaldehyde, acetone, or paraldehyde in excess of 0.1% will inhibit the color development. This can be overcome by extracting the developed color with chloroform. No other materials are known to interfere. Phenazopyridine has been reported to interfere.

REFERENCE†

Andryauskas, S., Matusiak, W., and Dal Cortivo, L. A., Ethchlorvynol in toxicological analysis, *Int. Microfilm J. Legal Med.*, 2, Card 4, 1967.

TYPE C PROCEDURE

Gerald Kananen

APPARATUS

1. Culture tubes, screw-capped, with Teflon®-faced liners (Kontes 45066 A), 16 × 125 mm
2. Multipurpose rotator (Model 150V)‡
3. Centrifuge
4. Graduated test tubes, conical (Kontes 41055)
5. Syringes (Hamilton 701-N), 10 μl
6. Gas chromatograph, dual column (F & M Model 402), equipped with a flame ionization detector, a 1 mV recorder (Minneapolis-Honeywell Model 15) with attached Disc

*For blood, this must be multiplied by 5 because a 2.0-ml aliquot of 10.0 ml was used.
†For an updated list of reference material, see References, p. 159.
‡Scientific Industries, Inc., Springfield, Mass.

integrator (Model 201b), and a glass column, 6′ × ¼″ o.d., packed with 1% Hi-Eff 3-BP (neopentyl glycol succinate) on 80/100 mesh Gas Chrom Q

Operating Conditions

Gas Flow Rates:
- nitrogen – 35 ml/min
- hydrogen – 25 ml/min
- air – 500 ml/min

Temperatures:
- column – 110°C
- injection port – 150°C
- detector – 190°C

Condition the column overnight at 140°C prior to use. Recondition the column for 1 hr at 140°C after the analysis of 20 biological samples or when necessary.

REAGENTS

All chemicals should be analytical reagent grade.

1. Acetone
2. Ethchlorvynol stock solution, 100 mg/100 ml
   Dissolve 100 mg of ethchlorvynol in a few milliliters of acetone. Dilute this solution to 100 ml with water.
3. Ethchlorvynol reference solutions
   Dilute 0.25, 1.0, 5.0, and 10.0 ml of the ethchlorvynol stock solution to 100 ml with water.
4. Ethyl acetate
5. GC-standardizing solution
   Dissolve 50.0 mg of ethchlorvynol in ethyl acetate. Dilute this solution to 100 ml with ethyl acetate.

PROCEDURE

1. Pipet 3.0 ml of specimen (blood, urine, stomach content, or the homogenate made from 3.0 g of tissue and 3.0 g of water) into a 15-ml screw-capped culture tube. Pipet 3.0 ml of the ethchlorvynol reference solution into a second tube.
2. Add 3.0 ml of ethyl acetate to each tube. Cap the tubes and place them for 10 to 15 min on the rotator.
3. Centrifuge the tubes for 5 min at 2,000 rpm.
4. Transfer a 2.0-ml aliquot of the supernatant ethyl acetate to a graduated conical test tube.
5. Concentrate the ethyl acetate to 0.2 ml by evaporation under a stream of dry nitrogen.*
6. Inject a 5.0-μl aliquot of the ethyl acetate concentrate into the gas chromatograph, making sure that the operating conditions stated above are met.

CALCULATION

Calculate the ethchlorvynol concentration in the specimen by the following formula:

$$C_S = C_R \times \frac{P_S}{P_R} \times \frac{V_F}{V_I} \times \frac{S_I}{S_F},$$

where

- C_S = ethchlorvynol concentration in the specimen;
- C_R = ethchlorvynol concentration in the GC-standardizing solution;
- P_S = peak area for ethchlorvynol in the specimen;
- P_R = peak area for ethchlorvynol in the reference solution;
- V_F = volume of ethyl acetate concentrate (0.2 ml);
- V_I = volume of the specimen;
- S_I = volume of ethyl acetate used for extraction;
- S_F = volume of the aliquot of ethyl acetate injected (0.5 μl).

INTERPRETATION (see p. 7)

Following oral ingestion of 200 mg of ethchlorvynol, the highest concentration in blood occurred within 1 to 2 hr and ranged up to 0.15 mg/100 ml. After 1 hr blood concentrations ranged from 0.06 to 0.15 mg/100 ml. The half-life of ethchlorvynol is estimated to be 1 hr. Blood concentrations following continuous therapeutic dosages rarely exceed 1.0 to 2.0 mg/100 ml. Blood concentrations higher than 5.0 mg/100 ml will almost

*This evaporation will result in a significant loss of ethchlorvynol unless done at room temperature or if the evaporation proceeds to a dry residue.

Specimen	Ethchlorvynol added, mg/100 ml	Number of determinations	% Recovery
Aqueous	0.25	4	72 ± 4.2
	1	3	80 ± 4.0
	5	3	94 ± 1.3
	10	3	96 ± 1.3
Urine	0.25	4	61 ± 1.6
	1	3	81 ± 2.3
	5	3	92 ± 2.1
	10	3	100 ± 3.6
Blood	0.25	4	60 ± 2.7
	1	3	79 ± 3.3
	5	3	98 ± 5.3
	10	3	99 ± 5.3
Liver	5	2	90 ± 3.2

certainly result in coma and can, without medical aid, cause death.

Fatal blood and liver concentrations vary greatly. When only ethchlorvynol is involved, blood concentrations are usually higher than 6.0 mg/100 ml; however, in conjunction with relatively small amounts of ethanol (0.05 to 0.15%), ethchlorvynol concentrations as low as 2.5 mg/100 ml can prove fatal. The complete circumstances of a fatality (particularly the victim's health before death and the time interval between ingestion and death) must be considered when judging the significance of blood and tissue concentrations. Following long coma, post-mortem blood concentrations are often lower than ante-mortem concentrations.

ACCURACY AND PRECISION

Recovery of ethchlorvynol from biological specimens is shown in the table above.

INTERFERING SUBSTANCES

Under these conditions, no other drugs were noted whose peaks could be construed to have the same retention time as the one due to ethchlorvynol.

REFERENCES

Cantrell, J. W., Hopkins, N. E., Queen, C. A., and Frings, C. S., Effect of phenazopyridine hydrochloride (Pyridrium®) on determination of ethchlorvynol, *Clin. Chem.*, 18, 591, 1972.

Cummins, L. M., Martin, Y. C., and Scherfling, E. E., Serum and urine levels of ethchlorvynol in man, *J. Pharm. Sci.*, 60, 261, 1971.

Evenson, M. A. and Poquette, M. A., Rapid GC method for quantitation of ethchlorvynol in serum, *Clin. Chem.*, 20, 212, 1974.

Gibson, P. F. and Wright, N., Ethchlorvynol in biological fluids: specificity of assay methods, *J. Pharm. Sci.*, 61, 169, 1972.

Maes, R., Hodnett, N., Landesman, H., Kananen, G., Finkle, B., and Sunshine, I., The gas chromatographic determination of selected sedatives (ethchlorvynol, paraldehyde, meprobamate, carisoprodol) in biological material, *J. Forensic Sci.*, 14, 235, 1969.

ETHOSUXIMIDE

PRINCIPLE

Ethosuximide is extracted from serum with toluene containing the internal standard. The toluene is subsequently extracted with ammonium hydroxide to remove the ethosuximide. The ammonium hydroxide is acidified with phosphoric acid, and the ethosuximide is extracted into dichloromethane. This solvent is evaporated at room temperature and the *N*-butyl derivative of ethosuximide is prepared by reaction with butyl iodide in *N,N*-dimethylacetamide. This derivative is quantitated relative to the internal standard by gas chromatography.

TYPE C PROCEDURE

Charles J. Least, Jr., George F. Johnson, and Harvey M. Solomon

APPARATUS

1. Eppendorf Pipets, 500 and 1,000 μl
2. Repipets®, 10 and 5 ml
3. Microliter syringe, 10 μl
4. Culture tubes, 16 X 125 mm, with Teflon®-lined screw caps
5. Centrifuge tubes, 13 ml, with Teflon®-lined screw caps
6. Concentratubes®,* 18 X 114 mm (nipple tubes)
7. Pasteur pipets
8. Centrifuge
9. Vortex mixer
10. Eberback shaker
11. Ultrasonic bath
12. Nitrogen evaporator
13. Gas chromatograph equipped with a flame ionization detector, 1 mV recorder and a glass column 4′ X 2 mm i.d., packed with 3% OV-1 on 100/120 Gas Mesh Chrom Q

Operating Conditions

Gas Flow Rate:
- nitrogen – 40 ml/min

Temperatures:
- column – post injection hold for 2 min at initial oven temperature of 100°C, programmed 100° to 120° at 8°/min, followed by a 2 min hold at 120°C.
- injection port – 200°C
- detector – 250°C

REAGENTS

All chemicals should be analytical reagent grade.

1. Phosphate buffer, 1*M*, pH 6.8
   (a) Prepare 1*M* K_2HPO_4: Dissolve 87.1 g of K_2HPO_4 in 500 ml of distilled water; (b) Prepare 1*M* KH_2PO_4: Dissolve 68.0 g of KH_2PO_4 in 500 ml of distilled water; (c) Using a pH meter, adjust the K_2HPO_4 with KH_2PO_4 to a pH of 6.8.
2. Stock ethosuximide standard, 100 μg/ml
   Dissolve 50 mg ethosuximide (Parke, Davis and Co.) in 1*M* phosphate buffer and dilute to 500 ml with 1*M* phosphate buffer.
3. Working ethosuximide standards
   Make appropriate dilutions of stock standard with 1*M* phosphate buffer to give working solutions of 10, 20, 40, 60 and 80 μg ethosuximide/ml of buffer.
4. Stock internal standard solution, 500μg/ml
   Dissolve 250 mg of α,α-dimethyl-β-methyl succinimide (Aldrich Chemical Co.) in toluene and dilute to 500 ml with toluene.
5. Working internal standard solution, 5 μg/ml
   Dilute 10 ml of the stock internal standard solution to one liter with toluene.
6. Dichloromethane, chromatoquality (Matheson, Coleman and Bell)
7. Toluene, chromatoquality (Matheson, Coleman and Bell)
8. *N,N*-dimethylacetamide, spectrophotometric grade (Aldrich Chemical Co.)

*Laboratory Research Co., P.O. Box 36509, Los Angeles, California.

9. Iodobutane, 99% (Aldrich Chemical Co.)
10. Tetramethylammonium hydroxide (TMH)
 Dilute the 24% in methanol solution (obtainable from Matheson, Coleman and Bell), 1:10 (V:V) with methanol. Store at 4°C.
11. Ammonium hydroxide, 0.5*M*
 Dilute 3.4 ml of concentrated NH_4OH to 100 ml with distilled water.
12. Sodium sulfate, anhydrous
13. Phosphoric acid, 5.7*M*
 Add 390 ml of 85% H_3PO_4 to distilled water and dilute to one liter with distilled water.

PROCEDURE

1. To 0.5 ml of patient's plasma or serum in a 16 X 125 mm screw-top culture tube with Teflon®-lined cap, add 1.0 ml of 1*M* phosphate buffer. For quantitate controls, add 1.0 ml of the appropriate working standard to 0.5 ml of drug-free plasma to yield standards of 10, 20, 40, 60 and 80 μg of ethosuximide.
2. Add 7.0 ml of the working internal standard solution to each tube.
3. Extract for 10 min on a shaker at 250 oscillations/min and centrifuge all tubes at 2,000 rpm for 5 min.
4. Transfer the toluene phase to a 13-ml screw-top centrifuge tube with a Teflon®-lined cap, and add 0.5 ml of 0.5*M* NH_4OH while holding each tube in an ultrasonic bath to disperse the base. A Vortex mixer is not an adequate substitute for the ultrasonic bath.
5. Extract for 10 min at 250 oscillations/min.
6. Centrifuge all tubes at 2,000 rpm for 5 min and remove the toluene phase by aspiration
7. Acidify the remaining aqueous phase with 100 μl of 5.7*M* H_3PO_4, mix by vortexing, and add 5 ml of dichloromethane to each tube.
8. Extract for 10 min on the shaker and centrifuge at 2,000 rpm for 5 min.
9. Remove the aqueous phase by aspiration and add about 0.5 g of Na_2SO_4.
 Mix well and centrifuge for 2 min at 2,000 rpm.
10. Decant the dichloromethane into nipple tubes and evaporate at room temperature to dryness.
11. To each tube add 40 μl of *N,N*-dimethylacetamide, 10 μl of dilute TMH solution and 10 μl iodobutane. Mix by vortexing after each addition and then let the tubes rest for 10 min vertically in a rack. Centrifuge at 1,000 rpm for 1 min and inject 1 μl of the supernatant into the gas chromatograph.
12. Measure the peak heights of the internal standards and the ethosuximide for the standard solutions and the specimens.

CALCULATION

1. Calculate the ratio of the peak height of ethosuximide to that of the peak height of the internal standard. Plot these ratios against the amount of ethosuximide in each of the internal standards.
2. Determine the quantity of ethosuximide in the samples by determining the amount of ethosuximide which corresponds to the calculated peak height ratio obtained from the analysis of the sample (12 above). Determine the concentration of ethosuximide in μg/ml by dividing this amount of ethosuximide by the volume of sample in milliliters.

INTERPRETATION (see p. 7)

Patients receiving an average daily dose of ethosuximide of 20.7 ± 5.8 mg/kg had an average plasma concentration of 40.0 ± 14.9 μg/ml with a range of 10.8 to 55.2 μg/ml. In a group of patients whose seizures were effectively controlled with ethosuximide, none had plasma levels of less than 30 μg/ml and only 9% had levels below 40 μg/ml. Although plasma concentrations of ethosuximide as high as 168 μg/ml have been observed, it has not been possible to establish a relation between toxicity and the plasma concentration of this drug.

ACCURACY AND PRECISION

Ethosuximide recovery from serum ranged from 95 to 105%. The limit of sensitivity of the procedure is 1 μg of ethosuximide/ml serum. The coefficient of variation of the assay at 40 μg/ml is 4% between runs.

INTERFERING SUBSTANCES

This procedure shows no interferences from

normal constituents of plasma or from the following anticonvulsant drugs: trimethadione, dimethadione, phenobarbital, diphenylhydantoin, primidone, methsuximide, phensuximide, mephenytoin, metharbital, and carbamazepine.

REFERENCES

Greeley, R. H., New approach to derivatization and gas chromatographic analysis of barbiturates, *Clin. Chem.*, 20, 192, 1974.

Kutt, H., Pharmacodynamic and pharmacokinetic measurements of antiepileptic drugs, *Clin. Pharmacol. Ther.*, 16, 243, 1974.

Sherwin, A. L., Robb, J. P., and Lechter, M., Improved control of epilepsy by monitoring plasma ethosuximide, *Arch. Neurol.*, 28, 178, 1973.

Solow, E. B. and Green, J. B., The determination of ethosuximide in serum by gas chromatography. Preliminary results of clinical application, *Clin. Chim. Acta*, 33, 87, 1971.

Solow, E. B., Metaxas, J. M., and Summers, T. R., Antiepileptic drugs: A current assessment of simultaneous determination of multiple drug therapy by gas liquid chromatography on column methylation, *J. Chromatogr. Sci.*, 12, 256, 1974.

Van der Kleijn, E., et al., GC determination of ethosuximide and phensuximide in plasma and urine of man, *J. Pharm. Pharmacol.*, 25, 4, 1973.

ETHYLENE GLYCOL

PRINCIPLE

The oxidation product of ethylene glycol reacts with Schiff's reagent to give a characteristic colored product whose absorbance is used to measure the ethylene glycol content of the sample (Procedure B). In Procedure C propylene glycol and ethylene glycol are determined by direct injection of blood and urine onto a polar column in a gas chromatograph equipped with a flame ionization detector. Tissue samples are treated first with 1.2*N* perchloric acid to precipitate protein and prepare them for GLC analysis.

TYPE B PROCEDURE

Edgar W. Kivela and Staff

APPARATUS

1. Brown bottle, glass-stoppered, 250 ml
2. Serological pipets, 0.25, 1.0, 5.00, and 10.0 ml
3. Erlenmeyer flasks, 25 and 250 ml
4. Glass funnels, small
5. Filter paper (Whatman #1), 9-cm circles
6. Test tubes, 10 and 15 ml
7. Clock or stopwatch
8. Spectrophotometer or photoelectric photometer with a 600-nm filter

REAGENTS

All chemicals should be analytical reagent grade.

1. Ethylene glycol stock solution, 100 mg/100 ml
   Dissolve 100 mg of ethylene glycol in water and dilute to 100 ml with water.
2. Ethylene glycol reference solutions
   Dilute 7.0, 5.0, 3.0, and 1.0 ml of the ethylene glycol stock solution to 10 ml with distilled water. The resulting solutions have ethylene glycol concentrations of 0.7, 0.5, 0.3, and 0.1 mg/ml, respectively.
3. Sodium tungstate, 10 g/100 ml
   Dissolve 10 g of sodium tungstate in water and dilute to 100 ml with water.
4. Sulfuric acid, 0.67*N*
   Add 1.86 ml of concentrated sulfuric acid (36*N*) to about 80 ml of distilled water and mix. Allow the solution to cool, then dilute it to 100 ml.
5. Periodic acid, 0.1*M*
   Dissolve 2.28 g of periodic acid (H_5IO_6) or 2.14 g of sodium periodate ($NaIO_4$) in 0.67*N* sulfuric acid and dilute to 100 ml with the acid.
6. Basic fuchsin, crystalline
7. Sodium metabisulfite ($Na_2S_2O_5$)
8. Hydrochloric acid, concentrated
9. Shiff's reagent
   To a 250-ml Erlenmeyer flask containing 120 ml of water heated to almost boiling, add 0.2 g of basic fuchsin. After the dye is dissolved, cool the contents of the flask to room temperature under running water. Dissolve 2 g of sodium metabisulfide in 20 ml of water and add this solution to the cooled fuchsin solution. Add 2 ml of concentrated hydrochloric acid and 60 ml water to the flask, mix thoroughly, then filter the mixture. Store the reagent in a glass-stoppered brown bottle in a refrigerator. This solution is stable for several months.

PROCEDURE

1. Dilute 1.0 ml of blood or urine with 7.0 ml of water in a 25-ml Erlenmeyer flask. Process 1.0 ml of each reference solution and 1.0 ml of water for a reagent blank in the same manner as the specimen.
2. Add 1.0 ml of the sodium tungstate solution to each flask.
3. With vigorous shaking, add 1.0 ml of 0.67*N* sulfuric acid, drop by drop, to each mixture. Stopper the flasks and shake well.

4. Filter the contents of each flask into 15-ml test tubes.
5. Place 1.0 ml of each filtrate in a 10-ml test tube. Add 4.0 ml of water.
6. Add 0.25 ml of the periodic acid reagent to each tube and mix. Let the mixtures stand for 10 min.
7. Add 2.0 ml of Schiff's reagent to each tube and mix. Let the mixtures stand for 25 min.
8. Determine the absorbances of the products obtained from the test sample and from each reference solution at 555 nm, using the processed water sample as the reference solution.

CALCULATION

Determine the concentration of ethylene glycol in the blood or urine sample by direct comparison of its absorbance with that of a reference solution of comparable value.

INTERPRETATION (see p. 7)

Harger and Forney[1] report that loss of ethylene glycol occurs on storage of the specimen. In one case they noted that the blood concentration dropped from 385 mg/100 ml to 80 mg/100 ml after storing the specimen in a refrigerator for 12 days.

Ethylene glycol concentrations of 5 mg/100 ml of blood and 2 mg/100 ml of urine have been reported in fatal cases. If death from ethylene glycol poisoning is rapid, concentrations of several hundred milligrams per 100 ml can be found in blood. If death is delayed for several days, the ethylene glycol concentrations in the blood will be very low, in some cases barely detectable. In the latter case, the concentration of oxalic acid should be determined, and the kidney should be investigated for the presence of oxalic acid crystals. (Oxalate crystals may be observed microscopically in polarized light in urine specimens. Oxalate may be quantitated indirectly by atomic absorption spectrophotometry by measuring total and free calcium in urine samples to which calcium has been added.)[2]

ACCURACY AND PRECISION

The standard curve, if plotted, would not follow the Beer-Lambert Law. All calculations should be made by direct comparison of solutions of similar concentration. Recovery of ethylene glycol from blood and urine is 100 ± 5%.

INTERFERING SUBSTANCES

Ethanol and methanol, if present, do not interfere. Tissues give high blank values, up to the equivalent of 35 mg of ethylene glycol/100 g of tissue. This method is, therefore, not recommended for tissue extracts. As blood specimens age, high blank values will develop. It is therefore, recommended that this procedure not be used on blood specimens more than 12 hr after collection from a live subject, or in fatal cases, more than 12 hr after death has occurred.

REFERENCES

1. **Harger, R. N. and Forney, R. B.,** A simple method for detecting and estimating ethylene glycol in body materials: analytical results in six fatal cases, *J. Forensic Sci.*, 4, 136, 1959.
2. **Menache, R.,** Routine micro determination of oxalic acid in urine by atomic absorption spectrophotometry, *Clin. Chem.*, 20, 1444, 1974.

TYPE C PROCEDURE

Naresh C. Jain and Robert Forney, Jr.

APPARATUS

1. Blender (Waring)
2. Centrifuge, large, 6″ head radius
3. Gas chromatograph, equipped with flame ionization detectors, a 1 mV recorder, and a glass column, 6′ × 1/4″ o.d. and 6′ × 1/8″ i.d., packed with 80 to 100 mesh Porapak Q (Water Associates, Framingham, Mass.)

Operating Conditions

Gas Flow Rates:
- helium – 50 ml/min
- air* – 300 ml/min
- hydrogen –

Temperatures:
- column–240°C
- injection part – 280°C
- detector – 280°C

Condition the column for 24 hr at 220°C.

REAGENTS

All chemicals should be analytical reagent grade.

1. Propylene glycol reference solutions
   Dissolve quantities of propylene glycol ranging from 100 to 200 mg in water and dilute each solution to 100 ml.
2. Ethylene glycol reference solution, 90 mg/100 ml
   Dissolve 90 mg of ethylene glycol in water and dilute to 100 ml.
3. Perchloric acid, 1.2*N*
   Dilute 10 ml of concentrated (70%) perchloric acid to 100 ml with water.
4. Potassium carbonate, saturated aqueous solution

PREPARATION OF SPECIMENS

Tissue

1. Place 20 g of tissue in chilled Waring blender cup.
2. Add 80 ml of 1.2*N* perchloric acid.
3. Homogenize the tissue for 2 min.
4. Immediately pour the homogenate into a 250-ml centrifuge bottle. Stopper the bottle and centrifuge it for 15 min at 3,000 rpm.

Stomach Content

1. Add to centrifuge tube a 5.0-ml aliquot of specimen and 20.0 ml of 1.2*N* perchloric acid.
2. Centrifuge the mixture for 15 min at 3,000 rpm.

Blood and urine do not require preparation.

PROCEDURE

1. Examine the gas chromatograph to be sure that all conditions stated above are met. Inject reference solutions. Retention times for propylene glycol and ethylene glycol should be approximately 2.7 and 1.8 min, respectively.
2. Place a 5.0-ml aliquot of the supernatant from the centrifuged specimen in a chilled centrifuge tube and carefully neutralize the perchloric acid with 0.5 ml of saturated solution of potassium carbonate.
3. After the evolution of carbon dioxide is completed, stopper the tube and centrifuge it for 5 min at 1,500 rpm.
4. Add 1.0 ml of the resulting supernatant fluid, blood or urine, to 1.0 ml of the appropriate internal control† solution and inject a 1- or 2-μl aliquot of this mixture into the gas chromatograph.

*Pure oxygen is used for increased sensitivity.

†Since ethylene glycol and propylene glycol can be used as internal standards for each other, use ethylene glycol as the internal control solution when assaying propylene glycol, and vice versa.

CALCULATION

Calculate the concentration of the unknown compound in the biological specimen preparation as follows:

$$C_X = C_S \times \frac{H_X}{R_X} \times \frac{R_S}{H_S},$$

where

C_X = concentration of the unknown;
C_S = concentration of the substance to be assayed in the reference solution;
H_S = peak height of the substance to be assayed in the reference mixture;
H_X = peak height of the specimen mixture at the retention time of the substance to be assayed;
R_S = peak height of the internal control in the reference mixture;
R_X = peak height of the internal control in the specimen mixture.

INTERPRETATION (see p. 7)

Harger and Forney[1] report that loss of ethylene glycol occurs on storage of the specimen. In one case they noted that the blood concentration dropped from 385 mg/100 ml to 80 mg/100 ml after storing the specimen in a refrigerator for 12 days.

Ethylene glycol concentrations of 5 mg/100 ml of blood and 2 mg/100 ml of urine have been reported in fatal cases. If death from ethylene glycol poisoning is rapid, concentrations of several hundred milligrams per 100 ml can be found in blood. If death is delayed for several days, the ethylene glycol concentrations in the blood will be very low, in some cases barely detectable. In the latter case, the concentration of oxalic acid should be determined, and the kidney should be investigated for the presence of oxalic acid crystals. (Oxalate crystals may be observed microscopically in polarized light in urine specimens. Oxalate may be quantitated indirectly by atomic absorption spectrophotometry by measuring total and free calcium in urine samples to which calcium has been added).[2]

Propylene glycol is metabolized in a manner similar to the carbohydrates and is less toxic than ethylene glycol. As much as 50% of a given dose may be recovered in the urine.

ACCURACY AND PRECISION

1. Known quantities of propylene glycol, when added to tissue homogenates and analyzed by the above method, gave recovery values ranging from 100 to 111%, with an average of 105%. Blank tissue homogenates similarly analyzed gave an average propylene glycol value of 6 mg/100 ml, which could be due to the fact that propylene glycol is normally present in biological tissues.
2. For ethylene glycol the recovery values ranged from 95 to 100%. Blank tissue homogenates contained no apparent ethylene glycol.

INTERFERING SUBSTANCES

No peaks are found to interfere with the quantitation of ethylene or propylene glycol when blank tissue homogenates are injected into the gas chromatograph.

REFERENCES

1. **Harger, R. N. and Forney, R. B.,** A simple method for detecting and estimating ethylene glycol in body materials: analytical results in six fatal cases, *J. Forensic Sci.*, 4, 136, 1959.
2. **Menache, R.,** Routine micro method for determination of oxalic acid in urine by atomic absorption spectrophotometry, *Clin. Chem.*, 20, 1444, 1974.

GENERAL REFERENCES

Balakhontseva, V. N. and Poltinina, R. M., Determination of glycols by gas chromatography, *Zh. Analit. Klin.*, 29, 757, 1964.

Brown, D. J., Jain, N. C., Forney, R. B., Hughes, F. W., and Richards, A. B., Gas-Chromatographic assay of glycol – ethanol combinations in biological materials, *J. Forensic Sci.*, 13, 537, 1968.

Davis, A., Roaldi, A., and Tufts, L. E., Detection of traces of glycol by gas chromatography, *J. Gas Chromatogr.*, 2, 306, 1964.

Harger, R. N., and Forney, R. B., A simple method for detecting and estimating ethylene glycol in body materials: analytical results in six fatal cases, *J. Forensic Sci.*, 4, 136, 1959.

Parry, M. F. and Wallach, R., Ethylene glycol poisoning, *Am. J. Med.*, 57, 143, 1974.

Pons, C. A. and Custer, R. P., Acute ethylene glycol poisoning, *Am. J. Med. Sci.*, 211, 544, 1946.

FLUORIDE

PRINCIPLE

Fluorides may be separated from their matrix by acidifying the sample and trapping the evolved hydrogen fluoride. Plastic Conway cells or petri dishes are very suitable for this purpose, and the evolved hydrogen fluoride can be trapped in appropriate reagents. The absorbance of the trapping reagent or the product formed by reacting it with a suitable chromophoric reagent can be used to determine fluoride concentrations (Procedures A and B). More simply, a specific ion electrode can be used to quantitate the fluoride content (Procedure C).

TYPE A PROCEDURE

Fredric Rieders

APPARATUS

1. Microdiffusion dishes, polypropylene, Öbrink modification*
   Clean the dishes before use with nitric acid and distilled water.

REAGENTS

All chemicals should be analytical reagent grade. All water used to prepare the reagents should be redistilled and free of fluorides.

1. Fluoride-liberating reagent I, sulfuric acid containing 0.025% Tergitol®
   To 25 ml of distilled water in a 500-ml Erlenmeyer flask, add 25 µl of Tergitol®. Place the flask into a shallow pan containing a mixture of ice and water. Add slowly, with intermittent swirling, 80 ml of concentrated sulfuric acid to the flask. Stopper the flask with a polyethylene plug. This solution is stable indefinitely. If a blood specimen is suspected to contain products of putrefaction, use the following liberating agent.
2. Fluoride-liberating reagent II, silver sulfate in concentrated perchloric acid, 0.25*M*
   Dissolve 4.0 g of silver sulfate in a mixture containing 2 ml of distilled water and 23 ml of concentrated perchloric acid. If necessary, heat the mixture to about 80°C to insure solution. After solution has been effected, add 75 ml of concentrated perchloric acid. Cool the mixture, then transfer it to an amber glass-stoppered bottle. If kept refrigerated, this solution is stable indefinitely.
3. Acetic acid, 0.25*M*
   Dilute 1.44 ml of glacial acetic acid to 100 ml with distilled water.
4. Sodium acetate, 0.25*M*
   Dissolve 34.02 g of sodium acetate ($CH_3COONa \cdot 3H_2O$) in distilled water. Dilute the solution to one liter with distilled water.
5. Acetate buffer, pH 5.4
   Mix 100 ml of 0.25*M* acetic acid with 457 ml of 0.25*M* sodium acetate. Adjust the pH to 5.4 by adding more acetic acid or sodium acetate as needed.
6. Alizarin Complexone®, 0.001*M*
   Dissolve 0.388 g of alizarin Complexone®† in pH 5.4 acetate buffer with gentle warming on a steam bath. Cool to room temperature, then dilute the solution to one liter with the buffer. This solution is stable for at least 6 months.
7. Lanthanum nitrate, 0.001*M*
   Dissolve 0.433 g of lanthanum nitrate ($La(NO_3)_3 \cdot 6H_2O$) in one liter of water. This solution is stable indefinitely.
8. Fluoride-trapping reagent
   Mix equal volumes of 0.001*M* alizarin Complexone® and 0.001*M* lanthanum nitrate just prior to use.
9. Fluoride-trapping reagent, alternate
   Dissolve 1.0 g of Amadac-F®‡ in 20 ml of distilled water. Add 30 ml of isopropyl alco-

*Available from A. H. Thomas Co., Cat. No. 4472-S, Size 68.
†3,5-Dihydroxy-2-anthraquinone methyl iminodiacetic acid dihydrate, Aldrich 12765-5.
‡3,5-Dihydroxy-2-anthraquinone methyl iminodiacetic acid hydrate, Aldrich 12765-5.

hol, then transfer the solution to a glass-stoppered bottle. If kept refrigerated, this solution is stable for at least 10 days.

10. Fluoride stock solution, 0.1 mg/ml
Dissolve 0.2210 g of sodium fluoride in distilled water and dilute to one liter. Store the solution in a polyethylene bottle.
11. Fluoride reference solution, 1 μg/ml
Dilute 1.0 ml of the fluoride stock solution to 100 ml with distilled water. Prepare fresh just before use.

PROCEDURE

1. Place approximately 2 ml of fluoride-liberating reagent (I or II) into the outermost (sealing) well of a microdiffusion dish.
2. Place 1 ml of the same liberating reagent on one side of the intermediate annular well.
3. Place 1 ml of the fluoride-trapping reagent in the center well.
4. Place a 1-ml sample of well-mixed unknown blood on the other side of the intermediate annular well, away from the liberating reagent.
5. Seal the microdiffusion dish by twisting the cover so that it makes a continuous liquid seal in the outer well.
6. Gently tilt the sealed dish back and forth to mix the blood sample with the liberating reagent and distribute this mixture over the entire surface of the intermediate annular well.
7. Prepare control samples by processing 1 ml of distilled water and 1 ml of the fluoride reference solution in the same manner as the specimen.
8. Place the microdiffusion dish containing the test sample next to the those containing the control samples and visually compare the colors in the center wells after 15 min, 1 hr, and 3 hr.
9. In the presence of 0.2 mg or more F^- per 100-ml sample, the color reagent in the cell containing the unknown attains a much stronger violet color than that of the reference solutions within less than an hour. At and above concentrations of 0.5 mg F^- per 100-ml sample, this color difference becomes noticeable in 15 min or less. If a larger excess of fluoride is present, the color reagent may bleach out. If the color of the test sample has not attained or exceeded the color of the reference samples after 3 hr, no abnormal fluoride concentration is present.

INTERPRETATION (see p. 7)

This procedure is designed to qualitatively determine if excess fluoride ions are present. Should this be so, a quantitative assay is required to assess the degree of hazard.

REFERENCES*

Frere, J. F., A microdiffusion method for the determination of fluorides, *Microchem. J.*, 6, 167, 1962.
Gettler, A. O. and Ellerbrook, L., The toxicology of fluoride, *Am. J. Med. Sci.*, 197, 625, 1939.
Waldbott, G. L., Fluoride in clinical medicine, *Int. Arch. Allergy Appl. Immunol.*, 20, 60, 1962.

TYPE B PROCEDURE

Irving Sunshine and Bryan S. Finkle

APPARATUS

1. Petri dishes, plastic, disposable (Falcon Plastics)
2. Oven, constant-temperature
3. Pasteur pipets, disposable
4. Volumetric flasks, 10 ml
5. Photometer, photoelectric, equipped with a 625-nm filter

REAGENTS

All chemicals should be analytical reagent grade.

1. Trapping agent
Dissolve 4.0 g of sodium hydroxide in 80% ethanol. Dilute this solution to 100 ml with 80% ethanol.
2. Fluoride stock solution, 10 mg/dl

*For an updated list of reference material, see General References, p. 172.

Dissolve 0.2210 g of sodium fluoride in water and dilute to one liter.

3. Fluoride reference solutions
   Dilute 1.0, 2.0, 4.0, and 6.0 ml of the fluoride stock solution to 100 ml with water to obtain solutions containing 1.0, 2.0, 4.0, and 6.0 μg of fluoride/ml, respectively.
4. Fluoride-liberating agent
   To a 250-ml Erlenmeyer flask add 4.0 g of silver sulfate, 2.0 ml of water, and 23.0 ml of 72% perchloric acid. Carefully heat this mixture to 80°C to dissolve the silver sulfate. Add 75.0 ml of 72% perchloric acid, cool, then pour the reagent into a dark Pyrex® bottle. This solution is stable for at least 6 months if stored in a refrigerator.
5. Phenolphthalein indicator solution
   Dissolve 1.0 g of phenolphthalein in 100 ml of 95% ethanol.
6. Ammonium acetate, 20 g/dl
   Dissolve 20.0 g of ammonium acetate in 100 ml of water
7. Hydrochloric acid, 2*M*
   Add 20.0 ml of concentration hydrochloric acid to 100 ml of distilled water.
8. Belcher reagent
   Dissolve 0.0479 g of alizarin Complexone®* in 4.0 to 6.0 ml of distilled water containing 0.1 ml of concentrated ammonium hydroxide and 1.0 ml of the ammonium acetate solution. Filter this mixture through Whatman #1 filter paper into a 200-ml volumetric flask containing 8.2 g of anhydrous sodium acetate, 6.0 ml of glacial acetic acid and enough water to dissolve the solid. Wash the filter paper with a small volume of water and add the washing to the flask. Slowly, with a swirling motion to ensure mixing, add 100 ml of acetone. In a separate beaker dissolve 0.0612 g of lanthanum chloride or 0.0714 g of lanthanum nitrate in 2.5 ml of 2*M* hydrochloric acid, using enough heat to ensure solution of the solid. Add this solution, with swirling, to the 200-ml volumetric flask. Dilute the flask contents to 200 ml with water and mix. Cool the solution to room temperature. Add more water, if necessary. Transfer the prepared reagent to a glass-stoppered brown bottle and store it in a refrigerator. The reagent is stable for at least 3 months if stored under these conditions.

PROCEDURE

1. Spread 0.1 ml of the 1.0*N* alcoholic sodium hydroxide solution inside each of a series of plastic petri dish covers. As the solution dries, be sure that it is spread evenly and covers an area of about 10 cm^2.
2. Pipet 1.0 ml of specimen (blood, urine, stomach content, or homogenized tissue) or 1.0 ml of each reference solution into the bottom sections of the petri dishes. Add 2.0 ml of the fluoride-liberating agent to each bottom section.
3. Cover each bottom section with a lid containing the dried sodium hydroxide spot.
4. Place the assembled dishes on a tray and keep them for 24 hr at 50°C in the constant-temperature oven.
5. At the end of the 24-hr period remove the tray from the oven and allow the petri dishes to cool to room temperature. Discard the bottom sections.
6. Dissolve the sodium hydroxide spots on the lids by washing each lid twice with 1.0 ml of water, using a clean, disposable Pasteur pipet. Pull the wash solution into the pipet, then discharge the liquid onto the lid. Repeat this several times with each wash solution to be sure that all the sodium hydroxide is dissolved and that the entire surface of the cover has been rinsed.
7. Transfer each washing to a 10-ml volumetric flask, using a Pasteur pipet. Rinse the Pasteur pipet, and add this washing to the others in the flask.
8. To check whether or not all the sodium hydroxide was dissolved, add 1 drop of phenolphthalein and 0.5 ml of water to each cover. If a distinct pink color develops, use the phenolphthalein solution to wash the lid once more, then transfer this washing to the volumetric flask and add 1 or 2 drops of acetic acid to eliminate the color. A very faint pink color may be disregarded.
9. Add 3.0 ml of the Belcher reagent to the

*3-Aminomethyl alizarin *N,N*-diacetic acid (Hopkins and Williams, Chadwell Heath, Essex, England).

solution in the flask, then dilute the mixture to volume. Let the flask stand for at least 2 hr in the dark at room temperature for color development. The developed color is stable for at least 24 hr.

10. After color development is completed, but before 24 hr have elapsed, determine the absorbance of each sample at 625 nm. Use a reagent blank (prepared by adding all the reagents to the water sample) as the photometric reference solution.

CALCULATION

Fluoride reference solutions with concentrations ranging from 1.0 to 6.0 μg/ml yield absorbance values that are linear functions of their concentrations.

INTERPRETATION (see p. 7)

Excretion of less than 4.0 mg of fluoride/liter of urine is seldom compatible with harmful exposure. If exposure results from drinking water only, the urinary fluoride concentration is of the same order of magnitude as that of the water supply. No fatal reactions to fluorides have been reported in which this method has been used for analyzing the specimens. In two men who died following an exposure to hydrofluoric acid, the blood fluoride concentration (determined by another method) was reported to be 0.4 mg/100 ml. Following death from fluoride ingestion, blood fluoride concentrations range up to 300.0 μg/ml.

ACCURACY AND PRECISION

A concentration of 1.0 μg of fluoride/ml of solution gives an absorbance value of 0.063 ± 0.003 in a 1-cm cuvette. Following the microdiffusion process, recovery of added fluoride is 95 to 100%.

REFERENCES*

Belcher, R. M., Leonard, A., and West, T. S., A new spot test for the detection of fluoride ion, *Talanta*, 2, 02, 1959.

Derryberry, O. M., Bartholomew, M. D., and Fleming, R. B. L., Fluoride exposure and worker health, *Arch. Environ. Health*, 6, 503, 1963.

Greendyke, R. M. and Hodge, H. C., Accidental death due to hydrofluoric acid, *J. Forensic Sci.*, 9, 383, 1964.

Rowley, R. J. and Farrah, G. H., Diffusion method for determination of urinary fluoride, *Am. Ind. Hyg. Assoc. J.*, 23, 314, 1962.

Singer, L. and Armstrong, W. D., Determination of fluoride based upon diffusion of hydrogen fluoride, *Anal. Biochem.*, 10, 495, 1965.

TYPE C PROCEDURE

Franklin D. Griffith and John R. Barnes

APPARATUS

1. Pasteur pipets
2. Beakers, 5 ml
3. Pipets, disposable, with 2-ml rubber bulbs
4. Microdish (Orion®)
5. Fluoride electrode (Orion®)
6. Calomel reference electrode, 4″
7. pH-Conductivity meter, expanded scale

REAGENTS

All chemicals should be analytical reagent grade.

1. Sodium hydroxide, 10*N*
   Using 25.0 ml of water, dissolve 40.0 g of sodium hydroxide pellets in a 100-ml beaker. Transfer this solution to a glass-stoppered 100-ml volumetric flask. After the sodium hydroxide is completely dissolved and the solution has cooled to room temperature, dilute it to volume with water. Store the solution in a polyethylene bottle.
2. Citrate buffer, 0.5*M*, pH 7.0
   Dissolve 96.06 g of citric acid in 500 ml of deionized water. Allow the solution to cool to room temperature, then adjust the pH to 7.0 with the 10*N* sodium hydroxide. Transfer the

*For an updated list of reference material, see General References, p. 172.

solution quantitatively to a glass-stoppered one-liter volumetric flask and dilute to the mark with water. Store the reagent at 4°C in a polyethylene bottle. Discard 1 week after preparation.

3. Fluoride stock solution, 1 mg F^-/ml
   Dissolve 2.2105 g of sodium fluoride, dried overnight at 100°C, in deionized water. Dilute this solution to one liter with deionized water. Transfer the solution to a polyethylene bottle and store in a refrigerator. This solution is stable for an indefinite period.
4. Fluoride reference solutions:

   Reference solution #1, 100 μg F^-/ml
   Allow the fluoride stock solution to come to room temperature. Transfer 10.0 ml to a glass-stoppered 100-ml volumetric flask and dilute to the mark with water. Transfer this solution to a polyethylene bottle and store in a refrigerator when not in use. Label the bottle, indicating its reference solution number and the concentration of fluoride ion it contains. Discard the contents after 1 week.

   Reference solutions #2 and #3
   Prior to performing an analysis, allow reference solution #1 to come to room temperature. Transfer the quantities indicated in the table below to glass-stoppered volumetric flasks of the size specified, then dilute each to the mark with water. Label each flask, indicating its reference solution number and the concentration of fluoride ion it contains.

Reference solution #	Concentration, μg F^-/ml	Solution #1, ml	Flask size, ml
2	20.0	2.0	10
3	10.0	5.0	50

   Reference solutions #4, #5, and #6
   Using reference solution #3, transfer the quantities indicated in the table below to glass-stoppered volumetric flasks of the size specified, then dilute each to the mark with water. Label each flask, indicating its reference solution number and the concentration of fluoride ion it contains.

Reference solution #	Concentration, μg F^-/ml	Solution #3, ml	Flask size, ml
4	5.0	5.0	10
5	2.0	2.0	10
6	1.0	5.0	50

   Reference solutions #7, #8, and #9
   Using reference solution #6, transfer the quantities indicated in the table below to glass-stoppered volumetric flasks of the size specified, then dilute each to the mark with water. Label each flask, indicating its reference solution number and the concentration of fluoride ion it contains.

Reference solution #	Concentration, μg F^-/ml	Solution #6, ml	Flask size, ml
7	0.5	5.0	10
8	0.2	2.0	10
9	0.1	1.0	10

PROCEDURE

1. Pipet 1.0 ml of buffer into a series of labeled 5-ml beakers. Add 1.0 ml of sample (fresh urine specimen and reference solutions) and mix.
2. Using a disposable pipet with a 2-ml rubber bulb, transfer each solution to an Orion® microdish and determine the potential to the nearest 0.1 mV. It usually takes about 10 min for the meter to reach its final reading, but experience is necessary to recognize the proper end point.
3. Before transferring the electrodes from one sample to another, rinse with water and dry with tissue paper.

CALCULATION

Plot the potential of the reference solutions against their respective fluoride concentrations on semilogarithmic paper (K & E No. 47-6010), using the horizontal axis for potential and the vertical axis for concentration. Draw a straight line through the points. Determine the fluoride concentration in the specimen by comparison with the calibration curve.

INTERPRETATION (see p. 7)

Excretion of less than 4.0 mg of fluoride/liter of urine is seldom compatible with harmful exposure. If exposure results from drinking water only, the urinary fluoride concentration is of the same order of magnitude as that of the water supply. No fatal reactions to fluorides have been reported in which this method has been used for analyzing the specimens. In two men who died following an exposure to hydrofluoric acid, the blood fluoride concentration (determined by another method) was reported to be 0.4/100 ml. Following death from fluoride ingestion, blood fluoride concentrations range up to 300.0 μg/ml.

PRECAUTIONS

The manufacturer's instructions should be followed closely to avoid problems with air bubbles inside the electrode and on the crystal. It is important to keep the distance between the fluoride electrode and the reference electrode constant. Operators must be well versed in this technique.

If urine specimens must be stored, the usual preservation precautions must be observed. Largent[1] (Reynolds Metals Company) uses 0.4*M* citrate buffer, adding 58 ml of 40% formaldehyde per liter of buffer. After adding 40 ml of this mixture to 100 ml of fresh urine, no change in F^- concentration was observed over a period of 10 weeks.

REFERENCE

1. **Largent, E. J.,** personal communication.

GENERAL REFERENCES

Frant, M. S. and Ross, J. W., Jr., Use of a total ionic strength adjustment buffer for electrode determination of fluoride in water supplies, *Anal. Chem.,* 40, 1169, 1968.

Gron, P., McCann, H. G., and Brundevold, F., The direct determination of fluoride in human saliva by a fluoride electrode: Fluoride levels in parotid saliva after ingestion of single doses of sodium fluoride, *Arch. Oral Biol.,* 13, 203, 1968.

Maduska, A. L., Serum inorganic fluoride levels in patients receiving enflurane anaesthesia, *Anesth. Anal.,* 53, 351, 1974.

Orion Research, Inc., *Instruction Manual for Fluoride Electrode Model 94-09,* Orion Research, Inc., Cambridge, 1966.

Singer, L. and Armstrong, W. D., Determination of fluoride in bone with the fluoride electrode, *Anal. Chem.,* 40, 613, 1968.

Singer, L., Armstrong, W. D., and Vogel, J. J., Fluoride determination by electrode potential measurements, *Abstr. 45th Gen. Meet. Int. Assoc. Dental Res.,* 1967, 77.

FLUOROCARBONS

PRINCIPLE

Fluorocarbon propellants are very volatile and may be detected by head-space analysis using gas chromatography (Procedure A). They are also quite soluble in hexane and thus can be extracted from the biological specimen. An aliquot of this extract can be analyzed by gas chromatography, preferably using an electron-capture detector (Procedure B).

TYPE A PROCEDURE

Robert H. Cravey

APPARATUS

1. Syringes, gastight
2. Flasks with airtight rubber diaphragms, 50 ml
3. Gas chromatograph, equipped with a hydrogen-flame ionization detector and a 6′ X 1/8″ i.d. stainless steel column packed with 42 to 60 firebrick containing 28% of a mixture of 15 parts Flexol 8N8, 10 parts diisodecylphthalate, and 3 parts Carbowax® 600 *

   Operating Conditions

   Gas Flow Rates:
   - helium – 10 ml/min
   - hydrogen – 25 ml/min

   Temperatures:
   - column – 30°C
   - injection port – 40°C
   - detector – 55°C

REAGENTS

1. CCl_3F (or CCl_2F_2) reference head-space gases Using a microliter syringe, add 1-μl to 10-μl volumes of the gas under investigation and to weighed samples of uncontaminated tissue in 50-ml flasks with airtight rubber diaphragms.

PROCEDURE[1]

To insure accurate determinations of tissue concentrations, caution must be exercised by the pathologist and the toxicologist to avoid undue loss of these highly volatile gases. The autopsy should be performed without delay, and the tissues should be taken without undue exposure to the atmosphere. Vacutainers provide an excellent means of obtaining blood for analysis. Other specimens should be sealed immediately in plastic bags or adequate glass containers and maintained at -20°C until analyzed if the analysis cannot be performed immediately upon receipt of the samples. The analyst should bear in mind that there is a possibility of contamination in the freezer if other fluorocarbons are stored in the same unit.

1. Inject 1.0-ml samples of the reference head-space gases into the gas chromatograph, making sure that the stated operating conditions are met.
2. Measure the peak heights.
3. Seal accurately weighed samples of frozen tissue in 50-ml flasks and allow them to equilibrate for several hours at room temperature.
4. Inject 1.0-ml samples of their head-space gases

*Column available from Beckman Instruments, Fullerton, California.

into the gas chromatograph under the same operating conditions.

5. Record the resulting peak heights.

CALCULATION

To estimate the concentration in the specimen, compare the peak heights of the reference gases with peak heights of the gases obtained from the unknown tissues.

INTERPRETATION (see p. 7)

Using their procedure, Baselt and Cravey[1] reported the following concentrations (μg/100 g wet weight) in a fatal case involving CCl_3F and CCl_2F_2:

Tissue	CCl_3F	CCl_2F_2	Tissue	CCl_3F	CCl_2F_2
Blood	0.86	0.05	Lung	5.78	9.23
Kidney	1.65	0.05	Liver	0.83	0.67
Brain	1.33	0.67	Stomach content	5.78	6.92

Bass[2] suggests that the mechanism of death in fatal cases results from severe cardiac arrhythmia. He has reviewed a number of reported cases.

ACCURACY AND PRECISION

Reference samples show a linear relationship between concentration and peak height.

INTERFERING SUBSTANCES

The flame ionization detector is not selective for halocarbons; therefore, other compounds may elute at the same retention times. A second gas-chromatographic analysis of the specimen utilizing a second column, Porapak S, chromasorb 102, or other suitable packing, will provide another parameter helpful in establishing identity.

REFERENCES

1. **Baselt, R. C. and Cravey, R. H.,** A fatal case involving trichloromonofluoromethane and dichlorodifluoromethane, *J. Forensic Sci.*, 13, 407, 1968.
2. **Bass, M.,** Sudden sniffing death, *JAMA*, 212, 2075, 1970.

GENERAL REFERENCES

Azar, A., et al., Blood levels of fluorocarbons related to cardiac sensitization, *Am. Ind. Hyg. Assoc. J.*, 34, 102, 1973.

Terrill, J. B., Determination of fluorocarbon propellants in blood and animal tissue, *Am. Ind. Hyg. Assoc. J.*, 33(11), 736, 1972.

Trochimowicz, H., et al., Blood levels of fluorocarbons related to cardiac sensitization, Part II, *Am. Ind. Hyg. Assoc. J.*, in press.

TYPE B PROCEDURE

James B. Terrill

APPARATUS

1. Chromatographic column: 4′ × 1/8″ od stainless steel packed with Porapak® Q (Water Associates)
2. Vacutainer® tubes, 10-ml heparinized (Becton-Dickinson)
3. Syringes: 5-ml liquid with 20 gauge needle and 10-μl gas chromatographic (Hamilton)
4. 100-ml volumetric flasks and a series of 1 to 10 ml pipets
5. Gas chromatograph equipped with electron-capture (EC) detector and strip chart recorder (the Hewlett-Packard Model 5700 with a linearized ^{63}Ni EC detector is recommended)

Operating Conditions

Gas Flow Rate:
5% methane in argon – 60 ml/min

Temperatures:
column – This depends upon the specific fluorocarbon to be analyzed. Retention times ranging up to about 5 min are given at 120 to 160°C. The upper limit of operation with this type of column is 225°C.
injection port – 150°C
detector – 250°C

Column Conditioning: New columns must be conditioned prior to use. Connect the column inlet side, but not the outlet. Use nitrogen carrier for 4 hr at 225°C oven temperature. After this period, cool the oven, connect the outlet and switch to 5% methane in argon carrier. The EC detector outlet must be vented to a hood.

REAGENTS

All chemicals should be analytical reagent grade.

1. Hexane, pesticide grade
2. Fluorocarbons, reagent grade or highest available purity
3. Sodium heparin, dissolve 10 gm in water and dilute to 100 ml
4. Dry ice

STANDARDIZATION OF THE GAS CHROMATOGRAPH

1. Fill to the mark three 100-ml volumetric flasks with room temperature hexane. Withdraw 1 ml from each flask and discard this 1 ml.
2. Chill each flask and three 1 ml pipets at -70°C (20 min in dry ice).
3. Gaseous fluorocarbons must be liquified by passing the gas through a coil of copper tubing covered with dry ice.
   (a) Keep the condensed fluorocarbon as cold as possible and, using a chilled pipet, transfer 1 ml to the chilled hexane remaining in the 100 ml flask. This is a 1 ml/dl solution. Mix by inversion.
   (b) Dilute the solution from (a) 1:100 to form a 100 μl/ml solution. Mix by inversion.
   (c) Use this 100-μl/ml solution to prepare a series of standards in the 1 to 100-μl/ml range. It is desirable, but not necessary, to use chilled hexane for the dilutions. Convert solution concentrations from μl/ml to μg/ml by multiplying by the density of the fluorocarbon. The density of each fluorocarbon mentioned above is:

Fluorocarbon 11	1.47 g/cc	25°C
Fluorocarbon 12	1.31 g/cc	25°C
Fluorocarbon 113	1.56 g/cc	25°C
Fluorocarbon 114	1.45 g/cc	25°C

   Other fluorocarbon densities are listed in handbooks such as *CRC Handbook of Chemistry and Physics.* *
4. Construct a calibration curve by plotting recorder response vs. fluorocarbon concentration, μg/ml (w/v). Use 4 μl for each injection.

*Weast, R. C., Ed., *Handbook of Chemistry and Physics*, 55th ed., CRC Press, Cleveland, 1974, E-34.

5. Repeat the preparation of standards starting with pure solutions until successive calibration curves agree within 10%.

PROCEDURE

1. Introduce 5.0 ml of hexane into each Vacutainer® tube. Heparinize one 5-ml syringe and needle prior to withdrawing 2 ml of blood. Add the blood to the tube which contains the hexane. Shake vigorously for 1 min. Place the upright tube in a freezer at -10°C. Allow the blood to solidify (approximately 30 min at -10°C).
2. Withdraw 4 μl of the hexane layer for chromatographic analysis. The volume of hexane should be the same as the volume used in the preparation of the calibration curve (see Figure 1).
3. If the concentration of fluorocarbon is outside the linear range of the EC detector, the hexane layer must be diluted.

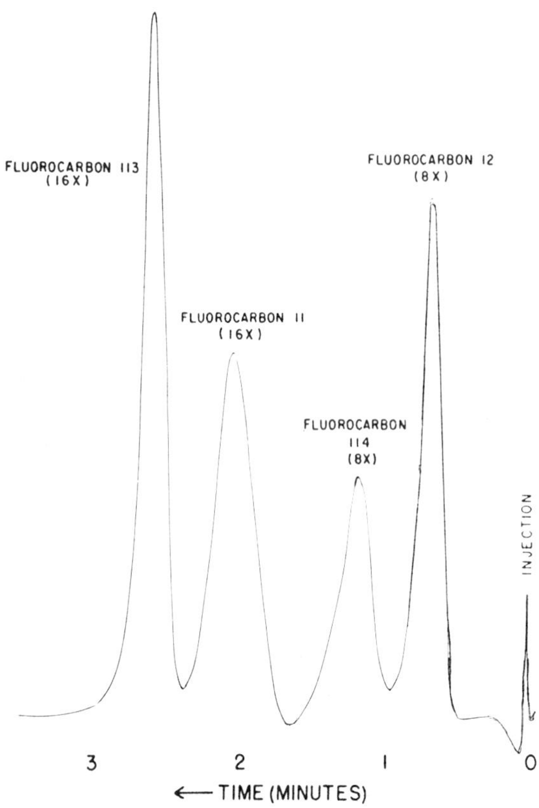

FIGURE 1. Chromatographic separation of four common fluorocarbons. Oven temperature was 150°C. All other chromatographic conditions are those stated under Operating Conditions.

CALCULATION

Determine fluorocarbon concentration in the 4-μl aliquot of the hexane extract by reference to the calibration curve. Multiply this value by 5/2 (hexane to blood ratio) in order to obtain the concentration of fluorocarbon per milliliter of blood. Report the results as microgram of fluorocarbon per milliliter of blood.

INTERPRETATION (see p. 7)

In an inhalation exposure to fluorocarbon propellants, equilibrium between arterial and venous blood is achieved in less than 10 min. Laboratory animals exposed to atmospheres containing approximately 1% fluorocarbon have blood fluorocarbon levels in the μg/ml range.[1,2] Specific levels depend on the kind of fluorocarbon and the concentration inhaled.

ACCURACY AND PRECISION

Using the procedure described above, the recovery of fluorocarbons added to blood ranged from 85 to 95%. There may be a drift in EC response, and a periodic check of standardization is advised. The major sources of error are loss of pure fluorocarbon in preparation of the 1% standard and changes in chromatographic response. These can be minimized by practice and frequent standardization checks.

Pure fluorocarbons should not be stored in the same quarters as hexane or any of the reference solutions. Contamination occurs easily. Stability of the blood-hexane solutions depends on the deterioration of the Vacutainer® stopper. The solution can be kept at -10°C for at least 1 week.

INTERFERING SUBSTANCES

Temperature programming may be necessary to improve chromatographic resolution. H_2O, CO_2, and O_2 are all retained to some degree on Porapak® Q, and the EC detector is responsive to these materials. They should not be confused in the analysis of fluorocarbons.

REFERENCES

1. **Azar, A., et al.,** Blood levels of fluorocarbons related to cardiac sensitization, *Am. Ind. Hyg. Assoc. J.*, 34, 102, 1973.
2. **Trochimowicz, H., et al.,** Blood levels of fluorocarbons related to cardiac sensitization, Part II, *Am. Ind. Assoc. J.*, in press.

GENERAL REFERENCES

Terrill, J. B., Determination of fluorocarbon propellants in blood and animal tissue, *Am. Ind. Hyg. Assoc. J.*, 33(11), 736, 1972.

GLUTETHIMIDE

PRINCIPLE

Glutethimide may be separated from a biological matrix by solvent extraction (Procedure B). If nonpolar solvents are used, inactive metabolites are not coextracted; if a polar solvent, such as a chlorinated hydrocarbon, is used, the inactive metabolites are coextracted. The drug and its metabolites have nonspecific UV absorbance characteristics; however, the products of alkaline hydrolysis have a useful absorbance at 230 nm and can be used to quantitate the extracted materials. The chloroform extract yields very high results which do not correlate well with the patients's clinical condition; opposite results occur with a petroleum ether extract, which is preferable. Either extract may be used for gas chromatography (Procedure C) because each of the compounds involved are well separated; thus, separation of glutethimide from its metabolites is feasible, and reliable quantitative data can be obtained.

TYPE B PROCEDURE

Bryan S. Finkle

APPARATUS

1. Serological pipets, 5 ml
2. Bottles, ground-glass-stoppered, 60 ml
3. Glass funnels
4. Measuring cylinders, ground-glass-stoppered, 50 ml
5. Beakers, 50 ml
6. Beakers, 10 ml
7. Volumetric flasks, 10 ml
8. Centrifuge
9. UV spectrophotometer

REAGENTS

All chemicals should be analytical reagent grade.

1. Glutethimide stock solution, 100 μg/ml
   Dissolve 100 mg of glutethimide in water and dilute to one liter.
2. Glutethimide reference solution, 10 μg/ml
   Dilute 10.0 ml of the glutethimide stock solution to 100 ml with water.
3. Chloroform, Mallinckrodt Nonograde
4. Petroleum ether
5. Sodium hydroxide, 0.45*N*
   Dissolve 18 g of sodium hydroxide in water and dilute to one liter.
6. Glass wool, acid-washed
7. Sodium sulfate, anhydrous
8. Ethanol, 95%
9. Potassium hydroxide, 0.2*N*
   Dissolve 0.11 g of potassium hydroxide in water and dilute to 100 ml.
10. Hydrochloric acid, 0.5*N*
    Dilute 10.0 ml of concentrated hydrochloric acid to 240 ml with water.

PROCEDURE[1,2]

1. Transfer 5.0 ml of whole blood or urine to a 60-ml ground-glass-stoppered bottle. If tissues are to be analyzed, prepare an aqueous homogenate, using 4.0 ml of water for each gram of tissue. Process a 5.0-ml sample of the glutethimide reference solution concurrently and in the same manner.
2. Extract each sample with 50 ml of chloroform.* Allow the phases to separate, then remove the aqueous phases by aspiration.
3. Add 5.0 ml of 0.45*N* sodium hydroxide and shake the mixtures. Allow the layers to separate (centrifuge, if necessary).
4. Separate the alkali from the chloroform. Save the alkali for determination of barbiturates, should this be required. Add 5.0 ml of water to the chloroform, mix, then separate and

*Available from Spex Industries, Inc., Metuchen, N.J.

discard the wash water. This should be done very promptly after the alkaline extraction.

5. Filter the washed chloroform through anhydrous sodium sulfate supported on glass wool in the neck of a funnel, collecting it in a 50-ml measuring cylinder.
6. Transfer 40 ml of the chloroform filtrate to a 50-ml beaker.
7. Evaporate the filtrate to approximately 5 ml, transfer it quantitatively to a 10-ml beaker, and continue the evaporation to dryness.
8. Dissolve each residue in 3.0 ml of water. Triturate the water and residues in the beaker to insure solution. Add 3.0 ml of ethanol to the water and proceed in the same manner. Transfer this solution to a 10-ml volumetric flask. Repeat this operation with 1.5 ml of water and 1.5 ml of ethanol, pool the solutions, then dilute to 10.0 ml.
9. Transfer 3.0 ml of each solution obtained in Step 8 to a cuvette. Add 1.0 ml of 0.2*N* potassium hydroxide and mix. *Note the exact time at which the alkali is added.* This is *zero time.*
10. Immediately determine the UV absorbance of each sample at 235 nm (A_0), using a mixture containing 3.0 ml of 95% ethanol and 1.0 ml of 0.2*N* potassium hydroxide as the reference solution.
11. If the absorbance of the test sample at 235 nm is too high, dilute another aliquot of the solution obtained in Step 8 and repeat Step 9 on the diluted solution. Note the dilution factor.
12. Record the absorbance of each solution after 10 min (A_{10}). At this time the alkaline hydrolysis of the glutethimide is complete. The final absorbance reading may be regarded as the reagent blank.

CALCULATION

1. Subtract the A_{10} from the A_0.
2. Extrapolate the semi-log plot to zero time in order to obtain the absorbance value at zero time.
3. Calculate the glutethimide concentration (μg/ml) in the specimen as follows:

$$\text{concentration} = \frac{(A_{10} - A_0) \text{ of specimen}}{(A_{10} - A_0) \text{ of reference}} \times 10.$$

INTERPRETATION (see p. 7)

The maximum blood concentration following a single dose of 1.0 g of glutethimide is approximately 7 μg/ml. This occurs about 2 hr after ingestion. At this concentration, symptoms of sleepiness and apparent intoxication can be expected in nontolerant subjects. The glutethimide is detectable in the urine for at least 48 hr following such an ingestion. Coma will generally result from blood concentrations of approximately 10 μg/ml or higher. Deep coma and death are consistent with concentrations of 25 μg/ml of blood or higher, although recoveries have been observed following blood concentrations of 40 μg/ml when prompt and expert medical treatment was instituted.

Glutethimide is lipid-soluble and only slowly absorbed from the stomach and small intestine. As a consequence, in acute overdose cases coma may be dangerously prolonged unless the stomach and upper gastrointestinal tract are promptly cleared of unabsorbed drug. In a comatose patient blood concentrations may reach a plateau at a relatively low level and remain steady for many hours. Concentrations ranging from 10 to 15 μg/ml should therefore not be regarded lightly or accepted simply at face value. A potentially fatal situation may exist. A series of determinations should be made to recognize whether a long coma is likely. If a series of determinations made at 6-hr intervals shows a relatively unchanging concentration over 18 to 24 hr, the situation is extremely dangerous. This method may detect some of the glutethimide metabolites. A more precise measure of glutethimide and its metabolites may be obtained using a gas-chromatographic method (Procedure C).

ACCURACY

Recovery of glutethimide is 95 to 100%.

INTERFERING SUBSTANCES

Neutral fats, as well as acidic and basic compounds, may be extracted and result in spurious absorbance values. These materials can be removed by washing the chloroform filtrate first with 0.5*N* sodium hydroxide and then with 0.5*N* hydrochloric acid or by extracting with petroleum ether. Bemegride has a maximum UV absorbance at approximately 232 nm, but is unaffected by alkaline hydrolysis.

REFERENCES*

1. **Goldbaum, L., Williams, M., and Koppanyi, T.,** Determination of glutethimide in biological fluids, *Anal. Chem.*, 30, 81, 1960.
2. **Knowlton, M. A., and Goldbaum, L.,** A rapid improved method for the determination of doriden in the blood, *Clin. Chem.* (Abstr.), 13, 683, 1967.
3. **Sunshine, I., Maes, R., and Faracci, R.,** Determination of glutethimide and its metabolites in biologic specimens, *Clin. Chem.*, 14, 595, 1968.

TYPE C PROCEDURE

Bryan S. Finkle

APPARATUS

1. Bottles, ground-glass-stoppered, 120 ml, or separatory funnels
2. Serological pipets, 5 ml
3. Glass funnels
4. Measuring cylinders, ground-glass-stoppered, 50 ml
5. Beakers, 50 ml
6. Conical evaporating tubes, disposable, 2 ml
   Cut Pasteur pipets to the desired lengths and seal the tips.
7. Graduated pipets, 50 μl
8. Melting point capillary tubing
9. Rubber bulb
10. Mortar and pestle – boron carbide,* mortar cavity – ½″ diameter, 5/32″ depth
11. Infrared lamp
12. Ultramicro die (Perkin-Elmer)
13. IR spectrophotometer (Perkin-Elmer Model 21), fitted with a double-beam condenser and variable scale expansion (from X ¼ to X 20)
14. Gas chromatograph, fitted with a flame ionization detector, and a U-shaped glass column, 6′ X ¼″ o.d., packed with 2.5% S.E. 30 on 80/100 Chromosorb G (AW-DMCS)

   Operating Conditions

   Gas Flow Rates:
   nitrogen (carrier gas) – 50 ml/min
   Temperature:
   column – 195°C
   injection port – 230°C
   detector – 220°

REAGENTS

All chemicals should be analytical reagent grade.

1. Chloroform, Mallinckrodt Nanograde
2. Glass wool, acid-washed
3. Sodium sulfate, anhydrous
4. Chloroform-ethanol mixture, 1:1
   Mix 50.0 ml of chloroform with 50.0 ml of absolute ethanol. Prepare this reagent just prior to use.
5. Internal standard, 100 mg/100 ml
   Dissolve 100 mg of *p*-dimethylaminobenzaldehyde in 100 ml of the chloroform-ethanol mixture. Discard the solution after 1 month.
6. Glutethimide reference solution, 5 μg/μl
   Dissolve 250 mg of glutethimide in 50.0 ml of the internal standard. Aliquots of 0.4, 0.8, and 1.6 μl of this solution are equivalent to 2, 4, and 8 μg of glutethimide, respectively.
7. Chloroform, dry
8. Potassium bromide, infrared quality (Harshaw Chemical Company)

PROCEDURE, QUANTITATIVE

1. Using a 120-ml ground-glass-stoppered bottle or a separatory funnel, extract 3.0 ml of specimen (blood, gastric content, urine, or 1.0 g of homogenized tissue) with 50.0 ml of chloroform. Process 3.0 ml of reference solution in the same manner. Allow the phases to separate.
2. Aspirate the aqueous phase. Filter the chloro-

*For an updated list of reference material, see References, p. 181.

form into a 50-ml ground-glass-stoppered measuring cylinder through anhydrous sodium sulfate supported by a glass wool plug in a small funnel.
3. Collect 40.0 ml of the chloroform filtrate in the cylinder.
4. Evaporate the chloroform filtrate to 1 or 2 ml in a 50-ml beaker.
5. Transfer the concentrate to a disposable 2-ml conical tube, then continue the evaporation to dryness.
6 Dissolve the residue in 25 μl of internal standard.
7. Inject 1 μl of the dissolved residue into the gas chromatograph, making sure that the operating conditions stated above are met. The retention times under these conditions are approximately 5.3 min for glutethimide and approximately 1.8 min for the internal standard.

CALCULATION

1. Calculate the $\frac{\text{peak height of glutethimide}}{\text{peak height of internal standard}}$
2. Calculate the weight of drug injected into the gas chromatograph by relating the ratio resulting from the glutethimide reference sample directly to the ratio obtained from the specimen.

INTERPRETATION (see p. 7)

The maximum blood concentration achieved following a single dose of 1.0 g of glutethimide is approximately 7 μg/ml. This occurs about 2 hr after ingestion. At this concentration, symptoms of sleepiness and apparent intoxication can be expected in nontolerant subjects. The glutethimide is detectable in the urine for at least 48 hr following such an ingestion. Coma will generally result from blood concentrations of 10 μg/ml or higher. Deep coma and death are consistent with concentrations of 25 μg/ml of blood or higher, although recoveries have been observed in patients with blood concentrations of 40 μg/ml when prompt and expert medical treatment was instituted.

Glutethimide is lipid-soluble and only slowly absorbed from the stomach and small intestine. As a consequence, in acute overdose cases coma may be dangerously prolonged unless the stomach and upper gastrointestinal tract are promptly cleared of unabsorbed drug. In a comatose patient, blood concentrations may reach a plateau at a relatively low level and remain steady for many hours. Concentrations ranging from 10 to 15 μg/ml should therefore not be regarded lightly or accepted simply at face value. A potentially fatal situation exists. A series of determinations should be made to recognize whether a long coma is likely. If a series of determinations made at 6-hr intervals shows a relatively unchanging concentration over 18 to 24 hr, the situation is extremely dangerous.

ACCURACY AND PRECISION

Using this procedure, recovery of glutethimide added to blood is approximately 90%. Drug concentrations of 2 μg/ml can be detected with ease. The method is accurate to ± 0.5 μg/ml in the range from 10 to 100 μg/ml. Any value in this range is reproducible within ± 2%.

INTERFERING SUBSTANCES

There is no major interference by known substances in this procedure. The two metabolites of glutethimide, α-phenyl-α-ethyl glutaconamide and α-phenyl glutarimide, have retention times of 5.3 and 4.2 min respectively.

REFERENCES

Finkle, B. S., The identification, quantitative determination and distribution of meprobamate and glutethimide in biological material, *J. Forensic Sci.*, 12, 509, 1967.

Hansen, A. R. and Fisher, L. J., GC simultaneous analysis for glutethimide and an active hydroxylated metabolite in tissues, plasma and urine, *Clin. Chem.*, 20, 236, 1974.

Rejient, T. A. and Klendshaj, N. C., Rapid determination of glutethimide in biological fluids, *Clin. Toxicol.*, 1(2), 143, 1968.

GOLD

PRINCIPLE

Since gold salts are used in the treatment of arthritis, the concentration of gold in blood or urine may be of critical interest. Gold may be measured by diluting the sample and aspirating the solution into the burner of an atomic absorption spectrophotometer. Absorption measurements are made at 242.8 nm using a suitable gold hollow-cathode lamp.

TYPE A PROCEDURE

Louis A. Williams and Joseph S. Annino

APPARATUS

1. Test tubes, 16 X 100 mm
2. Atomic absorption spectrophotometer with hollow-cathode lamp for gold

REAGENTS

All chemicals should be analytical reagent grade.

1. Stock standard, 1,000 mg/l
   Weight 100 mg of pure gold wire and place in a 100-ml volumetric flask. Add 2-ml concentrated nitric acid and 3-ml concentrated hydrochloric acid. Heat in a sand bath until the gold dissolves. Additional 1-ml amounts of hydrochloric acid may be added *cautiously* during the process, as required. Cool to room temperature, then dilute to 100 ml with water.
2. Intermediate standard, 100 mg/l
3. Working standards, 0, 1.0, 2.0, 4.0, and 6.0 mg/l
   To five 50-ml volumetric flasks, each containing 5 ml of a 30% human albumin solution, add 0, 0.5, 1.0, 2.0, and 3.0 ml of the intermediate standard, respectively. Dilute the contents of each flask to 50 ml with water. Store at 4°C.

PROCEDURE

Specimen Preparation

Serum

1. Add 1 ml of serum and 1 ml of water to a 16 X 100 mm test tube.
2. Set up each of the working standards in the same fashion.

Urine

A 24-hr urine specimen is desirable for this analysis.

1. Add 2 ml of urine, 1.8 ml of water, and 0.2 ml of 30% human serum albumin solution to a 16 X 100 mm tube.
2. Set up each of the working standards in the same way, using 2 ml of standard and 2 ml of water.

ATOMIC ABSORPTION SPECTROPHOTOMETER SETTINGS

Note: These specifications are for a Varian Techtron AA-5. Other instruments may work equally well, although different settings may be required.

Lamp current	4 mA	Damping	D
Wavelength	242.8 nm	Mode	Absorbance
Slit	100 u	Acetylene	3-m units
Expansion	9 x	Air	6-m units
		Aspiration	4 ml/min

Adjust the flame until luminescence just disappears. Adjust the spectrophotometer to the peak wavelength.

MEASUREMENT

Set absorbance at zero while aspirating water, then measure the absorbances of the standards and samples.

CALCULATION

1. Using linear graph paper, plot the absorbances of the standards against their respective concentrations. Plot the absorbance of the zero standard at zero concentration.
2. Determine the concentrations of the samples (mg/l) from the standard curve.
3. For urine, multiply mg/l by $\frac{24\text{h volume (ml)}}{1{,}000}$ to get mg/24h.

INTERPRETATION (see p. 7)

Normally gold is not present in body fluids unless it has been administered. Gold salts are used in the treatment of arthritis. The usual therapeutic dosages of 10 to 100 mg of gold per week usually result in levels of 2 to 10 mg/l in serum and 0.1 to 0.4 mg/l in urine; however, the correlations between dosage, blood level, and clinical effect are not well established. A comprehensive discussion of the clinical aspects of gold therapy has been published.[1]

PRECISION

The coefficient of variation on a day-to-day basis is approximately 4%.

INTERFERING SUBSTANCES

There is no published report of an interfering substance. If such a substance is found, it will no doubt be referred to as "fool's gold."

REFERENCE

1. **Hollander, J. L. and McCarthy, D. L.,** *Arthritis and Allied Conditions,* 8th ed., Lea & Febiger, Philadelphia, 1972.

GENERAL REFERENCES

Balazs, N. D. H., Pole, D. J., and Masarei, J. R., Determination of gold in body fluids by atomic absorption spectrophotometry, *Clin. Chim. Acta,* 40, 213, 1972.

Dietz, A. and Rubenstein, H. M., Serum gold by AA spectroscopy, *Ann. Rheum. Dis.,* 32, 2, 1973.

Dunckley, J. V., Estimation of gold in serum by atomic absorption spectroscopy, *Clin. Chem.,* 17, 992, 1971.

Harth, M., Serum gold levels during chrysotherapy with relation to urinary and fecal excretion, *Clin. Pharmacol. Ther.,* 15, 354, 1974.

Harth, M., Haines, D. S. M., and Bondy, D. C., A simple method for the determination of gold in serum, blood, and urine by atomic absorption spectroscopy, *Am. J. Clin. Pathol.,* 59, 423, 1973.

HALOGENATED HYDROCARBONS

PRINCIPLE

Halogenated hydrocarbons are adsorbed by toluene placed in the center wall of a microdiffusion cell. If halogenated hydrocarbons are present, the toluene reacts with pyridine and alkali to produce a red color.

TYPE A PROCEDURE

Milton Feldstein

APPARATUS

1. Conway microdiffusion dishes

REAGENTS

All chemicals should be analytical reagent grade.

1. Trichloromethane stock solution, 5 mg/ml
   Dilute 1.0 ml of trichloromethane to 300 ml with absolute ethanol.
2. Trichloromethane reference solutions, 5.0, 10.0, and 15 mg/100 ml
   To 1.0-ml samples of trichloromethane-free blood in the outer compartments of Conway cells add 10, 20, and 30 μl of the trichloromethane stock solution.
3. Toluene
4. Ucon® water-soluble grease (Union Carbide Corporation)
5. Pyridine
6. Sodium hydroxide, 20 g/100 ml
   Dissolve 20 g of sodium hydroxide in water and dilute to 100 ml.

PROCEDURE

1. Add 1.0 ml of specimen (oxalated blood or urine), 1.0 ml of each reference solution, and 1.0 ml of water for a reagent blank to each of the outer compartments of a series of Conway microdiffusion dishes. Add 1.0 ml of toluene to each center compartment.
2. Smear the cover plate of each dish with Ucon® and cover the dish with it, making sure that the seal is airtight. Let the dishes stand for 3 hr at room temperature to reach equilibrium.
3. Transfer 0.5 ml of the toluene from the center compartment of each sample to a test tube. Add 5.0 ml of the pyridine and 0.5 ml of the sodium hydroxide solution to each tube and mix.
4. Place the tubes for exactly 5 min in a boiling water bath. The presence of a red color in the pyridine layer is indicative of the presence of a halogenated hydrocarbon.
5. Cool the tubes in ice water, then transfer 4.0 ml of each pyridine layer to a cuvette. Add 1.0 ml of water to each sample to remove any turbidity.
6. Measure the absorbance of each sample at 530 nm, using the solution obtained by processing the water sample as the reference solution.
7. Prepare a standard curve from the data obtained by processing the trichloromethane reference solutions.

CALCULATION

Compare the absorbance of the specimen with those of the solutions obtained by processing the trichloromethane reference solutions. Other halogenated hydrocarbons may be used as reference solutions if indicated in a specific case.

INTERPRETATION (see p. 7)

Normally, halogenated hydrocarbons are not found in blood. Toxic concentrations vary with the specific substance present. Chloroform at 15.0

mg/100 ml of blood and trichloroethylene at 10.0 mg/100 ml of blood may result in anesthesia.

ACCURACY AND PRECISION

Replicate analyses agree within ±10% of the true value.

INTERFERING SUBSTANCES

Great care and control must be exercised in performing this analysis. Chlorinated hydrocarbons are ubiquitous in most toxicology laboratories and could interfere with the procedure. *A reagent blank must be processed with each series of analyses, to insure the reliability of the test result.*

REFERENCE

Feldstein, M., Microdiffusion analysis as applied to toxicology, in *Toxicology,* Vol. 1, Stewart, C. P. and Stolman, A., Eds., Academic Press, New York, 1960, 639.

HALOPERIDOL

PRINCIPLE

Haloperidol is extracted from an alkaline solution of the sample by chloroform. The chloroform extract is concentrated and an aliquot is analyzed by gas chromatography.

TYPE B PROCEDURE

Robert A. Maes

APPARATUS

1. Graduated cylinders, 10 and 100 ml
2. Separatory funnels, 250 ml
3. Evaporator reduced pressure, rotary (Büchi)
4. Syringes (Hamilton), 10 μl
5. Gas chromatograph (Varian Aerograph Model 1400), equipped with a flame ionization detector, a 1 mV recorder (Varian Aerograph Model 20) with attached Disc integrator, and a glass column, 6′ × 1/4″ o.d., containing a Pyrex® injector insert packed with 3% of a mixed phase of OV-25/OV-210 (2:1) on Gas Chrom Q, 80 to 100 mesh

   Operating Conditions

   Gas Flow Rates:
   - nitrogen – 63 ml/min
   - hydrogen – 35 ml/min
   - air – 200 ml/min

   Temperatures:
   - column – 220°C
   - injection port – 230°C
   - detector – 225°C

   Condition the column for 24 hr at 240°C and silanize it *in situ* with bistrimethylsilylacetamide.

REAGENTS

All chemicals should be analytical reagent grade.

1. Ammonium hydroxide, 3.7*N*
   Dilute 25.0 ml of concentrated ammonium hydroxide to 100 ml with water.
2. Haloperidol reference solutions
   Dissolve quantities of 0, 1.0, 2.0, 5.0, and 10.0 mg of haloperidol in 100 ml of urine.
3. Chlorpheniramine maleate internal-standard solution, 1 mg/100 ml
   Dissolve 1.0 mg of chlorpheniramine maleate in 100 ml of distilled water.
4. Chloroform
5. Glass wool
6. Sodium sulfate, anhydrous
7. Acetone

PROCEDURE

1. Adjust 50 ml of urine to a pH between 8 and 9 by adding small amounts of the ammonium hydroxide solution. Process the reference urine samples containing different concentrations of haloperidol in the same way.
2. Add 1.0 ml of the internal-standard solution and 30.0 ml of chloroform.
3. Extract each mixture using a separatory funnel. Allow the layers to separate.
4. Filter each chloroform layer into a flask through the neck of a funnel whose apex contains a plug of glass wool covered with about 2 g of anhydrous sodium sulfate.
5. Repeat the extractions twice, using 30.0 ml of chloroform each time.
6. Filter each of these extracts through the funnel containing the glass wool plug and sodium sulfate that was used for filtering the first extract. Pool the three extracts obtained from each sample.

7. Wash the sodium sulfate on each glass wool filter with 10.0 ml of chloroform and add this washing to the flask.
8. Evaporate each of the pooled chloroform extracts to dryness in the Büchi evaporator under vacuum (30 mm Hg) in a glycerine bath at 50°C.
9. Dissolve each residue in 0.5 ml of acetone.
10. Inject 10 μl of the dissolved residue from each sample into the gas chromatograph, making sure that the operating conditions stated above are met. The retention times for haloperidol and chlorpheniramine are 14 and 11 min, respectively.

CALCULATION

Determine the haloperidol concentration in the specimen by calculating the ratio of the peak height of haloperidol to that of chlorpheniramine maleate and relating this ratio to similarly obtained data from the analysis of the reference urine samples. Use the following formula:

$$C_U = \frac{C_S \times A_U \times P_S}{A_S \times P_U},$$

where

C_U = haloperidol concentration in the urine specimen;
C_S = haloperidol concentration in the reference solution;
A_U = peak height due to the haloperidol in the urine specimen;
A_S = peak height due to the haloperidol in the reference solution;
P_S = peak height due to the chlorpheniramine maleate in the reference solution;
P_U = peak height due to the chlorpheniramine maleate in the urine specimen.

INTERPRETATION (see p. 7)

Following a daily therapeutic dose of 5.0 mg haloperidol/70 kg body weight, only 8 to 10% of pure haloperidol is excreted in urine every 24 hr. Theoretically, this procedure can be applied to blood; in practice it is impossible since the blood concentrations resulting from therapeutic doses would be below the detection limit of the instrumentation.

ACCURACY AND PRECISION

1. With this procedure, 85 to 95% of the haloperidol added to urine is recovered.
2. Use of an internal control with extraction characteristics similar to those of haloperidol compensates for extraction losses.
3. The flame ionization detector shows a linear response for the concentration ranging from 0.2 to 100 μg/ml.

INTERFERING SUBSTANCES

Other drugs likely to be encountered in urine do not cause interference.

REFERENCE

Braun, G. A., Kade, C. F., and Roscoe, E. L., Metabolism of haloperidol in the rat, *Int. J. Neuropsychiat.*, 3, S22, 1967.

HALOTHANE

PRINCIPLE

A benzene extract of the sample is analyzed by gas chromatography using an electron-capture detector.

TYPE B PROCEDURE

Robert A. Maes

APPARATUS

1. Tubes, ground-glass-stoppered, 5 ml
2. Glass beads
3. Centrifuge
4. Syringes (Hamilton), 1 μl
5. Gas chromatograph (Aerograph Moduline 1520), equipped with an electron-capture detector (250-mCi tritium source), a 1 mV recorder (Honeywell) with attached Disc integrator, and a stainless steel column, 15″ × 1/8″ o.d., packed with Tide®*

   Operating Conditions

   Gas Flow Rate:
   nitrogen (carrier gas) – 25 ml/min

   Temperatures:
   column – 75°C
   injection port – 110°C
   detector – 130°C

   Condition the column for 8 hr at 200°C. A supplementary nitrogen supply of 25 ml/min directly to the detector inlet improves its output.

REAGENTS

All chemicals should be analytical reagent grade.

1. Benzene
2. Halothane stock solution, 200 μg/100 ml
   Dissolve 200 μg of halothane in 100 ml of benzene.
3. Halothane reference solutions
   Dilute 20, 40, 60, and 80 ml of the halothane stock solution to 100 ml with benzene to obtain concentrations of 40, 80, 120, and 160 μg halothane/100 ml solution, respectively.
4. Sodium sulfate, anhydrous

PROCEDURE

1. Introduce 2.0 ml of benzene and 30 to 50 μl of blood into a ground-glass-stoppered tube containing 4 glass beads. Shake the mixture manually for 3 min. Process comparable aliquots of each reference solution concurrently and in the same manner.
2. Add 0.5 g of anhydrous sodium sulfate to each tube. Centrifuge the tubes for 5 min at 1,500 rpm. At this point the samples may be kept for several days without loss of halothane content.
3. Inject 1 μl of each benzene extract into the gas chromatograph, making sure that the operating conditions stated above are met.

CALCULATION

Determine the blood halothane concentration by comparing the gas chromatographic response of the specimen to those of the reference solutions.

*Procter and Gamble, Cincinnati, Ohio.

INTERPRETATION (see p. 7)

Arterial, venous, and capillary blood specimens obtained 30 min after a therapeutic dose of halothane showed concentrations of 1.60, 0.66 and 1.03 mg of halothane/100 ml, respectively. The limit of detection is 10 mg of halothane/μl of blood.

ACCURACY AND PRECISION

Using the procedure described above, recovery of halothane added to blood ranges from 70 to 85%.

Because of change in the standing current of the electron-capture detector after prolonged use, reference samples must be analyzed with each injection.

INTERFERING SUBSTANCES

No other drugs or normal blood constituents interfere.

REFERENCE

Brachet-Liermain, A., Ferrus, L., and Caroff, J., Electron capture detection and measurement of fluothane (halothane) in blood, *J. Chromatogr. Sci.*, 9, 49, 1971.

HEXACHLOROPHENE

PRINCIPLE

Hexachlorophene (HCP) can be determined in blood by extraction with a mixture of ether and absolute ethanol (18 + 7), formation of the acetyl derivative of the HCP thus extracted, and subsequent identification by electron-capture gas chromatography.

TYPE C PROCEDURE

Robert A. Maes

APPARATUS

1. Graduated centrifuge tubes, glass-stoppered, 15 ml
2. Graduated test tubes, conical (Kontes 41055)
3. Pasteur pipets
4. Volumetric pipets, 1 ml
5. Centrifuge
6. Water bath
7. Syringe (Hamilton 701-N), 10 μl
8. Multipurpose rotator (model 150 V)*
9. Gas chromatograph (Varian Aerograph Model 1440), equipped with a ^{63}Ni electron-capture detector, a 1 mV recorder (Varian Aerograph Model 25) with attached Disc integrator and a glass column, 6′ × ¼″ i.d., packed with 3% OV-101 on 80 to 100 mesh Gas Chrom Q

   Operating Conditions

   Gas Flow Rate:
   nitrogen (carrier gas) – 120 ml/min

   Temperatures:
   column – 250°C
   injector port – 275°C
   detector – 300°C

   Prior to packing, pretreat the glass column with 5% dimethyldichlorosilane in toluene (v/v). Condition the packed column for 24 hr at 290°C under nitrogen at 10 to 20 ml/min prior to use.

REAGENTS

All chemicals should be analytical reagent grade.

1. Ether
2. Ethanol, absolute
3. Benzene
4. Acetic anhydride
5. Pyridine
6. Silica gel G (Merck)
7. Hexachlorophene stock solution 100 mg/dl
   Dissolve 100 mg of hexachlorophene in absolute ethanol and dilute to 100 ml with absolute ethanol. This solution is stable on storage under normal laboratory conditions for several months.
8. Hexachlorophene substock solution, 1 mg/dl
   Dilute 1.0 ml of the stock solution to 100 ml with absolute ethanol.
9. Hexachlorophene reference solutions
   Add 200, 50, 10, 5, 1, and 0.5 μl of the substock solution to 1-ml aliquots of hexachlorophene free blood.

PROCEDURE

1. Dilute 1 ml of each sample (test blood and hexachlorophene reference solution) with an equal volume of water in a 15-ml graduated glass-stoppered centrifuge tube.
2. Add 8 ml of the ether-absolute ethanol mixture and extract by mechanical mixing.

*Scientific Industries, Inc., Springfield, Mass.

3. Remove the upper solvent phase with a Pasteur pipet.
4. Repeat the extraction with an additional 8-ml portion of the solvent mixture.
5. Remove this solvent extract and add it to the one obtained in Step 3.
6. Add approximately 1 ml of water to the pooled extracts. Two phases result.
7. Separate the supernatant ether layer.
8. Evaporate it to dryness under a stream of nitrogen at 60°C with the addition of 1 ml of ethanol to hasten the process.
9. Dissolve the dried extract in 1.0 ml of benzene and 0.2 ml of a mixture of acetic anhydride-pyridine (1 +1).
10. Heat this mixture 15 min in a water bath at 60 to 70°C.
11. Evaporate the reaction mixture to dryness at 60°C under a stream of nitrogen. (The drying process should take 10 to 15 min and should not be prolonged, since the derivative may volatilize with longer exposure.)
12. Dissolve the residue in 1.0 ml of benzene.
13. Add approximately 0.1 g ($\leqslant$ 0.25 g) silica gel G. Mix the contents of the tube.
14. At 0 to 5°C centrifuge the mixture for 3 to 4 min.
15. Stopper the tubes and allow them to warm to room temperature.
16. Inject aliquots of 2 to 10 μl into the gas chromatograph. The retention time of the acetyl derivative of HCP is 3.4 min.
17. Determine the peak area of the acetyl derivative of HCP (P).

CALCULATION

Determine the concentration of HCP in the specimen by the following formula:

$$C_X = \frac{C_S \times P_X}{P_S}$$

where

C_X = concentration of HCP in the specimen;
C_S = concentration of HCP in the reference solution;
P_X = peak area of the acetyl derivative of HCP obtained from the specimen;
P_S = peak area of the acetylderivative of HCP obtained from the reference solution.

INTERPRETATION (see p. 7)

Values range from 0.38 μg/ml in an individual using a 3% HCP cleaner for whole body washing to less than 0.005 μg/ml in some individuals using 1 or 3% HCP cleansers for hand washing only. HCP concentrations resulting from prolonged use of a soap containing 0.75% HCP range from 0.02 to 0.14 μg/ml, while those resulting from the use of a mouthwash containing 0.5% HCP for 3 weeks ranged from 0.02 to 0.12 μg/ml.[1] The HCP concentration in the blood of a person whose death was caused by the ingestion of 200 cc of 3% HCP was 3.5 mg/100 ml.[2]

SENSITIVITY AND PRECISION

Using the procedure described above, recovery of HCP from samples of blood containing 0.1 μg/ml is 95%. Sensitivity for the determination is 0.005 μg/ml. Because of the change in the standing current of the electron-capture detector after prolonged use, reference samples must be analyzed with each injection.

INTERFERING SUBSTANCES

No significant gas-chromatographic response is observed from normal blood constituents that might be extracted by this procedure.

REFERENCES

1. **Ulsamer, A. G. and Marzulli, F. N.,** Hexachlorophene concentrations in blood associated with the use of products containing hexachlorophene, *Food Cosmet. Toxicol.*, 11, 625, 1973.
2. **Di Maio, V. J. M., Mullick, F. G., and Henry, L. D.,** Hexachlorophene poisoning, *J. Forensic Sci.*, 18, 303, 1973.

GENERAL REFERENCE

Ulsamer, A. G., The determination of hexachlorophene in mammalian tissues by gas-liquid chromatography, *J. Assoc. Off. Anal. Chem.*, 55, 1294, 1972.

IMIPRAMINE

PRINCIPLE

The simplest test for imipramine and its metabolites is its green oxidation product (Procedure A). When this test is carefully controlled, it can be quantitative (Procedure B). Another test depends on the fluorescence of the drug, which can be measured after extraction of the active agents from the biological fluid (Procedure C).

TYPE A PROCEDURE

George Cimbura

REAGENTS

All chemicals should be analytical reagent grade.
Caution! When preparing acid solutions, always add acid in small portions to water, constantly stirring.

1. Potassium dichromate, 200 mg/dl
   Dissolve 200 mg of potassium dichromate in 100 ml of water.
2. Sulfuric acid, 12*N*
   Dilute 30.0 ml of concentrated sulfuric acid to 100 ml with water.
3. Perchloric acid, 20 ml/dl
   Dilute 20.0 ml of concentrated perchloric acid to 100 ml with water.
4. Nitric acid, 8*N*
   Dilute 50.0 ml of concentrated nitric acid to 100 ml with water.
5. Forrest reagent
   Mix equal volumes of the above four reagents. Store the mixture in an amber glass bottle.

PROCEDURE

1. Add 1.0 ml of Forrest reagent to 1.0 ml of urine or stomach content. Shake the mixture gently.
2. Promptly observe if a green solution is produced.
3. If a purple color develops, repeat the test using 2.0 ml of Forrest reagent and 1.0 ml of urine or stomach content.

INTERPRETATION (see p. 7)

Absence of a green color indicates that imipramine is not present in the sample. A color ranging from olive to deep emerald green is an indication that imipramine (Tofranil®) and/or desipramine (Pertofrane®) and/or trimipramine (Surmontil®) may be present in the specimen. A clearly positive test is a good indication that imipramine and/or desipramine and/or trimipramine may be present. Definite identification requires further confirmatory tests. Development of a purple color may indicate the presence of phenothiazine derivatives.

REFERENCES

Forrest, F. M., Forrest, I. S., and Mason, A. S., A review of rapid urine tests for phenothiazine and related drugs, *Am. J. Psychiatr.*, 118, 300, 1961.
Forrest, I. S., Forrest, F. M., and Mason, A. S., A rapid urine color test for imipramine, *Am. J. Psychiatr.*, 116, 1021, 1960.

TYPE B PROCEDURE

George Cimbura

APPARATUS

1. Separatory funnel, 250 ml
2. Clinical centrifuge
3. Spectrophotometer, or photoelectric photometer

REAGENTS

All chemicals should be analytical reagent grade.

1. Potassium hydroxide, 6 g/dl
   Cautiously dissolve 30 g of potassium hydroxide in about 300 ml of water. Cool the solution to room temperature, then dilute to 500 ml with water.
2. *n*-Hexane, spectro grade
3. Sulfuric acid, 6*N*
   Cautiously add 168 ml of concentrated sulfuric acid 600 ml of water. Cool the solution to room temperature, then dilute it to one liter with water.
4. Sulfuric acid, 1*N*
   Cautiously add 28.0 ml of concentrated sulfuric acid to 100 ml of water. Cool the solution to room temperature, then dilute it to one liter with water.
5. Cerium (IV) sulfate, 200 mg/dl
   Dissolve 200 mg of cerium sulfate in the 1*N* sulfuric acid and dilute to 100 ml with 1*N* sulfuric acid.
6. Color-developing reagent
   Cautiously mix 30.0 ml of the cerium sulfate and 70.0 ml of concentrated sulfuric acid.
7. Imipramine hydrochloride stock solution, 100 mg/dl
   Dissolve 100 mg of imipramine hydrochloride in water and dilute to 100 ml.
8. Imipramine hydrochloride reference solutions
   Dilute 1.0, 5.0, and 10.0 ml of the imipramine hydrochloride stock solution to 100 ml with water to obtain solutions containing 10, 50, and 100 μg imipramine/ml, respectively.

PROCEDURE

1. Pipet 10.0 ml of blood, or appropriate samples of urine or tissue homogenate, into a 250-ml separatory funnel and make it alkaline with the potassium hydroxide solution.
2. Add 100 ml of *n*-hexane and shake the mixture for about 5 min. Allow the layers to separate (centrifuge, if necessary).
3. Filter the organic phase through filter paper into a 250-ml separatory funnel and wash with 10.0 ml of water. Discard the aqueous wash.
4. Add 5.0 ml of the 6*N* sulfuric acid and extract the washed *n*-hexane for 5 min.
5. Separate the acidic layer and centrifuge it.
6. Pipet 1.5 ml of the acidic extract into a cuvette and add 1.5 ml of the color-developing reagent.
7. Measure the intensity of the resulting blue color at 620 nm, using a mixture containing equal volumes of 6*N* sulfuric acid and color-developing reagent as the reference solution. Save the remainder of the acidic extract for additional tests (if required).

CALCULATION

1. Prepare a standard curve by adding accurately measured volumes of the imipramine hydrochloride reference solutions to drug-free blood to obtain final concentrations of 1 to 10 μg of imipramine/ml of blood. Place 10.0 ml of each blood sample with known imipramine concentration in a separatory funnel and follow the above procedure. Make duplicate determinations for each known concentration.
2. Determine the imipramine concentration in the specimen by comparing its absorbance with those of the reference samples.

INTERPRETATION (see p. 7)

These assays do not distinguish between imipramine and its metabolite desimipramine. Consequently in a case of imipramine poisoning, the concentration obtained is the total of the drug and its metabolite.

Patients on long-term therapy, receiving between 50.0 and 300 mg of imipramine/day, can be expected to have blood concentrations in the range from 5 to 60 μg/100 ml. Ingestion of toxic amounts of imipramine may result in blood concentrations between 0.1 and 0.5 mg/100 ml. Concentrations of the drug in liver tissue can be expected to be higher than those in blood and may be on the order of several mg/100 g tissue. Urine concentration in fatal cases may be relatively low.[1]

ACCURACY AND PRECISION

Analysis of ten drug-free blood specimens did not give false positive results. Variations in the triplicate determinations of the blood standard curve were not greater than ± 0.03 absorbance units. Average recovery of imipramine after in vitro addition to biological specimens is reported[1] to be 89.6% for blood, 74.4% for urine, and 84.7% for homogenized liver. The blue color produced is stable for at least 2 hr.

INTERFERING SUBSTANCES

Desipramine (Pertofrane®) and trimipramine (Surmontil®) will interfere. At high concentrations, thioridazine (Mellaril®) will also interfere. Desipramine is an active primary metabolite of imipramine. Further tests have to be carried out if it is necessary to differentiate between these drugs. Amitriptyline, phenothiazine derivatives, and a large number of other organic bases were found[2] not to interfere at a concentration of 10 μg in final solution.

REFERENCES

1. **Wallace, J. E., and Biggs, J. D.,** Colorimetric determinations of imipramine in biological specimens, *J. Forensic Sci.,* 14, 528, 1969.

GENERAL REFERENCE

Curry, A., *Poison Detection in Human Organs,* 2nd ed., Charles C Thomas, Springfield, 1969, 135.

TYPE C PROCEDURE

J. Grove and J. V. Halliwell

APPARATUS

1. Centrifuge tubes, glass-stoppered, 15 ml
2. Multipurpose rotator (Model 150V)*
3. Spectrofluorimeter (Aminco-Bowman), equipped with an X-Y recorder

REAGENTS

All chemicals should be analytical reagent grade.

1. Carbon tetrachloride, redistilled
2. Potassium hydroxide, 60 g/100 ml
   Dissolve 60 g of potassium hydroxide in water and dilute to 100 ml. Wash this solution with redistilled carbon tetrachloride.
3. Sodium hydroxide, 1*N*
   Dissolve 40 g of sodium hydroxide in water and dilute to one liter.
4. Sodium hydroxide, 10*N*
   Dissolve 400 g of sodium hydroxide in water and dilute to one liter.
5. Sulfuric acid, 1*N*
   Dilute 28 ml of sulfuric acid to one liter with water.
6. Sodium sulfate, anhydrous
   Purifiy this reagent by washing it with redistilled carbon tetrachloride prior to use.
7. Imipramine stock solution, 100 μg/ml

*Scientific Industries, Inc., Springfield, Mass.

Dissolve 50.0 mg of imipramine hydrochloride in 1*N* sulfuric acid. Dilute this solution to 500 ml with 1*N* sulfuric acid.

8. Imipramine reference solution, 2 μg/ml
   Dilute 2.0 ml of the imipramine stock solution to 100 ml with 1*N* sulfuric acid.

PROCEDURE

1. Place 5.0 ml of plasma in a 15-ml glass-stoppered centrifuge tube. Add 0.5 ml of the potassium hydroxide solution, 1.0 ml of distilled water, and 2.0 ml of redistilled carbon tetrachloride. Stopper the tube, shake it or place it on the rotator for 10 min, then centrifuge it for 5 min at 3,000 rpm.
2. Separate the organic phase and put it in a clean 15-ml glass-stoppered centrifuge tube. Leave the aqueous phase in the original tube.
3. Reextract the aqueous phase with 2.0 ml of redistilled carbon tetrachloride, then centrifuge it.
4. Aspirate and discard the aqueous phase. Add the carbon tetrachloride to the first extract in the second tube.
5. Wash the pooled carbon tetrachloride extracts twice with 1*N* sodium hydroxide, shaking and centrifuging as before.
6. Aspirate each aqueous wash completely and discard it. Add a spatula full of anhydrous sodium sulfate to the organic phase. Any emulsion present will separate.
7. Centrifuge the tube, then decant the organic solvent into a third tube.
8. Wash the sodium sulfate with 2.0 ml of redistilled carbon tetrachloride, then decant the washing into the third tube.
9. Add 5.0 ml of 1*N* sulfuric acid to the third tube. Stopper the tube, shake it for 10 min, then centrifuge it.
10. Transfer 2.0 ml of the supernatant to a quartz cuvette. Add 0.2 ml of 10*N* sodium hydroxide to the supernatant in the cuvette.
11. Measure the fluorescence of the solution at an excitation wavelength of 290 nm and an emission wavelength of 415 nm, using slit arrangement #5 at a sensitivity of 30.
12. Repeat Steps 10 and 11, using 2.0 ml of the imipramine reference solution instead of the supernatant.

CALCULATION

Use the following formula to calculate the imipramine (and desipramine) concentration in the specimen:

$$\frac{F_S}{F_R} \times C_R = C_S,$$

where

F_S = relative fluorescence of the specimen;
F_R = relative fluorescence of the reference solution;
C_R = concentration of the reference solution used;
C_S = concentration of the specimen.

INTERPRETATION (see p. 7)

These assays do not distinguish between imipramine and its metabolite desipramine. Consequently, in a case of imipramine poisoning, the concentration obtained is the total of the drug and its metabolite. Patients on long-term therapy receiving between 50.0 and 300 mg of imipramine/day, can be expected to have blood concentrations in the range from 5 to 60 μg/100 ml. Ingestion of toxic amounts of imipramine may result in blood concentrations between 0.1 and 0.5 mg/100 ml. Concentrations of the drug in liver tissue can be expected to be higher than those in blood and may be on the order of several mg/100 g tissue. Urine concentration in fetal cases may be relatively low.[1]

ACCURACY AND PRECISION

The relative fluorescence is proportional to concentration over the range from 0 to 2 μg/ml. Mean recovery of imipramine added to plasma is 90% ± 6%.

REFERENCE

1. **Curry, A.,** *Poison Detection in Human Organs,* 2nd ed., Charles C Thomas, Springfield, 1969, 135.

IRON

PRINCIPLE

Serum iron is separated from transferrin with an acid buffer and reduced with ascorbic acid. The color which results from the addition of sulfonated bathophenanthroline is proportional to the amount of iron present. Addition of a known amount of iron serves as an internal standard for each specimen. The color is stable and has a maximum absorbance at 535 nm (Procedure A). Serum iron may also be determined by atomic absorption spectrophotometry (Procedure B), using the 248.3 nm iron resonance line. The serum samples are diluted with an equal volume of trichloroacetic acid. The mixture is heated at 90°C for 15 min, then centrifuged. The purpose of this preparation is threefold. First, protein, which could clog the burner slot or change the absorbance of the sample, is precipitated. Second, about 95% of any hemoglobin iron, which could cause high readings, is removed. Third, dilution is held to a minimum, important because normal serum iron values range from about 50 to 150 μg/100 ml.

TYPE A PROCEDURE

Clifford B. Walberg

APPARATUS

1. Filter photometer (see Note 2) with 540-nm filter
2. Calibrated cuvettes for photometer
3. Vortex mixer
4. Serological pipets, 0.1 and 0.2 ml
5. Volumetric pipets, 1 and 4 ml

REAGENTS

All chemicals should be analytical reagent grade and as free of iron as possible.

1. Hydrochloric acid, 1*N*
   Dilute 83.3 ml of concentrated hydrochloric acid to one liter with iron-free water.
2. Ascorbic acid solution, 5 g/dl
   Prepare only small amounts because of the limited stability of this solution. Dissolve 250 mg of ascorbic acid in iron-free water and dilute to 5 ml with iron-free water. Store at 4°C. The solution may be used until it turns yellow (approximately 6 months if not exposed to light).
3. Glycine buffer, 0.2*M*, pH 1.9 ± 0.3, stock solution
   Dissolve 3.75 g of glycine in approximately 250 ml of water. Add 52 ml of 1*N* HCl. Mix well and dilute with water to one liter. Adjust to pH 1.9. This buffer is stable indefinitely when stored at 4°C.
4. Glycine buffer, working solution
   Prepare just prior to use. Mix 20 ml of glycine stock solution with 0.1 ml of the ascorbic acid solution.
5. Bathophenanthroline,* sulfonated (sodium salt), 0.4 g/dl
   Dissolve 0.4 g in water and dilute to 100 ml with water.
6. Iron stock solution, 100 mg/dl, Harleco Iron Standard #7558 (or equivalent)
7. Iron reference solution, 2.5 mg/dl
   Dilute 5.0 ml of iron stock solution to 200 ml with iron-free water.

PROCEDURE

A protein-free filtrate is not required. The entire procedure is carried out using a single cuvette for each specimen. The absorbance of each solution is determined using a reagent blank, and the net absorbance is used for the calculations.

1. Prepare a sufficient amount of glycine buffer-ascorbic acid mixture (Reagent 4) to deliver 4 ml into a sufficient number of test tubes for

*Available in sulfonated form from the G. Frederick Smith Co., Columbus, Ohio 43223.

each test sample, plus one control serum and one reagent blank (see Note 3).

2. Add 1.0 ml of sample (serum, control serum, and water) to 4.0 ml of the glycine buffer-ascorbic acid mixture. Mix well. Determine the absorbance of each sample after 2 min using the processed water sample as the reference solution (R_1).
3. Add 0.16 ml (see Note 1) of the bathophenanthroline solution to each cuvette including the water sample (reference). Mix well. The instrument should be rezeroed using the processed water sample as the reference solution. Determine the absorbance of each serum sample 5 min after mixing (R_2).
4. Add 0.08 ml of the iron reference solution to the serum samples only. *Do not* add it to the water sample. *Mix well immediately after adding the iron solution.* Determine the absorbance of each sample 5 min after mixing (R_3), using the processed water sample as the reference solution.

CALCULATION

$$\frac{R_2 - R_1}{R_3 - R_2} \times 200 = \mu\text{g iron/100 ml serum}$$

When this test is performed using the volumes shown, no corrections are necessary for small changes of volume when the color reagent and internal standard are added.

NOTES

1. Small volumes may be delivered most conveniently from a calibrated microliter syringe (Hamilton 725CH); however, 0.1- and 0.2-ml serological pipets may be used to deliver 0.08 and 0.16 ml, respectively. To prevent contamination, pour a sufficient amount of the reagent into a 5-ml beaker and dispense the reagent from this container.
2. This procedure is designed as a one-tube internal standard method using stable reagents and a simple photometer. The method requires no sample preparation and is simple and fast. The entire procedure must be done in a single tube. The procedure cannot be done on spectrophotometers which employ flow-through cuvettes or on any system which does not allow removal of the tube for making additions, shaking, and reinserting for successive readings. The absorbance of the water sample (reference) changes from Step 2 to Step 3 and thereafter remains constant. Rezeroing is not a problem on instruments such as the Klett filter photometer, Spectronic 20, Beckman Model DB, or similar instruments. If a spectrophotometer is used, the instrument should be set at 535 nm.
3. A commercial control serum with a known iron value should be run concurrently with the test to assure accuracy.

INTERPRETATION (see p. 7)

The method is applicable to low, normal, or elevated serum iron. The normal range for serum iron is 65 to 175 μg/100 ml. The values found in 51 cases of accidental ingestion of iron tablets in children ranged from 202 to 662 μg/100 ml.

PRECISION

The precision obtained on a control pool in the normal range was 81 ± 8 μg/dl (2 S.D.).

INTERFERING SUBSTANCES

This procedure is not affected by turbidity (eg., lipemia), icterus, or hemolysis as may be the case when using methods which do not employ an internal standard. The method also is not affected by the presence of Imferon®, an iron-dextran complex used in the treatment of iron-deficiency anemias, since this complex is not broken by the addition of any of the reagents. Methods using TCA filtrates or surfactants will give spuriously high levels if Imferon® is present.

REFERENCE

Beale, R. N., Bostrom, J. O., and Taylor, R. F., Improved rapid methods for the determination of iron content and binding capacity of serum, *J. Clin. Pathol.*, 15, 156, 1962.

TYPE B PROCEDURE

Frank J. Fernandez

APPARATUS

1. Polyethylene test tubes, 12 X 75 mm
2. Centrifuge
3. Vortex mixer
4. Heating block, 90°C (or water bath)
5. Spectrophotometer, atomic absorption (Perkin-Elmer Model 360), equipped with an iron hollow-cathode lamp, a three slot air-acetylene burner head, and a 10 in. strip-chart recorder

   Operating Conditions

   Wavelength: 248.3 nm
   Slit Width: 0.7 nm
   Flame: oxidizing, air-acetylene (blue flame)
   Air Flow: 65 div
   Acetylene Flow: 35 div
   Signal Mode: concentration
   Recorder Response: time constant #2

REAGENTS

All chemicals should be analytical reagent grade. All water should be deionized, then distilled.

1. Trichloroacetic acid (TCA) stock solution, 200 g/l
   Dissolve 200 g of TCA in water and dilute to 1 liter.
2. Hydrochloric acid, concentrated
3. Iron stock solution I, 1,000 μg/ml
   Dissolve 100 mg of Baker AR grade iron wire in 10 ml of concentrated hydrochloric acid and dilute to 100 ml with water.
4. Iron stock solution II, 5 μg/ml
   Dilute 5 ml of iron stock solution I to one liter with water.
5. Iron reference solutions, 25, 50, 75, and 100 μg/100 ml
   Pipet 5, 10, 15, and 20 ml of the iron stock solution II into 100-ml volumetric flasks. Add 50 ml of the TCA stock solution to each flask and dilute to volume with water.
6. Blank solution
   Add 50 ml of the TCA stock solution to a 100-ml volumetric flask and dilute to volume with water.

PROCEDURE

Sample Preparation

1. Transfer 2 ml of serum into a 12 X 75 mm polyethylene tube.
2. Add 2 ml of the TCA stock solution, cap the tube loosely, and mix.
3. Heat in a heating block at 90°C for 15 min.
4. Centrifuge at least 10 min (500 X g or greater).

Analysis

1. Allow spectrophotometer and burner system to warm up at least 10 min.
2. Set readout of the spectrophotometer and recorder to zero while aspirating blank solution.
3. Aspirate the iron reference solution (100 μg/100 ml) and adjust recorder response to 50% of full scale.
4. Establish calibration by aspirating the blank and the iron reference solutions for 10 sec, interspersing a 10-sec aspiration of water between reference solutions.
5. Aspirate sample supernatant directly from the 12 X 75 mm polyethylene tube and record concentration reading.

CALCULATION

1. Prepare a standard curve by plotting the recorder readings of the reference solutions against their respective concentrations.
2. Determine the iron concentration in the diluted serum sample by comparing the observed recorder reading and the standard curve. Multiply this value by 2 to obtain the iron concentration in the original serum sample. (Serum samples are diluted 1:1 with TCA.)

INTERPREATION (see p. 7)

According to Olson and Hamlin,[1] the normal value for iron is as follows:

serum (N = 57): mean = 109 μg/100 ml ± 51.4 μg/100 ml

ACCURACY AND PRECISION

Replicate analyses of a serum pool with a serum iron concentration of 83.5 μg/100 ml yielded a coefficient of variation of 3.4%.[1] Measurement of the recovery of iron added to serum averaged 96%.[1]

REFERENCE

1. **Olson, A. D. and Hamlin, W. B.,** A new method for serum iron and total iron-binding capacity by atomic absorption spectrophotometry, *Clin. Chem.*, 15, 438, 1969.

GENERAL REFERENCE

Yee, H. Y. and Goodwin, J. F., Simultaneous determination of copper and iron in a single aliquot of serum, *Clin. Chem.*, 20, 189, 1974.

ISONIAZID

PRINCIPLE

Isoniazid is extracted from an alkalinized serum sample and then reextracted into dilute acid. After reaction with *trans*-cinnamaldehyde, it can be identified and quantitated by spectrophotometry.

TYPE B PROCEDURE

Leslie Eidus and Anita M. T. Harnanansingh

APPARATUS

1. Erlenmeyer flasks, glass-stoppered, 250 ml
2. Mechanical shaker, horizontal
3. Test tubes, 16 X 150 mm
4. Centrifuge
5. Pasteur pipets
6. Lambda pipets
7. Spectrophotometer, equipped with a microcell unit
8. Heparinized Vacutainer®

REAGENTS

All chemicals should be analytical reagent grade.

1. Isoniazid stock solution, 10 mg/100 ml
   Dissolve 10 mg of isoniazid in water and dilute to 100 ml with water.
2. Isoniazid plasma reference solutions, 1, 2, 5, and 10 μg/ml
   Add 0.10, 0.20, 0.50, and 1.0 ml of the isoniazid stock solution to 10-ml volumetric flasks containing drug-free biological fluid (serum). Dilute the contents of each flask to 10 ml with the biological fluid.
3. Sodium hydroxide, 4*N*
   Dissolve 16 g of sodium hydroxide in 100 ml of water.
4. Ammonium sulfate
5. Extraction mixture, chloroform-butanol, 7:3
   Purify *n*-butanol and chloroform, each separately, by adding activated charcoal, mixing, then filtering it through 1 sheet of Whatman #1 filter paper. Add approximately 30 g of anhydrous sodium sulfate to one liter of each solvent to render it free of water, then filter it through 3 sheets of Whatman #1 filter paper. Mix 3 volumes of the purified *n*-butanol with 7 volumes of the purified chloroform.
6. Hydrochloric acid, 0.1*N*
   Dilute 8 ml of concentrated hydrochloric acid to one liter with water.
7. *trans*-Cinnamaldehyde, 0.04%
   Dissolve 1 ml of chlorine-free *trans*-cinnamaldehyde (Eastman Kodak Co.) in 100 ml of absolute ethanol. This solution may be stored for 3 weeks at 4°C. Prior to the isoniazid determination, dilute 1.0 ml of this solution to 25.0 ml with absolute ethanol.

SPECIMEN PREPARATION

Collect blood specimens in a heparinized Vacutainer®. Centrifuge and separate the plasma immediately. Store plasma frozen (−20°C) until the determination is performed.

PROCEDURE

1. Mix 2.0 ml of plasma or serum with 1 drop of 4*N* sodium hydroxide and 2.2 g of ammonium sulfate in a 250-ml glass-stoppered Erlenmeyer flask. Process in duplicate 2.0 ml of each reference solution and 2.0 ml of drug-free biological fluid in the same manner as the specimen. If a low isoniazid concentration is suspected, use 3.0 ml of plasma and 3.2 g of ammonium sulfate for increased sensitivity.
2. Add 20.0 ml of the extraction mixture, then shake the flask for 30 min on a horizontal shaker at 145 excursions/min.

3. Separate the organic extract and filter it through Whatman #1 filter paper.
4. Place 15.0 ml of the filtrate in a clean, 250-ml, glass-stoppered Erlenmeyer flask and add 1.0 ml of 0.1*N* hydrochloric acid. Shake the mixture for 15 min on a horizontal shaker at 145 excursions/min.
5. Transfer the contents to a 16 × 150 mm test tube and centrifuge for 10 min at 2,000 rpm.
6. Withdraw the aqueous supernatant, using a Pasteur pipet. Mix 0.5 ml of the supernatant with 150 μl of the alcoholic *trans*-cinnamaldehyde reagent. Add the latter with a lambda pipet.
7. Determine the absorbance of each sample at 340 nm, using 0.5 ml of the 0.1*N* hydrochloric acid and 150 μl of alcoholic *trans*-cinnamaldehyde as the reference solution.

CALCULATION

1. Determine the isoniazid concentration (μg/ml) in the specimen by the following formula:

$$C_r \times \frac{A_s}{A_r} = C_s$$

where

C_r = isoniazid concentration of the reference solution;
C_s = isoniazid concentration in the specimen;
A_s = absorbance of the specimen at 340 nm;
A_r = absorbance of the reference solution at 340 nm.

2. The absorbance has a linear relationship to isoniazid concentrations from 1.0 to 10 μg/ml. A specimen must be repeated, diluting prior to extraction, if its concentration is higher than 10 μg/ml.

INTERPRETATION (see p. 7)

Following usual therapeutic doses of 300 to 400 mg once a day, serum isoniazid concentrations range from 0.5 to 12 μg/ml.

ACCURACY AND PRECISION

During extraction, 85% of isoniazid added to drug-free biological fluid (serum) is recovered. This may vary with the quality of the organic solvents used. The sensitivity of this method is five times greater than that of other published procedures.

REFERENCE

Boxenbaum, H. G. and Riegelman, S., Determination of isoniazid and metabolites in biological fluids, *J. Pharm. Sci.*, 63, 1191, 1974.

Eidus, L. and Harnanansingh, A. M. T., A more sensitive spectrophotometric method for determination of isoniazid in serum or plasma, *Clin. Chem.*, 17, 492, 1971.

ISONIAZID PHENOTYPING

PRINCIPLE

Urine is collected in the 6 to 8 hr period following an oral test dose of 10 mg of INH/kg body weight. In one aliquot of this sample only acetylisoniazid is determined; in the other acetylisoniazid and INH, artificially acetylated (total hydrazines) are estimated by the same color reaction. The classification of slow and fast acetylators is based on the percentage of acetylisoniazid versus the total hydrazines.

TYPE B PROCEDURE

Leslie Eidus and Mary M. Hodgkin

APPARATUS

1. pH Meter
2. Centrifuge
3. Pasteur pipets
4. Test tubes, 20 ml
5. Serological pipets, 5 and 10 ml
6. Spectrophotometer or colorimeter

REAGENTS

All chemicals should be analytical reagent grade.

1. Hydrochloric acid, 0.5*N*
   Dilute 50.0 ml of standardized 1.00*N* hydrochloric acid to 100 ml with water.
2. Sodium hydroxide, 0.5*N*
   Dilute 50.0 ml of standardized 1.00*N* sodium hydroxide to 100 ml with water. Well-matched acid and base will ensure proper neutralization of the specimens.
3. Sodium hydroxide, 7*N*
   Cautiously dissolve 28 g sodium hydroxide in approximately 75 ml of water. Cool the solution to room temperature and dilute to 100 ml with water.
4. Acetic anhydride
5. Phosphate buffer, 0.5*M*, pH 6.0
   (A) Dissolve 43.54 g of anhydrous, potassium phosphate, and dibasic (K_2HPO_4) in water and dilute to 500 ml. (B) Dissolve 34.02 g of potassium phosphate monobasic (KH_2PO_4) in water and dilute to 500 ml. Prepare the buffer by mixing 87.7 ml of Solution B with 12.3 ml of Solution A. Check the pH and adjust to 6.0, if necessary, with either solution.
6. Potassium cyanide, 20 g/dl
   Dissolve 5 g in water and dilute to 25 ml with water. Prepare fresh daily. (This reagent is very toxic and requires care in handling, storage, and disposal.)
7. Chloramine-T (Eastman Kodak), 12.5 g/dl
   Dissolve 12.5 g in water and dilute to 100 ml with water. Prepare fresh daily.
8. Acetone

SPECIMEN PREPARATION

After a drug-free period of 48 hr, an oral test dose of 10 mg of isoniazid/kg body weight is administered. Six hr later the individual should empty his bladder completely, and this urine sample is discarded. The total urine excreted during the following 2 hr is collected, and an aliquot of it used for the analysis. If the test is not performed a few hours after collection, the sample should be stored in a deep freeze.

PROCEDURE[1-3]

1. Centrifuge 10 ml of urine for 10 min at 2,000 rpm.
2. Transfer 4.0 ml of clear urine to a clean test tube.
3. Add 2.0 ml of 0.5*N* hydrochloric acid, mix, and allow the mixture to stand at room temperature for 15 min.

4. From the acidified urine, transfer 2 aliquots of 1.5 ml each into separate test tubes labeled A and B.
5. Add 1 drop of acetic anhydride to Tube B and shake the mixture for 1 min; then, add 1 drop of 7*N* sodium hydroxide.
6. Add 2 drops of distilled water to Tube A to ensure that both tubes have equal volumes.
7. Add 0.5 ml of 0.5*N* sodium hydroxide to both aliquots 15 min after acidification and shake gently.
8. Dilute both aliquots with 8.0 ml of distilled water (equivalent to 1:10 final dilution of the urine). In general, this dilution is satisfactory; however, occasionally 1:5 or 1:20 may be optimal (e.g., 3.0 or 18.0 ml of water).
9. Transfer 2.0 ml of the diluted aliquots to clean test tubes and add 1.0 ml of 0.5*M* phosphate buffer. Add 2.0 ml of distilled water to another clean test tube. This will serve as a reagent blank.
10. Add 1.0 ml of the potassium cyanide reagent to each tube, followed by 4.0 ml of the chloramine-T solution, and mix.
11. After a waiting period of 90 sec, add 5.0 ml of acetone to each tube and mix well in order to dissolve the precipitate.
12. A small amount of the precipitate may not dissolve due to urine constituents. Should this ensue, centrifuge the tube at 2,000 rpm for 10 min and use the supernatant for Step 13.
13. Determine the absorbances of the solutions at 550 nm, using the processed water sample as the blank.

CALCULATION[3,4]

Determine the percentage of acetylisoniazid to total hydrazides by the following formula:

$$\%AC - INH = \frac{A_a}{A_b} \times 100$$

where

%AC - INH = percentage of acetylation;
A_a = absorbance of solution in Tube A (containing only acetylisoniazid);
A_b = absorbance of solution in Tube B (containing acetylisoniazid and isoniazid acetylated in vitro).

INTERPRETATION[3,4] (see p. 7)

Patients with a percentage less than 70 are classified as slow inactivators, while those with values over 70 are termed fast inactivators.

INTERFERING SUBSTANCES[3]

Interference from cycloserine and chlorpromazine is of no importance, as the patient should be drug-free 48 hr prior to phenotyping. For test doses only pyridoxine-free INH tablets should be used, as Vitamin B_6 may influence the result. Glucose in urine interferes with the acetylisoniazid estimation by suppressing the color development. Care, therefore, should be exercised in the interpretation of a phenotyping result of a diabetic.

REFERENCES

1. **Eidus, L. and Hodgkin, M. M.,** Screening of isoniazid inactivators, *Antimicrob. Agents Chemother.*, 3, 130, 1973.
2. **Eidus, L. and Hodgkin, M. M.,** Simplified screening test for phenotyping of isoniazid inactivators, *Int. J. Clin. Pharmacol.*, 7, 82, 1973.
3. **Hodgkin, M. M., Hsu, A. H. E., Varughese, P., and Eidus, L.,** Evaluation of a new method for phenotyping of slow and rapid acetylators, *Int. J. Clin. Pharmacol.*, 7, 355, 1973.
4. **Jessamine, A. G., Hodgkin, M. M., and Eidus, L.,** Urine tests for phenotyping slow and fast acetylators, *Can. J. Public Health.*, 65, 119, 1974.

LEAD IN BIOLOGICAL MATERIALS

PRINCIPLE

The classical yet still functional procedure for the determination of lead in biological materials requires that all the organic matter be removed. This may be done by a wet or dry digestion. The former technique is preferred and usually uses a mixture of strong oxidizing agents to digest the organic matter. Once removed, along with any excess oxidants, the lead in the residue can be determined by forming lead dithizonate, which forms a characteristic magenta solution in chloroform. This complex can be separated from other metal dithizonates by extraction at an optimal pH in the presence of other substances designed to remove potential interfering cations (Procedure B). A simpler, more direct method for the determination of lead depends on chelation with ammonium pyrrolidine dithiocarbamate, extraction of this chelate into methylisobutyl ketone, and aspiration of this solution into an atomic absorption spectrophotometer (Procedure C).

TYPE B PROCEDURE

Irving Sunshine

APPARATUS

1. Kjeldahl flasks, Pyrex,® 300 ml
2. Bottles, Pyrex,® glass-stoppered, 125 ml
3. Photometer, photoelectric

REAGENTS

All chemicals should be analytical reagent grade and low in lead content. All water used in the preparation of reagents and in the final rinsing of all glassware should be deionized. All glassware used, including sample bottles, must be lead-free. This is best achieved by thorough washing and a final rinse with 10% nitric acid.

1. Nitric acid, 1 ml/100 ml
   Dilute 10 ml of concentrated nitric acid to one liter.
2. Perchloric acid, concentrated (72%)
   Store in a refrigerator when not in use. **Caution!** This reagent is potentially explosive and requires great care in handling and storage.
3. Hydroxylamine hydrochloride, 20 g/100 ml
   Dissolve 20 g of hydroxylamine hydrochloride in water and dilute to 100 ml.
4. Citric acid, 50 g/100 ml
   Dissolve 50 g of citric acid in water and dilute to 100 ml.
5. Phenol red, 0.2 g/100 ml
   Dissolve 0.2 g of phenol red in water and dilute to 100 ml.
6. Potassium cyanide, 10 g/100 ml
   Dissolve 10 g of potassium cyanide in water and dilute to 100 ml. **Caution!** This reagent is very toxic and requires care in handling, storage, and disposal.
7. Dithizone stock solution, 40 mg/100 ml
   Dissolve 400 mg of dithizone in chloroform and dilute to one liter. Store in an amber bottle in a refrigerator.
8. Dithizone working solution, 0.8 mg/100 ml
   Dilute 2 ml of the stock solution to 100 ml with chloroform. Prepare as needed. Use within 6 hr and discard any unused solution.
9. Wash solution
   Mix 75 ml of concentrated ammonium hydroxide with 100 ml of potassium cyanide and dilute to 500 ml with water.
10. Lead stock solution, 1 mg/ml
    Dissolve 1.5984 g of lead nitrate in dilute nitric acid. Dilute this solution to one liter with additional dilute nitric acid.
11. Lead reference solution, 1 μg/ml
    Dilute 1.0 ml of the lead stock solution to one liter with dilute nitric acid. Use 10.0- and 20.0-ml aliquots of this solution for reference analyses.

SPECIMEN REQUIREMENTS

Unless adequate precautions have been taken, false positive results may occur due to lead contamination from many different sources. All urine specimens should be collected in specially cleaned, acid-rinsed Pyrex® or polyethylene containers. A specimen volume of 100 to 200 ml is desirable, but 50 ml will suffice. Blood specimens should be obtained in Vacutainer® tubes specially designated for lead analyses. No anticoagulants should be used. Alternatively, a suitably washed all-glass syringe (no metal Luer lock) with a disposable needle may be used to draw the blood specimen.

PROCEDURE

1. Pipet either 50.0 ml of urine, a specimen of clotted whole blood of recorded weight (approximately 10 g), or 10 g of homogenized tissue into a lead-free 300-ml Pyrex® Kjedahl flask. Process 10.0 ml of water (as a reagent blank) and 10 ml of the lead reference solution (as a standard) in the same manner as the specimen.
2. Add 2.0 ml of concentrated sulfuric acid and 15.0 ml of concentrated nitric acid to the flask. Heat the contents until charring just begins. *Do not allow all the liquid to boil away.* When reference solutions or aqueous samples are analyzed, cease heating when dense, rolling white fumes of sulfur trioxide appear in the bulb of the flask.
3. After the flask contents have cooled to room temperature, add 15.0 ml of concentrated nitric acid and 2.0 ml of concentrated (72%) perchloric acid. *Be certain that the flask is cool before adding the perchloric acid.* Reheat the flask until sulfur trioxide fumes appear in the bulb.
4. Cool the mixture, add 10.0 to 15.0 ml of water, then heat again until sulfur trioxide fumes appear. When this digest cools, it should be colorless and clear. If this is not so, repeat Steps 3 and 4. (If necessary, the procedure may be halted at this point and continued at another time. In that case it is advisable to add 10.0 to 20.0 ml of water to each flask.)
5. Add to the digest, in the order given, 2.0 ml of the hydroxylamine hydrochloride solution, 2.0 ml of the dilute citric acid, and 2 to 4 drops of phenol red indicator solution. To this mixture, now red in color, slowly add concentrated ammonium hydroxide. The solution will change to yellow, then back to red. When this end point is reached, add 1.0 ml of concentrated ammonium hydroxide.
6. Cool the flask to room temperature, then quantitatively transfer its contents to a 125-ml glass-stoppered Pyrex® bottle. Rinse the flask twice, using between 10.0 and 15.0 ml of deionized water each time. Transfer both washings to the Pyrex® bottle.
7. Cool the contents of the bottle to room temperature, then add 5.0 ml of the potassium cyanide solution.
8. Extract the lead from the aqueous phase by adding 10.0 ml of the dithizone working solution and shake vigorously for 5 min.
9. Examine the chloroform layer. If it is not green, add 10.0 ml more of the dithizone working solution, shake, then examine the chloroform layer again. (One 10.0-ml aliquot of the dithizone working solution is usually sufficient; additional 10.0-ml aliquots are required only when abnormally high lead concentrations are present.)
10. Remove the upper red aqueous layer by aspiration and discard it, exercising great care because this liquid has a high cyanide content.
11. Add 10.0 to 15.0 ml of wash solution to the chloroform remaining in the Pyrex® bottle and shake vigorously. This extracts any excess dithizone into the aqueous phase and leaves the red-colored lead dithizonate in the chloroform.
12. Remove the aqueous phase by aspiration and carefully discard it. (This aqueous phase frequently has a characteristic brown color due to the solubility of the removed dithizone.)
13. Repeat the wash procedure once more to get rid of any remaining dithizone in the chloroform extract.
14. Transfer the lead dithizonate to a cuvette and centrifuge it.
15. Determine the absorbance of the resulting clear red chloroform solution in a suitable photoelectric photometer at 505 nm, using the chloroform obtained by processing the water sample as the reference solution. Use this latter solution also as a reagent blank for measuring the absorbance of the 10-μg lead reference sample which was processed in the same manner.

CALCULATION

1. Determine the amount of lead in the processed specimen by comparing its absorbance with that obtained from the processed lead reference sample.
2. Calculate the lead concentration (mg/100 ml or mg/100 g) in the specimen by using the following formula:

$$C_S = \frac{A_S}{A_R} \times C_R \times \frac{100}{V_S},$$

where

C_S = lead concentration in the specimen;
C_R = lead concentration in the reference solution;
A_S = absorbance of the specimen at 505 nm;
A_R = absorbance of the reference solution at 505 nm;
V_S = volume or weight of the specimen.

INTERPRETATION (see p. 7)

A blood lead concentration below 0.06 mg/100 g is generally accepted as being within safe limits. Concentration above 0.10 mg/100 g is regarded as a significant indication of probable toxicity. If a patient has the latter blood lead concentration and displays symptoms compatible with lead intoxication, therapy should be considered. In the absence of symptomatology, removal from exposure to lead is mandatory for insuring the patient's safety. For an industrial worker this means removal to a lead-free area and job; for a child it means control of the source, usually old paint with high lead content, by resurfacing the offending areas with paint low in lead content.

A similar interpretation pertains to urine lead concentrations. The highest concentration usually considered to be compatible with a safe limit is 0.06 mg/liter. Higher values are usually indicative of excessive absorption. In some industrial workers chronically exposed over a long period, however, the upper limit of urine lead concentration compatible with safety is generally accepted as 0.15 mg/liter, because many exposed workers with urine lead concentrations between 0.08 and 0.15 mg/liter are asymptomatic. Since urinary excretion varies directly with the extent of exposure and liquid intake and output, diurnal variation may be large. A random spot urine will, therefore, not be as valuable as an indicator of excessive absorption as a larger sample collected over an extended period. A one-liter specimen is considered desirable. Obviously, this is not possible when young children are involved. In such cases random urine specimens are usually analyzed, if they are obtainable, and interpreted with due caution.

ACCURACY AND PRECISION

Blood: ±0.01 mg/100 g when the specimen is 10 g or more. Urine: ±0.01 mg/liter when the specimen is 50 ml or more.

REFERENCE*

Keenan, R. G., Byers, D. H., Saltzman, B. E., and Hyslop, F. L., The USPHS method for determining lead in air and in biological materials, *Am. Ind. Hyg. Assoc. J.*, 24, 481, 1963.

*For an updated list of reference material, see References, p. 209.

TYPE C PROCEDURE

B. Davidow, B. Searle, and W. Chan

APPARATUS

1. Vacutainer® tubes, heparinized (Becton-Dickinson No. L3200 XF 313)
2. Polyethylene bottles, screw-capped, 4 oz
3. Homogenizer (Sorvall Co. Omni-Mixer–OM, Model 17105), equipped with a 50-ml stainless steel chamber assembly (Model 17077)
4. Shaker (Eberbach Corp.)
5. Centrifuge tubes (Fisher Scientific Cat. No. 5-558 or 5-558-5), 50 ml
6. Centrifuge (International Model UV)
7. Spectrophotometer, atomic absorption (Perkin-Elmer Model 303), equipped with a lead intensitron lamp and digital reader (Perkin-Elmer Model DCR-1)

REAGENTS

All chemicals should be analytical reagent grade. All aqueous solutions are prepared with double-distilled water.

1. Ammonium pyrrolidine dithiocarbamate (APDC) (K and K Laboratories) Triton® X-100 (Rhom and Haas) reagent
   Dissolve 14 g of APDC in about 300 ml of distilled water. Add 280 ml of 5% Triton® X-100 and shake thoroughly. Add sufficient distilled water to make a total volume of 500 ml. Keep refrigerated.
2. MIBK (methylisobutylketone), water-saturated
   Saturate the solvent with distilled water prior to use.
3. Lead stock solution, 10 mg/100 ml
   Dissolve 0.1599 g of dried lead nitrate in distilled water containing 1.0 ml of concentrated nitric acid and dilute to one liter with water.
4. Lead reference solution, 1 mg/100 ml
   Dilute 10.0 ml of the lead stock solution to 100 ml with distilled water. Discard 7 days after preparation.

PROCEDURE

Preparation of the Specimen

1. Mark the exact level of the blood on the Vacutainer® tube in which the specimen has been received. A sample size of 3.0 to 5.0 ml is required.
2. Pour the entire blood specimen into a 4-oz plastic bottle. Note whether the specimen is clotted.
3. Rinse the collection tube by adding 5.0 ml of the APDC Triton® X-100 reagent and shaking it. Add the rinse to the blood in the plastic bottle.
4. Remove any remaining liquid in the blood collection tube, using a water aspirator.
5. Fill the tube with water-saturated MIBK to the mark designating the volume of blood (Step 1). Add the solvent to the plastic bottle, then shake the mixture for 10 min.
6. If the sample is clotted, transfer it and the MIBK to the homogenizer cup and homogenize for 5 min at 5,000 rpm.
7. Transfer the homogenized (6) or agitated (5) specimen into a suitable test tube. Stopper the tube.
8. Centrifuge the tube for 15 min to separate the layers.
9. Remove the upper layer, which contains the extracted lead-APDC chelate, from each sample and aspirate it into the flame of the spectrometer.

Preparation of Reference Samples

1. To each of four 4-oz plastic bottles, add the following reagents in the order listed on the following page.

Reagent	Reference lead concentration, μg/100 ml			
	0	30	60	120
Lead reference solution	0.0	0.6	1.2	2.4
Water	20.0	19.4	18.8	17.6
APDC Triton® X-100 reagent	4.0	4.0	4.0	4.0
Water-saturated MIBK	20.0	20.0	20.0	20.0

2. Shake each bottle for 5 to 10 min.
3. Transfer each solution to a 50-ml centrifuge tube.
4. Centrifuge the solutions for 15 min.
5. Remove the upper layer, which contains the extracted lead-APDC chelate, from each sample and aspirate it into the flame of the spectrometer.

Measurement of Unknown and Reference Samples

1. Set the controls of the atomic absorption spectrophotometer as follows:
   Slit: 4 (1 mm, 7A)
   Range: UV
   Gas Mixture: air flow 9, acetylene 9
   Wavelength: 283.3 nm
   Aspiration Rate: 5 ml/min
   Air Pressure: 30
   Averaging Switch: position 4X
   Noise Suppression: 2
   Scale: 1
   Allow a warm-up time of 1 hr for the instrument and 30 min for the flame. Adjust the amount of acetylene in the flame while aspirating a water-saturated solution of MIBK, so that there is a slightly visible orange tint in the flame.
2. Determine the absorbance of each specimen. After performing 25 analyses, check the absorbance of the reference samples and make any necessary corrections for instrumental drift or changes in the flame characteristics.
3. Plot the absorbances of the reference samples against their respective lead concentrations, then draw a standard curve from the data obtained.

CALCULATION

Determine the lead concentration in the specimen by comparing its absorbance with that of a suitable reference sample or a standard curve prepared from the reference samples suggested above.

INTERPRETATION (see p. 7)

A blood lead concentration below 0.06 mg/100 g is generally accepted as being within safe limits. Concentration above 0.10 mg/100 g is regarded as a significant indication of probable toxicity. If a patient has the latter blood lead concentration and displays symptoms compatible with lead intoxication, therapy should be considered. In the absence of symptomatology, removal from exposure to lead is mandatory for insuring the patient's safety. For an industrial worker this means removal to a lead-free area and job; for a child it means control of the source, usually old paint with high lead content, by resurfacing the offending areas with paint low in lead content.

A similar interpretation pertains to urine lead concentrations. The highest concentration usually considered to be compatible with a safe limit is 0.06 mg/liter. Higher values are usually indicative of excessive absorption. In some industrial workers chronically exposed over a long period, however, the upper limit of urine lead concentration compatible with safety is generally accepted as 0.15 mg/liter because many exposed workers with urine lead concentrations between 0.08 and 0.15 mg/liter are asymptomatic. Since urinary excretion varies directly with the extent of exposure and liquid intake and output, diurnal variation may be large. A random spot urine will, therefore, not be as valuable as an indicator of excessive absorption as a larger sample collected over an extended period. A one-liter specimen is considered desirable. Obviously, this is not possible when young children are involved. In such cases random urine specimens are usually analyzed, if they are obtainable, and interpreted with due caution.

ACCURACY AND PRECISION

In the range from 25 to 120 μg/100 ml, the relative error is on the order of 5%, with a standard deviation of approximately 4 μg/100 ml. Results obtained by this method and those obtained by the dithiozone procedure yield comparable data.

INTERFERING SUBSTANCES

At a wavelength of 283.3 nm there is no interference from other metal ions. Therapeutic blood concentrations of EDTA, used in the treatment of lead poisoning, also do not interfere with the lead determinations.

COMMENT

The method requires no pipeting, since all volumes used are based on the volume of blood collected. A technician can analyze up to 50 samples per day by this method, including preparation of solutions, calculations, and reporting of data.

REFERENCES

Barthel, W. F., et al., Modified delves cup atomic absorption determination of lead in blood, *J. Assoc. Off. Agric. Chem.*, 56, 1252, 1973.

Delves, H. T., A microsampling method for the rapid determination of lead in blood by atomic-absorption spectrophotometry, *Analyst*, 95, 431, 1970.

Hessel, D. W., A simple and rapid quantitative determination of lead in blood, *Atomic Absorption Newsletter* (Perkin-Elmer Corp.), 7, 55, 1968.

Hicks, J. M., Gutierrez, A. N., and Worthy, B. E., Evaluation of the delves micro system for blood lead analysis, *Clin. Chem.*, 19, 322, 1973.

Zinterhafer, L. J. M., Jatlow, P. I., and Fappiano, A., Atomic absorption determination of lead in blood and urine in the presence of EDTA, *J. Lab. Clin. Med.*, 78, 664, 1971.

LEAD IN PAINT CHIPS

PRINCIPLE

A solution of the sample is reacted with an iodide. If lead is present, insoluble lead iodide is formed and recognized by its characteristic yellow color.

TYPE A PROCEDURE

Irving Sunshine

APPARATUS

1. Test tube, Pyrex®, 13 × 100 mm
2. Water bath
3. Centrifuge

REAGENTS

All chemicals should be analytical reagent grade.

1. Sodium sulfate, 1 mg/100 ml
   Dissolve 1.0 mg of sodium sulfate in water and dilute to 100 ml.
2. Potassium iodide, 20 mg/100 ml
   Dissolve 20.0 mg of potassium iodide in water and dilute to 100 ml.

PROCEDURE

1. Place a 25.0-mg sample of paint scraping, free of wood, plaster, or other extraneous material, in the test tube. Add 3 drops of a 1:1 mixture of nitric acid and water.
2. Place the tube in a boiling water bath for 15 min.
3. Remove the tube from the water bath. Add 2.0 ml of the freshly prepared sodium sulfate solution.
4. Centrifuge the tube and its contents at low speed for 15 min.
5. Remove the tube from the centrifuge and place it for 5 min in a water bath at a temperature between 60 and 65°C.
6. Remove the tube from the water bath. Let 2 drops of the potassium iodide solution fall directly into the tube contents. Do not shake.

INTERPRETATION (see p. 7)

An immediate yellow precipitate indicates the presence of more than 1% lead in the original sample.

REFERENCE

Kaplan, E. and Shoull, R. S., Determination of lead in paint scrapings as an aid in the control of lead paint poisoning in young children, *Am. J. Public Health*, 51, 65, 1961.

LIDOCAINE

PRINCIPLE

Charcoal is used to adsorb the lidocaine, which is then eluted with chloroform. The concentrated eluate is then gas chromatographed (Procedure B). In Procedure C methadone is added, as an internal standard, to the alkalinized sample which is then extracted with ether. The ether is extracted with dilute acid which is then made alkaline and extracted with a small volume of chloroform. The concentration of lidocaine in the original sample is determined by gas-chromatographic analysis of an aliquot of the chloroform layer.

TYPE B PROCEDURE[1]

John M. Meola

APPARATUS

1. Glass-stoppered tubes, 15 ml
2. Pipets, 1 and 2 ml
3. Small glass tubes, Kimble 75 × 2 mm
4. Centrifuge
5. Vortex mixer
6. Manifold connected to a supply of compressed air for evaporation
7. Gas chromatograph (Perkin-Elmer Model 900) with FID and a Model 56 Recorder with a glass column 6′ × 0.08″ i.d. × ¼″ o.d., packed with 0.2% OV-17 on Corning GLC 110 textured glass beads 100 to 200 mesh. The OV-17 liquid phase was stabilized by the addition of 0.2% Silanox

   Operating Conditions

   Gas Flow Rate:
   - nitrogen – 20 ml/min

   Temperatures:
   - column – 220°C
   - injection port – 270°C
   - detector – 285°C

REAGENTS

All chemicals should be analytical reagent grade.

1. Norit® A, neutral charcoal*
2. Chloroform, Mallinckrodt®, analytical grade.
3. Bicarbonate-carbonate buffer, pH 11.0
   To a one-liter volumetric flask containing about 600 ml of distilled water, add 21.0 g of sodium carbonate (Na_2CO_3) and 420 mg of sodium bicarbonate. Mix well to dissolve, check the pH, and adjust, if necessary, to 11.0 ± 0.1 with 2*N* NaOH or 2*N* HCl. Dilute to one liter with water and mix well. Store at 4°C.
4. Lidocaine† stock solution, 100 mg/dl (as free base)
   Dissolve 29.25 mg of lidocaine hydrochloride in distilled water and dilute to 25 ml with water. Store at 4°C.
5. Lidocaine working standards, 0.5, 1.0, 1.5, and 2.0 mg/dl
   Dilute 0.5, 1.0, 1.5, and 2.0 ml of lidocaine stock solution, respectively, to 100 ml.
6. Carbocaine®† stock solution for internal standard, 40 mg/dl
   Transfer 10 mg of Carbocaine® to a 25-ml volumetric flask containing 2 ml of 1*N* hydrochloric acid. Dilute to volume with distilled water. Store at 4°C.
7. Carbocaine® working solution, 2 mg/dl
   Transfer 5.0 ml of Carbocaine® stock solution to a 100-ml volumetric flask and dilute to volume with distilled water

*Amed Drug & Chemical Co., Irvington, N.J. 07111.
†Available from Sterling-Winthrop Research Institute Rensselaer N.Y. 12144

PROCEDURE[2,3]

1. Transfer 1 ml of serum and 1 ml of distilled water to a 15-ml glass-stoppered centrifuge tube. Add 1 ml of the internal standard, the Carbocaine® working solution, and 2 ml of the carbonate-bicarbonate buffer. Add 5 mg of Norit® A neutral charcoal.
2. Standards are prepared by adding 1 ml of each working standard to 1 ml of drug-free serum or reconstituted serum (Hyland Normal) and proceeding as directed for serum samples under Step 1, except that the addition of 1 ml of distilled water is omitted.
3. Mix briefly on Vortex mixer. Centrifuge at 200 X g for 4 min. Remove and discard the supernatant by aspiration.
4. Disperse charcoal over the wall of the tube using a Vortex mixer to insure maximum dispersion.
5. Add 2 ml of chloroform and extract the charcoal. (Shake tube contents vigorously.)
6. Decant the solvent into a small glass tube and evaporate it to dryness at room temperature, using compressed air.
7. Dissolve the residue in 20 μl of chloroform and inject 1 μl into gas chromatography.
8. Measure the peak heights of the internal standard and lidocaine for both the serum samples and standards.
9. Determine the ratio of the peak height of the standard to that of the internal standard (S_r).
10. Determine the ratio of the peak height of the serum to that of internal standard (S_s).

CALCULATION

1. Plot the S_r values against their respective concentrations to form a standard curve.
2. Calculate the respective concentrations of each serum sample by comparing its S_s with the reference curve.
3. The drug concentration of the serum samples can also be calculated by the following formula:

$$\frac{S_r}{S_s} \times C_r = \text{Serum concentration}$$

where

C_r = the concentration of the reference standard, not above 2.0 mg/dl.

INTERPRETATION (see p. 7)

With the above procedure, 0.05 mg of lidocaine/100 ml can be easily detected. Treatment of cardiac arrest with lidocaine generally results in blood levels of 0.1 to 0.6 mg/100 ml[1] (e.g., 150 mg of lidocaine injected intravenously results in a blood concentration of 0.23 mg/100 ml 2 hr post injection). When used as a regional anesthetic, lidocaine levels in blood from the anaesthetised areas are between 1 and 2 mg/100 ml.[4]

SENSITIVITY AND PRECISION

The sensitivity for lidocaine is 0.5 mg/dl. The CV at all levels (from 0.5 to 2.0 mg/dl) is 5.0% for lidocaine.

REFERENCES

1. **Strong, J. M. and Atkinson, A. J., Jr.,** Simultaneous measurement of plasma concentrations of lidocaine and its desethylated metabolite by mass fragmentography, *Anal. Chem.*, 44, 2287, 1972.
2. **Meola, J. and Vanko, M.,** A simple system for drug analysis, *Clin. Chem.*, 17, 556, 1971.
3. **Meola, J. and Vanko, M.,** The use of charcoal in the qualitative and quantitative analysis of drugs, *Clin. Chem.*, 18, 579, 1972.
4. **Thorn-Alquist, A. M.,** Blood concentrations of local anaesthetics after intravenous regional anaesthetic, *Acta Anaesthesiol. Scand.*, 13, 229, 1969.

TYPE C PROCEDURE

Vijay Aggarwal and Raymond Bath

APPARATUS

1. Test tubes with Teflon®-lined screw caps, 50 ml
2. Conical centrifgue tubes, 15 ml
3. Centrifuge, International Equipment Co.
4. Pasteur pipets
5. Vortex mixer, Scientific Products #58223
6. Gas chromatograph, Bendix 2500, equipped with flame ionization detectors, a 1 mV Honeywell strip chart recorder and a U-shaped glass column 6′ X 1/8″ i.d., packed with 5% OV-7 on Chromosorb WHP 80/100 mesh

   Operating Conditions

   Gas Flow Rates:
   - nitrogen – 30 ml/min
   - hydrogen – 30 ml/min
   - air – 400 ml/min

   Temperatures:
   - column – 200°C
   - injection port – 250°C
   - detector – 250°C

REAGENTS

All chemicals should be analytical reagent grade.

1. Lidocaine stock solutions, 50 mg/dl
   Dissolve 57.3 mg lidocaine hydrochloride in water and dilute to 100 ml with distilled water.
2. Lidocaine reference solutions 1.0, 2.0, and 4.0 mg/100 ml
   Add 2.0, 4.0, and 8.0 ml of lidocaine stock solution to three separate 100-ml volumetric flasks and fill to the mark with distilled water.
3. Internal standard solution
   Dissolve 50 mg of tetracaine hydrochloride in 100 ml of distilled water.
4. H_2SO_4, 0.5*N*
   Dilute 1.4 ml of concentrated H_2SO_4 to 100 ml with distilled water.
5. NH_4Cl/NH_4OH buffer
   To a saturated solution of NH_4Cl add concentrated ammonium hydroxide to bring the pH to 9.3.
6. Diethyl ether
7. NaOH, 12*N*
   Dissolve 48 g of NaOH in water and dilute to 100 ml with water.
8. $CHCl_3$

PROCEDURE

1. To 10 ml of sample (blood, urine, tissue homogenate, or lidocaine reference solution) contained in a 50-ml test tube, add 1.0 ml of the internal standard solution.
2. Add 2.0 ml of NH_4Cl/NH_4OH buffer and 30 ml of ether to each tube, cap, and shake gently for 3 min or rotate on a mechanical rotator for 5 min.
3. Centrifuge the samples and transfer the ether layer to a clean test tube containing 5.0 ml of 0.5*N* H_2SO_4.
4. Cap the tubes and shake for 2 min. Centrifuge as above. Aspirate and discard the ether layer.
5. Gently warm each tube in hot water to expel any traces of ether from the aqueous phase, and then transfer the aqueous phase to a 15-ml conical centrifuge tube.
6. While vortexing the centrifuge tube, add 6 drops of 12*N* NaOH, 1.0 ml of NH_4Cl/NH_4OH buffer, and 200 μl of $CHCl_3$. Vortex each sample for 30 sec.
7. Centrifuge the samples and inject 3 μl of the $CHCl_3$ layer into the gas chromatograph.

CALCULATION

The amount of lidocaine in the sample is determined by using the following formula:

$$Ci = Cs \times \frac{Li}{Mi} \times \frac{Ms}{Ls}$$

where

Ci = concentration of lidocaine in the sample;

Cs = concentration of lidocaine in the lidocaine reference solution which was analyzed along with the sample;
Li = area of the lidocaine peak in the sample;
Mi = area of the tetracaine peak in the sample;
Ls = area of the lidocaine peak in the reference solution;
Ms = area of the tetracaine peak in the reference solution.

Either peak heights or peak areas may be used for the computation, but peak areas are generally more reproducible. Under the gas-chromatographic conditions given above, the retention time of lidocaine is 5.0 min and that of tetracaine is 11 min.

INTERPRETATION (see p. 7)

With the above procedure, 0.05 mg of lidocaine/100 ml can be easily detected. Treatment of cardiac arrest with lidocaine generally results in blood levels of 0.1 to 0.6 mg/100 ml[1] (e.g., 150 mg of lidocaine injected intravenously results in a blood concentration of 0.23 mg/100 ml 2 hr post injection). When used as a regional anaesthetic, lidocaine levels in blood from the anaesthetized areas are between 1 and 2 mg/100 ml.[2]

ACCURACY AND PRECISION

The ratio of the lidocaine peak area to the tetracaine peak area is a linear function of lidocaine concentration from 0.1 to 8 mg/100 ml. The coefficient of variation for ten replicate analyses of samples containing 0.4 mg/100 ml was 1.7%.

INTERFERING SUBSTANCES

Under the stated gas-chromatographic conditions, lidocaine is resolved from any other basic compounds which may be coextracted. The presence of lidocaine in a sample can be confirmed by comparing its retention times to those of authentic samples on different gas-chromatographic columns such as OV-1 or OV-3.

REFERENCES

1. **Strong, J. M. and Atkinson, A. J.,** Simultaneous measurement of plasma concentrations of lidocaine and its desethylated metabolite, *Anal. Chem.*, 44, 2287, 1972.
2. **Thorn-Alquist, A. M.,** Blood concentrations of local anaesthetics after intravenous regional anaesthetic, *Acta Anaesthesiol. Scand.*, 13, 229, 1969.

LITHIUM

PRINCIPLE

Lithium salts impart a characteristic color to a flame. The intensity of this color is a function of the sample's lithium content. It can be measured in a suitable flame photometer and thus quantitate the lithium present in the sample.

TYPE B PROCEDURE

Jesse A. Hancock, Jr.

APPARATUS

1. Flame photometer (Beckman DU)
2. Centrifuge tubes, 10 ml

REAGENTS

All chemicals should be analytical reagent grade.

1. Protein precipitant, trichloracetic acid, 5 g/100 ml
   Dissolve 5 g of trichloracetic acid in water and dilute to 100 ml.
2. Lithium stock solution, 20.0 meq/liter
   Dissolve 0.739 g of lithium carbonate in 100 ml of deionized water, add 1.0 ml of concentrated hydrochloric acid, then dilute with deionized water to one liter.
3. Lithium reference solutions
   Add 2.0 ml of the lithium stock solution to 8.0 ml of the protein precipitant and mix well. This will give a concentration of 4.0 meq Li^+/liter (Solution A). Further dilutions may be made if desired, although these two points should fall in a straight line passing through 0% transmission at zero lithium concentration.

SAMPLE REQUIREMENTS

1. Serum that is lithium-free, or a control serum such as Versatrol®
2. The unknown sera that are to be tested for lithium
   Make a second dilution by adding 5.0 ml of Solution A to 5.0 ml of the protein precipitant. This will give a concentration of 2.0 meq Li^+/liter (Solution B).
3. Lithium reference solution with a concentration of 2.0 meq/liter (Solution B)

PROCEDURE

Preparation of a Standard Curve

1. Adjust the flame photometer so that the slit width is 0.04 mm. Set the wave length at 670.8 nm. Use the sensitivity controls to adjust the instrument so that the protein-precipitant gives a reading of 0% transmission and the 2.0 meq/liter lithium reference solution gives a reading of 50% transmission. It may be necessary to readjust the slit width to achieve these conditions.
2. When these operating conditions are achieved, successively aspirate each of the lithium reference solutions.
3. Read the percent transmission obtained. Using semi-log coordinates, the relationship between these readings and the concentrations is linear over a range from 0.00 to 4.00 meq/liter.

Analysis

1. Mark three test tubes A, B, and C.
2. In test tube A place 0.50 ml of lithium-free serum or plasma and 4.50 ml of the protein-precipitant solution.
3. In test tube B place 0.50 ml of lithium-free serum, 0.50 ml of the 4.0 meq/liter lithium reference solution (Solution A), and 4.00 ml of the protein-precipitant solution. Shake well.
4. In test tube C place 0.50 ml of the serum specimen to be analyzed and 4.50 ml of the protein-precipitant. Shake well.

5. Centrifuge all the test tubes, then use the supernatants as described below.
6. Aspirate the supernatant from test tube A into the flame. Use the dark current control to balance the instrument at 0% transmission.
7. Replace supernatant A with supernatant B. Make this read 50% transmission, using the sensitivity adjustment or the slit width. This may necessitate going back to A and rezeroing the instrument.
8. Without changing any of the settings on the instrument, determine the percent transmission obtained when supernatant C is aspirated.
9. Determine the lithium concentration in the specimen by comparison with the standard curve obtained by analyzing the reference lithium solutions. This procedure will compensate for contamination in the serum by contaminants that appear to be lithium or unexplainable background contaminations.

INTERPRETATION (see p. 7)

The Li^+ concentration can be interpolated from the standard curve constructed as described above. Therapeutic doses of lithium carbonate usually produce a serum concentration of 1 meq/liter. Serum concentrations above 4 meq/liter are very dangerous and may be lethal.

ACCURACY AND PRECISION

While in most cases phosphate, sodium, potassium, sulfate, and chlorides do not interfere, there does seem to be some interference when calcium is found in variable amounts in different sera. The procedure as outlined will compensate for varying amounts of calcium and give correct results for lithium concentration. With the Beckman DU-2 with flame attachment and photomultiplier tube, the accuracy and precision is approximately 0.01 meq Li^+/liter.

REFERENCES

Crammer, J. L., Rosser, R. M., and Crane, G., Blood levels and management of lithium treatment, *Br. Med. J.*, 3, 650, 1974.

Hansen, J. L., The measurement of serum and urine lithium by atomic absorption spectrophotometry, *Am. J. Med. Technol.*, 34, 1, 1968.

Robertson, R., Fritz, K., and Grof, P., On the determination of lithium in blood and urine, *Clin. Chim. Acta*, 45, 25, 1973.

MANGANESE

PRINCIPLE

When vigorously oxidized, manganese salts form permanganates. This anion has a characteristic color, the absorbance of which can be used to indicate the manganese content of the sample.

TYPE A PROCEDURE

Jesse A. Hancock, Jr.

APPARATUS

1. Erlenmeyer flasks, 100 ml
2. Digestion rack and hood
3. Volumetric flasks, 100 ml
4. Spectrophotometer

REAGENTS

All chemicals should be analytical reagent grade.

1. Nitric acid, concentrated
2. Perchloric acid, concentrated (72%)
3. Sodium bisulfite
4. Phosphoric acid, concentrated
5. Potassium periodate
6. Potassium permanganate stock solution, 100 μg Mn/ml
   Dissolve 292.66 mg of potassium permanganate in water, add 50 ml of concentrated phosphoric acid, then dilute to one liter with water.
7. Potassium permanganate reference solutions
   Solution A, 10 μg/100 ml
   Dilute 1.0 ml of the stock solution to one liter with water.
   Solution B, 5 μg/100 ml
   Dilute 50 ml of Solution A to 100 ml with water.

PROCEDURE

1. Digest 1 g of specimen (tissue, blood, or urine) with a 1:1 mixture of concentrated nitric and perchloric acids in a 100-ml Erlenmeyer flask, adding more of the acid mixture as needed to oxidize all of the specimen. Heat until the mixture begins to fume.
2. If the solution should turn purple at this point, allow it to cool to room temperature, then add 50.0 mg of sodium bisulfite and reheat the mixture until it boils. Repeat this step if the solution is not colorless.
3. Add 40.0 ml of deionized water, 5.0 ml of concentrated phosphoric acid, and 0.5 g of potassium periodate. Boil the mixture gently for a few minutes, then allow it to cool to room temperature.
4. Dilute the cooled digest to 100 ml in a volumetric flask, using deionized water as the diluent. If there is any manganese present, the solution will have a perceptible purple tinge; if not, the specimen contains less than 20 μg of manganese/100 ml.
5. Determine the absorbance of the solution at 420 nm, using water as the reference solution. Compare this absorbance with the absorbances obtained from potassium permanganate reference solutions in phosphoric acid.

CALCULATION

The relationship between the absorbance of solutions containing manganese and their respective concentrations, ranging from 0.01 to 10 μg/100 ml, is linear.

INTERPRETATION (see p. 7)

Trace quantities of manganese are found in nearly all tissue and blood, usually in concentrations around 0.1 μg/ml. Concentrations up to 10 μg/ml are found in persons mining or crushing manganese dioxide ore, usually with no discernible clinical effects. Occasionally, a patient displaying a marked Parkinsonism syndrome has brown-speckled discolorations on the backs of the hands and around the facial areas; the manganese concentrations in these areas are usually above 5 μg/100 ml.

ACCURACY AND PRECISION

The accuracy, depending on the spectrophotometer, is approximately 0.1 μg/100 ml. Results are reproducible within ±10%.

INTERFERING SUBSTANCES

No interferences are apparent in the determination of manganese in tissue, blood, or urine by this method.

MEPROBAMATE

PRINCIPLE

Chemically, meprobamate is a neutral organic compound; hence it can be extracted from biological specimens with an organic solvent. This extract may be purified by aqueous acid and alkaline washes. Meprobamate can then be identified in the washed organic extract. One identification method involves concentrating the washed extract and applying an aliquot to a thin-layer chromatogram. After development, the meprobamate can be isolated by noting if a black spot forms on the chromatogram after it is sprayed with furfural (Procedure A). Another procedure, which is more tedious but quantitative, is based on the reaction of meprobamate with antimony trichloride. The absorbance of the resulting complex can be used to calculate the meprobamate concentration (Procedure B). The more elegant quantitative procedure (and the simplest, if the equipment is available) depends on the characteristic retention time of meprobamate after an aliquot of the extract is injected into a suitable gas chromatograph (Procedure C).

TYPE A PROCEDURE

Bette Hamman

APPARATUS

1. Centrifuge tubes, glass-stoppered, 15 ml
2. Centrifuge
3. Water bath
4. Thin-layer chromatography (TLC) equipment: (a) Micropipets; (b) Glass plates, 20 X 20 cm, precoated with silical gel G, without fluorescence indicator; (c) Developing tank; (d) Spray bottles

REAGENTS

All chemicals should be analytical reagent grade.

1. Chloroform-methanol mixture, 1:1
   Mix equal volumes of chloroform and methanol. Prepare this mixture just prior to use.
2. Meprobamate reference solution, 1 μg/10μl
   Dissolve 10.0 mg of meprobamate in the 1:1 mixture of chloroform and methanol. Dilute the solution to 100 ml with the same mixture.
3. Methylene dichloride
4. Sodium sulfate, anhydrous
5. Chloroform-methanol mixture, 9:1
   Mix 180 ml of chloroform with 20.0 ml of methanol. Prepare this mixture just prior to use.

PROCEDURE

1. Add duplicate 2.0-ml samples (plasma or urine specimen, and reference solution) and 10.0 ml of methylene dichloride to 15-ml glass-stoppered centrifuge tubes.
2. Shake each sample for 15 min, then allow the tubes to stand for 10 min.
3. Centrifuge the tubes for 5 min.
4. Remove the aqueous layer by aspiration. Add a few grains of anhydrous sodium sulfate to the extract to dry it.
5. Transfer 8.0 ml of the dry extract to a clean centrifuge tube.
6. Evaporate the solvent to dryness in a 60°C water bath with the aid of an air stream.
7. Place 200 ml of the 9:1 chloroform-methanol mixture in the bottom of a chromatographic developing tank.
8. Spot 10, 30, and 50 μl of the reference solution (1, 3, and 5 μg of meprobamate) 1.0 cm apart in a straight line 2 cm from the bottom of the TLC plate.
9. Reconstitute the residues obtained from the specimen in Step 6, one at a time, in the 1:1 chloroform-methanol mixture. If the residue is from a plasma specimen, use 100 μl of the solvent mixture; urine residues require 500 μl. Shake each solution so that it contacts the

entire lower two thirds of the tube, then allow it to stand for 1 min.

10. Withdraw an aliquot of the specimen solution and spot it immediately on the TLC plate, adjacent to the meprobamate reference spots. The diameter of the spot should not exceed 0.5 cm. One plate can accommodate the reference spots, 10 specimen extracts, a plasma blank, and a plasma containing 10 μg of added meprobamate.
11. Place the spotted plate in the previously prepared TLC tank and allow the solvent to ascend a distance of 15 cm.
12. Air-dry the plate for 15 min, then spray it with the furfural reagent. (A black spot indicates that meprobamate may be present.)

INTERPRETATION (see p. 7)

A black spot indicates that meprobamate may be present. This is only a qualitative presumptive test. All positive results should be confirmed by some other identification procedure (see Procedure B or C).

INTERFERING SUBSTANCES

Neither urine nor plasma samples free of meprobamate show visible spots in the meprobamate region of the chromatogram. Other carbamates will yield black spots if they are present, but their R_f values are different.

TYPE B PROCEDURE

Robert H. Cravey

APPARATUS

1. Test tubes, glass-stoppered, or centrifuge tubes
2. Water bath
3. Spectrophotometer, or photoelectric photometer

REAGENTS

All chemicals should be analytical reagent grade.

1. Sodium hydroxide, 0.5*N*
   Dissolve 20 g of sodium hydroxide in water and dilute to one liter.
2. Chloroform
3. Meprobamate stock solution, 100 mg/100 ml
   Dissolve 100 mg of meprobamate in 100 ml of water and dilute to 100 ml with water.
4. Meprobamate reference solution, 1 mg/100 ml
   Dilute 1.0 ml of the meprobamate stock solution to 100 ml with water.
5. AAA reagent
   Add 1 volume of glacial acetic acid to 3 volumes of acetone. This reagent is stable indefinitely if stored in a dark brown bottle.
6. DMB (*p*-dimethylaminobenzaldehyde) reagent, 1 g/100 ml
   Dissolve 1 g of *p*-dimethylaminobenzaldehyde in benzene. Dilute the solution to 100 ml with benzene. This reagent is stable for 1 month if stored in a dark brown bottle.
7. ATA reagent
   Combine 5 g of antimony trichloride with 20.0 ml of chloroform and 5.0 ml of acetic anhydride. Prepare fresh as needed.
8. Benzene

PROCEDURE

1. To 1.0 ml of specimen (serum, plasma, urine, or whole blood) in a glass-stoppered tube, add 0.1 ml of 0.5*N* sodium hydroxide and 10.0 ml of chloroform. Process 1.0 ml of water for a reagent blank and 1.0 ml of reference solution simultaneously and in the same manner as the specimen.
2. Shake each mixture vigorously, then allow the layers to separate.
3. Transfer an aliquot of each chloroform extract

to a second glass-stoppered test tube. Avoid transfer of any of the aqueous layer. For blood specimens containing an unknown amount of meprobamate, it is best to take both a 5.0 and a 0.5-ml aliquot.

4. Evaporate the aliquots of the chloroform extracts to dryness in a water bath.
5. Add 0.2 ml of the AAA reagent, 0.2 ml of DMB reagent, and 1.0 ml of ATA reagent, in that order, to each tube.
6. Place the tubes in a water bath set at 50°C. Heat them for 10 min, then cool them in a cold bath until they reach room temperature.
7. Add 2.0 ml of benzene to each tube.
8. Transfer the contents of each tube to a cuvette.
9. Determine the absorbance of each sample at 550 nm, using the reagent blank as the reference solution.
   Caution! when the analysis is completed, wash the cuvettes with acetone. Do *not* wash first with water.

CALCULATION

Use the following formula to calculate the meprobamate concentration in the specimen:

$$C_x = \frac{A_x}{A_R} \times C_R \times \frac{10}{V_a},$$

where

C_x = concentration of the specimen;
A_x = absorbance of the specimen;
A_R = absorbance of the reference solution;
C_R = concentrations of the reference solution;
V_a = aliquot of the chloroform extract used.

INTERPRETATION (see p. 7)

Therapeutic concentrations generally range from 1.0 to 2.0 mg/100 ml of blood. At a higher blood concentration the patient is difficult to rouse. Serious intoxication is associated with blood concentrations in excess of 100 mg/100 ml.[1] Gitelson[2] reports that the lowest dose expected to produce coma is 6 g, but in some cases investigation up to 40 g resulted only in drowsiness.

INTERFERING SUBSTANCES

The test is not specific for meprobamate, since any carbamate will react. Thin-layer chromatograpy is an easy, efficient means of determining which carbamate is present. Another aliquot of the chloroform extract obtained in Step 2 could be used for this purpose.

REFERENCES

1. **Maddock, R. K. and Bloomer, H. A.,** Meprobamate overdosage, *JAMA*, 201, 999, 1967.
2. **Gitelson, S.,** Methaqualone-meprobamate poisoning, *JAMA*, 201, 977, 1967.

GENERAL REFERENCE

Hoffman, A. J. and Ludwig, B. J., An improved colorimetric method for the determination of meprobamate in biological fluids, *J. Am. Pharm. Assoc.*, 48, 740, 1959.

TYPE C PROCEDURE

Bryan S. Finkle

APPARATUS

1. Bottles, ground-glass-stoppered, 120 ml, or separatory funnels
2. Serological pipets, 5 ml
3. Glass funnels
4. Measuring cylinders, ground-glass-stoppered, 50 ml
5. Beakers, 50 ml
6. Conical evaporating tubes, disposable, 2 ml
   Cut Pasteur pipets to the desired lengths and seal the tips.
7. Graduated pipets, 50 μl
8. Gas chromatograph, fitted with a flame ionization detector, and a U-shaped glass column, 6′ X ¼″ i.d., packed with 2.5% S.E. 30 or 3.0% O.V-17 on 80 to 100 mesh Chromosorb G (AW – DMCS)

   Operating Conditions

   Gas Flow Rate:
   nitrogen (carrier gas) - 50 ml/min

   Temperatures:
   column – 195°C
   injection port – 230°C
   detector – 220°C

REAGENTS

All chemicals should be analytical reagent grade.

1. Chloroform, Mallinckrodt Nanograde
2. Glass wool, acid-washed
3. Sodium sulfate, anhydrous
4. Chloroform-ethanol mixture, 1:1
   Mix 50.0 ml of chloroform with 50.0 ml of absolute ethanol. Prepare this reagent just prior to use.
5. Internal standard 100 mg/100 ml
   Dissolve 100 mg of *p*-dimethylaminobenzaldehyde in 100 ml of the chloroform-ethanol mixture. Discard the solution after 1 month.
6. Meprobamate reference solution, 5 μg/μl
   Dissolve 250 mg of meprobamate in the internal standard and dilute to 50.0 ml with the internal standard. Aliquots of 0.4, 0.8, and 1.6 μl of this solution are equivalent to 2, 4, and 8 μg of meprobamate, respectively.
7. Furfural, 10 ml/100 ml
   Dilute 10.0 ml of furfural to 100 ml with absolute ethanol. If the furfural stock solution is very black, it must be redistilled to a water-clear liquid. When not in use, store the solution in a glass-stoppered dark bottle at 4°C.
8. Hydrochloric acid, concentrated
9. Chloroform, dry

PROCEDURE, QUANTITATIVE

1. Using a 120-ml ground-glass-stoppered bottle or a separatory funnel, extract 3.0 ml of specimen (blood, gastric content, urine, or 1 g of homogenized tissue) with 50.0 ml of chloroform. Process 3.0 ml of the meprobamate reference solution in the same manner. Allow the phases to separate.
2. Aspirate the aqueous phase. Filter the chloroform into a 50-ml ground-glass-stoppered cylinder through anhydrous sodium sulfate supported by a glass wool plug in a small funnel. Do not use filter paper.
3. Collect 40.0 ml of the chloroform filtrate in the cylinder.
4. Evaporate the chloroform filtrate to 1 or 2 ml in a 50-ml beaker.
5. Transfer the concentrate to a disposable 2-ml conical tube and continue the evaporation to dryness.
6. Dissolve the residue in 500 μl of internal standard.
7. Evaporate, using low heat, to approximately 25 μl and inject 1 μl of the dissolved residue into the gas chromatograph, making sure that the operating conditions stated above are met. Under these conditions, the retention time for meprobamate is approximately 5.0 min and that for the internal standard is approximately 1.8 min.

8. Calculate the ratio of the peak height of meprobamate to that of the internal standard.

CALCULATION

Calculate the weight of drug injected into the gas chromatograph by relating the ratio resulting from the meprobamate reference sample directly to the ratio obtained from the specimen.

ACCURACY AND PRECISION

Using this procedure, recovery of meprobamate added to blood is approximately 90%. Drug concentrations of 2 μg/ml can be detected with ease. The method is accurate to ± 0.5 μg/ml, ranging from 10 to 100 μg/ml. Any value within this range is reproducible within ± 2%.

PROCEDURE, QUALITATIVE

Color Test

1. Spot an aliquot of the residual solution from the gas-chromatographic analysis (Step 6 of the quantitative procedure) onto a piece of filter paper. Allow it to air-dry.
2. Spray the spot lightly with the furfural reagent. Allow it to air-dry.
3. Expose the dried spot to hydrochloric acid and fumes. The development of a blue-black color is specific for a carbamate.

INTERPRETATION (see p. 7)

A single therapeutic dose of 400 mg of meprobamate results in a peak blood concentration of approximately 5 μg/ml. This occurs about 2 hr after ingestion. With continuous therapeutic dosage (e.g., 400 mg every 6 hr), maximum blood concentrations will range from 15 to 20 μg/ml. Symptoms of sleepiness and sedation are usually observed at these blood concentrations. In unhabituated, nontolerant subjects, coma is likely to result when the blood concentration is higher than 30 μg/ml. In tolerant subjects, blood concentrations may reach 60 to 70 μg/ml before coma ensues. In fatal cases, the concentrations found vary greatly with the physical and environmental circumstances of the death, particularly with the presence or absence of alcohol in the victim. Although with proper medical treatment recovery has been made from blood concentrations as high as 150 μg/ml, blood or liver concentrations in excess of 100 μg/ml or g, respectively, are consistent with death in most situations.

INTERFERING SUBSTANCES

There are no common drugs or poisons that will interfere with either the extraction or the gas-chromatographic quantitation of meprobamate when this method is used. The analyst should be aware that caffeine and α-phenyl glutarimide (the principal metabolite of glutethimide) have retention times close to meprobamate, but are easily resolved. In addition, meprobamate has a minor peak at 1.4 min. This is a breakdown product and aids in the qualitative identification; it may be ignored for purposes of quantitation.

REFERENCES

Bloomer, H. A., Maddock, R. K., Sheehe, J. B., *et al.*, Rapid diagnosis of sedative intoxication by gas chromatography, *Ann. Intern. Med.*, 72, 223, 1970.

Finkle, B. S., The identification, quantitative determination and distribution of meprobamate and glutethimide in biological material, *J. Forensic Sci.*, 12, 509, 1967.

Maddock, R. K. and Bloomer, H. A., Meprobamate overdosage: Evaluation of its severity and methods of treatment, *JAMA*, 201, 999, 1967.

Martis, L. and Lery, R. H., GLC determination of meprobamate in water, plasma, and urine, *J. Pharm. Sci.*, 63, 835, 1974.

MERCURY

PRINCIPLE

Classically, mercury is demonstrable in a sample if a clean copper wire, which has been dropped in the acidified test solution, is covered with a silver gray deposit. This wire can then be removed from the solution and the mercury thereon characterized by suitable reactions which produce characteristic colors (Procedure A). Quantitation can be realized by oxidizing away the organic matter in the sample and then determining the mercury remaining in the aqueous digest. This technique is effective, but the oxidation must be done at a low temperature to avoid volatilizing any mercury. The quantitation then depends on chelation with dithizone under proper conditions and can be performed by measuring the absorbance of the mercury dithizonate (Procedure B). Mercury can also be determined using a flameless atomic absorption spectrophotometer, since the mercury vapor can be carried into the detection system easily and thus measure the mercury content (Procedure C).

TYPE A PROCEDURE

Sidney Kaye

REAGENTS

All chemicals should be analytical reagent grade.

1. Hydrochloric acid, concentrated
2. Copper strips, 5 × 10 mm
3. Mercury stock solution, 1 mg/ml
   Dissolve 1.668 g of mercuric nitrate ($Hg(NO_3)_2 \cdot \frac{1}{2}H_2O$) in water containing 2.0 ml of nitric acid. Dilute this mixture to one liter with water.
4. Mercury reference solution, 10 μg/ml
   Dilute 1.0 ml of the stock solution to 100 ml with water.
5. Cuprous iodide reagent (according to Ganassini as reported by Gettler[1])
   Dissolve 5 g of copper sulfate and 3 g of ferrous sulfate in 10.0 ml of water. To this, while stirring continually, add a solution containing 7 g of potassium iodide in 50 ml of water. A precipitate of cuprous iodide is gradually formed. Filter this precipitate and wash it with water. Transfer the washed cuprous iodide to a brown bottle, keeping it in the form of a suspension with the aid of a little water. This suspension is quite stable.

PROCEDURE

1. Place the strip of copper in an Erlenmeyer flask of suitable size. Add the specimen (a 20.0-ml aliquot of stomach content, vomitus, or urine, or 10 g of kidney homogenized with 10.0 ml of water) and 4 ml of concentrated hydrochloric acid. Gently heat this mixture for 45 min. Maintain the volume by placing a watch glass on the lip of the Erlenmeyer flask.
2. Remove the copper strip, wash it with water, then dry it on filter paper. A dark discoloration may suggest arsenic, bismuth, or antimony. If mercury is present, the color of the deposit ranges from grayish to a shiny silver. This is faintly visible at about 50 μg and is very definitely silverish at 100 μg.
3. Estimate the amount of mercury deposited by comparison with suitable reference solutions processed in a similar manner.

Identification, Confirmation, and Estimation

The following operations should be performed even in the absence of a visible silvery deposit.

1. Place a small piece of filter paper on a watch

glass, then place 1 or 2 drops of cuprous iodide suspension on the filter paper.

2. Put the exposed copper strip on the spot of cuprous iodide and cover it with another watch glass.
3. Inspect the unit after 30 min. Mercury iodide develops a rose to salmon-pink color in the presence of trace amounts (30 μg) of mercury. Other quantities of mercury (25, 50, 75, and 100 μg), treated in a similar manner, may be used for comparison.

ACCURACY AND PRECISION

This test is sensitive to 30 μg of mercury, and estimates may be made at 25-μg intervals up to about 100 μg; however, if a more accurate quantitative determination is necessary, the dithizone procedure (B) should be used.

INTERFERING SUBSTANCES

This test is specific for mercury. All other metals that form a deposit on copper, when treated as outlined above, give negative results.

REFERENCE

1. **Gettler, A. O.,** Simple test for mercury in body fluids and tissues, *Am. J. Clin. Pathol. (Tech. Suppl.)*, 7, 13, 1937.

GENERAL REFERENCES

Gettler, A. O. and Kaye, S., A simple and rapid analytical method for mercury, bismuth, antimony, arsenic, selenium, and sulfides in biologic material, *J. Lab. Clin. Med.*, 35, 146, 1950.

Kaye, S., A rapid and specific method for the detection and estimation of mercury, bismuth and arsenic in body fluids, *Am. J. Clin. Pathol.*, 14, 83, 1944.

Kaye, S., Toxicology of mercury, *Bol. Assoc. Med. P.R.*, 60, 602, 1968.

Kevalo, P., Vesapar, A., and Bachman, B., Atomic absorption of mercury in fish using the Coleman MAS-50 mercury analyzer, *Anal. Chem.*, 46, 1814, 1974.

TYPE B PROCEDURE

Sidney Kaye

REAGENTS

All chemicals should be analytical reagent grade. All the water used to prepare the reagents must be redistilled in an all-glass apparatus.

1. Sulfuric acid, concentrated
2. Nitric acid, low in copper
3. Potassium permanganate, 5 g/100 ml
   Dissolve 5 g of potassium permanganate in 100 ml of water.
4. Hydroxylamine hydrochloride, 100 g/100 ml
   Dissolve 50 g of hydroxylamine hydrochloride in 50 ml of water.
5. Ammonium hydroxide, 9*N*
   Add 100 ml of concentrated ammonium hydroxide to 60 ml of water.
6. Dithizone stock solution, 2.5 mg/100 ml
   Dissolve 25 mg of dithizone in redistilled chloroform. Dilute this solution to one liter with redistilled chloroform. Do not use for at least 24 hr.
7. Dithizone reference solution, 625 μg/100 ml
   Add 75 ml of redistilled chloroform to 25 ml of the dithizone stock solution. Prepare fresh as needed.
8. Potassium cyanide
9. Mercury stock solution, 100 mg/100 ml
   Dissolve 1.668 g of mercuric nitrate ($Hg(NO_3)_2 \cdot ½H_2O$) in water containing 2.0 ml of nitric acid. Dissolve this mixture to one liter with water.
10. Mercury reference solutions, 10 μg/ml
    Dilute 1.0 ml of the stock solution to 100 ml with water.

PROCEDURE

1. To 50 ml of urine in a 500-ml Erlenmeyer

flask, while cooling under tap water, add 1 ml of sulfuric acid. Mix, then add 5 ml of nitric acid.

2. Place a watch glass on the lip of the flask as a lid, mix the contents of the flask, then heat the mixture gently to barely a simmer for about 5 min.
3. Remove the flask from the heat source and add 50 ml of potassium permanganate, a little at a time, to minimize foaming. Manganese dioxide will start to precipitate.
4. When all the permanganate is added, heat the mixture gently to barely a simmer for about 10 min. Use the watch glass as a lid. Swirl the contents gently from time to time.
5. Allow the mixture to cool to room temperature. Add 3 ml of the hydroxylamine hydrochloride, in small portions, to dissolve the manganese dioxide and to remove excess oxidizing agents.
6. Test for absence of oxidizing agents, using potassium iodide starch paper. If a blue-brown color forms, add more hydroxylamine hydrochloride.
7. Transfer the solution to a small Pyrex® separatory funnel. (If the specimen is vomitus or gastric lavage and contains fat, shake with 5.0 ml of carbon tetrachloride to remove the fat. Remove and discard the carbon tetrachloride.)
8. Make certain that the pH is between 1 and 2. Adjust, if necessary, with dilute ammonium hydroxide or sulfuric acid, checking with pH test paper.
9. Promptly add 10.0 ml of the dilute dithizone solution and shake the mixture vigorously. A yellow to peach-orange chloroform layer indicates that mercury is present in excess of 20 μg. Allow the phases to settle and separate.
10. Collect the lower dithizone extract. Add an additional 10.0 ml of the dithizone solution and shake the mixture vigorously.
11. Collect the dithizone extract and add it to the first extract. Repeat Step 10, if necessary, until all the mercury is extracted; this is indicated by a persistent green color of the final dithizone extract. Record how much dithizone was required to reach this point.
12. Shake the combined dithizone extracts with 25 ml of 9*N* ammonium hydroxide to remove excess dithizone.
13. Quickly separate and filter the chloroform phase through filter paper to remove droplets of water. Save the ammonium hydroxide for Step 15.
14. Determine the absorbance of the mercury-dithizone extract at 490 nm, using the dithizone solution as the reference solution. Compare this absorbance with those obtained from reference solutions containing 2 to 10 μg of mercury and processed in exactly the same manner as the specimen.
15. To rule out possible bismuth interference, add 50 mg of potassium cyanide to the ammonium hydroxide saved in Step 13. Add the mercury-dithizone extract (Step 14) to this mixture and shake. The color should instantly disappear. If bismuth is present, the orange color will persist.

INTERPRETATION (see p. 7)

Mercury is not a normal trace element in man. Normal concentrations range from 0 to about 20 μg/100 ml of blood or 1,000 ml of urine, depending upon a person's occupation. Absorption may occur by all portals, including inhalation of metallic vapors. If exposure is low-grade and chronic, the kidney will eliminate mercury in urine for many months after the last exposure without suffering damage.

For orally ingested mercuric chloride the MLD is approximately 7 mg/kg of body weight or 500 mg for a 150-lb man. Other inorganic mercury compounds vary in toxicity, depending upon their solubility. Phenyl mercuric salts or esters are almost as toxic as mercuric chloride, but are less corrosive.

REFERENCES

Kaye, S., Toxicology of mercury, *Bol. Assoc. Med. P.R.*, 60, 602, 1968.

Kevalo, P., Vesapar, A., and Bachman, B., Atomic absorption of mercury in fish using the Coleman MAS-50 mercury analyzer, *Anal. Chem.*, 46, 1814, 1974.

Natelson, S., *Microtechniques of Clinical Chemistry*, Charles C Thomas, Springfield, Ill., 1961, 294.

TYPE C PROCEDURE

A. Rathje

APPARATUS

1. Mercury detector assembly* (Figure 1)

REAGENTS

All chemicals should be analytical reagent grade.

1. Nitric acid, concentrated
2. Mercury stock solution, 50 μg/ml
   Weigh 0.1 g of metallic mercury accurately into a clean, dry 100-ml volumetric flask. Add 5 ml of concentrated nitric acid. Wait until all the mercury is dissolved, then dilute the flask contents to the mark with water. Calculate the volume of this solution, which is equivalent to exactly 50.0 mg of mercury. With the aid of a burette, transfer this volume to a one liter volumetric flask. Add 20 ml of concentrated nitric acid, then dilute the flask contents to the mark with water. This solution is stable for at least 6 months.
3. Mercury reference solution, 0.5 μg/ml
   Transfer 1.0 ml of the mercury stock solution to a 100-ml volumetric flask. Add 2.0 ml of concentrated nitric acid, then dilute the flask contents to 100 ml with water. Prepare this solution shortly before use.
4. Hydrochloric acid, 6*N*
   Dilute 50 ml of concentrated hydrochloric acid to 100 ml with water.
5. Stannous chloride, 20 g/100 ml
   Dissolve 20 g of stannous chloride in 100 ml of 6*N* hydrochloric acid.
6. Antifoaming solution
   Suspend 5 g of Antifoam 60† in 95 ml of water.

PROCEDURE

Preparation of a Standard Curve

1. Place 5 ml of concentrated nitric acid into a 100-ml round-bottom flask and dilute it to 50 ml with water at approximately 25°C.
2. Using an air of nitrogen line, gently blow out

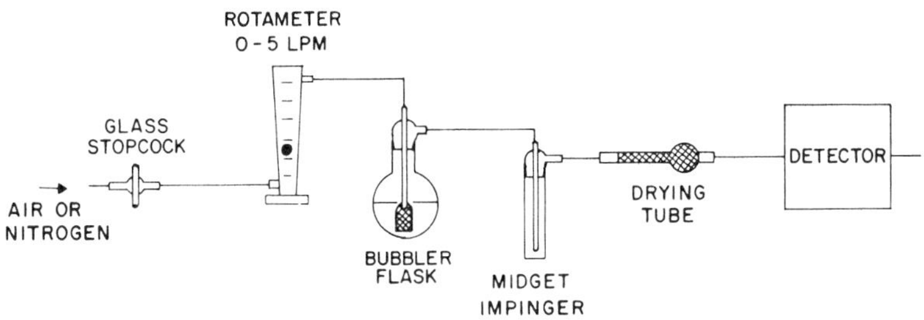

FIGURE 1. Mercury detector. (a) Glass stopcock; (b) Rotameter, 0 to 5 liter/min; (c) Bubbler flask – To a 100-ml round-bottom flask with a 24/40 ground glass neck, fit an all glass midget impinger stopper whose inlet tube has been cut off and replaced with a coarse fritted glass bubbler tube. The fritted glass bubbler should be approximately 1/8 in. from the bottom of the flask; (d) Drying tube packed with magnesium perchlorate; (e) Mercury detector – An atomic absorption spectrophotometer (Perkin-Elmer Model 303), modified so that the burner assembly is replaced by a Pyrex® tube 8″× 1¼″ in diameter, and equipped with quartz end windows and glass side-arm tubes near each end for passing the air stream in and out. A unit suitable for this purpose is now commercially available.

*An appropriate instrument to replace the component assembly described above is now commercially available.
†Available from Silicone Products Department, General Electric Company, Waterford, N.Y.

the mist that forms above the solution when water is added to the concentrated acid.

3. With the aid of a graduated 1-ml pipet add a measured quantity (between 0 and 1 ml) of the mercury reference solution to the flask.
4. Immediately add 1 ml of the stannous chloride solution and 1 drop of the antifoaming solution. Swirl the flask contents a few times.
5. Connect the flask to the fritted bubbler tube, which has previously been connected with tubing to the other parts of the generating train.
6. Turn on the stopcock and pass air or nitrogen through the system at a rate of 2 liters/min. (The pressure from the air or nitrogen line should be adjusted earlier, with only water in the flask, so that merely opening the stopcock gives the desired flow rate immediately.)
7. Observe and record the maximum arbitrary scale reading of the detector or recorder. If a Perkin-Elmer Model 303 with a digital concentration readout (DCR) is used, the noise suppression of the DCR should be set at "2", the averaging dial at "Repeat", and the mode dial on "Absorbance"; observe the readout counter carefully and record the maximum reading.
8. On the basis of the data obtained in this first run, repeat the calibration with appropriate quantities of mercury to cover the entire scale of the meter or a convenient working range. Both the degree of linearity and the full scale sensitivity depend on the particular instrument used for detection.

Analysis*

1. Transfer 2.0 ml of the urine specimen to the round bottom flask. If the urine contains a sediment, shake it well immediately before sampling and swirl it gently while withdrawing the sample.
2. Add 5 ml of concentrated nitric acid, then allow the mixture to stand at room temperature for 3 min. Longer standing is not necessary, but will do no harm.
3. Dilute the flask contents to 50 ml with water at 25°C.
4. Blow out any mist above the liquid with a gentle puff of air or nitrogen.
5. Add 1 ml of stannous chloride and 1 drop of the antifoaming solution. Swirl the flask contents a few times.
6. Connect the flask to the bubbler tube in the generating train.
7. Open the stopcock and pass air or nitrogen through the system at a rate of 2 liters/min, exactly as in the calibration procedure.
8. Observe and record the maximum scale reading. If the needle goes off scale, repeat the analysis with a smaller volume of the specimen.

CALCULATION

1. Refer to the standard curve to determine the mercury content (μg) in the urine sample.
2. Divide the value obtained by the sample volume (ml) to determine the mercury concentration (mg/liter) of the specimen.

The sensitivity of this method will depend primarily on the characteristics of the detector and the dimensions of the absorption cell used. With the Perkin-Elmer Model 303 and other detectors, as little as 6 ng of mercury can be detected with no difficulty. For a 2-ml urine specimen, this would correspond to a mercury concentration of 0.003 mg/liter.

INTERPRETATION (see p. 7)

The concentration of mercury in urine should be used only as a guide in evaluating the degree of exposure of individuals to elemental mercury vapor, not as a diagnostic tool. Individuals with no occupational exposure rarely show mercury excretion levels in excess of 0.010 mg/liter, and in many cases one cannot detect any mercury at all. As exposure increases, there is a corresponding increase in mercury excretion. There is no precise relationship, but various workers have reported a urine:air ratio of approximately 3; that is, at continued 8-hr exposures to concentrations of 0.1

*This method has been shown to work very well where the exposure has been to mercury vapor. It would probably also work well for exposure to soluble inorganic mercury compounds; however, some workers have indicated that the digestion procedure with nitric acid is indadequate where the exposure involves organic mercurials. For the latter, overnight digestion of a mixture of nitric acid, sulfuric acid, and potassium permanganate has been suggested.

mg of mercury/m^3 air, the excretion rate tends to be around 0.3 mg of mercury/liter of urine. Evidence indicates that, on a group basis, a concentration of 0.1 mg of mercury/m^3 air should correspond to an excretion rate of 100 to 300 μg of mercury/liter of urine. Individual variation, however, is very pronounced.

ACCURACY AND PRECISION

Recovery of mercury from urine samples containing known amounts of mercury is essentially 100%.

INTERFERING SUBSTANCES

This method has few, if any, interferences from substances that might normally be found in urine specimens. Metals such as gold or platinum, which alloy with mercury when reduced to the elemental state by stannous chloride, would interfere. The presence of such metals in urine is undoubtedly very rare, so that, for all practical purposes, such interference may be ignored. Certain organic solvents absorb 253.7-nm radiation, but these also are normally not present in sufficient quantity to cause a significant error. As much as 100 mg of the disodium salt of EDTA caused no interference.

COMMENTS

Inasmuch as the determination of mercury by this procedure is based on peak height rather than on the area under a curve, it is very important that all conditions of the analysis are carefully controlled and that identical test conditions are observed for the analysis of the specimen and the preparation of a standard curve. One or two known concentrations of mercury must be checked with each series of specimens, or whenever any of the reagents are changed. For best results, the temperature of the water used to dilute the specimen should be controlled to within 1°C.

Return of the meter to zero indicates that all the mercury has been removed from the sample. It is not necessary, therefore, to rinse off the bubbler tube when replacing one round-bottom flask with

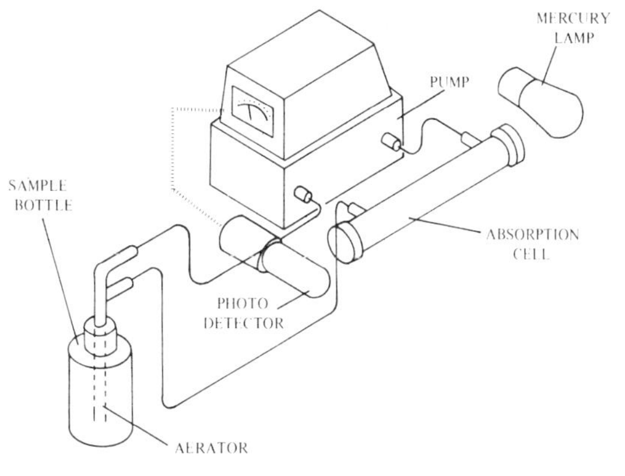

FIGURE 2. Model MAS-50 mercury analyzer system.

another containing a new sample. Thus, a series of samples can be analyzed in very rapid succession if a number of flasks are used. The peak meter reading occurs about 20 sec after bubbling has started, and the evolution of all mercury is generally complete in less than 2 min.

REFERENCES

Hatch, N. R. and Ott, W. L., Determination of submicrogram quantities of mercury by atomic-absorption spectrophotometry, *Anal. Chem.*, 40, 2085, 1968.

Rathje, A. O., A rapid ultraviolet-absorption method for the determination of mercury in urine, *Am. Ind. Hyg. Assoc. J.*, 30, 126, 1969.

Subcommittee for MAC Values (prepared at a symposium at the Karolinska Institute, Sweden, November 4–7, 1968), Maximum allowable concentrations of mercury compounds, *Arch. Environ. Health*, 19, 891, 1969.

APPENDIX

A commercial unit* designed to facilitate the analysis of various samples for their mercury content is available. The unit (Figure 2) contains a circulating pump, a mercury light source, an absorption cell, a photodetector, and a 5½-in. meter calibrated to read directly from 0 to 9 μg of mercury. A scale expansion unit provides reading from 0 to 28 μg, if required. Response time is less than 1 min over the full concentration range.

The system is designed to be trouble-free. The all plastic absorption cell with demountable quartz windows makes it easy to clean and inexpensive to

*Model MAS-50 Mercury Analyzer System is available from Coleman Instruments Division, Perkin-Elmer Corp., 2000 York Road, Oak Brook, Ill., 60521.

replace. All solid-state electronic circuits are mounted on plug-in circuit boards for easy maintenance.

PROCEDURE (Specific directions are provided with the instrument.)

Mercury in the sample is oxidized to mercuric ion with permanganate in a nitric acid/sulphuric acid medium. Hydroxylamine hydrochloride is then added to remove the excess permanganate before stannous chloride is added to reduce the mercury to metallic form. The sample is then connected to the analyzer and air is bubbled through it, evaporating the mercury and carrying it through the absorption cell. Some of the energy from the 253.7-nm mercury line emitted by the mercury lamp is absorbed by the vapor from the sample in proportion to its mercury concentration. The result is read on the 5½ meter directly in micrograms of mercury. The built-in peak-detection circuit will hold the meter needle at maximum deflection until the operator pushes the reset button to prepare the unit for the next analysis.

METHADONE

PRINCIPLE

Procedure A involves an alkaline extraction of methadone from biologic specimens with *n*-hexane and subsequent back-extraction into a solution of ceric sulfate-sulfuric acid. The acid extract is refluxed with *n*-heptane, oxidizing methadone to benzophenone which, in contrast to the unchanged drug, has a much higher UV molar absorbance. The resulting benzophenone can also be measured by gas-liquid chromatography. The underivatized drug and its metabolites are extractable from alkaline samples, and aliquots of this extract may be analyzed by gas-liquid chromatography (Procedure C). An Alternate Type C Procedure is available for the direct analysis of a biological specimen – immunoassay. The principles and procedures of this method are discussed subsequently.

TYPE A PROCEDURE

Jack E. Wallace and Horace E. Hamilton

APPARATUS

1. Separatory funnels, 125 ml
2. Filter paper (Whatman #541)
3. Graduated cylinders, glass-stoppered
4. Round-bottom flasks, 50 and 125 ml
5. Magnetic stirrers and Teflon® stirring bars
6. Reflux condenser
7. UV spectrophotometer, recording
8. Gas-liquid chromatograph with a glass column 2 m × 4 mm i.d., packed with 3% OV-17 on Supelcoport 100 to 120 mesh

   Operating Conditions

   Gas Flow Rate:
   nitrogen – 45 ml/min
   Temperatures:
   column – 200°C
   injection port – 260°C
   detector – 260°C

REAGENTS

All chemicals should be analytical reagent grade.

1. Methadone stock solution, 50 mg/dl
   Dissolve 55.9 mg of methadone hydrochloride in water and dilute to 100 ml with water.
2. Methadone reference solution, 1 mg/dl
   Dilute 1.0 ml of the methadone stock solution to 50.0 ml with water. Other appropriate dilutions of the stock solution may be prepared if a standard curve is desired.
3. Ceric sulfate-sulfuric acid reagent
   Add 76 ml of concentrated sulfuric acid, very slowly and with constant stirring, to a large beaker containing 6.25 g of ceric sulfate and 174 ml of water. Solution is facilitated by stirring the mixture for 30 min at 80 to 100°C. This solution is stable for 2 months at room temperature.
4. *n*-Hexane, spectrograde
5. *n*-Heptane spectrograde

PROCEDURE

1. Adjust each sample to pH 9 to 12.
2. Place 2 ml of each specimen (blood, urine, methadone reference solution, and water as a reagent blank) into a 125-ml separatory funnel containing 50 ml of *n*-hexane. Mix each vigorously for 3 min. Allow the phases to separate.
3. Filter the hexane layer into a graduated cylinder, using Whatman #1 filter paper or its equivalent. Retain a 35-ml aliquot.
4. Add 10.0 ml of the ceric sulfate-sulfuric acid reagent to the 35-ml aliquot of the *n*-hexane extract and shake the mixture for 3 min.
5. Transfer 9.0 ml of the aqueous layer to a 250-ml round-bottom flask.
6. Add 5.0 ml of *n*-heptane and a Teflon®-coated magnetic stirring bar to the flask.

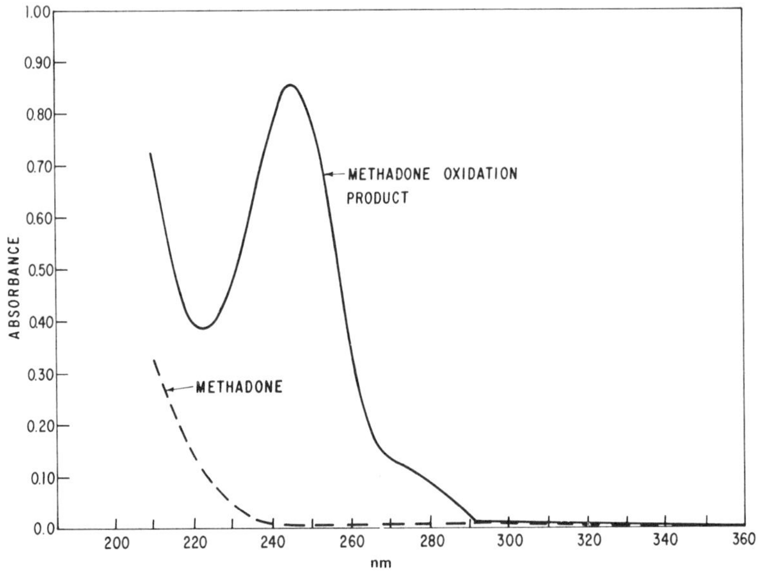

FIGURE 1. UV absorption spectra of methadone in 0.5*N* HCl and of the oxidation product in *n*-heptane, each corresponding to a methadone concentration of 20 μg/ml.

7. Attach a reflux condenser to each flask and place the assembled unit in a heating mantle.
8. Reflux the contents of the flask for 30 min.
9. After 30 min cool the mixture and separate the *n*-heptane from the aqueous layer.
10. Determine the absorbance of the *n*-heptane from 230 to 300 nm, using a solution of nonrefluxed *n*-heptane as the reference solution. Note the absorption maximum at 247 nm (Figure 1).
11. An aliquot of the *n*-heptane extract can be injected into the column of the gas chromatograph for a confirmatory analysis of the benzophenone.

CALCULATION

The absorbance of the reaction product at 247 nm has a linear relationship to the concentration of methadone in the specimen. The methadone concentration of the unknown is determined from the following equation:

$$C_u = C_s \times \frac{A_u}{A_s}$$

where

C_u = concentrations of unknown;
A_u = absorbance of unknown at 247 nm;
C_s = concentration of standard;
A_u = absorbance of standard at 247 nm.

If a standard curve is plotted, it is linear over the range from 1 to 100 μg/ml.

INTERPRETATION (see p. 7)

Methadone concentration in urine from addicts on maintenance doses of methadone generally ranges between 0.4 and 4.0 mg/dl; 98% of addict urines examined in a study by the authors resulted in a concentration less than 5.0 mg/dl.

Since methadone and its primary metabolite are effectively extracted from urine by *n*-hexane, the spectrophotometric method will detect both methadone and its metabolite; therefore, utilization of another technique in conjunction with the spectrophotometric method is needed to provide specificity for methadone. Gas-liquid chromatography can be used to differentiate between methadone and its metabolite as well as to quantitate each. Under the operating conditions stated above, relative retention times for methadone as compared to its metabolite, 1,5-demethyl-3,3-diphenyl-2-ethylidene pyrolidine, are 1.44 min on the OV-1 column and 1.42 min on the OV-17 column.

PRECISION

Since the spectrophotometric procedure measures both methadone and its primary metabolite, this technique is best used as a qualitative test. No measure of precision is relevant.

INTERFERING SUBSTANCES

Other diphenyl-substituted alkaline extractable drugs are susceptible to ceric sulfate oxidation.

REFERENCES*

Beckett, A. H., Taylor, J. F., Casy, A. F., and Hasson, M. M. A., The biotransformation of methadone in man: synthesis and identification of a major metabolite, *J. Pharm. Pharmacol.*, 20, 754, 1968.

Hamilton, H. E., Wallace, J. E., and Blum, K., Improved methods for the quantitative determination of methadone, *J. Pharm. Sci.*, 63, 741, 1974.

Mulé, S. J., Determination of narcotic analgesics in human biological materials: Application of ultraviolet spectrophotometry, thin layer and gas liquid chromatography, *Anal. Chem.*, 36, 1907, 1964.

Rickards, J. C., Boxer, G. E., and Smith, C. C., Studies on the distribution and metabolism of methadone in normal and tolerant rats by a new colorimetric method, *J. Pharmacol. Exp. Ther.*, 98, 380, 1950.

Robinson, A. E. and Williams, F. M., The distribution of methadone in man, *J. Pharm. Pharmacol.*, 23, 353, 1971.

Wallace, J. E., Biggs, J. D., Merritt, J. H., Hamilton, H. E., and Blum, K., A sensitive thin-layer chromatographic technique for determining morphine in urine, *J. Chromatogr.*, 71, 135, 1972.

Wallace, J. E., Hamilton, H. E., Payte, J. T., and Blum, K., Sensitive spectrophotometric method for determining methadone in biological specimens, *J. Pharm. Sci.*, 61, 1397, 1972.

TYPE C PROCEDURE

Philip C. Reynolds

APPARATUS

1. Extraction tubes, 15 × 125 mm fitted with Teflon® or Polyseal† linear caps
2. Mechanical shaker
3. Centrifuge tubes, 5 ml
4. Thin-layer chromatography (TLC) (Brinkmann Instruments): (a) micropipets, (b) glass plates coated with silica gel G, (c) developing tanks, (d) spray bottles

   injection port – 240°C
   detector and manifold – 240°C

5. Gas chromatograph (Perkin-Elmer 900) equipped with dual flame ionization detectors, two 1 mV recorders, and two glass columns 6′ × 1/4″ o.d. and 6′ × 1/8″ i.d., packed, respectively, with 3% SE 30 Ultraphase and 3% OV 17 on Chromosorb W (HP), 80 to 100 mesh

Operating Conditions

Gas Flow Rates:
air, nitrogen and hydrogen – adjusted for maximum response per manufacturer's instructions.

Temperatures:
injection port – 240°C
detector and manifold – 240°C

REAGENTS

All chemicals should be analytical reagent grade.

1. Drug stock solutions, 100 mg/dl in methanol
Dissolve 28.3 mg of the hydrochloride salt of each drug (methadone and methapyriline) in methanol and dilute to 25 ml with methanol.
2. Drug reference solutions in whole blood, 1 mg/dl

*For an updated list of reference material, see General References, p. 235.

†Scientific Products, 1430 Wawkegon Rd., McGraw Park, Ill. 60085.

Dilute 0.5 ml of the stock drug solutions to 50 ml with drug-free whole blood. (Retain a portion of the drug free blood for future dilutions.) Place on a magnetic stirring apparatus for at least 3 hr for equilibration, then store at 4°C.

3. Working reference solutions, 0.5 and 0.2 mg/dl in blood
   Dilute 2.5 and 1.0 ml of the equilibrated blood reference solutions to 5 ml with drug-free whole blood. Use these solutions when each set of unknowns is analyzed.
4. Internal standard stock solution, trihexylphenidyl hydrochloride, 100 mg/dl
   Dissolve 20 mg of trihexylphenidyl HCl in 20 ml of methanol (stable if refrigerated).
5. Internal control trihexylphenidyl working solution, 10.0 mg/dl
   Dilute the stock trihexylphenidyl solution 1:10 with water.
6. 1-Chlorobutane (Mallinckrodt® # 1872)
7. Hydrochloric acid, 0.5*N*
   Dilute 4.0 ml of concentrated HCL to 100 ml with water.
8. Sodium hydroxide, 5 *N*
   Dissolve 200 g of NaOH in water and dilute to one liter.
9. Chloroform (Baker E921)
10. TLC developing solution[1]
    Solution A: methanol-ammonium hydroxide, 100: 1.5 (v/v)
11. Iodoplatinate spray reagent
    Dissolve 10 gm of potassium iodide in 240 ml of water. Add 10 ml of a 10% (w/v) platinum chloride solution, then dilute the mixture to 500 ml with water.

PROCEDURE[2]

1. To 5 ml of each sample (unknown blood, 50% tissue slurry, working reference solutions, and blank blood), add 0.5 ml of the trihexylphenidyl internal standard solution and 10 ml of 1-chlorobutane. Shake the mixture for 5 min.
2. Centrifuge the samples and transfer most of the supernatant to clean tubes. Discard the aqueous layer.
3. Add 5 ml of 0.5*N* HCL to all samples, and shake for 5 min.
4. Centrifuge the samples, then aspirate and discard the top solvent layer.
5. To the remaining NCl layer add 0.5 ml of 5*N* NaOH and 3 ml of chloroform. Shake for 5 min. Aspirate all the upper aqueous phase, and pour the remaining chloroform solvent into 5-ml centrifuge tubes.
6. Place the tubes in an approximately 50°C water bath. Evaporate the solvent just to dryness with the aid of a well-filtered air stream.
7. Dissolve the residue in about 50 μl of methanol and inject 1 to 2 μl into each column of the gas chromatograph.
8. Record the retention distance of each peak eluting, measuring from the solvent front.

CONFIRMATION

Spot the remainder of the extracts from the unknowns and reference samples about 2 cm from the bottom of a silica gel TLC plate. Place in solvent tank and allow to develop approximately 10 cm. Dry the plate with a warm air blower for about 30 min, then spray with iodoplatinate and observe the characteristic spots.

CALCULATION

Compare the peak height ratio of the unknown relative to trihexylphenidyl with that of a suitable drug reference solution relative to trihexylphenidyl. The gas-chromatographic response ratios are linear in the range of 0.1 to 1.0 mg/dl of original solution.

INTERPRETATION (see p. 7)

Methadone concentration in urine (from addicts on maintenance doses of methadone generally ranges between 0.4 and 4.0 mg/dl; 98% of addict urines examined in a study by the authors resulted in a concentration less than 5.0 mg/dl.

Since methadone and its primary metabolite are effectively extracted from urine by *n*-hexane, the spectrophotometric method will detect both methadone and its metabolite; therefore, utilization of

Table 1
CHROMATOGRAPHIC DATA FOR METHADONE AND RELATED DRUGS

Compound	RRT on SE-30	RRT on OV-17	$R_f \times 100$
Caffeine	.29	.44	–
Cyclizine (Marezine®)	.50	.52	–
Methapyriline	.47	.51	75
Methadone	.74	.71	70
Methaqualone	.73	1.20	–
Cocaine	.82	1.19	–
Propoxyphene	.82	.83	85
Amitriptyline	.85	.83	76
Nortriptyline	.93	1.12	50
Doxepin	.95	1.11	74
Trihexylphenidyl*	1.00	1.10	83

* GLC retention times relative to trihexylphenidyl

another technique in conjunction with the spectrophotometric method is needed to provide specificity for methadone. Gas-liquid chromatography can be used to differentiate between methadone and its metabolite as well as to quantitate each. Under the operating conditions stated above, relative retention times for methadone as compared to its metabolite, 1,5-dimethyl-3,3-diphenyl-2-ethylidene pyrolidine, are 1.44 on the OV-1 column and 1.42 on the OV-17 column.

ACCURACY AND PRECISION

Use of fortified blood reference solutions affords essentially 100% relative recovery.

INTERFERING SUBSTANCES

Extreme care in cleaning glassware and selecting reagents free from interfering GLC peaks is essential.

Table 1 gives the relative retention times in the GLC systems and the R_f values in the TLC system for common basic drugs likely to be present in poisoning incidents. Using the TLC confirmation method when necessary, the detection and quantitation is achieved with ease at the levels encountered in overdose and death.

REFERENCES

1. **Sunshine, I.,** Use of TLC in diagnosis of poisoning, *Am. J. Clin. Pathol.,* 40, 576, 1962.
2. **Wolen, R. L. and Gruber, C. M.,** Determination of propoxyphene in human plasma by gas chromatography, *Anal. Chem.,* 40(8), 1242, 1968.

GENERAL REFERENCES

Garriott, J. C., Sturner, W. Q., and Mason, M. F., Toxicologic findings in six fatalities involving methadone, *Clin. Toxicol.,* 6, 163, 1973.

Henderson, G. L. and Wilson, K. B., Excretion of methadone and metabolites in human sweat, *Res. Comm. Chem. Pathol. Pharm.,* 5, 1, 1973.

Inturrsi, C. E. and Verebely, K., A gas chromatographic method for the quantitative determination of methadone in human plasma and urine, *J. Chromatogr.,* 65, 361, 1972.

Inturrisi, C. E. and Verebely, K., Disposition of methadone in man after a single oral dose, *Clin. Pharmacol. Ther.,* 13, 923, 1972.

Inturrisi, C. E. and Verebely, K., The levels of methadone in the plasma in methadone maintenance, *Clin. Pharmacol. Ther.,* 13, 633, 1972.

Niyogi, S. K., Drug levels in cases of poisoning, *J. Forensic Sci.,* 2, 67, 1973.

Pohland, A., Boaz, H. E., and Sullivan, H. R., Synthesis and identification of metabolites resulting from the biotransformation of DL-methadone in man and the rat, *J. Med. Chem.,* 14(3), 194, 1971.

Robinson, A. E. and Williams, F. M., The distribution of methadone in man, *J. Pharm. Pharmacol.,* 23, 353, 1971.

Sullivan, H. R. and Due, S. L., Urinary metabolites of methadone in maintenance subjects, *J. Med. Chem.,* 16, 909, 1973.

ALTERNATE TYPE C PROCEDURE IMMUNOASSAY

Details for the EMIT procedure will be found on p. 401. Details for the RIA procedure will be found on p. 403.

METHANOL

PRINCIPLE

A commonly available volatile alcohol, methanol may be distilled from any matrix. Being miscible with water, it is also present in protein-free filtrates. It can be identified by determining the absorbance of its reaction product with chromotropic acid after first oxidizing the methanol to formaldehyde with a suitable oxidant (Procedures A and B). More simply and elegantly, a microliter of diluted sample may be injected into a gas chromatograph and thus the methanol concentration may be determined (Procedure C).

TYPE A PROCEDURE

Robert V. Blanke

REAGENTS

All chemicals should be analytical reagent grade.

1. Trichloroacetic acid, 20 g/100 ml
   Dissolve 20 g of trichloroacetic acid in water and dilute to 100 ml.
2. Potassium permanganate, 3 g/100 ml
   Add 3.0 g of potassium permanganate to a solution of 15 ml of 85% phosphoric acid diluted to 100 ml with water.
3. Sodium bisulfite
4. Chromotropic acid (1,8-dihydroxynaphthalene-3,6-disulfonic acid)
5. Sulfuric acid, concentrated

PROCEDURE

1. Do not use heparin or EDTA as an anticoagulant for blood specimens. To 2.0 ml of blood, serum, or urine, add 4.0 ml of the trichloroacetic acid solution. Shake the mixture thoroughly, then filter it as a reagent blank. Add 2.0 ml of water and 4.0 ml of the trichloroacetic acid solution. Mix thoroughly and filter, if necessary.
2. Label three small test tubes "Blank," "Oxidized Filtrate," and "Unoxidized Filtrate," respectively.
3. Pipet 1.0 ml of specimen filtrate into each tube labeled Oxidized Filtrate and Unoxidized Filtrate, respectively. Pipet 1.0 ml of the reagent blank mixture into tube labeled Blank.
4. Add 2 drops of potassium permanganate solution to the Blank and Oxidized Filtrate tubes. (Do *not* add potassium permanganate solution to the Unoxidized Filtrate tube.) Wait exactly 2 min.
5. To each of the three tubes add approximately 10 mg of sodium bisulfite to decolorize (reduce) the excess permanganate. Mix thoroughly. If some permanganate color remains, add more sodium bisulfite, but avoid a large excess.
6. Add approximately 2 mg of chromotropic acid to each of the three tubes. Mix thoroughly.
7. Carefully underlay the solution in each tube with 3.0 ml of sulfuric acid by inclining the tube and flowing the acid down the side of the inclined tube. A purple ring at the interface may be a positive test for methanol.
8. Shake the tube to diffuse the purple color. The color is fully developed after about 20 min.

INTERPRETATION (see p. 7)

A blood concentration higher than 80 mg/100 ml is dangerous to life. Equal amounts of color in both oxidized and unoxidized filtrates would be considered a negative test.

ACCURACY AND PRECISION

This method is very sensitive and will detect about 10 mg of methanol/100 ml of sample.

INTERFERING SUBSTANCES

An aqueous control, which will remain essentially colorless, should always be processed in parallel with each batch of samples in order to ensure lack of contamination of reagents. Formalin, heparin, methenamine, and EDTA also give positive tests. The dehydrating effect of concentrated sulfuric acid can produce formaldehyde from appropriate organic compounds and, hence, false positive results. This interference is occasionally observed in patients with severe acidosis. For this reason, an unoxidized portion of the filtrate is run for comparison purposes.

REFERENCE

Kaye, S., *Handbook of Emergency Toxicology,* 3rd ed., Charles C Thomas, Springfield, 1970, 314.

TYPE B PROCEDURE

Robert V. Blanke

APPARATUS

1. Spectrophotometer

REAGENTS

All chemicals should be analytical reagent grade.

1. Methanol stock solution, 785 mg/100 ml
   Dilute 10.0 ml of absolute methanol to one liter with distilled water.
2. Methanol reference solutions
   Dilute 1.0, 2.0, 4.0, and 8.0 ml of the methanol stock solution to 100 ml with water to obtain concentrations of 7.85, 15.7, 31.4, and 62.8 mg/100 ml, respectively.
3. Sodium tungstate, 10 g/100 ml
   Dissolve 10 g of sodium tungstate in water and dilute to 100 ml with water.
4. Sulfuric acid, approximately $2/3N$
   Dilute 2.0 ml of concentrated ($36N$) sulfuric acid to 100 ml with water.
5. Ethanol, 7.85 g/100 ml
   Dilute 10.0 ml of absolute ethanol to 100 ml with distilled water.
6. Phosphoric acid, concentrated (85%)
7. Oxidant solution
   Add 15.8 g of potassium permanganate to 14.0 ml of concentrated (85%) phosphoric acid and dilute to 500 ml with distilled water.
8. Phosphoric acid, 2.8 g/100 ml
   Dilute 14.0 ml of concentrated (85%) phosphoric acid to 500 ml with distilled water.
9. Sodium bisulfite, 5 g/100 ml
   Dissolve 5.0 g of sodium bisulfite in water and dilute to 100 ml. Prepare fresh every day.
10. Chromotropic acid (CTA), 1.5 g/100 ml
    Dissolve 150 mg of the sodium salt of 1,8-dihydroxynaphthalene-3,6-disulfonic acid in water and dilute to 10.0 ml with distilled water. Prepare just prior to use.
11. Sulfuric acid, concentrated (95%)

PROCEDURE

1. Prepare a 1:10 tungstic acid filtrate of each sample (specimen of blood, urine, or stomach content, water for a reagent blank, and reference solutions) as follows:
   a. Dilute 1.0 ml of sample to 7.0 ml with distilled water.
   b. Add 1.0 ml of the tungstic acid solution to the sample. Mix well.
   c. Slowly, while stirring, add 1.0 ml of the dilute sulfuric acid. Mix well. Allow the mixture to stand for 5 min.

   d. Filter the mixture through Whatman #1 filter paper.
2. Each sample must have its own control. Place duplicate 1.0-ml aliquots of the filtrates obtained from the specimen and the reference solutions in two tubes. Designate one tube of each set as the sample and the other as the sample control.
3. Pipet a 1.0-ml aliquot of the filtrate obtained from the reagent blank into another tube.
4. Pipet 1.0 ml of the dilute ethanol into each tube. Mix well.
5. Add 5.0 ml of the oxidant solution to the tubes designated as samples and to the reagent blank. Add 5.0 ml of the dilute phosphoric acid to the sample control tube. Mix the contents of each tube. Allow the tubes to stand for 10 min, accurately timed, at room temperature.
6. Add 2.5 ml of the sodium bisulfite solution to each tube, followed by 0.5 ml of concentrated (85%) phosphoric acid. Agitate each mixture until it is colorless.
7. Pipet 1.0 ml of each reaction mixture into a clean, appropriately labeled tube.
8. Carefully add 1.0 ml of CTA solution and 8.0 ml of concentrated sulfuric acid to each tube. Mix the tube contents carefully.
9. Place the tubes in a boiling water bath for 5 min then remove and cool them to room temperature.
10. Determine the absorbance of each solution at 570 nm, using the solution obtained from the reagent blank as the reference solution.
11. Determine the difference in absorbance between the sample and the sample control.

CALCULATION

Determine the methanol concentration in the specimen by the following formula:

$$C_X = \frac{A_X}{A_R} \times C_R,$$

where

C_X = methanol concentration of the specimen;
A_X = difference in absorbance between sample and sample control for the specimen;
A_R = difference in absorbance between sample and sample control for the methanol reference solution;
C_R = methanol concentration of the reference solution.

INTERPRETATION (see p. 7)

A blood concentration higher than 80 mg/100 ml is dangerous to life.

ACCURACY AND PRECISION

Methanol concentrations lower than 1.0 mg/100 ml of blood can be detected by this method, even in the presence of ethanol.

INTERFERING SUBSTANCES

The procedure described is empirical, and the set conditions must be established and adhered to rigidly before quantitative results can be achieved. A minor drawback of a chromotropic acid procedure for the determination of methanol is the use of concentrated sulfuric acid for the development of the final color. The dehydrating effect of concentrated sulfuric acid can produce formaldehyde from appropriate organic compounds and, hence, false high results. This interference is occasionally observed in patients with severe acidosis. For this reason, a sample control must always be run to avoid this error.

REFERENCES

Blanke, R. V., Toxicology – methanol, in *Fundamentals of Clinical Chemistry,* Tietz, N. W., Ed., W. B. Saunders, Philadelphia, 1970, 845.

Hindberg, J. and Weith, J. O., Quantitative determination of methanol in biologic fluids, *J. Lab. Clin. Med.,* 61, 355, 1963.

TYPE C PROCEDURE

Robert V. Blanke

APPARATUS

1. Diluter (Hobbs No. 015-Spec) designed to accept 0.40 ml and then wash the sample with 3.60 ml of diluent (1:10 dilution), including a wash cycle to insure no carry-over from one sample to the next*
2. Gas chromatograph (Pye Model 104, Phillips Electronics, Inc.), equipped with a flame ionization' detector, a 1 mV recorder with attached Disc integrator, and a glass column, 5' X 1/4" o.d. packed with 10% PEG 400 on 100 to 120 Anakrom SD

Operating Conditions

Gas Flow Rates:
carrier – 70 ml/min
hydrogen – 70 ml/min
air – 600 ml/min

Temperatures:
column – 85°C
injection port – 110°C
detector – 125°C

Place a small plug of glass wool in the end of the column nearest the injection port to trap solids. The plug is easily removed and should be replaced periodically with a clean plug.

REAGENTS

All chemicals should be analytical reagent grade.

1. Diluent stock solution, 241 mg/100 ml
   Dilute 3.0 ml of 1-propanol to one liter with water.
2. Diluent working solution, 24 mg/100 ml
   Dilute 10.0 ml of the diluent stock solution to 100 ml with water.
3. Methanol stock solution, 785 mg/100 ml
   Dilute 10.0 ml of absolute methanol to one liter with distilled water.
4. Methanol reference solutions
   Dilute 1.0, 2.0, 4.0, and 8.0 ml of the methanol stock solution to 100 ml with water to obtain concentrations of 7.85, 15.7, 31.4, and 62.8 mg/100 ml, respectively.

PROCEDURE

1. Dilute the specimen 1:10 with diluent working solution. The Hobbs diluter may be used or 1.0 ml of specimen may be added to a 10-ml volumetric flask and diluted to volume with the diluent working solution.
2. Inject duplicate 1-μl aliquots of the prepared samples into the gas chromatograph, making sure that the stated operating conditions are met. Calculate the ratio of the peak area of the methanol in the specimen to that of the diluent.
3. Inject comparable aliquots of each methanol reference solution, suitably diluted with the diluent working solution. Calculate the peak area ratios as above.

CALCULATION

Compare the peak area ratio obtained from the specimen with that obtained from a methanol reference solution of comparable concentration. The peak area ratios obtained from the methanol reference solutions are a linear function of their methanol concentrations from 0 to 400 mg/100 ml.

INTERPRETATION (see p. 7)

A blood concentration higher than 80 mg/100 ml may be life-threatening.

*This dilutor is not necessary, but is very useful if a large number of samples are to be analyzed.

ACCURACY AND PRECISION

This method can easily detect concentrations of 10.0 mg methanol/100 ml of blood. Lower concentrations can be detected by injecting larger volumes of the diluted specimen into the gas chromatograph. The standard error of the method is ± 3.0 mg/100 ml.

INTERFERING SUBSTANCES

Under the above conditions, 1-propanol has a retention time of about 6 min. The retention times for other volatile substances relative to 1-propanol are as follows: methanol, 0.585; ethanol, 0.654; acetone, 0.418; isopropanol, 0.609.

REFERENCE

Curry, A. S., Walker, G. W., and Simpson, G. S., Determination of ethanol in blood by gas chromatography, *Analyst,* 91, 742, 1966.

METHAQUALONE

PRINCIPLE

Methaqualone has a characteristic UV spectrum which can be used for both qualitative and quantitative analyses (Procedure B). It is very soluble in organic solvents and hence is easily extracted by most solvents. Specificity is obtained by using a solvent which is sufficiently nonpolar so that the polar metabolite is not extracted concomitantly with the methaqualone. If one prefers, the organic extract may be concentrated and an aliquot of this can then be analyzed by gas chromatography (Procedure C).

TYPE B PROCEDURE

David N. Baily and Peter I. Jatlow

APPARATUS

1. Centrifuge tubes, glass-stoppered, 15 ml
2. Centrifuge
3. Serological pipets, 1 ml
4. Volumetric pipets, 1, 3, and 5 ml
5. Pasteur pipets
6. Recording spectrophotometer, UV

REAGENTS

All chemicals should be analytical reagent grade.

1. Methaqualone stock solution, 100 mg/100 ml
   Transfer 115 mg of methaqualone (Quaalude®*) hydrochloride (equivalent to 100 mg of methaqualone base) to a 100-ml volumetric flask, dilute it in methanol, and dissolve to volume with methanol. Place the solution in a brown glass bottle and store it at 4°C.
2. Methaqualone reference solution, 1 mg/100 ml
   Transfer 1.0 ml of the methaqualone stock solution to a 100-ml volumetric flask and dilute it to 100 ml with pooled drug-free serum.
3. Sodium hydroxide, 1.0*N*
   Dissolve 40 g of sodium hydroxide in water and dilute it to one liter with water. Store the solution in a polyethylene bottle.
4. Sodium hydroxide, 0.45*N*
   Dissolve 18 g of sodium hydroxide in water and dilute it to one liter with water. Store the solution in a polyethylene bottle.
5. Hydrochloric acid, 1.0*N*
   Dilute 83.0 ml of concentrated hydrochloric acid to 1,000 ml with water.
6. Hexane
   Either redistilled or spectrophotometric grade hexane may be used.

PROCEDURE

1. Transfer 1.0 ml of serum to a 15-ml glass-stoppered centrifuge tube. Transfer 1.0 ml of methaqualone reference solution to a second centrifuge tube.
2. To each tube add 0.2 ml of 1*N* sodium hydroxide and 5.0 ml of hexane. Stopper the tubes and shake them for 3 min. Centrifuge the tubes for about 5 min to enhance separation of phases.
3. With a Pasteur pipet transfer as much of the upper (hexane) layer as possible to a second centrifuge tube. Save the lower (serum) phase because, if positive, it will be reextracted in Step 5 below.
4. Determine the UV absorption spectrum of each hexane extract, using hexane in the reference cuvette. If the typical spectrum of

*Available from William H. Rorer, Inc., Fort Washington, Pa.

methaqualone is not detected, the analysis may be discontinued at this point. If the spectral data indicate that methaqualone may be present, return each hexane extract to the centrifuge tube from which it was obtained and continue the procedure with Step 5.

5. Reextract the appropriate sera (lower phase, Step 3 above) with a second 5.0 ml of hexane, centrifuge the tubes and combine the upper phases with their respective extracts from Step 4.
6. Add 3.0 ml of 0.45*N* sodium hydroxide to each pooled hexane extract.
7. Shake the hexane-sodium hydroxide mixture for 2 min. Allow the layers to separate.
8. With a Pasteur pipet, remove and discard the lower (sodium hydroxide) layer.
9. Add 3.0 ml of 1*N* hydrochloric acid to the alkali-washed hexane extracts.
10. Shake the hexane-hydrochloric acid mixture for 2 min. Centrifuge for about 5 min. Separate the hydrochloric acid extracts from the hexane.
11. Determine the ultraviolet absorption spectrum of each hydrochloric acid fraction 190 to 390 nm, using 1*N* hydrochloric acid in the reference cuvette.
12. Remove the hydrochloric acid extract from the sample cuvette and replace it with 1*N* hydrochloric acid. Determine the baseline using the same reference cuvette as used in Step 11.
13. Calculate the methaqualone concentration (mg/100 ml) in the specimen by the following formula:

$$\text{concentration} = \frac{A_s - A_{HCl}}{A_r - A_{HCl}} \times C_r,$$

where

A_s = the absorbance of the specimen at 235 nm;

A_r = the absorbance of the reference sample at 235 nm;

A_{HCl} = the absorbance of the 1*N* hydrochloric acid at 235 nm (obtained from the baseline); and

C_r = the concentration of the reference solution in mg/100 ml.

Note: The wavelength used is the wavelength of maximum absorption of methaqualone (235 nm) in 1*N* hydrochloric acid. The absorbance of the 1*N* hydrochloric acid should be substracted from the absorbance of both the specimen and the reference before the calculation is performed. Note that methaqualone has a distinctly different spectrum in hexane.

INTERPRETATION (see p. 7)

Serum concentrations of unchanged methaqualone after use of therapeutic doses of the drug range from 0.2 to 0.3 mg/100 ml. Concentrations greater than 0.8 mg/100 ml are consistent with coma.

ACCURACY, PRECISION, AND SENSITIVITY

The UV absorption spectra of methaqualone (Figure 1) in hexane and in hydrochloric acid are specific for methaqualone. The recovery of methaqualone from serum by this method is 50 to 55%. The coefficient of variation both within day and between days is 6.0%. The correlation coefficient between concentrations of methaqualone in serum determined by this method and concentrations determined by a gas-liquid chromatography reference method is 0.90. Concentrations lower than 0.2 mg/100 ml may be difficult to determine with this procedure.

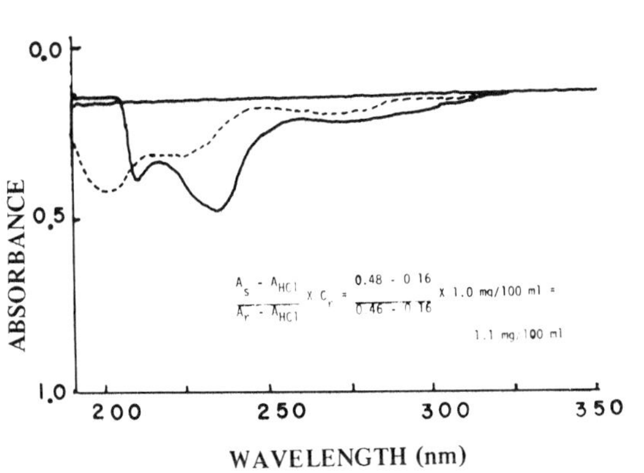

FIGURE 1. UV spectra of methaqualone in hexane (dotted line) and in 1*N* hydrochloric acid (solid line) obtained from the extraction of the serum from a patient who had taken methaqualone (1.1 mg/100 ml).

INTERFERING SUBSTANCES

Methaqualone has at least one metabolite which has the same UV spectrum as the unchanged drug. This metabolite is extractable into chloroform but not into hexane. Since the described method employs hexane, it measures only the unchanged methaqualone. Diazepam (Valium®), certain antihistamines such as tripelennamine (Pyribenzamine®) and chlorpheniramine (Chlor-Trimeton®), and any other basic drugs which are extractable into hexane and which reach sufficiently high concentrations in serum theoretically will interfere. They will show their own characteristic spectra, however, and will not be confused with methaqualone.

REFERENCES*

Bailey, D. N. and Jatlow, P. I., Methaqualone overdose: Analytical methodology, and the significance of serum drug concentrations, *Clin. Chem.,* 19, 615, 1973.

Berry, D. J., Gas chromatographic determination of methaqualone, 2-methyl-3-*o*-tolyl-4(3H)-quinazolinone, at therapeutic levels in human plasma, *J. Chromatogr.,* 42, 39, 1969.

Curry, A., *Advances in Forensic and Clinical Toxicology,* Chemical Rubber Co., Cleveland, Ohio, 1972, 91.

Morris, R. N., Gunderson, G. A., Babcock, S. W., and Zarolinski, J. F., Plasma levels and absorption of methaqualone after oral administration to man, *Clin. Pharmacol. Ther.,* 13, 719, 1972.

TYPE C PROCEDURE

D. J. Berry

APPARATUS

1. Gas chromatograph, dual column (Pye 104, Model 24), equipped with a 1mV recorder (Honeywell), a flame ionization detector, and a coiled glass column, 7′ × 1/4″ o.d., packed with 3% CDMS (cyclohexanedimethanol succinate, Perkin-Elmer Corporation) on Diatomite Q, 85/100 mesh

   Operating Conditions

   Gas Flow Rates:
   nitrogen – 55 ml/min
   hydrogen – 45 ml/min
   air – 400 ml/min
   Temperatures:
   column – 205°C
   injection port – 240°C
   detector – 205°C

REAGENTS

All chemicals should be analytical reagent grade.

1. Sodium hydroxide, 1*N*
   Dissolve 40 g of sodium hydroxide in water and dilute to one liter with water.
2. Hexane
3. Sodium sulfate, anhydrous
   Heat the anhydrous sodium sulfate for 24 hr at 650°C to remove water and all traces of organic material.
4. Butobarbituric acid stock solution, 100 mg/100 ml
   Dissolve 100 mg of butobarbituric acid in ether and dilute to 100 ml with ether.
5. Butobarbituric acid reference solution, 2 mg/100 ml
   Dilute 2.0 ml of the butobarbituric acid stock solution to 100 ml with water.
6. Ethanol, absolute
7. Butobarbituric acid in ethanol, 200 mg/liter
   Dissolve 200 mg of butobarbituric acid in absolute ethanol. Dilute this solution to one liter with absolute ethanol.
8. Methaqualone stock solution, 100 mg/100 ml
   Dissolve 100 mg of methaqualone in the ethanol solution of butobarbituric acid and dilute to 100 ml with the same solution.

*For an updated list of reference material, see References, p. 244.

9. Methaqualone reference solutions
Dilute 2.0, 5.0, 10.0, and 20.0 ml of the methaqualone stock solution to 100 ml with the ethanol solution of butobarbituric acid. The resulting solutions contain the equivalents of 2, 5, 10, and 20 μg of methaqualone extracted from each specimen.

Note: The methaqualone reference solutions are *not* taken through the extraction procedure; they are used only to prepare a standard curve.

PROCEDURE

1. Place 5.0 ml of plasma or urine together with 1.0 ml of 1*N* sodium hydroxide in a 30-ml centrifuge tube.
2. Add 15.0 ml of hexane. Shake the mixture gently for 10 min, then centrifuge the tubes.
3. Transfer the hexane layer to a tube containing approximately 3 mg of anhydrous sodium sulfate. Save the aqueous phase for reextraction (Step 4).
4. Add 10.0 ml of hexane to the alkalinized aqueous phase. Extract by shaking for 5 min, then centrifuge the tube.
5. Add the hexane layer to the first extract (Step 3). Shake the pooled hexane thoroughly with the sodium sulfate. Allow the layers to separate for 10 min, then centrifuge the tube.
6. Separate all of the clear hexane layer. Evaporate it to dryness under a stream of nitrogen in a 25-ml conical centrifuge tube to which 1.0 ml of butobarbituric acid reference solution has been added. This can be done in a water bath at 60°C.
7. Carefully dissolve the residue in 100 μl of absolute ethanol.
8. Inject 5 μl of the dissolved residue into the gas chromatograph. The relative retention time of methaqualone with respect to butobarbituric acid is 2.14.
9. Calculate the ratio of the peak height of methaqualone to that of butobarbituric acid.

CALCULATION

1. Inject 5 μl of each methaqualone reference solution into the gas chromatograph. Prepare a standard curve, plotting the ratio of the peak height of methaqualone to that of butobarbituric acid for each concentration against the methaqualone concentration of each sample.
2. Determine the amount of methaqualone in the specimem by comparison of the ratio obtained in Step 9 of the procedure with similar ratios plotted on the standard curve. The ratios of the peak heights of methaqualone to the peak heights of butobarbituric acid are a linear function of the methaqualone concentration ranging up to 20 μg of methaqualone/100 μl of ethanol.

INTERPRETATION (see p. 7)

Serum concentrations of unchanged methaqualone after use of therapeutic doses of the drug range from 0.2 to 0.3 mg/100 ml. Concentrations greater than 0.8 mg/100 ml are consistent with coma.

ACCURACY AND PRECISION

The mean recovery of methaqualone added to plasma was 96% with a standard deviation of 3.3%.

INTERFERING SUBSTANCES

No interfering peaks in the same regions as those due to methaqualone or butobarbituric acid were found in extracts of bloods and urines obtained from patients known not to have taken these drugs prior to collection of the specimens.

REFERENCES

Berry, D. J., Gas chromatographic determination of methaqualone, 2-methyl-3-*o*-tolyl-4(3H)-quinazolinone, at therapeutic levels in human plasma, *J. Chromatogr.*, 42, 39, 1969.

Brown, S. S. and Goenechea, S., Methaqualone: metabolic, kinetic, and clinical pharmacologic observations, *Clin. Pharmacol. Ther.*, 14(3), 314, 1973.

Clifford, J. M., Cookson, J. H., and Wickham, P. E., Absorption and clearance of secobarbital, heptabarbital, methaqualone, and ethinamate, *Clin. Pharmacol. Ther.*, 16, 376, 1974.

Evenson, M. A. and Lensmeyer, G. L., Qualitative and quantitative determination of methaqualone in serum by gas chromatography, *Clin. Chem.*, 20, 2, 1974.

Walberg, C. B., Lundberg, G. D., and Michaels, A. D., The toxicology of methaqualone with clinical correlation, *Am. J. Clin. Pathol.*, 62, 133, 1974.

METHEMOGLOBIN

PRINCIPLE

Methemoglobin has an absorption peak at 630 nm, whereas cyanmethemoglobin demonstrates minimal absorption at this wavelength. Addition of sodium cyanide to a hemolysate converts any methemoglobin present to cyanmethemoglobin. The absorbance of the hemolysate is measured at 630 nm before and after the addition of sodium cyanide. The difference (decrease) in absorbance is proportional to the concentration of methemoglobin. To determine total hemoglobin, NaCN is added to the solution, thus forming cyanmethemoglobin.

TYPE B PROCEDURE

Method of Evelyn and Malloy[1] as Modified by Henry[3]

Peter I. Jatlow

APPARATUS

1. Centrifuge tubes, conical, 12 ml
2. Centrifuge
3. Spectrophotometer with 1-cm cuvettes

REAGENTS

All chemicals should be analytical reagent grade.

1. Phosphate buffer, 1/60*M*, pH 6.6
   Dissolve 1.2 g of Na_2HPO_4 in water and dilute to 500 ml with water. Dissolve 1.1 g of KH_2PO_4 in water and dilute to 500 ml with water. To 500 ml of KH_2PO_4 add Na_2HPO_4 until the pH of the mixture is 6.6.
2. Sodium cyanide (NaCN), 10 g/100 ml
   Dissolve 10 g of NaCN in water and dilute to 100 ml with water.
3. Acetic acid, 2*M*
   Dilute 12 ml of glacial acetic acid to 100 ml with water.
4. Neutralized cyanide solution
   Mix equal volumes of the NaCN and 2*M* acetic acid solutions. Prepare in a hood within 1 hr prior to use.
5. Potassium ferricyanide ($K_3Fe[CN]_6$), 20 g/100 ml
   Dissolve 20 g of $K_3Fe[CN]_6$ in water and dilute to 100 ml with water.

PROCEDURE

1. Place 9.8 ml of buffer in a 12-ml conical centrifuge tube.
2. Add 0.2 ml of heparinized of EDTA treated blood.
3. Mix and let stand for 5 min.
4. Centrifuge for 10 min, decant, and save the entire hemolysate.
5. Measure the absorbance of the hemolysate at 630 nm (A_1), using water as a reference solution, and return the solution to the test tube.
6. Add one drop of neutralized cyanide solution to the hemolysate.
7. Mix and let stand for 2 min. Again determine the absorbance at 630 nm (A_2).
8. In a test tube mix 2 ml of the solution from Step 7, 8 ml of phosphate buffer, and 0.1 ml of $K_3Fe[CN]_6$. At the same time prepare a blank using 2 ml of water similarly treated.
9. After 2 min add one drop of 10% NaCN to the sample and to the blank.
10. Mix, wait 10 min, and determine the absorbance at 540 nm, using the blank as the reference solution (A_3).

STANDARDIZATION

1. Dilute 2 ml of whole blood 1:50 with phosphate buffer.

2. Centrifuge and save the clear hemolysate.
3. Dilute 1, 2, 4, and 8 ml of the hemolysate to 10 ml with phosphate buffer.
4. Add 0.1 ml of $K_3Fe[CN]_6$ to the undiluted hemolysate and to each diluted solution. This oxidizes all hemoglobin to methemoglobin.
5. After 10 min determine the absorbance of each solution at 630 nm (A_1) and then return the solution to the test tube.
6. Convert the methemoglobin in each sample to cyanmethemoglobin by adding one drop of the NaCN solution to the hemolysate. Again determine the respective absorbances at 630 nm (A_2).
7. To 1 ml of each standard dilution from Step 6, add 4 ml of the phosphate buffer and determine the absorbance at 540 nm (A_3).
8. Calculate the hemoglobin concentration as follows:

$$\text{Hb (g/100 ml)} = 36.81 \times A_3$$

9. Prepare a standard curve by plotting hemoglobin concentration (in g/100 ml) against (A_1 - A_2). Since the curve is linear, a constant may be determined as follows:

$$K = \frac{\text{Hb}}{(A_1 - A_2)}$$

Since all of the Hb was oxidized to methemoglobin (Step 4 above), the hemoglobin concentration, calculated in Step 8 above, is equal to the methemoglobin concentration determined by (A_1 - A_2). Constant (K*) may, therefore, be used for calculation of the methemoglobin in unknown specimens (below).

CALCULATION

g/100 ml metHb = K × (A_1 - A_2) or determine the methemoglobin concentration from standard curve.

$$\text{Percent metHb} = \frac{K \times (A_1 - A_2)}{36.8 \times A_3}$$

INTERPRETATION (see p. 7)

The blood of healthy people averages about 0.5% methemoglobin and should not contain more than 3%.

ACCURACY

The initial centrifugation will be adequate to prevent turbidity in most instances. If turbidity persists, it will not affect the absolute value of methemoglobin which is determined by absorbance difference. It can elevate the total hemoglobin and, therefore, reduce the calculated value of percent hemoglobin. In such cases, high speed centrifugation (10,000 rpm) of the hemolysate may be helpful.

The methemoglobin concentration changes upon standing. Analyses should be performed within an hour after the sample is taken if reliable data are to be obtained. Buffering is critical in that the absorbance of methemoglobin at 630 nm is pH dependent. A more sensitive modification using a 1:5 dilution of blood has been described.[2]

REFERENCES

1. **Evelyn, K. A. and Malloy, H. T.,** Microdetermination of oxyhemoglobin, methemoglobin and sulfhemoglobin in a single sample of blood, *J. Biol. Chem.*, 126, 655, 1938.
2. **Hegesh, E., Gruener, N., Cohen, S., Bochkovsky, R., and Shuval, H. I.,** A sensitive micromethod for the determination of methemoglobin in blood, *Clin. Chim. Acta*, 30, 679, 1970.
3. **Henry, R., Cannon, D. C., and Winkleman, J. W.,** *Clinical Chemistry, Principles and Practice,* Harper and Row, N.Y., 1974, 1149.

*Derived from molar absorptivity of cyanmethemoglobin.

N-METHYLBARBITURIC ACIDS

PRINCIPLE

The drug in a sample is extracted into an organic solvent and then reextracted into alkali. If the characteristic UV spectrum of an *N*-methylbarbiturate is obtained, the solution is acidified and the UV spectrum is obtained again. The resulting spectra can be used to qualitatively suggest and quantitatively measure the drug concentration.

TYPE B PROCEDURE

Raymond Bath and Gerald Kananen

APPARATUS

1. Pasteur pipets
2. Bottles, glass-stoppered, 60 ml, or separatory funnels, 100 ml
3. Filter paper (E & D #615)
4. UV spectrophotometer, recording

REAGENTS

All chemicals should be analytical reagent grade.

1. *N*-Methylbarbituric acid stock solution, 50 mg/100 ml
   Dissolve 50 mg of the *N*-methylbarbituric acid in question in water and dilute to 100 ml. If the free acid is used, add a trace of alkali to help dissolve the solid, add 50 ml of water, then acidify the solution and dilute to 100 ml with water.
2. *N*-Methylbarbituric acid reference solution, 5 mg/100 ml
   Dilute 1.0 ml of the stock solution to 10.0 ml with water. Store this solution in a glass-stoppered bottle at 4°C. If enough acid is added to bring the pH to 4 or lower, this solution is stable for at least 2 months.
3. Sodium hydroxide, 0.45*N*
   Dissolve 18 g of sodium hydroxide in water and dilute to one liter. Store the solution in a polyethylene bottle.
4. Chloroform
   All chloroform should be obtained in glass containers. An aliquot of each new lot should be extracted with 0.45*N* sodium hydroxide. The absorbance of this alkaline solution should be compared with that of 0.45*N* sodium hydroxide. There should be no significant absorption between 240 and 300 nm. If there is, the chloroform must be washed with dilute alkali, dilute acid, and water.
5. Sodium hydroxide, 0.1*N*
   Dissolve 4 g of sodium hydroxide in water and dilute to one liter.
6. Potassium dihydrogen phosphate, 0.1*M*
   Dissolve 13.6 g of potassium dihydrogen phosphate in water and dilute to one liter.
7. Phosphate buffer, pH 7.0
   Add 30 ml of 0.1*N* sodium hydroxide to 50 ml of 0.1*M* potassium dihydrogen phosphate. Dilute the mixture to 100 ml with distilled water. Any other pH 7.0 buffer will suffice.
8. Sulfuric acid, concentrated

PROCEDURE

1. Pipet 3.0 ml of specimen (whole blood, serum, plasma, urine, or stomach content) into a 60-ml glass-stoppered bottle or 100-ml separatory funnel. Include a 3.0-ml sample of reference solution and a 3.0-ml sample of water for a reagent blank in each series of analyses.
2. Adjust the pH of all samples other than whole blood to 6.5.
3. Add 50 ml of chloroform to each sample, then shake the container for 3 min.
4. Remove and discard the aqueous layers from all samples other than whole blood by aspira-

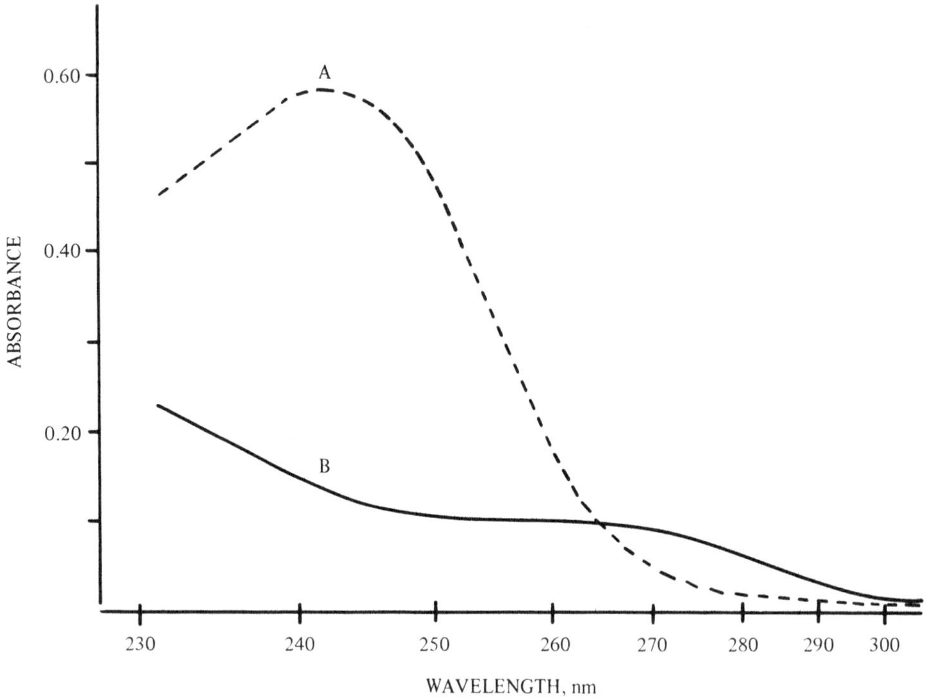

FIGURE 1. Absorption curves for N-methylbarbituric acids. A = in 0.45*N* NaOH, B = in acid.

tion. If whole blood was used, filter the extract through E & D #615 filter paper.

5. Shake the chloroform extract with 5.0 ml of pH 7.0 phosphate buffer. Allow the layers to separate.
6. Aspirate and discard the aqueous wash solution. Filter the washed chloroform through E & D #615 filter paper.
7. Place 40 ml of the washed chloroform extract into a clean 60-ml glass-stoppered bottle. Add 5.0 ml of 0.45*N* sodium hydroxide, then shake the mixture for 3 min.
8. Pipet the aqueous alkaline layer into a test tube and centrifuge it. The residual chloroform may be discarded, or it can be reserved for a determination of any neutral drugs it may contain.
9. Place 3.0 ml of the aqueous alkaline layer into a quartz cuvette and determine its UV absorbance from 340 to 230 nm (Curve B of Figure 1), using the extract of the water sample as the reference solution.
10. Add 1 or 2 drops of concentrated sulfuric acid to each cuvette, mix thoroughly, then determine the absorbance from 340 to 230 nm (Curve A of Figure 1).

CALCULATION

1. Subtract the absorbance of the acidified solution (A_A) at 243 nm from that of the alkaline solution (A_B) at 243 nm and compare the result with the difference in the absorbances of a reference solution analyzed in the same manner. For 5 mg of hexobarbital/100 ml, (A_B−A_A) approximates 0.480.
2. Determine the drug concentration in the specimen by the following formula:

$$\frac{(A_B - A_A)_{specimen}}{(A_B - A_A)_{reference}} \times C_R = C_S,$$

where

C_R = concentration of the reference solution;
C_S = concentration of the specimen.

INTERPRETATION (see p. 7)

Blood concentrations of hexobarbital in patients receiving a dose of 10 mg/kg body weight range from 0.5 mg/100 ml at 30 min to 0.08 mg/100 ml at 4 hr after ingestion. In a fatal case, blood and urine hexobarbital concentrations were 6.1 mg/100 ml and 3.0 mg/100 ml, respectively.

ACCURACY AND PRECISION

An accuracy of 92 + 3% can be achieved with this procedure.

INTERFERING SUBSTANCES

Several weakly acid drugs whose UV absorbance is significant at 235 nm can interfere, if present. Diphenylhydantoin (Dilantin®) is the most common. Megimide® and Ritalin®, "sulfa" drugs, and high concentrations of salicylic acid are also possible interferences. Except for Dilantin®, however, these drugs are seldom present concomitant with barbiturate poisonings.

REFERENCE

Bush, M. T., et al., Ultrashort-acting barbiturates as oral hypnotic agents in man, *Clin. Pharmacol. Ther.*, 7, 373, 1966.

3,4-METHYLENEDIOXYAMPHETAMINE (MDA)

PRINCIPLE

3,4-Methylenedioxyamphetamine (MDA) is extracted from alkalinized specimens into chloroform and back-extracted into 0.1*N* sulfuric acid for quantitation by UV spectroscopy. To confirm its identity, the drug is reextracted from the sulfuric acid extract into chloroform, acetylated, and subjected to a gas-chromatographic analysis on two different columns.

TYPE A PROCEDURE

G. Cimbura

APPARATUS

1. Separatory funnels, 125 and 250 ml
2. Centrifuge tubes, 10 to 15 ml
3. Centrifuge
4. Evaporating dishes
5. Conical evaporating tubes, 5 ml
6. Recording spectrophotometer and suitable 1.0-cm quartz cuvettes.
7. Gas chromatograph, equipped with a flame ionization detector and two columns – one a 3′ × 1/4″ o.d. coiled aluminum column packed with 3% OV-17 on 80/100 Varaport 30, and the other a 4′ × 1/4″ o.d. U-shaped glass column containing 1.5% FFAP on Varaport 30 (Varian).

Operating Conditions

	3% OV-17	1.5% FFAP
Gas Flow Rates:		
nitrogen –	50 ml/min	50 ml/min
hydrogen –	25 ml/min	25 ml/min
air –	300 ml/min	300 ml/min
Temperatures:		
column –	170°C	215°C
injection port –	280°C	280°C
detector –	280°C	280°C

REAGENTS

All chemicals should be analytical reagent grade.

1. Sodium hydroxide, 20 g/dl (20%)
   Dissolve 20 g of sodium hydroxide in water and dilute to 100 ml with water.
2. Sodium hydroxide, 2 g/dl (2%)
   Dissolve 2 g of sodium hydroxide in water and dilute to 100 ml with water.
3. Chloroform, double distilled
4. Sulfuric acid, 0.1*N*
   Cautiously add 2.8 ml of concentrated sulfuric acid to 100 ml of water. Cool and dilute to one liter with water.
5. Acetic anhydride
6. Methanol
7. MDA hydrochloride*
8. MDA hydrochloride stock solution, 1 mg/ml
   Dissolve 100 mg MDA hydrochloride in water and dilute to 100 ml with water.
9. MDA hydrochloride blood reference solution for quantitation – 0.5 mg/100 ml, 2.0 mg/100 ml. Add 0.5 and 2.0 ml of the MDA hydrochloride stock solution to each of two 100-ml volumetric flasks and dilute to volume with drug-free blood.
10. Acetylated MDA reference solution (qualitative)

    a. Make 10 ml of the MDA hydrochloride stock solution distinctly alkaline with the 20% sodium hydroxide solution, and extract it with 100 ml of chloroform.
    b. Filter (paper) the chloroform phase into an evaporating dish, add 4 drops of acetic anhydride and 3 drops of methanol, and carefully (see Step 4 of the procedure for

*Obtained from the Health Protection Branch, Department of Health and Welfare, Ottawa, Canada.

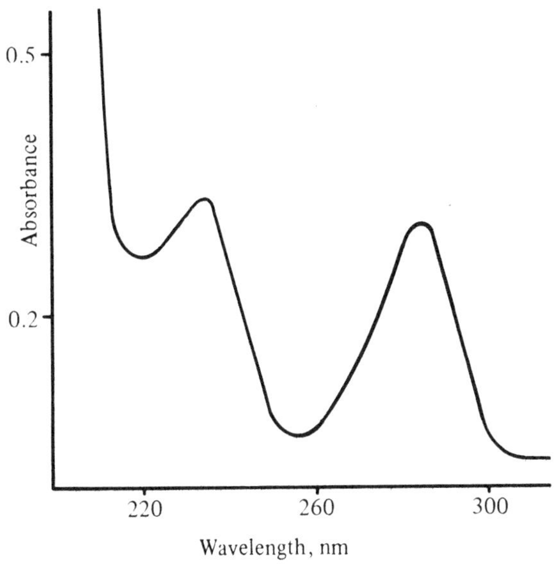

FIGURE 1. UV spectrum of MDA HCl in 0.1*N* sulfuric acid (ca. 1.6 mg/100 ml).

"Confirmation" below) evaporate almost to dryness.

c. Dissolve the residue in 10 ml of ethanol. Each microliter will contain approximately 1 μg of acetylated MDA.

PROCEDURE, QUANTITATIVE

1. In a 250-ml separatory funnel, make 10.0 ml of the specimen (blood, bile, urine, or fluid gastric content and MDA blood reference solution) distinctly alkaline with the 20% sodium hydroxide solution.
2. Extract twice with 100 ml of chloroform for 5 min and combine the chloroform layers in a second 250-ml separatory funnel.
3. Wash the combined chloroform layers first with 10 ml of the 2% sodium hydroxide solution and then with 20 ml of water. Discard the aqueous phases.
4. Filter (paper) the chloroform into another 250-ml separatory funnel, add 5.0 ml of the 0.1*N* sulfuric acid, and extract for about 5 min.
5. Separate the sulfuric acid layer and centrifuge it.
6. Place 3 ml of the sulfuric acid extract into a quartz cuvette and, using 0.1*N* sulfuric acid in the reference cell, record the UV spectrum of the extract between 340 and 220 nm. The presence of MDA is indicated by two absorption maxima, one at 285 nm and the other at 234 nm* (Figure 1). Save the remainder of the acid extract for the confirmation procedure (see Step 1 below).
7. Measure the absorbance at 285 nm, and retain the sulfuric acid extract.

CALCULATION

Calculate the concentration of MDA by comparison with the result from the reference solution whose absorbance value is closest to that of the sample.

$$C_S = \frac{A_S}{A_R} C_R$$

where

A_S = absorbance of the specimen at 285 nm
A_R = absorbance of the reference solution at 285 nm
C_R = concentration of the reference solution
C_S = concentration of the sample.

CONFIRMATION (Gas Chromatography)

1. Place an aliquot of the sulfuric acid extract (from Step 5 of the "Procedure") in a 125-ml separatory funnel and make it distinctly alkaline with the 20% sodium hydroxide solution.
2. Add 100 ml of chloroform and extract for 5 min.
3. Filter (paper) the chloroform phase into an evaporating dish, add 4 drops of acetic anhydride and 3 drops of methanol, and carefully evaporate the chloroform to about 1 to 2 ml.
4. Transfer this chloroform to a suitable conical evaporating tube, and carefully continue the evaporation at room temperature, using a current of air, to almost dryness.
5. Add 20.0 μl of chloroform to the residue, and inject 2 to 5 μl into the gas chromatograph, using the column packed with OV-17 at approximately 170°C. If blood is analyzed, inject 5 μl of the extract and use the highest acceptable instrumental sensitivity. The reten-

*Particularly at low MDA concentrations, the absorption peak at 234 nm may be masked by coextracted impurities.

tion time for acetylated MDA is approximately 3.5 min.

6. If MDA is indicated, rechromatograph 2 to 5 μl in the column packed with 1.5% FFAP at approximately 215°C. The retention time of acetylated MDA is approximately 8 min.

INTERPRETATION (see p. 7)

Blood concentrations associated with intoxication and impairment (in drivers) could be expected to be in the order of 0.1 to 0 07 mg/100 ml. In fatalities attributed to MDA poisoning, blood concentrations of MDA were found to range between 0.25 and 2.7 mg/100 ml. Higher concentrations of MDA were found in urine (3.7 to 16 mg/100 ml).

ACCURACY, PRECISION, AND SENSITIVITY

Blood samples containing 1.0, 2.0, and 4.0 mg of MDA hydrochloride/100 ml were analyzed in duplicate by the UV procedure. An average of 86.2% (from 83 to 89%) of the drug added was recovered. The results of each duplicate analysis were within ± 0.1-mg MDA/100 ml. The sensitivity of the UV procedure is approximately 0.25-mg MDA/100 ml of specimen. Lower concentrations can be detected by the gas-chromatographic procedure.

INTERFERING SUBSTANCES

1. An UV spectrum similar to that of MDA indicates that MDA may be present. Interference from other basic substances with a similar UV absorption is possible. For example, codeine, 2-5-dimethoxy-4-methylamphetamine (STP), flurazepam, and diazepam absorb in the region of 285 nm.
2. Confirmation on the two different GLC columns constitutes an identification with a reasonable degree of certainty.

REFERENCE

Cimbura, G., 3,4-Methylenedioxyamphetamine (MDA): Analytical and forensic aspects of fatal poisoning, *J. Forensic Sci.*, 17(2), 329, 1972.

N-METHYLFORMAMIDE (MMF) AND *N*-METHYLACETAMIDE (MMAC)

PRINCIPLE

The amides may be determined by direct injection of the urine sample into the chromatograph or by injecting an aliquot of a urine sample which has been adsorbed on a cellulose column and eluted with dichloromethane.

TYPE A PROCEDURE

J. R. Barnes and N. W. Henry III

APPARATUS

1. Graduate cylinders, 25 ml
2. Porcelain dish (Coors No. 6)
3. Soxhlet extraction apparatus, 125-ml flask
4. Chromatographic column, 300 × 10 mm
5. Capillary pipet
6. Glass wool
7. Erlenmeyer flasks, 25 ml
8. Vials, screw caps, 1 dram
9. Gas chromatograph (Hewlett-Packard 5750) equipped with flame ionization detector and a stainless steel column 5′ × 1/8″ o.d., packed with Chromosorb 103, 80 to 100 mesh

   Operating Conditions

   Gas Flow Rates:
   - helium (carrier gas) – 45 ml/min, 50 psig
   - hydrogen – 25 ml/min, 8 psig
   - air – 500 ml/min, 33 psig

   Temperatures:
   - column – 170°C
   - injection port – 200°C
   - detector – 200°C

REAGENTS

All chemicals should be analytical reagent grade.

1. Powdered cellulose (Whatman CFI)
2. Alumina (Fisher A-540, 80 to 200 mesh)
   Dry at 100°C for 3 hr, transfer to glass-stoppered bottle, and store in a desiccator.
3. Dichloromethane
   Add 100 g of anhydrous sodium sulfate to a 4- to 5-kg bottle of dichloromethane, shake for several minutes, allow to settle, and decant into a distilling flask. Distill the dichloromethane, collecting the fraction boiling at 40°C and store in a glass-stoppered bottle.
4. Methanol
   Redistill the methanol, collecting the fraction boiling at 65°C. Store in a glass-stoppered bottle.
5. 3.5% Methanol in dichloromethane
   Measure 3.5 ml of redistilled methanol into 100-ml volumetric flask and dilute to volume with dichloromethane.
6. 10% Methanol in dichloromethane
   Measure 50 ml of redistilled methanol into a 500-ml volumetric flask and dilute to volume with dichloromethane.
7. MMF or MMAC reference solutions, 10, 20, 50, and 100 µl/l
   For the direct injection method measure 10 µl of the amide into 1,000-, 500-, 200-, and 100-ml volumetric flasks, respectively, and dilute to volume with distilled water.
   For the urine extract method reference solutions will contain 0, 2, 4, 6, and 8 µl/liter. Collect at least 150 ml of urine from one or more persons who have not been exposed to dimethylformamide or dimethylacetamide. Measure 5 µl of the amide into a 10-ml volumetric flask and dilute to volume with the urine. Pipet 0.0, 0.1, 0.2, 0.3, and 0.4 ml of this solution into 25-ml volumetric flasks and dilute to volume with the urine. Transfer the solutions to porcelain dishes and carry out the procedure described below for samples.

PROCEDURE, DIRECT INJECTION

1. A 2-μl aliquot of urine is withdrawn from the collecting bottle with a microliter syringe and injected directly into the sampling port of the instrument.
2. The metabolite MMF or MMAC is identified by its retention time. Unidentified normal components of the urine will elute before and after the metabolite.
3. The next sample or reference solution can be injected when the last component has eluted, usually after 25 min.

PROCEDURE, URINE EXTRACT

1. Add 25 ml of the urine specimen to a porcelain dish and concentrate it to 1 to 2 ml by evaporation in a stream of air.
2. Mix the urine residue with 4 to 5 g of powdered cellúlose and transfer the mixture to a 25 × 80 mm extraction thimble.
3. Extract the urine residue-cellulose mixture with dichloromethane for 4 hr in a soxhlet extractor.
4. Concentrate the extract to 5 ml by evaporation.
5. Prepare a chromatographic column by mixing 5 g of activated alumina with sufficient dichloromethane to form a slurry. Pour the slurry into the chromatographic tube and wash it with 10 ml of dichloromethane.
6. Transfer the urine concentrate (Step 4) to the column with a capillary pipet containing a plug of glass-wool in its apex to serve as a filter which will remove any entrained solids.
7. Wash the extraction flask twice with 2-ml portions of dichloromethane and add the washings to the column.
8. Wash the column with 10 ml of dichloromethane followed by 2 ml of 3.5% methanol in dichloromethane. Discard both wash solutions.
9. Elute the MMF or MMAC with 15 ml of 10% methanol in dichloromethane. Collect the elute in a 25-ml Erlenmeyer flask.
10. Evaporate the eluate by carefully heating the flask on a hotplate.
11. Dissolve the residue containing the amide in 0.5 ml of redistilled water and transfer it to a glass vial.
12. A 2-μl aliquot is injected into the sampling port of the gas chromatograph.

CALCULATION, DIRECT INJECTION

1. Measure the area under the peak for the standard solutions.
2. Calculate the slope(s) by the method of least squares, for the increase in peak area (A_s) with increase in concentration of amide (C_s) in the standards.
3. Measure the area under the peak for the urine specimen.
4. $C_u = A_u \times s$

where

C_u = urine concentration of amide;
A_u = peak area of amide in the urine;
s = slope (C_s/A_s) from the calibration.

CALCULATION, URINE EXTRACT

1. Measure the area under the peak for the standard solutions.
2. Plot concentration in μl/l against peak area.
3. Measure the area under the peak for the urine specimens.
4. Read the concentration in the sample equivalent to the peak area from the calibration curve.

INTERPRETATION (see p. 7)

In 3 to 4% of the samples from unexposed individuals, a concentration of <1 μl/l of the amides may be found using the procedure described. In exposed individuals the concentration of amide will be >1 μl/l, depending on the degree of exposure and the interval of time between the exposure and sample collection.

PRECISION

Procedure	μl/liter	μl/liter
Direct injection		
MMF	5–500	20 ± 0.5
MMAC	10–500	10 ± 0.9
Extraction		
MMF	0.5–10	0.5 ± 0.05
MMAC	0.2–10	0.2 ± 0.02

INTERFERING SUBSTANCES

Following an exposure to dimethylformamide or dimethylacetamide, the metabolites MMF or MMAC are found in the urine. Small peaks with the same retention time as MMF or MMAC may appear in the urine of unexposed individuals. The identity of either amide may be confirmed by repeating the analysis on a second column. A 10 foot column packed with 10% Carbowax 20M on Haloport F operated under the same conditions is suitable.

REFERENCE

Barnes, J. R. and Ranta, K. E., The metabolism of dimethylformamide and dimethylacetamide, *Toxicol. Appl. Pharmacol.*, 23, 271, 1972.

METHYLPHENIDATE AND RITALINIC ACID IN URINE

PRINCIPLE

Methylphenidate is extracted from an alkaline sample of urine and determined by gas chromatography. Its principal metabolite, ritalinic acid, is methylated, and the methylphenidate thus formed is then determined.

TYPE A PROCEDURE

Rhondda Wells, Keith B. Hammond, and Denis O. Rogerson

APPARATUS

1. Glass-stoppered centrifuge tubes, 17 × 136 mm
2. Lang-Levy micro pipets, 100, 250, and 500 μl
3. Transfer pipets, 1, 2, 4, and 5 ml
4. Serological pipets, 5 and 10 ml
5. Volumetric flasks, 5 ml
6. Mechanical shaker (Model 5-500)*
7. Freeze-Dryer (Model 10-131)†
8. Centrifuge
9. Fume hood
10. Dry ice
11. Polyethylene-stoppered bottle, 125 ml
12. Nitrogen supply
13. pH indicator paper, wide-range
14. Hamilton microsyringe, series 700, 10 μl
15. Gas chromatograph, Perkin-Elmer Model 900, fitted with flame ionization detector, and glass column, 6′ × 0.08″ i.d., packed with a 3% O.V. 17 on 100 to 120 mesh Gas Chrom Q

Operating Conditions

Gas Flow Rate:
nitrogen – 25 to 30 ml/min

Temperatures:
column – 170°C
injection port – 300°C
defector – 300°C

REAGENTS

All chemicals should be analytical reagent grade.

1. Hydrochloric Acid, 2*N*
2. Sodium hydroxide, 5*N*
   Dissolve 20 g of sodium hydroxide in water and dilute to 100 ml with water.
3. Chloroform, G.C. spectrophotometric grade
4. Absolute ethanol
5. Diethyl ether, anhydrous
6. Potassium hydroxide
   Dissolve 60 g/100 ml in distilled water and dilute to 100 ml with water.
7. *N*-Methyl-*N*nitro-*N*nitrosoguanidine‡
8. Etherial diazomethane
   Prepare fresh daily by bubbling nitrogen through a mixture containing 5 ml of diethyl ether, 5 ml of the potassium hydroxide solution, and 200 ml of *N*methyl-*N*-nitro-*N*-nitrosoguanidine. The diazomethane evolved is bubbled into 50 ml of diethyl ether in a bottle surrounded by solid carbon dioxide. This procedure should be carried out in a well-ventilated fume hood since diazomethane is very toxic, and the diazomethane should not be stored in bottles with ground-glass-stoppers. It is not necessary to purify the reagent by distillation, a procedure made dangerous by its explosive potential.
9. Methylphenidate hydrochloride (Ritalin®‡, 20 mg/dl

*Kraft Apparatus, Inc., Queens, N.Y. 11419.
†The Virtis Co., Inc., Route 208, Gardiner, N. Y. 12525.
‡Aldrich Chemical Co., Inc., 2371 N. 30th St., Milwaukee, Wisc. 53215.
‡Ciba-Geigy Corp., Ardsley, N.Y. 10502.

Dissolve 20 mg in water and dilute to 100 ml with water.

10. Ritalinic acid,* 20 mg/dl
    Dissolve 10 mg in water and dilute to 50 ml with water.
11. Diphenhydramine,† 20 mg/dl
    Dissolve 20 mg in water and dilute to 100 ml with water.

PROCEDURE

There is some evidence that at least part of the conversion of methylphenidate to ritalinic acid occurs in vitro in stored urine, most rapidly at alkaline pH and slowest at a pH of about 2.9.[4] For this reason it is recommended that all urines be acidified as soon as possible after collection and stored frozen until assayed.

A. Methylphenidate

1. Prepare two standards by adding 100 μl (0.02 mg) and 250 μl (0.05 mg), respectively, of methylphenidate hydrochloride solution to 2-ml aliquots of drug-free urine. **Note:** Working standards are equivalent to 1 mg of methylphenidate hydrochloride/100 ml of urine and 2.5 mg of methylphenidate hydrochloride/100 ml of urine, respectively.
2. Acidify these standard solutions and 2 ml of each urine to be assayed to pH 2 with 2*N* hydrochloric acid. (Wide-range pH indicator paper is sufficiently accurate.)
3. Extract the urines with 6 ml of diethyl ether in glass-stoppered centrifuge tubes by shaking by hand for 30 sec.
4. Centrifuge to separate the layers and aspirate and discard the ether (top) layer.
5. Adjust the pH of the aqueous layer to pH 11 with 5*N* sodium hydroxide.
6. Add 100 μl of the diphenhydramine internal standard.
7. Extract for 5 min on a mechanical shaker with 10 ml of chloroform and centrifuge to separate the layers.
8. Transfer the aqueous (top) layer to a clean, stoppered tube and save it for the ritalinic acid determination.
9. Dry the chloroform layer with anhydrous sodium sulfate and transfer 5 ml to a clean centrifuge tube.
10. Evaporate the 5 ml chloroform extract under a stream of nitrogen at room temperature. (Elevated temperatures may decrease the recovery of methylphenidate).
11. Dissolve the residue in 50 μl of ethanol.
12. Inject a 4-μl aliquot onto the chromatographic column.
13. Measure the peak heights for the peaks corresponding to methylphenidate hydrochloride and the internal standard to the nearest millimeter (Figure 1).
14. Calculate the ratio of the peak height of methylphenidate to the peak height of diphenhydramine for the standards (R_s) and for each sample (R_x).

B. Ritalinic Acid

1. Prepare two standards by adding 250-μl (0.05 mg) and 500-μl (0.1 mg), respectively, of ritalinic acid solution to 1-ml aliquots of drug-free urine. **Note:** Working standards are equivalent to 2.5 mg of ritalinic acid/100 ml of urine and 5.0 mg of ritalinic acid/100 ml of urine, respectively.
2. Acidify the aqueous layer remaining from the assay for methylphenidate hydrochloride (Step 8 above), and the urine standards (Step 1) to pH 3.
3. Freeze in solid carbon dioxide and evaporate under reduced pressure.
4. Resuspend the residue in 2 ml of absolute ethanol and add freshly prepared diazomethane solution until a persistent yellow color is obtained.
5. Evaporate the mixture under nitrogen at room temperature and redissolve the residue in 1.5 ml of water. Proceed as for the methylphenidate hydrochloride procedure described above starting with Step A2.

CALCULATION

$$C_s \times \frac{R_x}{R_s} = \text{mg methylphenidate hydrochloride/100 ml.}$$

*Ciba-Geigy Corp., Ardsley, N.Y. 10502.

†Parke-Davis and Co., Detroit, Mich., 48232.

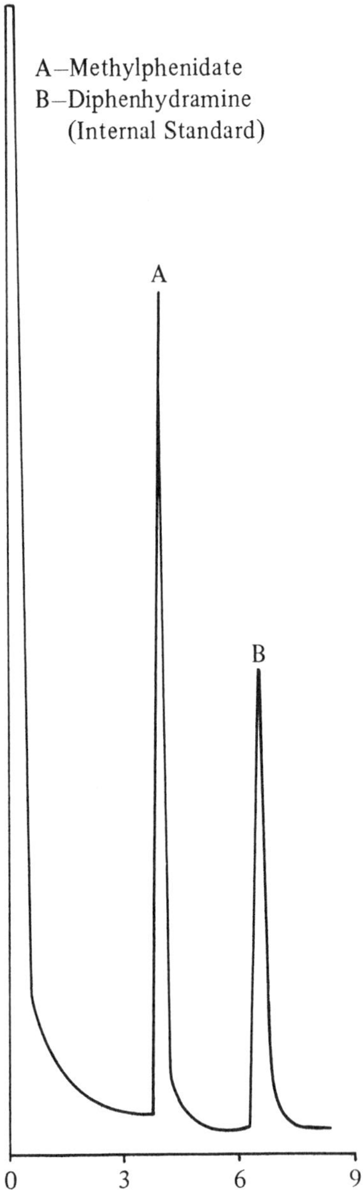

FIGURE 1. Chromatogram of a mixture of methylphenidate hydrochloride and the internal standard, taken through the assay procedure. (From Wells, R., Hammond, K. B., and Rodgerson, D. O., Gas-liquid chromatographic procedure for measurement of methylphenidate hydrochloride and its metabolite, ritalinic acid, in urine, *Clin. Chem.*, 20, 440, 1974. With permission.)

where R_x and R_s are the peak height ratios obtained following Procedure A, and C_s is the concentration of the standard solution.

$$C_s \times \frac{R_x}{R_s} = \text{mg ritalinic acid/100 ml}$$

where R_x and R_s are ratios obtained following Procedure B, and C_s is the concentration of the standard solution.

INTERPRETATION (see p. 7)

Methylphenidate hydrochloride is rapidly and extensively metabolized to ritalinic acid.[1,2] Consequently, the measurement of ritalinic acid is a much more sensitive and reliable index of ingestion than is measurement of methylphenidate alone. In six hyperkinetic children given a single 10-mg dose of Ritalin®, between 35 and 98% of the ingested dose (3.5 to 9.8 mg) was recovered from the urine excreted during the 6 hr after the dose. Of the total amount excreted by these patients, 0.8 to 11.0% was recovered as unchanged methylphenidate (mean, 5.7%), the remainder being excreted as ritalinic acid.[3]

SENSITIVITY AND PRECISION

1. Methylphenidate hydrochloride can be measured with a coefficient of variation of ± 3.2% within one run at a concentration of 2 mg/100 ml.
2. Recovery of ritalinic acid added to normal urine is 94% (range, 90 to 98%) with a coefficient of variation of ± 12.8%.
3. The response of the flame-ionization detector is linear over the range 0 to 7 mg of methylphenidate/100 ml urine.
4. The limit of detection is 0.125 mg of methylphenidate/100 ml.

INTERFERING SUBSTANCES

Neither normal constituents of urine nor other drugs have been found to interfere with this assay.

REFERENCES

1. **Sheppard, H., Tsien, W. H., Rodegker, W., and**

Plummer, A. J., Distribution and elimination of methylphenidate-C^{14}, *Toxicol. Appl. Pharmacol.*, 2, 353, 1960.

2. **Bernhard, K., Buhler, U., and Bickel, M. H.,** Zum Biochemischen Verhalten Eines Psychoanalepticums, des Phenyl-piperidyl-essigsaure-methylesters, *Helv. Chim. Acta,* 42, 802, 1959.
3. **Wells, R., Hammond, K. B., and Rodgerson, D. O.,** Gas-liquid chromatographic procedure for measurement of methylphenidate hydrochloride and its metabolite, ritalinic acid, in urine, *Clin. Chem.,* 20, 440, 1974.
4. **Siegel, S., Lachman, L., and Malpeis, L. J.,** A kinetic study of the hydrolysis of methyl *dl*-α-2-piperidylacetate, *J. Am. Pharm. Assoc., Sci. Ed.,* 48, 431, 1959.

METHYPRYLON (NOLUDAR®)

PRINCIPLE

Methyprylon is extracted into chloroform. This extract is evaporated to dryness and the residue is reacted with Folin-Ciocalteau reagent. The resulting colored solution can be used to determine the methyprylon concentration (Procedure B). Alternatively, the chloroform may be concentrated and an aliquot of this concentrate can be analyzed by gas chromatography (Procedure C).

TYPE B PROCEDURE

Edgar W. Kivela and Staff

APPARATUS

1. Bottles, glass-stoppered, 60 ml, or separatory funnels
2. Mechanical shaker
3. Centrifuge
4. Spectrophotometer, or photoelectric photometer equipped with a 600-nm filter

REAGENTS

All chemicals should be analytical reagent grade.

1. Methyprylon stock solution, 100 μg/ml
   Dissolve 10 mg of methyprylon (Noludar®) in water and dilute to 100 ml with water.
2. Methyprylon reference solutions
   Prepare solutions containing 5-, 10-, 20-, 50-, and 100 μg of methyprylon/ml, respectively, by making appropriate dilutions of the methyprylon stock solution with water.
3. Sodium hydroxide, 5*N*
   Dissolve 200 g of sodium hydroxide in water and dilute to one liter.
4. Chloroform
5. Sodium hydroxide, 0.5*N*
   Dilute 5*N* sodium hydroxide 1:10 with distilled water.
6. Sodium sulfate, anhydrous
7. Phenol regent of Folin-Ciocalteau[1]
   Introduce 100 g of sodium tungstate ($Na_2WO_4 \cdot 2H_2O$), 25 g of sodium molybdate ($Na_2MoO_4 \cdot 2H_2O$), 700 ml of water, 50 ml of 85% phosphoric acid, and 100 ml of concentrated hydrochloric acid into a 1,500-ml Florence flask. Reflux the mixture gently for 10 hr. Detach the condenser. Add 150 g of lithium sulfate, 50 ml of water, and a few drops of bromine to the flask. Boil the mixture for 15 min to remove any excess bromine. Cool the solution, then dilute it to one liter and filter it. The reagent should be free of any greenish tint. Protect it from dust during storage. Alternatively, the reagent may be purchased from Fisher Scientific Co. (Cat. No. So-P-24). For use, dilute 1 ml of the reagent with 2.5 ml of water.

PROCEDURE

1. Place 5.0 ml of specimen (blood,* plasma, urine, or stomach content) in a 60-ml glass-stoppered bottle or a separatory funnel. Prepare corresponding samples of appropriate reference solutions and distilled water for a reagent blank. Add 1.0 ml of 5*N* sodium hydroxide and 40 ml of chloroform to each sample. Shake the mixtures for 15 min on a mechanical shaker. Allow the layers to separate.
2. Remove the aqueous layers by aspiration and discard them. Shake each chloroform layer with 5 ml of 0.5*N* sodium hydroxide for 10 min.
3. Remove the aqueous layers and discard them. Dry each chloroform layer with anhydrous

*When blood is to be analyzed, a 5.0-ml sample of drug-free blood should be included in the series (see Accuracy and Precision, p. 261.)

sodium sulfate by either shaking it with 1 g of the salt or by filtering the extract through the salt supported on glass wool in the apex of the funnel.

4. Remove a 20.0-ml aliquot of each dried chloroform extract and evaporate it to dryness on a steam bath. Retain the rest of each extract for subsequent analysis in the event that the concentration of drug is very high.
5. Dissolve each residue in 3.0 ml of water, then add 1.0 ml of the diluted phenol reagent and 1.0 ml of the 5*N* sodium hydroxide to each solution. If the addition of the 5*N* sodium hydroxide causes turbidity, centrifuge the solution until it is clear (about 5 min at 2,000 rpm in a No. 2 centrifuge).
6. Determine the absorbance of each sample at 600 nm, using the extract obtained from the water sample as the reference solution.

CALCULATION[2]

1. Determine the methyprylon concentration in the specimen by comparing its absorbance with corresponding absorbances of reference solutions processed in the same way as the specimen.
2. Calculate the methyprylon concentration (μg/ml) in the specimen as follows:

$$C_S = \frac{A_S}{A_R} \times C_R,$$

where

C_S = concentration of the specimen;
C_R = concentration of the reference solution;
A_S = absorbance of the specimen at 600 nm (minus absorbance of the blank when blood is analyzed);
A_R = absorbance of the reference solution at 600 nm minus absorbance of the blank.

INTERPRETATION (see p. 7)

A serum methyprylon concentration of 7 mg/100 ml is compatible with coma. At a concentration of 3 mg/100 ml the patient should be rousable and able to respond to questions. Therapeutic blood concentrations probably do not exceed 1.0 mg/100 ml. Following a single oral dose of 650 mg in adults, the maximum plasma concentration of approximately 1.0 mg/100 ml is reached after 2 hr.[3] In fatal cases, blood concentrations in excess of 9.0 mg/100 ml have been reported.

ACCURACY AND PRECISION

The sensitivity of the method is about 5μg/ml. A blank sample of biological fluid must be analyzed because small amounts of reducing substances are extracted by the chloroform from the alkaline medium. The method is not specific for methyprylon. Other compounds with similar configurations and properties may give the same results. Phenol and phenolic compounds will not interfere, however. When methyprylon was added to water, blood, or urine in quantities of 150 to 600 μg/ml, and added amounts were recovered with an accuracy of ±6%.[4]

INTERFERING SUBSTANCES

Evidence is presented that one of the metabolites of methyprylon is a dehydrogenation product[4] which is designated as Ro 1-6462. The chemical formulae of methyprylon and its metabolite are as follows:

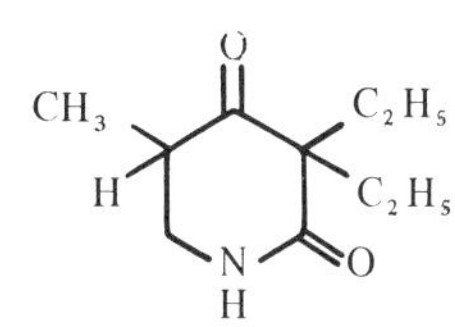

Methyprylon (Nodular® 1-6463
(3,3-diethyl-2,4-dioxo-5-methyl-piperidine)

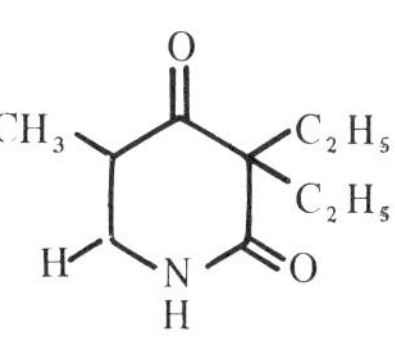

Ro 1-6462
(3,3-diethyl-2,4-dioxo-5-methyl-1,2,3,4-tetrahydropyridine)

The presence of Ro 1-6462 does not interfere in the method because there is no reaction of the phenol reagent with the metabolite.[4]

REFERENCES

1. **Folin, O. and Ciocalteau, V.,** On tyrosin and tryptophane determination in proteins, *J. Biol. Chem.,* 73, 627, 1927.
2. **Xanthaky, G., Freireich, A., Matusiak, W., and Lukash, L.,** Hemodialysis in methyprylon poisoning, *JAMA,* 198, 1212, 1966.
3. *Roche Laboratories Product Reference Manual,* Roche Laboratories, Nutley, N. J. 1970.
4. **Randall, L. O., Iliev, V., and Brandman, O.,** Metabolism of methyprylon, *Arch. Int. Pharmacodyn. Ther.,* 106, 388, 1956.

TYPE C PROCEDURE

Edgar W. Kivela and Staff

APPARATUS

1. Separatory funnels with Teflon® stopcocks, 60 ml
2. Glass funnels, small
3. Filter paper (Whatman #1), 9.0-cm circles
4. Round-bottom flasks, Pyrex®, with 24/40 ground glass neck, 100 ml
5. Rotary evaporator with 24/40 male flask connection
6. Water bath
7. Centrifuge tubes, graduated, 15 ml
8. Syringes (Hamilton), 10μl
9. Gas chromatograph (Barber Coleman 6,000 or a suitable substitute), equipped with a flame ionization detector, a 5 mV recorder (Sargent Model SRLG or a suitable substitute), and a U-shaped glass column, 6′ × ¼″ i.d., packed with 3% OV-22 on Gas Chrom Q, 80 to 100 mesh

   Operating Conditions

   Gas Flow Rates:
   - nitrogen – 60 ml/min
   - air – 500 ml/min
   - hydrogen – 40 ml/min

   Temperatures:
   - column – 180°C
   - injection port – 220°C
   - detector – 260°C

10. Graduated cylinders glass-stoppered, 25 ml

REAGENTS

All chemicals should be analytical reagent grade.

1. Methyprylon stock solution, 300 mg/100 ml
   Disolve 300 mg of methyprylon (Noludar®) in 100 ml of water.
2. Methyprylon reference solution, 30 μg/ml
   Dilute 1.0 ml of the methyprylon stock solution to 100 ml with water.
3. Chloroform
4. Ammonium hydroxide, concentrated
5. Preludin® stock solution, 100 mg/100 ml
   Dissolve 100 mg of Preludin® in 100 ml of chloroform.
6. Preludin® internal control solution, 200 μg/ml
   Dilute 20 ml of the Preludin® stock solution to 100 ml with chloroform.
7. Ethanol, absolute
8. Sulfuric acid, 0.1*N*
   Dilute 2.78 ml of concentrated sulfuric acid to one liter with distilled water.

PROCEDURE

Preparation of a Standard Curve

1. Add 1.0, 2.0, and 3.0 ml of the methyprylon reference solution to 60-ml flasks, each containing 25 ml of chloroform.
2. Make the aqueous layers basic with 1 or 2 drops of ammonium hydroxide.
3. Shake each sample for 5 min. Alow the layers to separate.
4. Drain the chloroform layers through filter paper into rotary evaporator flasks.
5. Reextract the water layers remaining in the separatory funnels twice by shaking with 5.0 ml of chloroform each time. Drain each chloroform wash into the corresponding evaporator flask, using the same filter paper that was used in Step 4.
6. Evaporate each combined chloroform extract to dryness on a rotory evaporator under

reduced pressure, immersing the flasks partially in a 50°C water bath.

7. Transfer each residue to a 15-ml centrifuge tube, using three 2.0-ml washings with chloroform.
8. Add 0.5 ml (100 µg) of the Preludin® internal control solution, mix throughly, then evaporate the chloroform to dryness under a stream of air.
9. Add 8 to 10 drops of absolute ethanol to each residue. Shake the tubes to dissolve the residues.
10. Inject 2 to 4 µl of each dissolved residue into the gas chromatograph, as needed to produce 50% to 90% full-scale response for the highest peak. The retention time of Preludin® is about 3 min; that of methyprylon is about 5 min.
11. Make a graph by plotting the ratio of the peak height of methyprylon to the peak height of Preludin® against the concentration of methyprylon.

Analysis of the Specimen

1. Place 10.0 ml of urine in a 60-ml separatory funnel and make it basic by dropwise addidion of ammonium hydroxide. Use indicator paper to check the pH.
2. Add 25 ml of chloroform and extract the specimen. Allow the layers to separate.
3. Drain the chloroform layer into a 25-ml graduated cylinder.
4. Wash the chloroform extract with 5.0 ml of 0.1*N* sulfuric acid by shaking for 3 min. This removes any organic bases that may be present.
5. Aspirate the acid and discard it. Record the volume of chloroform.
6. Process the chloroform solution in exactly the same way as the reference solutions, starting with Step 4 of the preparation of the standard curve.

CALCULATION

Calculate the methyprylon concentration (µg/ml) in the specimen by the following formula:

$$C_X = C_R \times \frac{H_U}{I_U} \times \frac{I_K}{H_K} \times R,$$

where

C_X = methyprylon concentration in the specimen;
C_R = methyprylon concentration in the reference solution;
H_U = peak height of methyprylon in the specimen;
H_K = peak height of methyprylon in the reference solution;
I_U = peak height of the internal control in the specimen;
I_K = peak height of the internal control in the reference solution;
R = correction for chloroform recovery, ie., $\frac{25}{\text{ml of chloroform recovered in Step 5}}$

INTERPRETATION (see p. 7)

A serum methyprylon concentration of 7 mg/100 ml is compatible with coma. At a concentration of 3 mg/100 ml the patient should be rousable and able to respond to questions. Therapeutic blood concentrations probably do not exceed 1.0 mg/100 ml. Following a single oral dose of 650 mg in adults, the maximum plasma concentration of approximately 1.0 mg/100 ml is reached after 2 hr.[1] In fatal cases, blood concentrations in excess of 9.0 mg/100 ml have been reported.

ACCURACY AND PRECISION

Recovery values of methyprylon from urine are 100 ± 5%. Urine concentrations of 30 µg/100 ml or higher can be detected by this method.

INTERFERING SUBSTANCES

No interfering gas-chromatographic peaks have been encountered.

REFERENCES

1. *Roche Laboratories Product Reference Manual,* Roche Laboratories, Nutley, N.J., 1970.
2. **Clarke, E. G. C.,** *Isolation and Identification of Drugs,* Pharmaceutical Press, London, 1969, 426.

GENERAL REFERENCE

Bailey, D. and Jatlow, P., Methyprylon overdose: Interpretation of serum drug concentrations, *Clin. Toxicol.,* 6, 563, 1974.

METRONIDAZOLE

PRINCIPLE

Metronidazole is extracted from alkalinized plasma into methylene chloride. The extracted drug is silylated and the derivatized compound is determined by gas chromatography.

TYPE C PROCEDURE

K. K. Midha, I. J. McGilveray, and J. K. Cooper

APPARATUS

1. Centrifuge tubes, glass-stoppered, 42 ml
2. Centrifuge tubes, glass-stoppered, 45 ml
3. Conical tubes, glass-stoppered, 3 ml
4. Reciprocating shaker (Eberbach), tube angle 30°
5. Oscillating mixer
6. Gas chromatograph (F/11 Perkin-Elmer) equipped with a flame ionization detector and a glass coiled column, 6′ × 0.06″ i.d., packed with a mixed stationary phase consisting of 0.5% OV-7, 0.5% SE-30, and 1.0% Apiezon-L on Chromosorb W, high performance, 80/100 mesh

   Operating Conditions

   Gas Flow Rate:
      nitrogen (carrier gas) – 80 ml/min
   Temperatures:
      column – 135°C
      injection port – 210°C
      detector – 210°C
   Chart Speed: 5 mm/min

REAGENTS

All chemicals should be analytical reagent grade.

1. Metronidazole* stock solution, 100 μg/ml
   Dissolve 10 mg of metronidazole in 100 ml of water (prepared weekly).
2. Metronidazole working standard solutions 0.25 to 16 μg/ml
   Dilute stock solution daily with drug-free plasma to prepare working standard solutions in the indicated range of concentrations.
3. Internal standard stock solution, 1-β-hydroxy ethyl-2-methoxy-5-nitroimidazole,† 100 μg/ml
   Dissolve 10 mg of internal standard in 100 ml of water (prepared weekly).
4. Internal standard working solution, 1-β-hydroxyethyl-2-methoxy-5-nitroimidazole, 15 μg/ml
   Dilute 15 ml of stock solution daily to 100 ml with water.
5. Carbonate-bicarbonate buffer pH 9.0 , 0.1*M*
6. Diethyl ether, glass distilled
7. Methylene chloride, glass distilled
8. Acetonitrile, silylation grade‡
9. Tri-Sil® concentrate‡
10. Calcium chloride, anhydrous

PROCEDURE

1. Transfer 1 ml of sample (plasma and drug-free plasma containing metronidazole) to a 42-ml glass-stoppered centrifuge tube containing 1 ml of internal standard solution (15 μg/ml) and 4 ml of 0.1*M* carbonate-bicarbonate buffer pH 9.0.
2. Mix on an oscillating shaker for 30 sec and add 15 ml of a mixture of diethyl ether and methylene chloride (14:11).
3. Extract on a reciprocating shaker at an angle of 30° for 30 min.

*Available from Delmar Chemicals, Lachine, Canada.
†Available from Hoffman-La Roche Inc., Nutley, N. J.
‡Tri-Sil® and silylation grade acetonitrile available from Pierce Chemical Co., Rockford, Ill.

4. Centrifuge for 5 min at 3,000 rpm.
5. Pipet 13.0 ml of the upper organic layer into a conical glass-stoppered centrifuge tube.
6. Repeat the extraction twice with two 15.0-ml portions of the solvent mixture and combine these extracts with the first extract.
7. Evaporate the combined extracts to approximately 1 ml on a water bath at 60°C under a stream of dry nitrogen.
8. Add a small crystal of anhydrous calcium chloride and swirl the tube gently.
9. Transfer the extract to a 3-ml glass-stoppered conical tube by means of a Pasteur pipet with the aid of two 0.5-ml portions of methylene chloride.
10. Evaporate the combined extracts and washings to dryness in a water bath at 60°C under a stream of dry nitrogen.
11. Add 50 μl of acetonitrile and 30 μl of Tri-Sil® concentrate to the evaporated extracts in the tube.
12. Stopper the tubes, mix for 30 sec, and leave overnight at room temperature in a desiccator.
13. Evaporate at room temperature to dryness under a stream of dry nitrogen and redissolve the residue in 50 μl of acetonitrile by carefully washing the sides of the tube and mixing for 1 min.
14. Inject 2 μl into the gas chromatograph under the conditions described. The retention times of the TMS ethers of metronidazole and 1-β-hydroxyethyl-2-methoxy-5-nitroimidazole are approximately 5 and 11 min, respectively.

CALCULATION

1. Measure the ratio of the peak heights of the silylated metronidazole and internal standard in the specimen.
2. Compare these with those for the reference plasma samples.
3. Calculate the concentration of metronidazole in the plasma specimen by comparison of these ratios.

INTERPRETATION (see p. 7)

Therapeutic doses (200 to 250 mg) of metronidazole yield peak plasma levels of *ca* 5 μg/ml in 2 to 3 hr. About 50% is excreted unchanged in urine with 2-methyl-5-nitroimidazol-1-yl acetic acid and other metabolites.[1] The major toxic effects have been noted in association with alcohol, as a disulfuram type reaction may ensue.[2] Large doses of metronidazole given over 2 years to mice showed an increase in tumors, which was not observed in rats or hamsters treated in a similar way.[3]

ACCURACY AND PRECISION

Recovery of metronidazole and 1-β-hydroxyethyl-2-methoxy-5-nitroimidazole approximately 100 and 99%, respectively. The overall precision of the assay in the range of 0.25 to 16.0 μg/ml is 4.0%.

INTERFERING SUBSTANCES

No interference on GLC is observed under the conditions described.

REFERENCES

1. **Stambaugh, J. E., Fe, L. G., and Manthei, R. W.,** The isolation and identification of the urinary oxidative metabolites of metronidazole in man, *J. Pharmacol. Exp. Ther.*, 161, 373, 1968.
2. **Taylor, J. R. T.,** Metronidazole – a new agent for combined somatic and psychic therapy of alcoholism, *Bull. Los Angeles Neurol. Soc.*, 29, 158, 1964.
3. **Nida, F. R.,** FDA Talk Paper., T74-56, Nov. 4, 1974.

GENERAL REFERENCE

Midha, K. K., McGilveray, I. J., and Cooper, J. K., Determination of therapeutic levels of metronidazole in plasma by gas-liquid chromatography, *J. Chromatogr.*, 87, 491, 1973.

MORPHINE

PRINCIPLE

In Procedure A morphine is extracted with a mixed organic solvent from the biological fluid which is brought to pH 8.5 to 9.0. The organic extract is evaporated to dryness. Concentrated H_2SO_4 is added, the pH is adjusted to approximately 9 to 10 by the addition of H_2O and concentrated NH_4OH, and the mixture is autoclaved. The morphine fluorophor is then measured spectrophotofluorometrically. Gas chromatography is used to identify and quantitate the extracted morphine in Procedure C. Morphine, the principle metabolite of heroin, and codeine are excreted in the urine primarily as conjugates in the form of glucoronides. These conjugates are highly water-soluble and consequently extremely difficult to extract into organic solvents, whereas unconjugated opiates (free morphine and codeine) are readily extracted. More than 90% of the excreted drugs are converted into glucoronides; only a fraction of the metabolized drug is excreted in free form.

Hydrolysis with acid catalysis cleaves off the glucoronide group, liberating the free unconjugated opiates which are then easily extracted by organic solvents. Morphine and codeine as amphoteric compounds are best extracted from urine specimens at pH 9. Because of their large molecular structures, opiates even in their free forms are not easily gas chromatographed. They generally require high column temperatures and produce tailing and long retention times. Conversion of morphine and codeine to their acetate derivatives by reaction with acetic anhydride in pyridine allows them to be gas chromatographed readily on 3% OV-25 and 3% Poly-A 103 columns. The use of the two different types of columns will eliminate false positives, while the use of nalorphine as an internal standard eliminates false negatives and allows accurate quantitation.

An Alternate Type C Procedure is available for the direct analysis of a biological specimen – immunoassay. The principles and procedures of this method are discussed subsequently.

TYPE A PROCEDURE

Joseph Monforte and Robert F. Turk

APPARATUS

1. Spectrophotofluorometer (Perkin-Elmer Model MPF-2A)
2. Separatory funnels, 250 and 50 ml
3. Beakers, 30 ml
4. Steam bath
5. Autoclave (A pressure cooker will suffice.)
6. Filter paper, Whatman #41
7. Graduated cylinders, 100 and 10 ml
8. pH Meter or narrow range (8 to 10) pH paper
9. Centrifuge
10. Pipets, 1-ml volumetric and 1-ml graduated
11. Test tubes, screw-capped, 125 × 16 mm
12. Multipurpose rotator (Model 150V)*
13. Capillary tubes, sealed
14. Centrifuge tubes, 15 ml

REAGENTS

All chemicals should be analytical reagent grade.

1. Morphine stock solution, 50 mg/100 ml of water
   Dissolve 62.5 mg of morphine sulfate in distilled water. Dilute to 100 ml with distilled water.

*Scientific Industries, Inc., Springfield, Mass.

2. Morphine reference solutions
   (A) Blood: 50, 25, and 10 μg/ml – Using a volumetric pipet, add 0.50 ml of the morphine stock solution to a 100-ml volumetric flask and dilute to the mark with distilled water. Add 1.0, 0.5, and 0.2 ml of this solution (0.25 mg/100 ml) to three 5-ml aliquots of blood known to contain no drugs. (B) Urine: 0.1 mg/100 ml – Add 0.20 ml of the morphine stock solution to a 100-ml volumetric flask and dilute to the mark with urine known to contain no drugs.
3. Sulfuric acid, 0.5*N*
   Slowly add 7.0 ml of concentrated sulfuric acid to approximately 450 ml of distilled water. Cool this solution, and dilute to 500 ml with distilled water.
4. Buffer solution
   Dissolve 53.5 g of ammonium chloride in 950 ml of water. Add 18 ml of concentrated ammonium hydroxide. Adjust the pH to 8.5 by adding either ammonium hydroxide or hydrochloric acid.
5. Chloroform-isopropyl alcohol mixture, 3:1
   Add 1 volume of isopropyl alcohol to 3 volumes of chloroform.
6. Chloroform-methanol, 4:1
   Add 200 ml of methanol to 800 ml of chloroform.

PROCEDURE

Blood

1. To 5.0 ml of sample (blood and each morphine working solution) in a 30-ml beaker, add 0.25 ml of concentrated ammonium hydroxide and a spatula tip of sodium bicarbonate. Mix these. It is not necessary to measure the final pH.
2. Transfer the samples to 250-ml separatory funnels which contain 100 ml of chloroform-methanol (8:2). Ensure complete transfer of the samples by washing the beakers with small portions of distilled water.
3. Extract the samples for 2 min. Allow the phases to separate.
4. Filter the chloroform-methanol (lower) layers into clean 250-ml separatory funnels. Discard the aqueous (upper) layers.
5. Add 5 ml of distilled water and extract the chloroform-methanol layers for 1 min. Allow the phases to separate.
6. Filter the chloroform-methanol (lower) layers into 100-ml graduated cylinders and record the volumes. Discard the aqueous (upper) layers.
7. Transfer the chloroform-methanol (lower) layers to clean 250-ml separatory funnels. Add 5.0 ml of 0.5*N* H_2SO_4 to each sample and extract them for 2 min. Allow the phases to separate.
8. Discard the chloroform-methanol (lower) layers and transfer the aqueous (upper) layers to centrifuge tubes. Centrifuge for 5 min at 2,500 rpm.
9. Adjust the pH of the aqueous layers to 8.5 to 9.0 by adding a spatula tip of sodium bicarbonate and concentrated ammonium hydroxide dropwise. The pH of these solutions must be measured with either a pH meter or narrow range (8 to 10) pH paper.
10. Transfer the aqueous solutions (pH 8.5 to 9.0) to clean 50-ml (or smaller) separatory funnels. Add 10.0 ml of chloroform-methanol (8:2) and extract each sample for 1 min. Allow the phases to separate.
11. Filter the chloroform-methanol (lower) layers into 10-ml graduated cylinders and record their volumes.
12. Transfer the chloroform-methanol layers into 30-ml beakers and place them on a steam bath.
13. When the solvent is evaporated to dryness, add 0.2 ml of concentrated H_2SO_4 to each sample, rotate the beakers to ensure contact with the acid, and allow them to stand at room temperature for 15 min.
14. Carefully add 2.0 ml of distilled water and agitate the mixtures.
15. Carefully add 2.0 ml of concentrated ammonium hydroxide to each sample and again agitate the mixtures.
16. Autoclave the samples for 30 min at 18 psi and 120°C, cool them to room temperature, then transfer the solutions to cuvettes for fluorometry.
17. Excite the samples at approximately 392 nm and record their emission spectra from 380 to 440 nm. Observe their fluorescence at 420 nm. The fluorophor produced by the reaction described in the procedure shows a maximum fluorescence at approximately 420 nm (uncorrected). When this reaction is applied to an

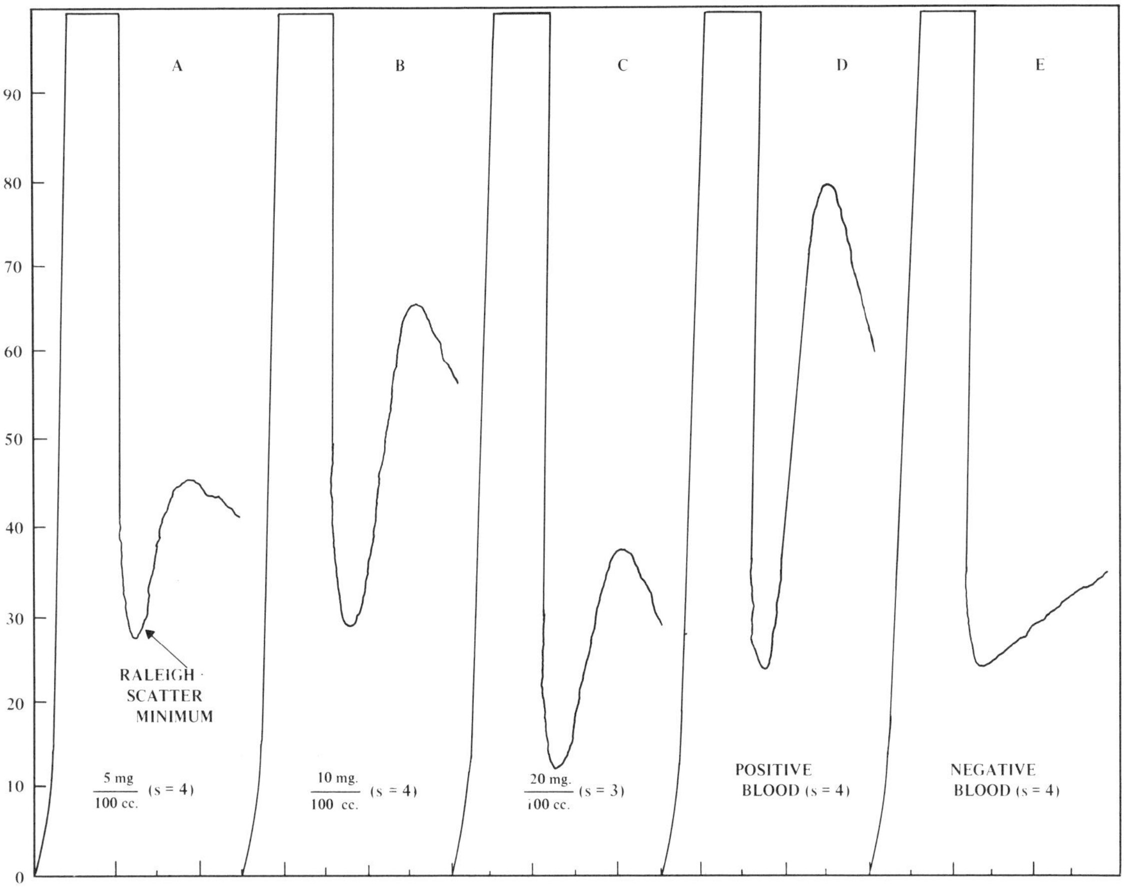

FIGURE 1. Fluorescence spectrum of morphine in blood. Curves A, B, and C illustrate blood samples to which morphine was added at concentrations of 5, 10, and 20 μg/100 ml of blood, respectively. Curve D represents a positive blood sample from a medical examiner's case. Curve E represents a negative blood sample represent 420 nm.

extract of blood, the resulting fluroescence spectrum will be as shown in Figure 1.

Urine

1. To 2.0 ml of sample (urine specimen, reference solution, or water for a reagent blank) in a screw-capped test tube, add 1.0 ml of buffer solution.
2. Add 4.0 ml of the chloroform-isopropyl alcohol mixture to each test tube and place the tubes on the rotator. Rotate the test tubes for approximately 15 min.
3. Centrifuge the test tubes for 2 min at approximately 1,500 rpm. Aspirate the upper (aqueous) layers.
4. Decant the organic layers into 30-ml beakers. Place the sealed end of a capillary tube in each wide-mouth tube (to prevent bumping).
5. Evaporate each organic layer to dryness on a water bath. Proceed to Step 13 of the procedure for blood (see above).
6. The resulting spectra are used for the qualitative identification of morphine in urine (Figure 2).

Note: Morphine and quinine may be detected in the same urine specimen by doubling the specimen and reagent volumes and dividing the chloroform-isopropyl alcohol extract in half. The analysis for morphine is performed by completing Steps 4 to 10 above. The analysis for quinine is performed by completing Steps 5 to 9 in the quinine procedure.*

*See p. 336.

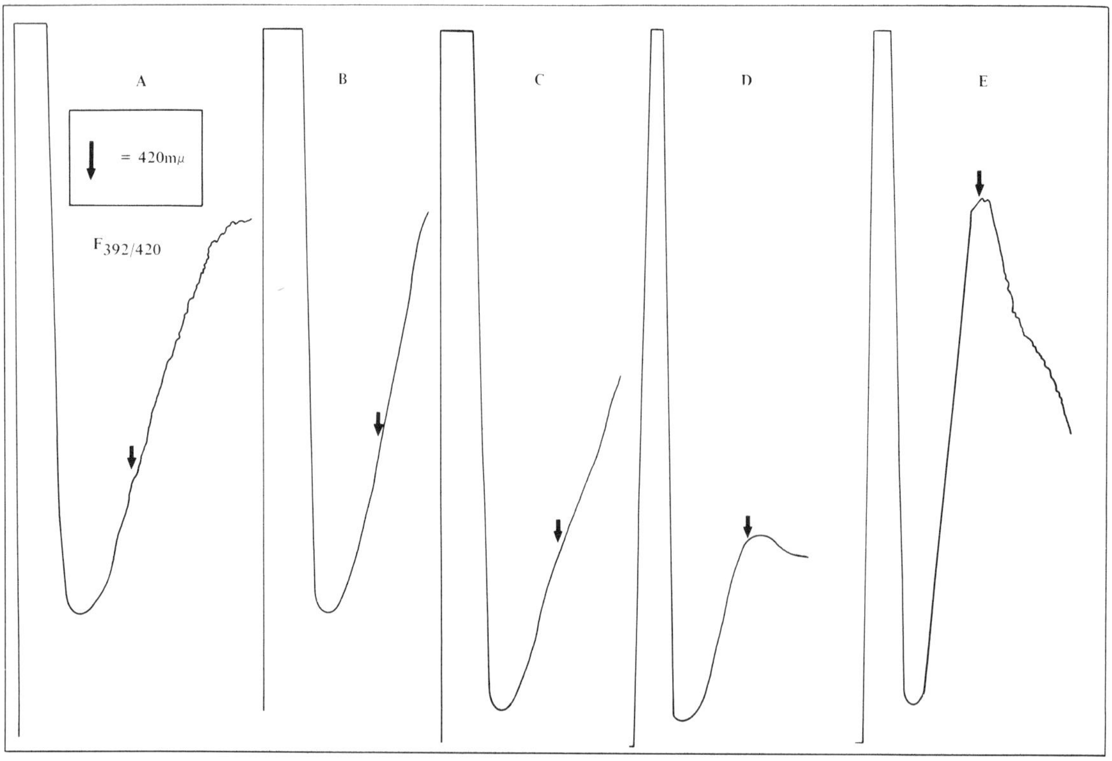

FIGURE 2. Fluorescence spectrum of morphine in urine. Curves A and B indicate that no morphine is present in the urine. Curve C is obtained when approximately 50 to 100 ng of morphine is present. Curve D indicates that a relatively high concentration of morphine (the fluorescence maximum at 420 nm) as well as some other fluorescent material is present in the urine. Curve E indicates a high concentration of morphine. Positive results (Curves D and E) should be confirmed by another technique to assure that morphine is the substance producing the observed fluorescence at 420 nm.

CALCULATION

To obtain the relative fluorescence of each blood sample, subtract the minimum value obtained after the Raleigh scatter peak (see Figure 1, Curve A) from the fluorescence maximum (approximately 420 nm). If the volumes of solvent recovered in Steps 6 and 11 are very different, then the relative fluorescence of each sample should be adjusted accordingly to compensate for this. Using the three processed working solutions and the original, plot their relative fluorescence vs their concentration in μg/100 ml. Draw the best straight line through these points. Obtain the concentration of each sample in μg of morphine/100 ml of blood from this calibration curve.

INTERPRETATION (see p. 7)

In acute heroin fatalities the concentration of morphine in blood ranges from 10 to 93 μg/100 ml (survival time less than 3 hr) to less than 10 μg/100 ml (survival time 3 to 24 hr). The highest concentration of morphine observed in a nonfatal case[1] was 14 μg/100 ml of blood.

SENSITIVITY AND PRECISION

The calibration curve is linear up to 50 μg of morphine/100 ml of blood. This procedure will detect approximately 2 μg of morphine/100 ml of blood. Replicate samples dissolved in the chloroform-methanol mixture and taken through the fluorophor producing steps (Steps 12 to 16 above) have a variation of approximately ±5%. The variation of the same blood sample analyzed on consecutive days is 1 to 2 μg of morphine/100 ml of blood.

INTERFERING SUBSTANCES

Pentazocine, quinine, Percodan®, meperidine, propoxyphene, chlorphentermine, methamphetamine, amphetamine, methaqualone, methapyrilene, and methadone do not interfere in the fluorometric procedure for morphine. Codeine will not interfere, but since morphine is a metabolite of codeine, a positive fluorescence spectrum may result. Normorphine, nalorphine, and apomorphine will yield the same fluorescence peak as morphine.

REFERENCE

1. **Robinson, A. E. and Williams, F. M.**, Post-mortem distribution of morphine in heroin addicts, *Med. Sci. Law*, 11, 135, 1971.

GENERAL REFERENCES

Fujimoto, J. M. and Way, E. L., Isolation and crystallization of bound morphine from urine of human addicts, *J. Pharmacol. Exp. Ther.*, 121, 340, 1957.

Fulton, C. C., Sulfomorphid – the purple fluorescence test, a new derivative test for morphine, *J. Am. Pharm. Assoc.*, 26, 726, 1937.

Garriott, J. C. and Sturner, W. Q., Morphine concentrations and survival periods in acute heroin fatalities, *N. Engl. J. Med.*, 289, 1276, 1973.

Kupferberg, H. J., Berkhalter, A., and Way, E. L., A sensitive fluorimetric assay for morphine in plasma and brain, *J. Pharmacol. Exp. Ther.*, 145, 247, 1964.

Matusiak, W. and Dal Cortivo, L. A., 156th Nat. Meet. Am. Chem. Soc., Atlantic City, September 1968.

Mulé, S. J. and Hushin, P. L., Semi-automatic fluorometric assay for submicrogram quantities of morphine and quinine in human biological material, *Anal. Chem.*, 43, 708, 1971.

Nadeau, G. and Sobolewski, G., Fluorescence assay of heroin and morphine, *Can. J. Biochem. Physiol.*, 36, 625, 1937.

Udenfriend, S., *Fluorescence Assay in Biology and Medicine*, Academic Press, N.Y., 1962, 423.

Yoshimura, H., Oguri, K., and Tsukamoto, H., in Drug Abuse: Basic Researches, I., Summarized Reports on Basic Researches, U.S.-Japan Cooperative Research Program, 1966–1968, 203.

TYPE C PROCEDURE

Naresh C. Jain, Robert D. Budd, and Thomas C. Sneath

APPARATUS

1. Round-bottom, glass-stoppered centrifuge tubes (Corning Cat. No. 8424), 50 ml
2. Racks to hold these tubes
3. Variable speed reciprocating shaker (Eberback Corp., Model 6000)
4. pH Meter
5. Polypropylene funnels (VWR Scientific Cat. No. 30231-046), 65 mm
6. Phase separating filter paper (Whatman #1 PS 12.5 cm)
7. Conical centrifuge tubes with glass stoppers (Kimble Cat. No. 45197), 40 ml
8. Serological pipets, 25, 10, 5, and 1 ml
9. Hamilton syringe, 10 μl
10. Water bath, adjustable to 70°C (VWR Cat. No. 13472-523)
11. Autoclave
12. Gas chromatograph, (Varian Model 2700) dual column with dual differential electrometer, two flame ionization detectors, and connected to a dual pen recorder and Autolab System IV Integrator (Spectra-Physics Cat. No. 21600-01). The gas chromatograph is equipped with the following two columns: (A) 3′ × 2 mm i.d. glass column containing 3% OV-25 on HP Chrom W (AW + DMCS) 80/100 mesh (Varian Cat. No. 82-001541-00); (B) 2′ × 2 mm i.d. glass column containing 3% Poly-A 103 on Gas Chrom Q 100/120 mesh (Applied Science Lab., Cat. No. 08258).

Operating Conditions (for both columns)

Gas Flow Rates:
- nitrogen (carrier gas) – 50 ml/min
- hydrogen – 30 ml/min
- air – 300 ml/min

Temperatures:
- column – 240°C
- injection port – 280°C
- detector – 280°C

REAGENTS

All chemicals and solvents should be analytical reagent grade.

1. Nalorphine HCl (Merck Sharp and Dohme), 5 mg/ml
2. Hydrochloric acid, 4.5*N*
   To 1,000 ml of distilled water add 756 ml of concentrated HCl, then dilute to 2,000 ml with distilled water.
3. Internal standard solution, nalorphine in 4.5*N* HCl, 15 μg/ml
   To 1,000 ml of 4.5*N* hydrochloric acid add 3.36 ml of 5 mg/ml of nalorphine HCl (Reagent 1). Nalorphine should be carefully measured because 3.36 ml gives a factor of 1 using the volumes of urine and internal standard acid solution as described (see Calculation).
4. *tert*-Butanol/chloroform, 10% v/v
   To 900 ml of $CHCl_3$ add 100 ml of *tert*-butanol.
5. Chloroform, spectrograde
6. Butyl acetate
7. Basic solution
   Dissolve 700 g of KOH and 1,300 g of K_2CO_3 in 1,500 ml of distilled water, then dilute to 2,000 ml. **Caution** – Prepare in a cool water bath or in an ice bath, as considerable heat is generated.
8. Pyridine
9. Acetic anhydride, anhydrous (Matheson, Coleman and Bell, Cat. No. AX85)
   This reagent should be periodically redistilled.
10. Sodium hydroxide, 6*N*
    Dissolve 240 g of NaOH in distilled water and dilute to 1,000 ml.
11. Standard reference solution, acetylated morphine, acetylated codeine, and acetylated nalorphine in spectrograde chloroform, 100 μl/ml of each
    Dissolve 13.17 mg of morphine hydrochloride and 13.14 mg of codeine sulfate in 2 ml of water. Add 2.24 ml of nalorphine hydrochloride (5 mg/ml) and dilute the mixture to 10 ml with distilled water. Adjust the pH of the solution to 9 with the addition of sufficient basic solution. Extract the mixture twice with 20-ml portions of spectrograde chloroform, and filter each of the chloroform extracts into the same dry 50-ml centrifuge tube. Evaporate the chloroform to dryness in a 70°C water bath, using a stream of nitrogen. Add 1.0 ml of pyridine and 1.0 ml of acetic anhydride to the tube. Cap the tube and place it in a 70°C water bath for 30 min. Remove the cap and evaporate the contents to dryness in the 70°C water bath, using a stream of nitrogen. Quantitatively transfer the acetylated drugs into a 100-ml volumetric flask by washing the tube with several 10-ml aliquots of spectrograde chloroform, and then dilute it to 100 ml with chloroform. Store in a glass-stoppered container. The reagent is stable and does not require refrigeration.

PROCEDURE

1. Label one 50-ml round-bottom centrifuge tube for each specimen and place in a rack.
2. To each labeled tube add 2.0 ml of the internal standard solution (Reagent 3). (This acid concentration is more than sufficient to hydrolyze the opiates.)
3. Add 15 ml of urine to an appropriately labeled tube.
4. Autoclave the tubes for 15 min.
5. Gradually reduce the pressure and remove the autoclaved tubes, placing them in an ice water bath for 5 min to cool them down to room temperature. (The tubes will not break.)
6. Add 10 ml of butyl acetate to each tube.
7. Cap the tubes and shake them at 150 cpm in a horizontal position on a platform shaker for 5 min.
8. Aspirate and discard the top organic layer. *Do not* remove any of the aqueous layer. (Centrifuge, if necessary.)
9. Evaporate the remaining traces of butyl acetate by placing the tubes in a 70°C water bath under a stream of nitrogen for 5 min.
10. Let the tubes cool to room temperature.
11. Add 1.3 ml of basic solution (Reagent 7) to each tube. Using a pH meter, adjust the pH of each specimen to 9.0 ± 0.2 by adding dropwise 4.5*N* HCl or 6*N* NaOH.
12. Add 25 ml of 10% v/v *tert*-butanol/chloroform (Reagent 4) to each tube.
13. Cap and shake the tubes at 150 cpm in a horizontal position on a platform shaker for 5 min.
14. Aspirate and discard the top aqueous layer.

15. Label one 40-ml tapered centrifuge tube for each specimen and place in a rack.
16. Place a 65-mm polypropylene funnel in each centrifuge tube.
17. Place one folded 12.5-cm Whatman #1 PS phase separating filter paper in each funnel.
18. Filter the solvent layer from the round-bottom tubes into an appropriately labeled centrifuge tube.
19. Evaporate the solvent in the centrifuge tubes to dryness in a 70°C water bath, using a stream of nitrogen.
20. To each centrifuge tube add 0.5 ml of pyridine and 0.5 ml of acetic anhydride.
21. Stopper the tubes and place them in a 70°C water bath for 30 min.
22. Remove the stopper and evaporate any excess pyridine and acetic anhydride to dryness in a 70°C water bath under a stream of nitrogen.
23. Dissolve the residue in each tube in 100 μl of spectrograde chloroform.
24. Inject 1 μl of the known standard reference solution (Reagent 11) containing acetylated derivatives of codeine, morphine, and nalorphine on both columns. The retention times (RT) of the acetylated opiates on the two columns are shown below:

Opiate	RT on Poly-A 103 column (min)	RT on OV-25 column (min)
Codeine	2.73	2.54
Morphine	3.57	3.12
Nalorphine	5.07	4.36

25. Inject 1 μl of the chloroform solution of each unknown specimen to be tested (Step 23) in the 3% Poly-A 103 column. Compare the retention times of the sample's peaks with those of the standard. Determine the peak areas to quantitate the positive samples (see Calculation).
26. Inject 1 μl of the chloroform solution (of those unknown specimens found positive for either morphine or codeine on the 3% Poly-A 103 column in Step 25) on the 3% OV-25 column for confirmation. Compare the retention times of the sample's peaks with those of the standard. Determine the peak areas to quantitate the positive samples (see Calculation).

CALCULATION

Calculate the morphine and codeine concentration (μg/ml) in the specimen by the following formula:

$$C_x = C_s \times \frac{A_u}{I_u} \times \frac{I_s}{A_s} \times R,$$

where

- C_x = morphine or codeine concentration in the specimen;
- C_s = internal standard (nalorphine) concentration in the acid, 15 μg/ml (Step 3);
- A_u = peak area of morphine or codeine in the specimen;
- A_s = peak area of morphine or codeine in the standard reference solution;
- I_u = peak area of the internal standard in the specimen;
- I_s = peak area of the internal standard in the standard reference solution;
- R = volume correction factor for internal standard concentration, i.e.,

$$\frac{\text{ml acid (Step 2)}}{\text{ml urine (Step 3)}}$$

INTERPRETATION (see p. 7)

Positive Specimen

A positive specimen for morphine or codeine must contain peaks for the internal standard (nalorphine) and peaks for morphine or codeine of identical concentrations on both columns.

Negative Specimen

A negative specimen for morphine and/or codeine must contain an internal standard (nalorphine) peak and no peaks for either morphine or codeine on the Poly-A 103 column. If a peak is found on the Poly-A 103 column which corresponds to either morphine or codeine, but no corresponding peak is found on the OV-25 column, then this must be considered a negative. A peak produced only on one column could possibly be due to an interfering substance present in the specimen.

Proper Sample Preparation

A peak for the internal standard must appear on both columns, even when the specimen is negative for morphine or codeine. If an internal standard peak does not appear on a column, it is an indication that the specimen has not been prepared properly, and the procedure must be repeated.

SENSITIVITY AND PRECISION

The method is sensitive to 0.1 μg/ml of morphine and codeine. The quantitation is precise to ±8% if an electronic integrator is used. The precision is significantly lower if peak areas are manually calculated because slight variations in measurements of peak heights and widths produce large errors.

INTERFERING SUBSTANCES

The analysis of acetylated opiates on two very different columns virtually eliminates false positive results. Several thousand specimens have been analyzed, and the results have not indicated any substances present in urine or other drugs which interfere with the analysis of morphine and codeine on both gas-chromatographic columns.

REFERENCES

Mulé, S. J., Identification of narcotics, barbiturates, amphetamines, tranquilizers and psychotomimetics in human urine, *J. Chromatogr.*, 39, 302, 1969.

Payte, J. T., Wallace, J. E., and Blum, K., Hydrolysis: a requisite for morphine detection in urine, *Curr. Ther. Res.*, 13, 412, 1971.

Schmezler, E., Yu, W., Hewitt, M. I., and Greenblatt, I. J., Gas chromatographic determination of codeine in serum and urine, *J. Pharm. Sci.*, 55, 155, 1966.

Wallace, J. E., Biggs, J. D., and Blum, K., Gas-liquid and thin-layer chromatographic determination of morphine in biologic specimens, *Clin. Chim. Acta*, 36, 85, 1972.

Wallace, J. E., Biggs, J. D., Merritt, J. H., Hamilton, H. E., and Blum, K., A sensitive thin-layer chromatographic technique for determining morphine in urine, *J. Chromatogr.*, 71, 135, 1972.

ALTERNATE TYPE C PROCEDURE IMMUNOASSAY

Details for the EMIT procedure will be found on p. 401. Details for the RIA procedure will be found on p. 403.

NICKEL

PRINCIPLE

Addition of trichloroacetic acid to serum dissociates nickel from serum proteins and simultaneously precipitates the proteins. Nickel in the protein-free supernatant fraction is converted to a pyrrolidine dithiocarbamate complex and is reextracted into methylisobutylketone. The concentration of nickel in the methylisobutylketone extract is measured by atomic absorption spectrometry. The same technique is applicable to analyses of nickel in whole blood, urine, and tissues, except that organic constituents of these destroyed by preliminary acid digestion.

TYPE C PROCEDURE

F. William Sunderman, Jr.

APPARATUS

1. Acid-washed plastic syringes coated with Teflon® catheter needles (Becton-Dickenson #6745)
2. Centrifuge tubes, 50 ml
3. Mechanical shaker
4. Centrifuge
5. Mixer (Vortex)
6. pH meter
7. Pasteur pipets
8. Spectrometer, atomic absorption (Perkin-Elmer Model 403), fitted with a nickel hollow cathode lamp, a Boling three-slot acetylene-air burner, and 10″ strip-chart recorder.

Operating Conditions

Gas Flow Rates:
acetylene – 4.2 liters/min
air – 23 liters/min
Wavelength: 232 nm
Nickel Lamp Current: 20 mA
Range: UV
Filter Settings: out
Entrance Slit Position: 3
Recorder Response Position: 2
Recorder Setting: 0.25 A, full scale
Concentration Dial Setting: 75
Curvature Correction: 0

REAGENTS

All concentrated acid and base reagents are Ultra Pure grade.* All water is deionized and then distilled in an all-glass still.

1. Nickel stock solution, 50 μg/ml
   Place 50 mg of powdered nickel in a 50-ml beaker and dissolve it in a mixture containing 5.0 ml of concentrated nitric acid and 5.0 ml of water, applying heat. Transfer the solution quantitatively to a one-liter volumetric flask and dilute it to the calibration mark with water.
2. Nickel reference solutions, 0.025 μg/ml, 0.05 μg/ml
   Transfer 1.0 ml portions of the nickel stock solution into 2- and 1-liter volumetric flasks, respectively then dilute to the calibration marks with water.
3. Trichloroacetic acid (TCA), 15 g/100 ml
   Dissolve 150 g of metal-free trichloroacetic acid† in one liter of water. Store the solution at 4°C. Prepare fresh every 2 weeks.
4. Hydrochloric acid, 1*N*
   Dilute 8.0 ml of concentrated (36%) hydrochloric acid to 100 ml with water.
5. Phthalate buffer solution, pH 2.5
   In a one-liter volumetric flask, dissolve 10.2 g of potassium hydrogen phthalate in 39 ml of

*Manufactured by E. Merck Co., Darmstadt, West Germany; available from Brinkman Instrument Co., Westbury, N. Y.
†Available from Distillation Products Division, Eastman Chemical Co., Rochester, N. Y., Catalog No. X-259.

1*N* hydrochloric acid added to approximately 400 ml of water. Dilute to the calibration mark with water, then transfer the contents to a 2-liter separatory funnel. Test the pH of the solution with a pH meter and adjust it, if necessary, to 2.5 by addition of either potassium hydrogen phthalate or hydrochloric acid.

6. Sulfuric acid-nitric acid mixture, 1:5
   Mix 1 volume of concentrated (96%) sulfuric acid with 5 volumes of concentrated (65%) nitric acid.
7. Perchloric acid, concentrated (70%)
8. Hydrochloric acid, 1.2*N*
   Dilute 10.0 ml of concentrated hydrochloric acid to 100 ml with water.
9. Methylisobutylketone (MIBK) (Fisher Scientific Co.)
10. Ammonium hydroxide, concentrated (25%)
11. Ammon.um hydroxide, 1.5*N*
    Di'ute 1).0 ml of concentrated ammonium hydroxide to 100 ml with water.
12. Ammonium pyrrolidine dithiocarbamate (APDC), 2 g/100 ml
    Dissolve 1 g of ammonium pyrrolidine dithiocarbamate* in 50 ml of water. Extract the solution twice, using 5.0 ml of MIBK each time. Prepare this reagent fresh each day.
13. MIBK saturated with TCA
    Place 400 ml of MIBK and 100 ml of TCA solution into a one-liter separatory funnel. Shake the mixture and allow it to stand for 1 hr at 4°C. Remove the MIBK phase, then centrifuge it to eliminate all traces of the aqueous phase. Prepare this reagent fresh each week. This solution is used to establish the spectrometer baseline.
14. MIBK-APDC solution
    Place 10.0 ml of the TCA solution in a 50-ml centrifuge tube. Adjust the pH of the solution to 2.5 by dropwise addition of concentrated (25%) ammonium hydroxide. Add 5.0 ml of the APDC solution and 30 ml of MIBK. Mix the contents of the tube with a Vortex mixer, then cool the tube in an ice bath. Centrifuge the tube for 15 min at 900 × g. Remove the MIBK phase. Store the MIBK phase in a refrigerator for up to 1 week. This solution is used daily to remove traces of nickel from the burner system.

PROCEDURE

Sample Preparation

Serum

1. Transfer duplicate 5.0-ml serum samples to 50-ml centrifuge tubes. Into additional duplicate sets of 50-ml centrifuge tubes place 1.0 ml of each nickel reference solution and 4.0 ml of water. These reference samples are equivalent to 0.5 and 1.0 μg nickel/100 ml serum. Place duplicate 5.0-ml water samples in 50-ml tubes to serve as the reagent blanks.
2. Constantly mixing, add 6.0 ml of TCA solution slowly to each tube.
3. Agitate the tubes for 30 min in a mechanical shaker, then centrifuge them for 15 min at 900 × g.
4. Decant the protein-free supernatant phases into clean 50-ml centrifuge tubes. Add 4.0 ml of TCA solution to each of the original tubes.
5. Resuspend the precipitated proteins by means of a Vortex mixer, then recentrifuge the suspensions for 15 min at 900 × g.
6. Combine the protein-free washings with the corresponding original supernatant fluids, add 2.0 ml of the phthalate buffer to each combined protein-free extract, then proceed with the analysis.

Urine, Whole Blood, and Tissues

1. Transfer the specimen (50 ml of urine, 10.0 ml of heparinized whole blood, or 10.0 ml of a 20% tissue homogenate) to duplicate 125-ml Erlenmeyer flasks. Add 10.0 ml of the sulfuric acid-nitric acid mixture to each flask. Process corresponding samples of each reference solution and of water for reagent blanks in the same manner as the specimen.
2. Heat the flasks gently on a hot plate, intermittently swirling, until the contents are clear, then continue the digestion with increased heat until charring occurs and white fumes of sulfur trioxide are generated. Allow the flasks to cool.
3. Add 2.0 ml of the sulfuric acid-nitric acid mixture and 0.5 ml of concentrated perchloric acid,

*Available from K and K Laboratories, Inc., 121 Express Street, Plainview, N. Y.

then continue the digestion until white fumes of sulfur trioxide appear. Allow the flasks to cool.

4. Add 1.0 ml of the sulfuric acid-nitric acid mixture and 0.25 ml of concentrated perchloric acid, then continue the digestion for 20 min after the samples have become practically colorless. The final volume of the digestion mixture should be less than 2.0 ml.
5. When using a urine specimen, cool the flasks and transfer their contents quantitatively with four washes of water to 50-ml centrifuge tubes. Adjust the volumes to approximately 20 ml by addition of water. When using whole blood or homogenates of tissues (such as muscle or liver) which contain appreciable amounts of iron, cool the flasks and add 5.0 ml of 1.2*N* hydrochloric acid. Heat the flasks to boiling, then allow the contents to cool. Add 6.0 ml of MIBK and shake the flasks to extract the iron. After the phases have separated, aspirate and discard the MIBK layer. Transfer the residual aqueous phases quantitatively with four washes of water to 50-ml centrifuge tubes. Adjust the volumes to approximately 15 ml by addition of water, then centrifuge the tubes for 5 min at 900 × g. Aspirate and discard any remaining traces of MIBK.
6. Add 2.0 ml of the phthalate buffer, then proceed to the analysis.

Analysis

1. Add concentrated (25%) ammonium hydroxide drop by drop to each sample, constantly mixing, until the pH reaches approximately 2.0. Monitor this with a pH meter. Gradually adjust the pH to 2.5 (2.4 to 2.6) by dropwise addition of 1.5*N* ammonium hydroxide.
2. Add 2.0 ml of the APDC solution to each sample and mix.
3. Add 2.0 ml of MIBK and mix for 20 sec, using a Vortex mixer.
4. Place the sample containers for 10 min in an ice bath, then centrifuge them for 10 min at 900 × g.
5. Using Pasteur pipets, transfer each MIBK extract to a small stoppered test tube, exercising care to avoid transfer of the aqueous phase.
6. Aspirate MIBK reagent into the burner of the atomic absorption spectrometer. Adjust the flame to a dark blue color, with a bright blue segment (5 mm high) immediately above the burner. Allow the MIBK to aspirate for 20 min in order to stabilize the flame conditions. Verify the absolute stability of the recorder baseline by aspirating MIBK saturated with TCA for 10 min while the strip-chart recorder is operating. Finally, aspirate the MIBK-APDC solution for 1 min to remove any residue of nickel from the burner system. The spectrometer is now ready for analysis.
7. Aspirate the MIBK extracts into the burner and record the absorbances of all samples.
8. Measure the heights of the absorbance peaks.
9. Determine the nickel concentration in the specimen by comparing the heights of the absorbance peaks of its extracts with those of the reference samples.

INTERPRETATION (see p. 7)

The following are normal concentrations of nickel in serum, urine, feces, hair, and sweat:[1–6]

serum nickel (N = 40)	mean	– 0.26 μg/100 ml, S.D. ±0.08
	range	– 0.11 to 0.46 μg/100 ml
urine nickel (N = 26)	mean	– 0.23 μg/100 ml, S.D. ± 0.14
	range	– 0.10 to 0.52 μg/100 ml
	mean	– 2.4 μg/day, S.D. ± 1.1
	range	– 1.0 to 5.6 μg/day
fecal nickel (N = 10)	mean	– 3.3 μg/g (wet), S.D. ± 0.8
	range	– 2.1 to 4.4 μg/g (wet)
	mean	– 14.2 μg/g (dry), S.D. ± 2.7
	range	– 10.8 to 18.7 μg/g (dry)
	mean	– 258 μg/day, S.D. ± 126
	range	– 80 to 540 μg/day
hair nickel (N = 29)	mean	– 0.22 μg/100 ml, S.D. ± 0.08
	range	– 0.13 to 0.51 μg/g
sweat nickel (N = 33)	mean	– 5.2 μg/100 ml, S.D. ± 3.6
	range	– 0.7 to 18.0 μg/100 ml
(N = 150)	mean	– 13.1 μg/100 ml, S.D. ± 6.5
	range	– 3.9 to 27.0 μg/100 ml

According to Sunderman et al.[3] the normal nickel concentrations in human lung, liver, and heart average 8.6, 3.2, and 2.3 μg/100 g (dry weight), respectively. The nickel content per 100 g tissue (dry weight) in a man who died 5 days after accidental inhalation of nickel carbonyl was as follows: lung, 115 μg; kidney, 80 μg; brain, 60 μg; testicle, 45 μg; spleen, 31 μg; liver, 20 μg; and bone, 17 μg.

ACCURACY AND PRECISION

As a measure of the day-to-day variability of the method, the coefficient of variation for 17 consecutive daily measurements of nickel concentration in a pooled specimen of serum was 9.9%. As measures of within-run variability, the coefficient of variation for duplicate analyses of nickel in 91 sera was 8.7%, and the coefficient of variation for duplicate analyses of nickel in 32 specimens of whole blood was 11.3%. The coefficient of variation for duplicate analyses of nickel in 50 urine specimens was 10.3%. The recovery of nickel added to serum, blood, urine, and tissues in a concentration of 2.5 μg/100 ml or per 100 g wet weight averaged 101, 102, 100, and 98%, respectively.[1]

INTERFERING SUBSTANCES

Cadmium and gold salts can cause slight inhibition in the atomic absorption of nickel due to the absorption of nickel upon insoluble complexes of cadmium or gold with pyrrolidine dithiocarbamate. Such interference would be detectable only when the concentrations of cadmium and gold exceed 10 and 25 μg/100 ml, respectively.

REFERENCES

1. **Nomoto, S. and Sunderman, F. W., Jr.,** Atomic absorption spectrometry of nickel in serum, urine, and other biological materials, *Clin. Chem.,* 16, 477, 1970.
2. **Nomoto, S., McNeely, M. D., and Sunderman, F. W., Jr.,** Isolation of a nickel α_2-macroglobulin from rabbit serum, *Biochemistry,* in press.
3. **Sunderman, F. W., Jr., Nomoto, S., and Nechay, M. W.,** Measurements of nickel in human tissues, in *Trace Substances in Environmental Health,* Hemphill, D. D., Ed., University of Missouri Press, Columbia, 1971.
4. **Horak, E. and Sunderman, F. W., Jr.,** Fecal nickel excretion by healthy adults, *Clin. Chem.,* 19, 429, 1973.
5. **Nechay, M. W. and Sunderman, F. W., Jr.,** Measurements of nickel in hair by atomic absorption spectrometry, *Am. Clin. Lab. Sci.,* 3, 30, 1973.
6. **Hohnadel, D. C., Sunderman, F. W., Jr., Nechay, M. W., and McNeely, M. D.,** Atomic absorption spectrometry of nickel, copper, zinc, and lead in sweat collected from healthy subjects during sauna bathing, *Clin. Chem.,* 19, 1288, 1973.

NICOTINE

PRINCIPLE

Nicotine base in alkaline solution is volatile with steam. Advantage is taken of this fact to affect a transfer of the drug from stomach contents to dilute acid, whence a general alkaloidal reagent is used to detect its presence (Procedure A). Specificity is low. Like many organic bases, nicotine can be extracted from an alkalinized biological specimen into a suitable immiscible organic solvent. The drug can then be reextracted from the solvent into dilute sulfuric acid (Procedure B). Its characteristic spectrum in the UV region can be used for quantitation if no interfering substances are present. The drug can be further purified by reextraction from the original solvent into dilute aqueous acid, which is then made alkaline. An organic solvent extract of this solution is evaporated to a small volume. An appropriate internal standard is added, and an aliquot of the resultant mixture is then injected onto a suitable gas-chromatographic column (Procedure C).

TYPE A PROCEDURE

Edgar W. Kivela and Staff

APPARATUS

1. Steam-distillation apparatus, all glass

REAGENTS

All chemicals should be analytical reagent grade.

1. Sodium hydroxide, 2.5*N*
   Dissolve 10 g of sodium hydroxide in water and dilute to 100 ml.
2. Hydrochloric acid, 1.2*N*
   Dilute 10.0 ml of concentrated hydrochloric acid to 100 ml with water.
3. Silicotungstic acid, 12 g/100 ml
   Dissolve 12 g of silicotungstic acid in water and dilute to 100 ml.

PROCEDURE

1. Make 10.0 ml of specimen (stomach content, urine, or blood) basic with 2.5*N* sodium hydroxide and steam-distill this mixture directly into a small test tube containing a drop of 1.2*N* hydrochloric acid. Collect about 2 ml of the distillate.
2. Add a small amount of the silicotungstic acid reagent to the distillate and observe the mixture for a cloudy precipitate.

INTERPRETATION (see p. 7)

A white, cloudy precipitate indicates the possible presence of nicotine. The value of this procedure is obtaining a negative result. If a positive result is obtained, the Type B Procedure or the Type C Procedure must be performed.

ACCURACY AND PRECISION

In fatal cases, nicotine is detectable in the urine by this test. Nicotine resulting from smoking is not detectable by this test.

INTERFERING SUBSTANCES

Other volatile alkaloidal drugs may cause a similar precipitate; therefore, this test should only be used as an indication of the possible presence of a volatile organic base. Its identity must be established by other physical or chemical tests.

REFERENCES*

Herwitz, W., *Official Methods of Analysis of the Association of Official Agricultural Chemists,* 9th ed., Assoc. of Off. Agric. Chem., Washington, D.C., 1960, 40.

McNally, W. D., Industrial exposure – and worker as affected thereby, *Ind. Med.*, 6, 270, 1937.

*For an updated list of reference material, see References, p. 283.

TYPE B PROCEDURE

Edgar W. Kivela and Staff

APPARATUS

1. Separatory funnels, 60 ml
2. UV spectrophotometer

REAGENTS

All chemicals should be analytical reagent grade.

1. Nicotine stock solution, 100 μg/ml
   Dissolve 10 mg of nicotine in water and dilute to 100 ml with water.
2. Nicotine reference solutions
   Dilute the nicotine stock solution with water to concentrations of 10.0, 7.5, 5.0, and 2.5 μg/ml.
3. Ammonium hydroxide, concentrated
4. Chloroform
5. Sulfuric acid, 0.1*N*
   Dilute 27.8 ml of concentrated sulfuric acid to one liter with water.

PROCEDURE

1. Place 10.0 ml of samples (urine or blood specimen, reference solutions, and water for a reagent blank) into 60-ml separatory funnels and make them basic by adding 2 drops of concentrated ammonium hydroxide.
2. Add 25 ml of chloroform and shake for 5 min.
3. Allow the layers to separate, then drain the chloroform layer through a plug of glass wool in the stem of the funnel. Record the volume recovered.
4. Add 4.0 ml of 0.1*N* sulfuric acid to the chloroform extract and shake for 5 min.
5. Allow the layers to separate, then aspirate the acid layer into a cuvette.
6. Determine the absorption spectrum of the acid extract, using the solution obtained from processing the water sample as the reference solution (Figure 1).

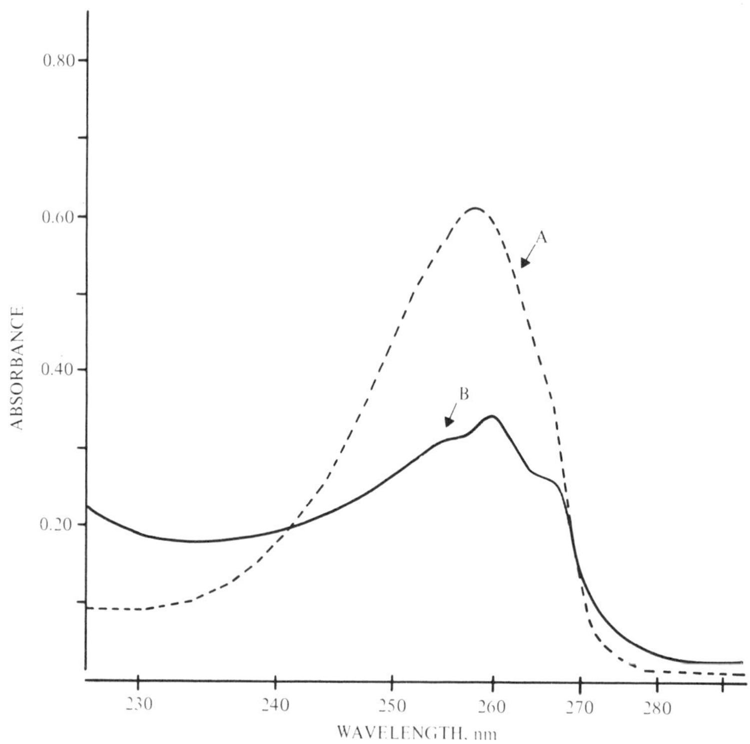

FIGURE 1. UV absorbance spectrum for nicotine. A = 20 μg/ml of acid; B = 20 μg/ml of base.

CALCULATION

Determine the nicotine concentration in the sample by comparing the absorbance of the specimen at 259 nm with those obtained from reference solutions with known concentrations of nicotine.

INTERPRETATION (see p. 7)

Urine of smokers may contain nicotine in amounts of 0.2 to 0.3 mg/100 ml. Blood nicotine concentrations of 1.0 mg/100 ml or higher can be considered toxic. Concentrations of 2.0 mg/ml of blood or higher are compatible with a lethal exposure.

ACCURACY AND PRECISION

By using this extraction method, 0.25 mg of nicotine/100 ml of specimen can be detected. However, much lower concentrations can be detected by using larger specimens or smaller volumes of 0.1*N* sulfuric acid. About 95% of the nicotine in the specimen is recovered by this procedure.

INTERFERING SUBSTANCES

Any organic base that has a similar ultraviolet absorption spectrum will interfere. Nicotinamide gives this spectrum and is frequently present in most urine specimens.

REFERENCE*

Goldbaum, L. R. and Domanski, T. J., An approach to the analysis of biological specimens in basic drugs, in *Progress in Chemical Toxicology*, Vol. 2, p. 229, Stolman, A., Ed., Academic Press, N.Y., 1965, 229.

TYPE C PROCEDURE

Edgar W. Kivela and Staff

APPARATUS

1. Syringe (Hamilton), 10 μl
2. Separatory funnels with Teflon® stopcocks, 125 ml
3. Rotary evaporator (evaporation under vacuum created by water aspirator pump)
4. Round bottom flasks with standard taper 24/40 neck (Pyrex®), 100 ml
5. Graduated cylinders, 25 ml
6. Gas chromatograph (Barber-Coleman 5000 or suitable substitute), equipped with flame ionization detector, a 5 mV recorder, and a U-shaped glass column, 6′ × ¼″, i.d., packed with 3% OV-22 on Gas Chrom Q, 80 to 100 mesh

   Operating Conditions

   Gas Flow Rates:
   - nitrogen – 60 ml/min
   - air – 500 ml/min
   - hydrogen – 40 ml/min

   Temperatures:
   - column – 180°C
   - injection port – 260°C
   - detector – 270°C

REAGENTS

All chemicals should be analytical reagent grade.

1. Chloroform
2. Nicotine stock solution, 0.1 mg/ml

   Dissolve 10 mg of nicotine in chloroform and dilute to 100 ml with chloroform.
3. Nicotine control solution, 0.1 mg/ml

   Dissolve 10 mg of nicotine in water to which 0.2 ml of concentrated sulfuric acid has been added and dilute to 100 ml with water.
4. Sodium hydroxide, 0.045*N*

   Dissolve 18.0 g of sodium hydroxide pellets in distilled water. Cool the solution to room temperature, then dilute it with distilled water.

*For an updated list of reference material, see References, p. 283.

Dilute 10 ml of this reagent to 100 ml with distilled water just prior to use in the procedure below.

5. Methyprylon stock solutions, 3 mg/ml
Dissolve 300 mg of methyprylon (Nodular®) in chloroform and dilute to 100 ml with chloroform.
6. Methyprylon control solution, 3 mg/ml
Dissolve 300 mg of methyprylon (Nodular®) in water and dilute to 100 ml with water.
7. Methyprylon internal control solutions, 0.1 mg/ml
Dilute each of the methyprylon stock solutions 1:30 with 0.045*N* sodium hydroxide.
8. Ammonium hydroxide, concentrated

PROCEDURE

1. Examine the gas chromatograph to be sure that all conditions stated above are met. Inject the stock solutions. The retention time for nicotine is approximately 2 min, and that for methyprylon is approximately 5.4 min.
2. To a 125-ml separatory funnel add 10 to 20 ml of specimen (blood, urine, stomach content, and nicotine control solution) and make it basic with 2 or 3 drops of concentrated ammonium hydroxide. Add 100 ml of chloroform and shake for 5 min. Allow the layers to separate.
3. Drain the chloroform layer through a plug of glass wool in the stem of the funnel into a second 60-ml separatory funnel. Discard the water layer.
4. To wash the chloroform extract, add 5 ml of 0.045*N* sodium hydroxide and shake for 5 min.
5. Drain the chloroform extract through a plug of glass wool in the stem of the funnel into a glass-stoppered graduated cylinder and record the volume. Discard the sodium hydroxide wash.
6. Add 1.0 ml of the aqueous methyprylon internal control solution directly to the chloroform extract in the cylinder and shake. Allow the layers to separate.
7. Remove any residual sodium hydroxide by aspiration and discard it.
8. Filter the chloroform layer into a 100-ml round-bottom flask equipped with a ground glass neck. Attach the flask to a rotary evaporator.
9. Evaporate the filtrate almost to dryness under reduced pressure at room temperature.
10. Rinse the residue into a small test tube with 2 or 3 ml of chloroform, then evaporate it in air to 1 or 2 drops.
11. Inject 4 μl of the residue into the gas chromatograph.
12. Determine the peak heights of the internal control and of the nicotine in both the specimen and the aqueous reference solution.

CALCULATION

Calculate the nicotine concentration (mg/100 ml) in the specimen by the following formula:

$$N_X = N_S \times \frac{A_X}{A_S} \times \frac{R_S}{R_X},$$

where

N_X = nicotine concentration in the specimen;
N_S = nicotine concentration in the control solution;
A_X = peak height of the specimen at the retention time of nicotine;
A_S = peak height of nicotine control solution;
R_S = peak height of methyprylon in nicotine control solution;
R_X = peak height of methyprylon in the specimen.

INTERPRETATION (see p. 7)

Urine of smokers may contain nicotine in amounts of 0.2 to 0.3 mg/100 ml. Blood nicotine concentrations of 1.0 mg/100 ml or higher can be considered toxic. Concentrations of 2.0 mg/ml of blood or higher are compatible with a lethal exposure.

ACCURACY AND PRECISION

Recovery of nicotine has been 102 ± 7%. Experience with the method could give less variation.

INTERFERING SUBSTANCES

The normal metabolites of nicotine have different retention times than nicotine itself and therefore do not interfere.

REFERENCES

Goldbaum, L. R. and Domanski, T. J., An approach to the analysis of biological specimens in basic drugs, in *Progress in Chemical Toxicology,* Vol. 2, Stolman, A., Ed., Academic Press, N.Y., 1965, 229.

Isaac, P. F. and Rand, M. J., Cigarette smoking and plasma levels of nicotine, *Nature,* 236, 308, 1972.

Rehling, C. J., *Registry of Human Toxicology,* Auburn, Alabama, 1968.

p-NITROPHENOL

PRINCIPLE

The hydrolyzed urine sample is extracted with an organic solvent which in turn is reextracted with alkali. This alkaline solution is reacted with *o*-cresol and titanium trichloride to yield a solution whose absorbance is a function of the *p*-nitrophenol concentration (Procedure B). The alkaline extract obtained previously may also be acidified and reextracted with an organic solvent. This, when concentrated and silated, may be gas chromatographed and used for the *p*-nitrophenol determination (Procedure C).

TYPE B PROCEDURE

Arthur J. Fisk

APPARATUS

1. Round-bottom flasks with glass 14/20 standard taper joints, 500 ml
2. Condensers, water cooled, with glass 14/20 standard taper joints
3. Electric hot plate or other source of gentle heat
4. Separatory funnels, 250 ml
5. Centrifuge tubes, glass-stoppered, 15 ml
6. Spectrophotometer

REAGENTS

All chemicals should be analytical reagent grade.

1. *p*-Nitrophenol stock solution, 10 mg/dl
   Dissolve 10.0 mg of *p*-nitrophenol in distilled water and dilute to 100 ml.
2. *p*-Nitrophenol reference solutions
   Dilute appropriate volumes of the *p*-nitrophenol stock solution to obtain concentrations of 20, 40, 100, and 200 μg/100 ml.
3. Hydrochloric acid, concentrated
4. Ethyl ether-benzene mixture, 20:80
   Mix 20 parts ethyl ether with 80 parts benzene.
5. Sodium sulfate, anhydrous
6. Sodium hydroxide, 0.5*N*
   Dissolve 20 g of sodium hydroxide in 100 ml of distilled water.
7. Acetonitrile
8. Ammonium hydroxide, 0.5*N*
   Dilute 25.0 ml of concentrated ammonium hydroxide to 100 ml with distilled water.
9. Sodium hydroxide, 0.2*N*
   Dissolve 8 g of sodium hydroxide in distilled water and dilute to one liter.
10. *o*-Cresol reagent
    Dissolve 1 g of *o*-cresol in 0.2*N* sodium hydroxide. Dilute the solution to 50.0 ml with 0.2*N* sodium hydroxide.
11. Titanium trichloride reagent
    Add 1.0 ml of 20% (w/v) titanium trichloride to 16.0 ml of distilled water. Prepare this reagent immediately prior to use.

SPECIMEN REQUIREMENTS

The urine specimen shoud contain a minimum of 10 μg of *p*-nitrophenol. Hence, the specimen size depends on the concentration of *p*-nitrophenol expected.

PROCEDURE

1. Place 100 ml of urine (or less if a high concentration of *p*-nitrophenol is anticipated) into a 500-ml round-bottom flask. Fit the flask to the water-cooled condenser. Include additional flasks containing 100 ml of suitable *p*-nitrophenol reference solution and 100 ml of water for a reagent blank, respectively, in each series of analyses.

2. Add 20 ml of concentrated hydrochloric acid to each flask. (Use proportionately less acid if a smaller sample was used.) Reflux the flask contents gently 1 hr, then cool.
3. Transfer the contents of each flask to 250-ml separatory funnels. Add 60.0 ml of the ethyl ether-benzene mixture and shake for 5 min.
4. Discard the aqueous layers. Add 5 g to 10 g of anhydrous sodium sulfate to each organic layer (ethyl ether-benzene mixture).
5. Filter 50.0 ml of each organic phase into another 125-ml separatory funnel. Add 5.0 ml of the 0.5*N* sodium hydroxide solution and shake for 5 min.
6. Discard the organic phases. Transfer each sodium hydroxide phase into a 15-ml glass-stoppered centrifuge tube. A dark yellow color indicates that the *p*-nitrophenol concentration is high. If this is so, use a smaller aliquot and account for this in the calculation.
7. Rinse each separatory funnel with 5.0 ml of acetonitrile and add the rinse solutions to the corresponding centrifuge tubes containing the sodium hydroxide.
8. Shake the tubes for 2 min, then centrifuge them to effect clear separation of layers.
9. Aspirate the sodium hydroxide layer from each sample and transfer it to another centrifuge tube.
10. Add 5.0 ml of 3*N* ammonium hydroxide and 1.0 ml of *o*-cresol reagent to each tube and mix. (The appearance of a blue color at this point indicates the presence of interfering amino compounds; however, in the course of performing numerous tests with this procedure, the presence of amino compounds has not been noted.)
11. Add 1.0 ml of titanium trichloride reagent to each tube and shake it until the dark precipitate disappears (about 15 sec).
12. Allow color development to proceed for 30 min. (The color remains stable for several hours.)
13. Centrifuge the tubes for 5 min, then transfer the mixtures to cuvettes.
14. Determine the absorbance of each sample at 620 nm, using the solution obtained by processing the water sample as a reference.

CALCULATION

Determine the *p*-nitrophenol content in the specimen from the absorbance data of the concomitantly processed *p*-nitrophenol reference solutions.

INTERPRETATION (see p. 7)

In the diagnosis of acute poisonings due to the absorption of organic phosphates, demonstration of the presence of urinary *p*-nitrophenol is valuable. Organic phosphates that have *p*-nitrophenol as a urinary metabolite are parathion, chlorothion, dicapthon, EPN, and methyl parathion. Its concentration can be used as a measure of exposure to these organic phosphates. Studies have shown urine *p*-nitrophenol to be a significantly more sensitive indicator of intoxication than blood cholinesterase when parathion is the offending agent. This is true even under optimal conditions and when the individual's preexposure cholinesterase level is known.

ACCURACY

This method yields 70 to 75% recovery.

INTERFERING SUBSTANCES

Of all the substances tested, only dinitro-*o*-cresol (DNOC) interfered in the analysis. Dinitro-*o*-cresol produces a yellow color in the blank solution.

REFERENCES

Davis, J. H., Davies, J. E., and Fisk, A. J., Occurrence, diagnosis and treatment of organophosphate pesticide poisoning in man, *Ann. N.Y. Acad. Sci.*, 160, 383, 1969.

Elliott, J. W., Walker, K. C., Penick, A. E., and Durham, W. F., A sensitive procedure for urinary *p*-nitrophenol determination as a measure of exposure to parathion, *J. Agric. Food. Chem.*, 8, 111, 1960.

TYPE C PROCEDURE

Irving Sunshine

APPARATUS

1. Test tubes, 15 ml, with 14/20 ground glass joints
2. Reflux condenser, equipped for water cooling, with 14/20 ground glass joints
3. Dri-Bath® heating block (Thermolyne)
4. Gas chromatograph (Micro-Tek MT-220, or its equivalent), equipped with a ^{3}H-foil or ^{63}Ni electron-capture detector, and U-shaped glass columns, 6′ × ¼″, i.d., packed with 3% DC 200 on 80 to 100 mesh Gas Chrom Q (or any of several other silicone liquid phases, including OV-1, OV-17, or OV-210; polar liquid phases, such as Versamid or DEGS, are not suitable)

Operating Conditions

Gas Flow Rate:
nitrogen – 50 ml/min
Temperatures:
column – 140°C
injection port – 220°C
detector – 205°C (^{3}H foil)
Electron-Capture Dectector: 17 V

It may be necessary in some instances to condition the column by injecting 5 μl of a 100 pg/μl solution of *p*-nitrophenol in hexamethyldisilazane-hexane (10:90, v/v) until a constant peak height is obtained for the silated *p*-nitrophenol.

REAGENTS

All chemicals should be analytical reagent grade.

1. Hydrochloric acid, concentrated
2. Sodium hydroxide, 0.1*N*
   Dissolve 4 g of sodium hydroxide in water and dilute to one liter.
3. Sodium hydroxide, 0.5*N*
   Dissolve 20 g of sodium hydroxide in water and dilute to 100 ml.
4. Benzene, Mallinckrodt Nanograde
5. Ether, Mallinckrodt Nanograde
6. Benzene-ether mixture, 80:20
   Mix 80 volumes of benzene with 20 volumes of ether. Prepare this mixture just prior to use.
7. Sodium sulfate, anhydrous powder
8. Hexamethyldisalazane reagent, 20 g/dl
   Dissolve 20 g of hexamethyldisilazane in 100 ml of hexane.
9. *p*-Nitrophenol stock solution, 100 mg/dl
   Dissolve 100 mg of *p*-nitrophenol in 100 ml of the hexamethyldisilazane reagent.
10. *p*-Nitrophenol reference solution, 10 mg/dl
    Dilute 10.0 ml of the *p*-nitrophenol stock solution to 100 ml with the hexamethyldisilazane reagent.

PROCEDURE

1. Place a 2.7-ml urine specimen in a 15-ml ground-glass test tube fitted to a stoppered water-cooled condenser.
2. Add 0.3 ml of concentrated hydrochloric acid, then reflux the mixture for 1 hr, using a Dri-Bath® heating block. During reflux, the condenser must be stoppered and cooled with cold water.
3. Rinse the condenser with 2.0 ml of 0.1*N* sodium hydroxide. Add the rinse to the hydrolyzed urine.
4. Cool the hydrolyzed urine, then adjust it to a pH of 11 or higher by adding approximately 0.4 ml of 0.5*N* sodium hydroxide solution.
5. Extract the alkaline urine twice, using 5.0 ml of the benzene-ether mixture each time. Discard each benzene-ether extract.
6. Acidify the urine with concentrated hydrochloric acid to pH 2 or lower, then extract it with 6.0 ml of the benzene-ether extract.
7. Remove 5.0 ml of the benzene-ether extract and dry it by adding sodium sulfate.
8. Remove a 1.0-ml aliquot of the dried benzene-ether extract and add to this 1.0 ml of the hexamethyldisilazane reagent.
9. Inject a 5-μl aliquot of this mixture into the gas chromatograph. The retention time of PNP

trimethylsilyl ether under the stated conditions is approximately 5 min.

CALCULATION

Compare the peak heights obtained from the urine samples with those obtained from the PNP reference solutions.

INTERPRETATION (see p. 7)

In the diagnosis of acute poisonings due to the absorption of organic phosphates, demonstration of the presence of urinary *p*-nitrophenol is valuable. Organic phosphates that have *p*-nitrophenol as a urinary metabolite are parathion, chlorothion, dicapthion, EPN, and methyl parathion. Its concentration can be used as a measure of exposure to these organic phosphates. Studies have shown urine *p*-nitrophenol to be a significantly more sensitive indicator of intoxication than blood cholinesterase when parathion is the offending agent. This is true even under optimal conditions and when the individual's preexposure cholinesterase level is known.

ACCURACY AND PRECISION

Recoveries of the PNP added to urine range from 85 to 100%. Comparison of six replicate analyses of four urine samples gave the following results:[1]

Sample number	Mean, ppb	Range, ppb	Standard deviation, ppb
1	55	53–56	1.1
2	111	106–114	2.6
3	300	280–315	13.4
4	415	400–440	15.0

INTERFERING SUBSTANCES

The specificity of the method is as good as any gas-chromatographic procedure, coupled with selective extraction and clean-up. Compounds that are acidic in nature and are extracted by benzene-ether from strongly acid but not from strongly alkaline aqueous solutions will be included on the gas chromatogram. The chromatographic conditions reported will separate *o*-, *m*-, and *p*-nitrophenol, chlorine-substituted nitrophenols, and chlorine-substituted phenols to the extent that they will not be confused with *p*-nitrophenol. An unknown compound with a retention time similar, but not identical, to that of PNP on a DC-200 column has been found in a small percentage of the samples examined.[1,2] When interferences of this type are found, confirmatory tests should be carried out on a column with a different liquid phase.

REFERENCES

1. **Cranmer, M. F. and Peoples, A.,** Determination of *p*-nitrophenol in urine by gas-liquid chromatography, *Bull. Environ. Contam. Toxicol.*, 5, 329, 1969.
2. **Elliott, J. W., Walter, K. C., Penick, A. E., and Durham, W. F.,** A sensitive procedure for urinary *p*-nitrophenol determination as a measure of exposure to parathion, *J. Agric. Food Chem.*, 8, 111, 1960.

GENERAL REFERENCES

Arterberry, J. D., Durham, W. F., Elliott, J. W., and Wolfe, H. R., Exposure to parathion, *Arch. Environ. Health*, 3, 476, 1961.

Waldman, R. K., Leiben, J., and Krause, L., Physiological responses to parathion exposure, *AMA Arch. Ind. Hyg. Occup. Med.*, 9, 37, 1954.

ORGANIC THIOPHOSPHATE ESTERS

PRINCIPLE

The organic thiophosphate esters can be extracted with pentane. In Procedure A these extracts are concentrated and aliquots are chromatographed on alumina plates. After the plates are developed, the spray reaction for identification is based on the release of naphthol from 2-naphthylacetate by human esterase. This reacts with Echtblausalz B to form a colored complex. The inhibiting pesticides show up on the chromatogram as white spots on a rose-violet background. Other aliquots of the pentane extract can be analyzed by gas chromatography (Procedure B).

TYPE A PROCEDURE

Robert A. Maes

APPARATUS

1. Separatory funnels, 100 ml
2. Shaker, mechanical
3. Beakers, 100 ml
4. Water bath
5. Watchglass (ϕ 5 cm)
6. Micropipets
7. Oven
8. Thin-layer chromatography (TLC) equipment: (a) glass plates coated with aluminum oxide G; (b) developing tanks; (c) spray bottle

REAGENTS

All chemicals should be analytical reagent grade.

1. Aluminum oxide G (E. Merck, Darmstadt)
2. Bromine
3. Echtblausalz B (Fast Blue B) (E. Merck, Darmstadt)
4. 2-Naphthylacetate
5. Ethanol
6. Sodium sulfate, anhydrous
7. Pentane
8. TLC developing solvents
   (a) Solvent 1 – Mix 50.0 ml of pentane with 10.0 ml of acetone and 10.0 ml of toluene. (b) Solvent 2 – Mix 20.0 ml of pentane with 20.0 ml of acetone, 10.0 ml of toluene, and 10.0 ml of ethyl acetate. Solvent 1 is used to separate the less polar, while Solvent 2 separates the more polar compounds.
9. Spray reagents
   (a) Human plasma; (b) Substrate solution – Dissolve 20 mg of 2-naphthylacetate in 8 ml of ethanol. Dissolve 50 mg of Echtblausalz B in 32 ml of water. Mix both solutions immediately before use. The solution obtained must be clear.
10. Organic thiophosphate ester stock solution, 1 mg/ml
    Dissolve 25 mg of parathion, methyl parathion, Phosdrin®, Diazinon®, Bidrin®, Gardona®, Guthion®, Ethyl Guthion®, ethion, Trithion®, and Methyl Trithion® in pentane, respectively, and dilute to 25 ml with pentane.
11. Organic thiophosphate ester reference solutions, 1 μg/ml
    Dilute each stock solution with pentane to a concentration where 1 to 10 μl of the pesticide can be applied to the plate.

PROCEDURE

1. Blend 2 g of the specimen (blood, urine, stomach content, or tissue) with 6 g of anhydrous sodium sulfate in a 100-ml separatory funnel.
2. Extract the mixture with 60 ml of pentane for

20 min on a mechanical shaker. Allow the layers to separate.
3. Filter the pentane layer through a plug of glass wool into a 100-ml beaker.
4. Evaporate the filtrate gently to approximately 0.1 ml on a water bath.
5. Apply 25-μl aliquots of the extract on a thin-layer chromatographic aluminum oxide G phase.
6. Spot about 10 μl of suitable organic thiophosphate reference solutions on the same plate, and chromatograph in saturated developing tanks using either developing Solvent 1 or 2 at room temperature. Allow the solvent front to rise 15 cm.
7. Remove the plate from the developing tank and dry it at room temperature.
8. Place the plate for 30 sec in a developing tank containing a beaker into which 0.1 ml of bromine has been pipeted.
9. Remove the plate from the developing tank and let the bromine evaporate (25 to 30 min).
10. Spray the plate with human plasma and place it in an oven at 37°C for 30 min.
11. Spray the plate with the substrate solution and again place it in an oven at 37°C for 30 min. The organic thiophosphate esters appear as stable white spots on a rose-violet background. The R_f values of some of these compounds are listed in Table 1.

INTERPRETATION (see p. 7)

The method provides a qualitative and semiquantitative analysis of the different organic thiophosphate esters.

SENSITIVITY

For all compounds listed the detection limit is 0.1 to 1 ng, with the exception of Guthion®, methyl parathion and Methyl Trithion®. For these esters, the detection limit is 20 to 50 ng.

Table 1

R_f VALUES (× 100) OF COMMON ORGANIC THIOPHOSPHORUS ESTERS

Pesticide	Solvent system 1	Solvent system 2
Parathion	70	82
Methyl Parathion	55	75
Phosdrin®	0, 10	60, 70
Diazinon®	82	90
Bidrin®	5	25
Gardona®	35	80
Guthion®	40	83
Ethyl Guthion®	45	87
Ethion	75	92
Trithion®	80	95
Methyl Trithion®	70	85

INTERFERING SUBSTANCES

No significant spots are observed from the analysis of a thiophosphate pesticide-free biological specimen. No drugs or other pesticides interfere.

REFERENCES

Bäumler, J. and Rippstein, S., Gaschromatographische Bestimmung Von Insecticiden im Blut mit dem Halogen-Phosphor Detektor, *Arch. Toxikol.*, 25, 57, 1969.

Winterlin, W., Walker, G., and Frank, H., Detection of cholinesterase-inhibiting pesticides following separation on thin-layer chromatograms, *J. Agric. Food Chem.*, 16, 808, 1968.

TYPE B PROCEDURE

Robert A. Maes

APPARATUS

1. Separatory funnels, 100 ml
2. Shaker, mechanical
3. Beakers, 100 ml
4. Water bath
5. Syringes (Hamilton), 10 μl
6. Gas chromatograph (Perkin-Elmer Model F 20), equipped with a halogen phosphorus (HP) detector, a 1 mV recorder (Leeds and Northrup Speedomax H) with attached Disc integrator, and a glass column 6′ × 1/8″ o. d., packed with 5% silicone fat (Merck) on Chromosorb G (DMCS-AW), and equipped with Pyrex® injector insert

Operating Conditions

Gas Flow Rates:
nitrogen (carrier gas) – 40 ml/min

Temperatures:
column – 220°C
injection port – 240°C
detector – 220°

Condition the column for 24 hr at 240°C

REAGENTS

All chemicals should be analytical reagent grade.

1. Sodium sulfate, anhydrous
2. Pentane
3. Methylstearate stock solution, 100 mg/dl
   Dissolve 100 mg of methylstearate in pentane. Dilute this solution to 100 ml with pentane.
4. Methylstearate internal control solution, 10 mg/dl
   Dilute 10.0 ml of the methylstearate stock solution to 100 ml with pentane. The retention time of the methylstearate should be 6.25 min.
5. Organic thiophosphate ester stock solution, 100 mg/dl
   Dissolve 100 mg of the substance under investigation (parathion, phenkapton, etc.) in 100 ml of water.
6. Organic thiophosphate ester reference solutions
   Add appropriate quantities of the stock solution to measured volumes of uncontaminated blood to obtain concentrations of 0.02, 0.05, 0.07, 0.10, 0.15, and 0.20 mg/dl.

PROCEDURE

1. Blend 1 g of blood with 3 g of anhydrous sodium sulfate in a 100-ml separatory funnel.
2. Extract the mixture with 50 ml of pentane for 20 min on a mechanical shaker. Allow the layers to separate.
3. Filter the pentane layer through a plug of glass wool into a 100-ml beaker.
4. Evaporate the filtrate gently to approximately 0.1 ml on a water bath.
5. Add 0.1 ml of the internal control solution to the concentrate.
6. Inject 1 or 2 μl of the mixture into the gas chromatograph, making sure that the operating conditions stated above are met.
7. Extract reference blood samples containing different concentrations of the organic thiophosphate ester in question and analyze them in the same manner as the specimen.

CALCULATION

Determine the concentration in the specimen by using the following formula:

$$C_U = \frac{C_S \times P_U \times H_S}{P_S \times H_U},$$

where

C_U = concentration of organic thiophosphorus ester in the specimen analyzed;
C_S = concentration of organic thiophosphorus ester in the reference solution;
P_U = peak height of the specimen;
P_S = peak height of the reference solution;
H_U = peak height of the internal control in the specimen;
H_S = peak height of the internal control in the reference solution.

INTERPRETATION (see p. 7)

The blood concentration depends on the dose and on the survival time of the substance involved. In some cases of intoxication, parathion concentrations from 0.1 to 0.2 mg/100 ml of blood and phenkapton concentrations from 0.04 to 0.08 mg/100 ml of blood were encountered.

ACCURACY AND PRECISION

Depending on the compound, a recovery of approximately 80% can be obtained from blood when the procedure described above is used.

INTERFERING SUBSTANCES

No drugs or other pesticides interfere. The high selectivity and sensitivity (10^{-9}g) of the HP detector for this group of compounds is of great advantage in this technique.

REFERENCE

Bäumler, J. and Rippstein, S., Gaschromatographische Bestimmung von Insecticiden im Blut mit dem Halogen-Phosphor Detektor, *Arch. Toxikol.*, 25, 57, 1969.

PARAMETHOXYAMPHETAMINE (PMA)

PRINCIPLE

Paramethoxyamphetamine is separated from its biological matrix by solvent extraction of an alkalinized sample. The extract is then evaporated to dryness, acetylated, and the acetylated derivative is identified by its gas-chromatographic properties on two differently packed glass columns.

TYPE C PROCEDURE

G. Cimbura and D. W. Robinson

APPARATUS

1. Centrifuge
2. Vortex Mixer (Vortex-Genie, Fisher Scientific)
3. Centrifuge tubes, 15 ml
4. Pasteur pipets
5. Reacti-vials, 1 ml (Chromatographic Specialties Ltd., Brockville, Ontario)
6. Gas chromatograph, equipped with a flame ionization detector and two 4′ × ¼″ o. d. U-shaped, glass columns; one packed with 3% Poly A-103 (Applied Science Labs) on 80/100 mesh Varaport 30 (Varian), and the other with 3% OV-1 on 80/100 mesh Varaport 30 (Varian)

Operating Conditions

	3% Poly A-103	3% OV-1
Gas Flow Rates:		
nitrogen –	50 ml/min	50 ml/min
hydrogen –	25 ml/min	25 ml/min
air –	300 ml/min	300 ml/min
Temperatures:		
column –	210°C	160°C
injection port –	280°C	280°C
detector –	280°C	280°C

REAGENTS

All chemicals should be analytical reagent grade.

1. Isopropyl ether
2. Sodium hydroxide, 4*N*
   Dissolve 16 g of sodium hydroxide in water and dilute to 100 ml with water.
3. Acetylating solution
   Add 0.2 ml of acetic anhydride to 10 ml of isopropyl ether and mix by swirling.
4. Chloroform
5. PMA stock solution, 50 µg/ml
   Dissolve 30.45 mg *para*-methoxyamphetamine hydrochloride* in water and dilute to 500 ml with water.
6. PMA reference solution, 0.5 µg/ml
   Dilute 1.0 ml of the stock solution to 100 ml with water.

PROCEDURE

1. Add 4 drops of 6*N* sodium hydroxide to 6.0 ml of isopropyl ether in a 15-ml centrifuge tube.
2. While vortexing the mixture, add to each tube dropwise 2.0 ml of specimen (blood, urine, bile, and the PMA reference solution). Continue to vortex for approximately 3 min.
3. Let the tubes stand for approximately 10 min. If an emulsion develops or if there is an inadequate separation between blood and isopropyl ether, centrifuge the mixture.
4. Transfer the isopropyl ether layer to a glass-stoppered centrifuge tube and wash it with 1 ml of water. After the layers separate, aspirate the water and discard it.
5. Transfer a 5-ml aliquot of the organic layer to another 15 ml centrifuge tube.
6. Add 0.4 ml of the acetylating solution to the isopropyl ether, mix by vortexing, and evapor-

*Obtained from the Health Protection Branch, Dept. of Health and Welfare, Ottawa, Canada.

Table 1

RELATIVE RETENTION TIMES FOR ACETYLATED AMPHETAMINES AND RELATED COMPOUNDS

Compound	3% Poly A-103 at 210°C*	3% OV-1 at 160°C*
Methamphetamine	0.57	0.63
Amphetamine	0.62	0.46
Phenylethylamine	0.74	0.46
Phenylpropanolamine	1 (3.75 min)	1 (3.75 min)
Phencyclidine†	1.13	2.11
Phenmetrazine†	1.44	1.47
para-Methoxyamphetamine	1.63	1.27
3,4-Methylenedioxyamphetamine	2.69	1.84

* Glass columns, 4′ × ¼″ o.d., U-shaped.
† These drugs will not form acetylated derivatives.

ate the mixture, under a current of nitrogen at room temperature, to just near dryness.

7. Dissolve the residue in isopropyl ether and transfer it to a 1-ml reacti-vial. Carefully (see Step 6) evaporate just to dryness.
8. Add 20.0 μl of chloroform to the residue, and inject a 2- to 5-μl aliquot into the gas chromatograph using the Poly A-103 column at approximately 210°C. If blood is analyzed, inject 5 μl of the extract and use the highest acceptable instrumental sensitivity.
9. If PMA is indicated by the appearance of a peak whose retention time is similar to that of the reference's, then chromatograph 2 to 5 μl of the chloroform solution (Step 8) in the column packed with OV-1 at approximately 160°C.

CALCULATION

Compare the peak heights of the samples with the one corresponding to PMA in the reference solution. The peak heights of the sample and the reference solution should be obtained by using the same instrumental attenuation.

INTERPRETATION (see p. 7)

In nine fatalities of young people attributed to PMA,[1] the PMA concentrations were found to be as follows:

Blood	0.03– 0.19 mg/100 ml
Urine	0.6 –17.5 mg/100 ml
Bile	0.04– 0.3 mg/100 ml
Liver	0.05– 1.03 mg/100 g

ACCURACY AND PRECISION

The quantitative analysis of blood for PMA is within ± 0.01 mg/100 ml in the concentration range of 0.02 to 0.2 mg/100 ml. Recoveries from blood are approximately 70%, and from urine better than 95%. The procedure is sensitive to approximately 0.01 mg/100 ml.

INTERFERING SUBSTANCES

Other amphetamine derivatives do not interfere with the gas-chromatographic identification of PMA (Table 1).

REFERENCE

1. **Cimbura, G.,** PMA deaths in Ontario, *Can. Med. Assoc. J.*, 110(11), 1221, 1974.

PARAQUAT

PRINCIPLE

Because prompt therapy may be lifesaving, tests for paraquat should be done very quickly. Procedure A describes a simple color test which can be performed in minutes directly on a urine sample. Quantitation and confirmation of paraquat require separation from the urine by ion exchange chromatography. The adsorbed paraquat is easily eluted and the eluate then may be checked for its paraquat content by spectrophotometry (Procedure B).

TYPE A PROCEDURE

D. J. Berry and J. Grove

REAGENTS

All chemicals should be analytical reagent grade.

1. Sodium hydroxide, 1*N*
   Dissolve 40 g of sodium hydroxide in water and dilute to one liter.
2. Sodium dithionite, 1 g/100 ml
   Dissolve 1 g of sodium dithionite in 100 ml of *N*-sodium hydroxide immediately prior to use. This reagent should be discarded after 2 hr.

PROCEDURE

1. Pipet 10 ml of urine into a 15-ml stoppered test tube.
2. Add 2 ml of dithionite reagent, stopper, and invert tube twice (do not shake).
3. Observe the color. The formation of blue color due to the paraquat-free radical is extremely sensitive, and inexperienced observers can detect 1 μg/ml.

INTERPRETATION (see p. 7)

The reaction is an "early warning" test and is influenced by urine volume and the time after ingestion. If a negative result is obtained, it is imperative that Procedure B be employed as confirmation.

INTERFERING SUBSTANCES

Urine pigments can cause difficulty in detecting very low concentrations of paraquat. If a questionable color change is observed, the ion-exchange method (Procedure B) should be employed.

REFERENCES

Berry, D. J. and Grove, J., The determination of paraquat (1,1′-dimethyl-4,4′-bipyridylium cation) in urine, *Clin. Chim. Acta*, 34, 5, 1971.

Copland, G. M., Kolin, A., and Shulman, H. L., Fatal pulmonary intraalveolar fibrosis after paraquat ingestion, *N. Engl. J. Med.*, 291, 290, 1974.

TYPE B PROCEDURE

D. J. Berry and J. Grove

APPARATUS

1. Burette, 25 ml
2. Volumetric flask, 50 ml
3. UV spectrophotometer

REAGENTS

All chemicals should be analytical reagent grade.

1. Ion-exchange column (Dowex 50 AGW-X8), 50 to 100 mesh
   Using water, wash 3 g of resin into a 25-ml burette in which a glass wool pad has been placed near the stopcock.
2. Hydrochloric acid, 1*N*
   Dilute 82.5 ml of concentrated hydrochloric acid to one liter with water.
3. Ammonium chloride, dilute, 2.5 g/100 ml
   Dissolve 25 g of ammonium chloride in water and dilute to one liter.
4. Ammonium chloride, saturated aqueous solution
5. Sodium hydroxide, 1*N*
   Dissolve 40 g of sodium hydroxide in water and dilute to one liter.
6. Sodium dithionite, 1 g/100 ml
   In a 100-ml volumetric flask, dissolve 1 g of sodium dithionite in 1*N* sodium hydroxide and dilute to 100 ml with 1*N* sodium hydroxide. Prepare this reagent just prior to use; it must be used within 1.5 hr of its preparation. (Solid sodium dithionite should be stored in a desiccator.)
7. Paraquat stock solution, 250 μg/ml
   Dissolve 86.4 mg of paraquat dichloride in saturated ammonium chloride solution. Dilute the solution to 250 ml with saturated ammonium chloride solution. Paraquat dichloride is hygroscopic and should be dried at 100°C before use
8. Paraquat substock solution, 10 μg/ml
   Dilute 10.0 ml of the paraquat stock solution to 250 ml with saturated ammonium chloride solution.
9. Paraquat reference solutions, 0.25, 0.5, 0.75, and 1.0 μg/ml
   Measure 2.5, 5.0, 7.5, and 10.0 ml of the substock paraquat stock solution into 100-ml volumetric flasks. Dilute the contents of each flask to 100 ml with saturated ammonium chloride solution.

PROCEDURE

1. Pass 50 to 200 ml of urine through the ion-exchange column at a rate of 5 ml/min.
2. Wash the column successively with: (a) 100 ml of water; (b) 100 ml of 1*N* hydrochloric acid; and (c) 100 ml of dilute ammonium chloride.
3. Elute paraquat from the column with the saturated ammonium chloride solution at a flow rate of 1 to 2 ml/min. Collect the first 50 ml.
4. Pipet 10.0 ml of the sample (eluates and each reference solution) into a stoppered test tube. Add 2.0 ml of dithionite solution and mix by inverting twice.
5. Place an aliquot of the mixture in a 4-cm glass cuvette and within 3 min measure the absorbance of the solution at 392, 396, 400, and 401 nm, using an aliquot of a mixture of 10.0 ml of saturated ammonium chloride and 2.0 ml of dithionite solution in the reference cuvette. Designate these absorbances as E_{392}, E_{396}, E_{400}, and E_{401}.
6. Add 2.0 ml of sodium dithionite to 10.0 ml of each reference solution, then measure their absorbances at 396 nm.

CALCULATION

1. Correct the absorbance at 396 nm (E_{396}) of the sample solution for irrelevant absorption by means of Equations 1 and 2. Designate the corrected absorbances as E_{396} (corrected 1) and E_{396} (corrected 2), respectively.

$$E_{396} \text{ (corrected 1)} = 2.91\ E_{396} - 1.61\ E_{392} - 1.28\ E_{401} \quad (1)$$

$$E_{396} \text{ (corrected 2)} = 1.68\ (2\ E_{396} - E_{392} - E_{400}) \quad (2)$$

2. Determine the average of E_{396} (corrected 1) and E_{396} (corrected 2). Designate this as E_{396} (mean corrected) and use it to determine the concentration of paraquat in the effluent by comparing it to the prepared standard curve. The recovery from aqueous samples is virtually 100%.

INTERPRETATION (see p. 7)

After ingestion of paraquat, 90% is excreted unchanged in the first 48 hr. It may still be detected as long as 3 weeks later.

ACCURACY

Solutions of paraquat obey Beer's law. The mean recovery of paraquat added to urine was 86 ± 4% in the range from 0.04 to 2.0 μg/ml.

INTERFERING SUBSTANCES

All interferences from background absorption have been eliminated by using the equations based on the method of Morton and Stubbs.[1] Paraquat-free urines carried through this procedure do not give any measurable absorbance.

REFERENCE

1. **Morton, R. A., and Stubbs, A. L.,** Photoelectric spectrometry applied to the analysis of mixtures and Vitamin A oils, *Analyst*, 71, 348, 1946.

GENERAL REFERENCES

Berry, D. J. and Grove, J., Analysis of paraquat (1,1′-dimethyl-4,4′-bipyridylium cation) in urine, *Clin. Chim. Acta*, 34, 5, 1971.

Copland, G. M., Kolin, A., and Shulman, H. L., Fatal pulmonary intraalveolar fibrosis after paraquat ingestion, *N. Engl. J. Med.*, 291, 290, 1974.

PHENCYCLIDINE (PCP)

PRINCIPLE

Phencyclidine, like many organic bases, can be extracted from a biological specimen by a suitable organic solvent, provided the original sample is alkaline. The drug can be further purified by reextraction from the original solvent into dilute aqueous acid, which is then made alkaline. An organic solvent extract of this alkaline solution is then evaporated to a small volume. An aliquot is then injected onto a suitable gas chromatographic column to determine if phencyclidine is present.

TYPE B PROCEDURE

H. R. Wetherell

APPARATUS

1. Separatory funnels with Teflon® stopcocks, 125 ml
2. Small glass funnels
3. Glass-stoppered graduated cylinders, 100 and 25 ml
4. Silanized, acid-washed glass wool
5. Pipets
6. Disposable Pasteur pipets
7. Centrifuge tubes, graduated, 15 ml
8. Microliter syringes, 10 μl
9. Gas chromatograph (Varian 2700 or equivalent) equipped with a flame ionization detector and a silanized glass column, 6′ × ¼″ o.d., packed with 2.5% SE-30 on 80/100 mesh Chromosorb G (AW-DMCS)

   Operating Conditions

   Gas Flow Rates:
   - nitrogen (carrier gas) – 30 ml/min
   - air – 300 ml/min
   - hydrogen – 30 ml/min

   Temperatures:
   - column – 220° C
   - injection port – 265° C
   - detector – 275° C

REAGENTS

All chemicals should be analytical reagent grade.

1. Sulfuric acid, 0.1*N*
   Dilute 2.8 ml of concentrated sulfuric acid to one liter with distilled water.
2. Sodium hydroxide, 1.0*N*
   Dissolve 40 g of sodium hydroxide in distilled water and dilute to one liter with water.
3. Sodium sulfate, anhydrous, granular
4. Chloroform
5. Heptane-isoamyl alcohol solvent mixture
   Add 15 ml of isoamyl alcohol to 985 ml of heptane.
6. Methanol, absolute
7. Silanizing reagent
   Add 5 ml of dimethyldichlorosilane to 95 ml of toluene.
8. Ketamine hydrochloride stock solution, 100 μg/ml of free base
   Dissolve 115 mg of ketamine hydrochloride (Parke-Davis & Co.) in water and dilute to one liter with distilled water
9. Ketamine hydrochloride internal standard solution, 1.0 μg/ml
   Dilute 10 ml of the ketamine hydrochloride stock solution to one liter with distilled water.
10. Phencyclidine hydrochloride stock solution, 100 μg/ml of free base
    Dissolve 115 mg of phencyclidine hydrochloride in distilled water and dilute to one liter with distilled water.
11. Phencyclidine hydrochloride reference solutions, 0.02, 0.05, 0.10, and 0.20 μg/ml
    Dilute 0.2, 0.5, 1.0, and 2.0 ml of the phencyclidine hydrochloride stock solution to one liter with distilled water, respectively.

PROCEDURE

The inner surfaces of all glassware should be silanized by placing them in contact with the silanizing reagent for 30 min. Drain the silanizing reagent and immediately rinse the glassware with anhydrous methanol. Allow the glassware to air dry.

Preparation of a Standard Curve

1. Add 10 ml of sample (blood and each phencyclidine hydrochloride reference solution) to 125-ml separatory funnels, each containing 50 ml of heptane-isoamyl alcohol solvent mixture. Add 1.0 ml of ketamine hydrochloride internal standard solution and 1.0 ml of 1.0*N* sodium hydroxide solution to each funnel.
2. Shake each funnel for 3 min. Allow the layers to separate.
3. Discard the lower aqueous phase, and pour the organic phase through a small amount of anhydrous sodium sulfate, supported by a pledget of silanized glass wool, in the apex of a small glass funnel. Collect this organic filtrate in a 100-ml glass-stoppered graduated cylinder.
4. Add 5-ml 0.1*N* sulfuric acid to each sample and extract for 3 min. Allow the phase to separate.
5. Remove as much of the lower acid phase as possible with a pipet and transfer it to a 25-ml glass-stoppered graduated cylinder. Add 10 ml of chloroform and 1.0 ml of 1.0*N* sodium hydroxide solution. Shake the cylinders for 3 min. Allow the phases to separate.
6. Remove and discard the upper aqueous phase with a Pasteur pipet. Filter the chloroform through a small amount of sodium sulfate supported on a pledget of silanized glass wool in the apex of a small glass funnel. Collect the filtrate in a 15-ml conical centrifuge tube.
7. Evaporate the solvent to approximately 10 μl in a stream of dry air.
8. Inject 2 μl of each extract into the gas chromatograph, and measure the heights of the ketamine and phencyclidine peaks in each extract. Ketamine has a retention time of approximately 4.8 min, while phencyclidine has a retention time of approximately 5.8 min.
9. Calculate R, the ratio of the peak height of phencyclidine to that of ketamine. Prepare a graph by plotting R_s (the ratio of the peak height of phencyclidine to the peak height of ketamine) against each concentration of phencyclidine.

CALCULATION

From the ratio of the peak height of phencyclidine in the unknown to the peak height of ketamine R_v, determine the amount of phencyclidine in the unknown from the standard curve.

INTERPRETATION (see p. 7)

Concentrations of phencyclidine in the blood, in fatal cases where no other drugs were detected, have been found to be between 0.2 to 6.0 μg/ml.[1]

ACCURACY AND PRECISION

The standard curve is linear over the range of phencyclidine concentrations from 0.02 to 0.3 μg/ml. Recoveries of phencyclidine added to blood at a concentration of 0.08 μg/ml averaged 80 ± 4% of an aqueous solution of the same concentration.

INTERFERING SUBSTANCES

As with any gas-chromatographic method, confirmation of the identity of the substance causing the detector response is desirable. Confirmation of phencyclidine has been obtained by means of its characteristic mass spectrum.[2]

REFERENCES

1. **Reed, D., Cravey, R. H., and Sedgwick, P. R.,** *Bull. Int. Assoc. Forensic Toxicol.*, p. 7, June 1972.
2. **Finkle, B. S., Taylor, D. M., and Bonelli, E. J.,** A GC/MS reference data system for the identification of drugs of abuse, *J. Chromatogr. Sci.*, 10, 312, 1972.

GENERAL REFERENCE

Kessler, G. F., Demers, L. M., and Berlin, C., Phencyclidine and fatal status epilepticus, *N. Engl. J. Med.*, 291, 979, 1974.

PHENOLS

PRINCIPLE

The phenol is separated from the biological matrix by steam distillation. Reactions with Millon's reagent and the Lux test are used to indicate qualitatively that phenols are present. Quantitative analysis requires bromination and a redox titration to determine the phenol content.

TYPE A PROCEDURE

Naresh C. Jain

REAGENTS

All chemicals should be analytical reagent grade.

1. Tartaric acid, 10 g/100 ml
   Dissolve 10 g of tartaric acid in water and dilute to 100 ml.
2. Sodium hydroxide, 1.25*N*
   Dissolve 5.0 g of sodium hydroxide in water and dilute to 100 ml.
3. Millon's reagent
   Dissolve 3 ml of mercury in 27 ml of cold fuming nitric acid. Dilute this solution with an equal volume of water.
4. Ammonium hydroxide, 1.5*N*
   Dilute 10 ml of concentrated ammonium hydroxide with water to 100 ml.
5. Bromine water, saturated aqueous solution
6. Sodium hypochlorite, 10 g/100 ml
   Dissolve 10 g of sodium hypochlorite in water and dilute to 100 ml.
7. Bromide-bromate solution, 0.1*N*
   Dissolve 2.784 g of potassium bromate and 15 g of potassium bromide in one liter of water.
8. Potassium iodide, 10 g/100 ml
   Dissolve 10 g of potassium iodide in water and dilute to 100 ml. Prepare fresh as needed.
9. Sodium thiosulfate, 0.1*N*
   Dissolve 24.8 g of sodium thiosulfate in one liter of water. Check the titer of this solution against the 0.1*N* bromide-bromate solution before use. Alternatively, check its normality against a standard 0.1*N* potassium dichromate solution.
10. Potassium dichromate, 1*N*
    Dissolve 4.903 g of potassium dichromate in water and dilute to 100 ml.
11. Sodium starch glycollate, 1 g/100 ml
    Dissolve 5.0 g of sodium starch glycollate in water and dilute to 100 ml. Dilute 20.0 ml of this solution to 100 ml with water.

SPECIMEN REQUIREMENTS

1. Acidify a 50-g biological specimen with the tartaric acid solution.
2. Steam-distill the sample. Collect the distillate in a 50-ml volumetric flask containing 5 ml of 1.25*N* sodium hydroxide.

PROCEDURE

Qualititative Determination

1. Millon's reagent test
   To 1 or 2 ml of the distillate, add 1 or 2 drops of Millon's reagent. Boil the mixture. A red color indicates the presence of phenol. This test is very sensitive, but not specific.
2. Fluckinger or Lex test
   To 1 or 2 ml of the distillate, add a few drops of 1.5*N* ammonium hydroxide and an excess of bromine water. A pale-yellow precipitate of tribromophenol indicates the presence of phenol. Cresol or other compounds with a phenolic structure will give a yellow color.
3. Hypochlorite test
   To 1 or 2 ml of the distillate add 2 drops of 1.5*N* ammonium hydroxide and 2 to 4 drops of freshly prepared sodium hypochlorite solution. Warm the mixture gently. The formation

of a blue color indicates the presence of phenol. In dilute solutions, phenol may give only green to blue-green coloration. Cresol or other compounds containing a phenolic group will also interfere with this test.

Quantitative Determination

1. Place 25 ml of the distillate in a 250-ml stoppered Erlenmeyer flask.
2. Titrate with 0.1*N* bromide-bromate solution until a permanent yellow color persists. Note the quantity of bromide-bromate reagent added and add 10% of this volume in excess.
3. Stopper the flask and shake it well for 1 min.
4. Add 5.0 ml of the potassium iodide solution. Titrate the liberated iodine with 0.1*N* sodium thiosulfate solution, using 1 ml of the sodium starch glycollate solution as the indicator.
5. Repeat Steps 1 to 4 on a 25-ml sample of distilled water. The resulting solution will serve as a reagent blank. Be sure to add to the reagent blank the same volume of bromide-bromate solution as to the specimen (Step 2).
6. The difference in the volume of sodium thiosulfate titrated against the distillate of the specimen and that titrated against the reagent blank is a measure of the phenol present.

CALCULATION

One milliliter of 0.1*N* sodium thiosulfate solution represents 1.6 mg of phenol. If the sodium thiosulfate solution was not exactly 0.1*N*, calculate the equivalent volume from the titer with the potassium dichromate solution.

INTERPRETATION (see p. 7)

In normal urine the total quantity of mixed phenol and cresols excreted in 24 hr ranges from 15 to 30 mg. In cases of phenol poisoning the urine is usually very dark in color.

REFERENCES

Autenreith, W., *Laboratory Manual for Detection of Poisons,* 6th ed., translated by William H. Warren, Blakiston, Philadelphia, 1946.

Bamford, F., *Poisons – Their Isolation and Identification,* 3rd ed., Blakiston, Philadelphia, 1951.

Dirmilius, S. M. and Darbre, A., GLC of simple phenols for urinalysis, *J. Chromatogr.,* 94, 169, 1974.

PHENOTHIAZINES

PRINCIPLE

In the presence of a suitable oxidizing agent, the phenothiazines develop a characteristic color that can be used for a qualitative determination.

TYPE A PROCEDURE

Irving Sunshine

REAGENTS

All chemicals should be analytical reagent grade.

1. Ferric chloride, 5 g/100 ml
   Dissolve 5 g of ferric chloride in 100 ml of water.
2. Perchloric acid, 20% (v/v)
   Dilute 20.0 ml of 70% perchloric acid to 100 ml with water.
3. Nitric acid, 7.5*N*
   Dilute 50 ml of concentrated nitric acid to 100 ml with water.
4. FPN reagent
   Mix 5 ml of the ferric chloride solution with 45 ml of 20% perchloric acid and 50 ml of 7.5*N* nitric acid.

PROCEDURE

1. Add 2 drops of FPN reagent to 1 drop of specimen (urine or stomach content).
2. Observe the intensity and color produced in 10 sec. Disregard any change that takes place after 10 sec.

INTERPRETATION (see p. 7)

If a blue, purple, or red color forms within 10 sec, this may be an indication that phenothiazines are present. The color and its intensity vary with the particular phenothiazine involved. After use of therapeutic doses of the more potent phenothiazines or fluorinated derivatives, false negatives may occur. Thus, this test may not be optimal as an indication of whether or not a patient is taking a prescribed phenothiazine. It is a good indication, however, of gross overdosage, and seldom yields false negatives following the ingestion of relatively large amounts of the drug. The limits of detection are such that the test is not useful on blood specimens.

REFERENCE

Forrest, I. S. and Forrest, F. M., Urine color test for the detection of phenothiazine compounds, *Clin. Chem.,* 6, 11, 1960.

PHENYLBUTAZONE (BUTAZOLIDIN®) AND OXYPHENBUTAZONE

PRINCIPLE

Phenylbutazone, a weak acid, is extracted into an organic solvent from a sample whose pH is 2 to 3. Aliquots of this extract can be tested with classical spot tests or by thin-layer chromatography for typical reactions that are characteristic of phenylbutazone or its metabolite, oxyphenbutazone (Procedure A). More elegant procedures depend on reextracting the organic solvent with alkali. The UV spectrum of this alkaline solution and its acidified counterpart can be used for the qualitative identification and quantitation of the drugs (Procedure B). If the alkaline solution is oxidized with potassium permanganate, an azobenzene derivative is formed; this can be extracted from the aqueous reaction mixture by heptane. The UV absorption of the heptane extract can then be used for qualitative and quantitative analysis. Procedure C is based on selective extraction of the drug and its metabolites and subsequent gas-chromatographic analysis of concentrates of the extracts.

TYPE A PROCEDURE

John J. McHugh and Marjorie Q. Swift

APPARATUS

1. Separatory funnels, 100 or 125 ml
2. Spot plate, porcelain
3. Steam bath
4. Thin-layer chromatography (TLC) equipment: (a) micropipets, disposable; (b) chromatogram sheet, silica gel G (Eastman #6061 or equivalent); (c) developing jars, screw-capped, 3″ X 6″ (d) spray bottles

REAGENTS

All chemicals should be analytical reagent grade.

1. Sulfuric acid, 3.6*N*
   Dilute 10.0 ml of concentrated sulfuric acid to 100 ml with water.
2. Chloroform
3. Sodium sulfate, anhydrous
4. Nitric acid, concentrated
5. Potassium hydroxide, alcoholic, 4 g/100 ml
   Dissolve 4 g of potassium hydroxide in absolute ethanol. Dilute the solution to 100 ml with absolute ethanol.
6. Ammonium molybdate, 0.5 g/100 ml
   Dissolve 0.5 g of ammonium molybdate in water and dilute to 100 ml.
7. Ammonium vanadate, 0.5 g/100 ml
   Dissolve 0.5 g of ammonium vanadate in water and dilute to 100 ml.
8. Phenylbutazone reference solution, 100 mg/100 ml
   Dissolve 100 mg of phenylbutazone in chloroform. Dilute the solution to 100 ml with chloroform.
9. Oxyphenbutazone reference solution, 100 mg/100 ml
   Dissolve 100 mg of oxyphenbutazone in chloroform. Dilute the solution to 100 ml with chloroform.
10. Chloroform-methanol developing solution, 9:1
    Mix 9 parts chloroform with 1 part methanol.
11. Ethyl acetate-methanol-ammonium hydroxide developing solution, 85:10:5
    Mix 85 parts ethyl acetate, 10 parts methanol, and 5 parts ammonium hydroxide.
12. Potassium permanganate, 1 g/100 ml
    Dissolve 1 g of potassium permanganate in water and dilute to 100 ml.
13. Potassium ferricyanide, 1 g/100 ml
    Dissolve 1 g of potassium ferricyanide in 100 ml of water.
14. Hydrochloric acid, 0.5*N*
    Dilute 20 ml of concentrated hydrochloric acid to 500 ml with water.
15. Ferric chloride, 2 g/100 ml
    Dissolve 2 g of ferric chloride in 0.5*N* hydrochloric acid. Dilute the solution to 100 ml with 0.5*N* hydrochloric acid.

PROCEDURE

Specimen Extraction

1. Pour 5 ml of urine into a separatory funnel.
2. Add 2 drops of 3.6*N* sulfuric acid.
3. Extract the mixture with 20 ml of chloroform.
4. Separate the chloroform, then dry it with anhydrous sodium sulfate.
5. Evaporate the chloroform to 2 or 3 ml for the following spot tests.

Spot Tests for Phenylbutazone and Oxyphenbutazone

Vitali's Screening Test

1. Place 2 drops of the chloroform extract on a spot plate.
2. Add 2 drops of concentrated nitric acid.
3. Evaporate the mixture to dryness on a steam bath.
4. Cool the residue, then add 1 drop of alcoholic potassium hydroxide.
5. Observe the color development. An orange to brown or black color indicates the possible presence of phenylbutazone or a metabolite thereof. If a positive result is obtained, continue the analysis with other tests. If the result is negative, no appreciable quantity of the drug is present.

Ammonium Molybdate Test

1. Add a drop of the ammonium molybdate solution to a drop of the test solution.
2. Evaporate the mixture to dryness on a steam bath.
3. Moisten the residue with a drop of sulfuric acid.
4. Observe the color development. An orange-yellow color indicates the presence of oxyphenbutazone.

Ammonium Vanadate Test

1. Add a drop of ammonium vanadate solution to a drop of the test solution.
2. Evaporate the mixture to dryness on a steam bath.
3. Moisten the residue with a drop of sulfuric acid.
4. Observe the color development. A dull purple color indicates the presence of phenylbutazone.

Thin-Layer Chromatography

1. Using micropipets, spot aliquots of the chloroform extract and of the phenylbutazone and oxyphenbutazone reference solutions (in chloroform) on a silica gel chromatogram sheet (Eastman #6061).
2. Develop the sheets in the chloroform-methanol (9:1) solution or in the ethyl acetate-methanol-ammonium hydroxide (85:10:5) solution.
3. After the developing solution has migrated 12 cm, remove the sheet from the tank and air-dry it.
4. Visualize the phenylbutazone and oxyphenbutazone spots by spraying the sheet with potassium permanganate. Positive spots appear yellow on a purple background. The background color fades quickly.
5. Alternatively, mix equal volumes of the potassium ferricyanide solution and the ferric chloride solution. Spray the sheet with this mixture. Positive spots appear bright blue on a yellow background. The background color quickly turns blue.
6. Typical R_f values for phenylbutazone and oxyphenbutazone are given below.

Compound	R_f in 9:1 chloroform-methanol	R_f in 85:10:5 ethyl acetate-methanol-ammonium hydroxide
Phenylbutazone	0.80–0.90	0.35–0.45
Oxyphenbutazone	0.65–0.75	0.15–0.25

INTERPRETATION (see p. 7)

The metabolism of phenylbutazone has been extensively studied. Two principal metabolites have been noted. The most common metabolite is *p*-hydroxyphenylbutazone (oxyphenbutazone), which is now marketed as a pharmaceutical product.

ACCURACY AND PRECISION

The spot tests are sensitive (1 μg) but not specific, since comparable colors may be obtained with several alkaloids; however, most alkaloids are separated and discarded in the procedure described above. Thin-layer chromatography will confirm the presence of 10 μ of either drug if the R_f values agree with those obtained from the reference solutions in two different developing systems.

INTERFERING SUBSTANCES

Nothing should interfere if the complete procedure is carried out. The spot tests, if negative, are sufficient to rule out the presence of the drugs, and further analysis of these specimens is not necessary. Another metabolite of phenylbutazone is unstable and unlikely to be noted.

REFERENCE*

Burns, J. J., Rose, R. K., Goodwin, S., Reichenthal, J., Horning, E. C., and Brodie, B. B., Metabolic fate of phenylbutazone (Butazolidin) in man, *J. Pharmacol. Exp. Ther.*, 113, 481, 1955.

TYPE B PROCEDURE

John J. McHugh and Marjorie Q. Swift

APPARATUS

1. Separatory funnels, 100 or 125 ml
2. Centrifuge
3. UV spectrophotometer (Unicam SP 800 or equivalent)

REAGENTS

All chemicals should be analytical reagent grade.

1. Hydrochloric acid, concentrated
2. *n*-Heptane
3. Sodium hydroxide, 0.1*N*
   Dissolve 4 g of sodium hydroxide in water and dilute to one liter.
4. Ethylene dichloride
5. Citrate-phosphate buffer, pH 4.8, 0.15*M*
   Dissolve 14.5 g of disodium phosphate in 200 ml of distilled water. Dissolve 4.5 g of citric acid in 200 ml of distilled water. Mix equal volumes of both solutions.
6. Sulfuric acid, 0.5*N*
   Dilute 15 ml of concentrated sulfuric acid to one liter with water.

PROCEDURE[1,2]

Separation

1. To 5.0 ml of specimen (plasma, urine, or 5 g of homogenized tissue) add 1.5 ml of concentrated hydrochloric acid. Extract the mixture with 15.0 ml of *n*-heptane, centrifuge, then separate the two phases. Save both phases. Process a 5.0-ml water sample for a reagent blank in the same manner as the specimen.
2. To the heptane obtained in Step 1, add 5.0 ml of 0.1*N* sodium hydroxide. The phenylbutazone, if present, is extracted into the alkali.
3. Extract the aqueous layer obtained in Step 1 with 30 ml of ethylene dichloride.
4. Wash the ethylene dichloride obtained in Step 3 with an equal volume of 0.15*M* citrate-phosphate buffer, pH 4.8. Discard the wash liquid.
5. To the washed ethylene dichloride obtained in Step 4 add 5.0 ml of 0.1*N* sodium hydroxide. The oxyphenbutazone, if present, is extracted into the alkali.

*For an updated list of reference material, see General References, p. 308.

UV Absorbance Measurements

6. Determine the absorbance of phenylbutazone in alkaline solution (Step 2) from 220 to 300 nm after bubbling nitrogen through the aqueous phase to remove the solvent. Use the alkaline solution obtained by processing the water sample as the reference solution.
7. Add 1.0 ml of 0.5*N* sulfuric acid to 2.0 ml of each solution, then determine the absorbance of the acidified solution from 220 to 300 nm.
8. To correct for dilution of the material by the acid, multiply the 265-nm absorbance in the acid solution by 1.5.
9. Determine the absorbance of oxyphenbutazone (metabolite I) in alkaline solution (Step 5) from 220 to 300 nm. Use the alkaline solution obtained by processing the water sample as the reference solution.
10. Add 1.0 ml of 0.5*N* sulfuric acid to 2.0 ml of each solution, then determine the absorbance of the acidified solution from 220 to 300 nm.
11. To correct for dilution of the material by the acid, multiply the 253-nm absorbance in the acid solution by 1.5.

CALCULATION

1. Determine the phenylbutazone concentration (μg/ml) in urine by the following formula:

$$C_p = (A_B - A_A) \times 19,$$

where

C_p = concentration of phenylbutazone in the specimen;
A_B = absorbance at 265 nm in basic solution;
A_A = corrected absorbance at 265 nm in acid solution (Step 8).

2. Determine the oxyphenbutazone (metabolite I) concentration (μg/ml) in urine by the following formula:

$$C_M = (A_B - A_A) \times 19,$$

where

C_M = concentration of oxyphenbutazone (metabolite I) in the specimen;
A_B = absorbance at 253 nm in basic solution;
A_A = corrected absorbance at 253 nm in acid solution (Step 11).

INTERPRETATION (see p. 7)

The identification of the parent drug, phenylbutazone, is necessary to confirm the use of this drug. If both phenylbutazone and oxyphenbutazone are found in the extracts, the administration of the parent compound is confirmed. If only oxyphenbutazone is found, its presence may be due either to separate administration of this substance or to metabolism of phenylbutazone. The results can be confirmed by thin-layer chromatography (Type A Procedure.)*

A single 400-mg oral dose of phenylbutazone resulted in a peak level of 60 μg/ml of unchanged drug 1 hr past administration, while a plateau level of 10 μg/ml of oxyphenbutazone was observed from 72 to 144 hr. No γ-hydroxy metabolite was detected. Multiple doses at the 200 mg b.i.d. level gave plateau levels at about 120 μg/ml of phenylbutazone by the seventh day with 10 to 15 μg/ml of oxyphenbutazone and 10 to 20 μg/ml of γ-hydroxyphenylbutazone by the seventh day. The dose dependent metabolism of phenylbutazone complicates interpretation.[2] Normal therapeutic levels are 50 to 100 μg/ml.[3]

ACCURACY AND PRECISION

Pure phenylbutazone exhibits an absorbance maximum at 265 nm and a minimum at 227 nm in alkaline solutions. In dilute (25 μg/ml) acid solutions it shows a maximum at 237 nm and a minimum at 225 nm. In more concentrated acid solutions the drug may precipitate. Oxyphenbutazone (metabolite I) in alkaline solution has an absorbance maximum at 253 nm, and in acid solution at 234 nm. Mixtures of phenylbutazone and its metabolite will show a maximum in alkaline solution between 253 and 265 nm, which shifts to about 235 nm in acid solution. On the

*See p. 302.

basis of these absorption characteristics and confirmation by spot and thin-layer chromatography tests, accurate identification and quantitation of phenylbutazone and its metabolite can be obtained.

INTERFERING SUBSTANCES

Metabolite II, which is hydroxylated on the butyl side chain, is less stable and is unlikely to interfere in the separation.

REFERENCES

1. **Burns, J. J., Rose, R. K., Goodwin, S., Reichenthal, J., Horning, E. C., and Brodie, B. B.,** Metabolic fate of phenylbutazone (Butazolidin) in man, *J. Pharmacol. Exp. Ther.,* 113, 481, 1955.
2. **Curry, A. S.,** Ed., *Methods of Forensic Science,* Vol. 4. Interscience Publications, John Wiley & Sons, N. Y. 1965.
3. **Steentoft, A.,** Poisoning due to phenylbutazone, *Bull. Int. Assoc. Forensic Toxicol.,* Central Research Establishment, Aldermaston, England, 4, 4, 1967.

GENERAL REFERENCE*

Curry A., *Poison Detection in Human Organs,* 2nd ed., Charles C Thomas, Springfield, Ill., 1969, 1974.

TYPE C PROCEDURE

K. K. Midha, I. J. McGilveray, and C. Charette

APPARATUS

1. Centrifuge tubes, Teflon®-lined screw caps, 20 ml
2. Evaporating tubes, Teflon®-lined screw caps, narrow bore base (tip 50 μl), total capacity 10 ml
3. Rotating mixer
4. Oscillating mixer
5. Gas chromatograph (F/11 Perkin-Elmer), equipped with a flame ionization detector and a stainless steel column 8′ × 1/8″ o.d., packed with 5% OV-7 on Chromosorb W high performance, 80/100 mesh

   Operating Conditions

   Gas Flow Rates:
   - nitrogen (carrier gas) – 40 ml/min
   - Hydrogen and compressed air flow rates were adjusted to give maximum response.

   Temperatures:
   - column – 260°C
   - injection port – 310°C
   - detector – 300°C

REAGENTS

All chemicals should be analytical reagent grade.

1. Distill diethyl ether and *n*-heptane in glass prior to use.
2. Prepare stock solutions of phenylbutazone† containing 100 μg/ml[1] and dilute with 0.2*M* phosphate buffer (pH 7.4) to the concentrations required (2 to 60 μg/ml) before use.
3. Prepare stock solutions of oxyphenbutazone† containing 16 μg/ml in ether daily and dilute to the required range (1 to 16 μg/ml).
4. Prepare stock solutions of γ-hydroxyphenylbutazone‡ containing 50 μg/ml and dilute to the required concentrations with methanol.
5. Solution 1
   Prepare stock solutions of 1-(*o*-chlorophenyl)-1-(*p*-chlorophenyl)-2,2,2-trichloroethane‡ containing 50 μg/ml in *n*-heptane daily and use as such.
6. Solution 2
   Prepare stock solutions of 5-(4-hydroxyphenyl)-5-phenylhydantoin‡ containing 22.2 μg/ml in 0.01*N* NaOH weekly and dilute to 1.11 μg/ml with 0.01*N* NaOH daily before use.

*For an updated list of reference material, see General References, p. 308.
†Ciba-Geigy, Canada.
‡Dr. A. Sallmann, Ciba-Geigy, Switzerland.
‡Aldrich Chemical Co., Milwaukee, Wis.

7. Phosphate buffer (pH 11.2), 0.2*M*
8. Hydrochloric acid, 1 and 2*N*
9. Methanolic solution of trimethylanilinium hydroxide (TMAH), 0.2*M*

PROCEDURE

Extraction of Phenylbutazone

1. Place 1 ml of plasma sample in a centrifuge tube. Include in each series of analyses 1-ml aliquots of a sufficient number of each reference compound.
2. Add 1 ml of diluted Solution 2 (1.11 μg/ml), 2 ml of 1*N* HCl, and 5 ml of ether.
3. Extract the sample for 10 min using a rotating mixer at 19 rpm. Centrifuge the tubes at 2,500 rpm for 10 min.
4. Transfer 4.0 ml of the ether layer to another centrifuge tube containing 5 ml of phosphate buffer (pH 11.2). Save the aqueous layer for Step 5.
5. Repeat the extraction of each mixture with 7 ml of ether and transfer 7 ml of the organic layer to the previous extract.
6. Roto-mix the combined extracts with the phosphate buffer (10 min), centrifuge (10 min), and discard the ether layer.
7. Acidify the aqueous phosphate solution with 2 ml of 2*N* HCl and extract with 2- to 5-ml portions of *n*-heptane. (Mix for 10 min and centrifuge for 10 min.)
8. Transfer 4 and 5 ml, respectively, of the *n*-heptane layers in Step 7 into an evaporating tube containing 1 ml of Solution 1 (50 μg/ml). Save the acidified phosphate buffer and any remaining hexane for Step 12.
9. Evaporate the *n*-heptane extract to dryness at 60°C under a stream of dry nitrogen.
10. Add 50 μl of TMAH to the residue.
11. Inject 1 to 2 μl into the gas chromatograph. Flash-heater methylated phenylbutazone and the reference compound in Solution 1 give retention times of 7.1 and 4.0 min, respectively.

Extraction of Oxyphenbutazone and γ-Hydroxyphenylbutazone

12. Remove with a disposable pipet any remaining *n*-heptane in the solution obtained in Step 8. Add 2 ml of *n*-heptane, swirl the tubes gently by hand, and remove the *n*-heptane with another disposable pipet.
13. Extract the washed aqueous acid with 2- to 5-ml portions of ether using a roto-mixer (15 min each) followed by centrifugation (10 min each).
14. Remove 4 and 5 ml, respectively, of the ether extracts in Step 13 into an evaporating tube.
15. Evaporate the pooled ether extracts to dryness under a stream of dry nitrogen at 40°C.
16. Add to the residue 20 μl of TMAH and mix on an oscillating mixer.
17. Inject 2 μl into the gas chromatograph. Flash-heater methylated oxyphenbutazone, γ-hydroxyphenylbutazone, and the reference substance in Solution 2 give retention times of 15.2, 10.5, and 12.6 min, respectively.

CALCULATION

1. Peak height ratios are calculated by dividing the peak height of the phenylbutazone methyl derivative by that of the Solution 1 methyl derivative.
2. Peak height ratios are calculated by dividing the peak height of the oxyphenbutazone methyl derivative or γ-hydroxyphenylbutazone methyl derivative by that of the Solution 2 methyl derivative.
3. Concentration of phenylbutazone or any of its metabolites is obtained by comparing the peak height ratios of the compound and the internal standard in unknown specimens with those obtained for the reference samples.

INTERPRETATION (see p. 7)

The identification of the parent drug, phenylbutazone, is necessary to confirm the use of this drug. If both phenylbutazone and oxyphenbutazone are found in the extracts, the administration of the parent compound is confirmed. If only oxyphenbutazone is found, its presence may be due either to separate administration of this substance or to metabolism of phenylbutazone.

The results can be confirmed by thin-layer chromatography (Type A Procedure.)*

A single 400-mg oral dose of phenylbutazone resulted in a peak level of 60 μg/ml of unchanged drug 1 hr post administration, while a plateau level of 10 μg/ml of oxyphenbutazone was observed from 72 to 144 hr. No γ-hydroxy metabolite was detected. Multiple doses at the 200 mg b.i.d. level gave plateau levels at about 120 μg/ml of phenylbutazone by the seventh day with 10 to 15 μg/ml of oxyphenbutazone and 10 to 20 μg/ml of γ-hydroxyphenylbutazone by the seventh day. The dose dependent metabolism of phenylbutazone complicates interpretation.[2] Normal therapeutic levels are 50 to 100 μg/ml.[3]

ACCURACY AND PRECISION

1. The overall recoveries of phenylbutazone, oxyphenbutazone, γ-hydroxyphenylbutazone, and Standard 2 from plasma are 93.42 ± 2.9%, 24.59 ± 0.55%, 20.8 ± 0.9%, and 69.72 ± 2.37%, respectively, by this method.
2. The overall coefficient of variation for concentrations of phenylbutazone in the range 2 to 64 μg/ml was found to be 4.65%.
3. The overall coefficient of variation for concentrations of oxyphenbutazone in the range 1 to 16 μg/ml was determined to be 3.5%.
4. The overall coefficient of variation for concentrations of γ-hydroxyphenylbutazone in the range 1 to 10 μg/ml was found to be 3.5%.

INTERFERING SUBSTANCES

1. Flash-heater methylation of phenylbutazone with TMAH gives two peaks with retention times of 7.1 and 14.9 min. The major peak (7.1 min) is used for quantitation.
2. Flash-heater methylation of oxyphenbutazone with TMAH gives two peaks with retention times of 15.2 and 31 min. The major peak, used for quantitation, elutes at 15.2 min.
3. Flash-heater methylation of γ-hydroxyphenylbutazone with TMAH gives four peaks with retention times of 10.5, 14.2, 24.2, and 28.5 min. The major peak, eluting at 10.5 min, is used for quantitation.
4. Oxyphenbutazone and γ-hydroxyphenylbutazone do not interfere with the assay of phenylbutazone because they are extracted with *n*-heptane only to the extent of 7% and have different retention times.
5. Phenylbutazone does not interfere in the oxyphenbutazone and γ-hydroxyphenylbutazone because it is removed by partitioning into *n*-heptane.
6. Oxyphenbutazone and γ-hydroxyphenylbutazone do not interfere with each other because they have different retention times.

*See p. 302.

REFERENCES

1. **McGilveray, I. J., Midha, K. K., Brien, R., and Wilson, L.**, The assay of phenylbutazone in human plasma by a specific and sensitive GLC procedure, *J. Chromatogr.*, 89, 17, 1974.
2. **Burns, J. J., Rose, R. K., Goodwin, S., Reichenthal, J., Horning, E. C., and Brodie, B. B.**, The metabolic fate of phenylbutazone (butazolidin) in man, *J. Pharmacol. Exp. Ther.*, 113, 481, 1955.
3. **Steentoft, A.**, Poisoning due to phenylbutazone, *Bull. Int. Assoc. Forensic Toxicol.*, 4, 4, 1967.

GENERAL REFERENCES

Bruce, R. B., Maynard, J. W. R., Jr., and Dunning, L. K., Oxyphenbutazone and phenylbutazone determination in plasma and urine by GLC, *J. Pharm. Sci.*, 63, 447, 1974.

Midha, K. K., McGilveray, I. J., and Charette, C., GLC determination of γ-hydroxyphenylbutazone in plasma, *J. Pharm. Sci.*, 63, 1751, 1974.

Midha, K. K., McGilveray, I. J., and Charette, C., GLC determination of plasma concentration of phenylbutazone and its metabolite oxyphenbutazone, *J. Pharm. Sci.*, 63, 1234, 1974.

PHOSPHORUS

PRINCIPLE

Volatilized phosphorus is trapped in silver nitrate, and its presence therein is indicated by reaction with ammonium molybdate.

TYPE B PROCEDURE

S. K. Niyogi

APPARATUS

1. Filter paper (Whatman #1)
2. Gas-washing unit as shown in Figure 1 (Corning No. 1760)
3. Glass wool
4. Steam bath
5. Hair dryer
6. Capillary tubes

REAGENTS

All chemicals should be analytical reagent grade.

1. Silver nitrate, saturated methanol solution
   Saturate 80% methanol with silver nitrate.
2. Phosphorus stock solution, 1 μg/μl
   Dissolve 100 mg of yellow phosphorus in 100 ml of absolute ethanol.
3. Phosphorus reference solutions, 0.2, 0.4, and 0.8 μg/ml
   Dilute 200, 400, and 800 μl of the phosphorus stock solution to 100 ml to obtain concentrations of 0.2, 0.4, and 0.8 μg/μl solution.
4. Basic lead acetate, saturated aqueous solution
5. Nitrogen gas
6. Chlorine gas
7. Ammonium molybdate solution
   Dissolve 5 g of ammonium molybdate in 100 ml of distilled water, then add 35 ml of concentrated nitric acid.
8. Benzidine, 50 mg/dl
   Add 10.0 ml of glacial acetic acid to 50 mg of benzidine, then dilute the mixture to 100 ml with distilled water.
9. Ammonium hydroxide, concentrated

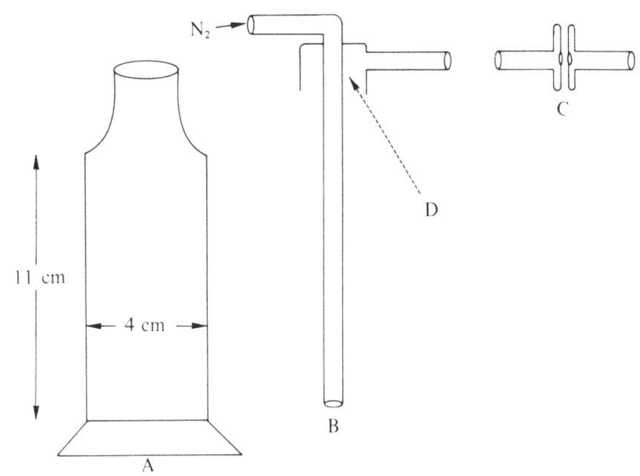

FIGURE 1. Gas-washing unit. (A) Glass jar. (B) Glass tube equipped with a head that fits into the neck of the jar A and a nitrogen input arm. (C) Paper holder with glass flanges measuring 2.5 cm in diameter and apertures 3.5 mm in diameter. Paper is held between the flanges by a pinch clamp (Arthur H. Thomas Co., Catalog No. 28). (D) Glass wool treated with basic lead acetate. Tygon plastic tubing (U.S. Stoneware, Inc., Akron, Ohio) is used for connections. The unit is similar to Corning No. 1760 (bottle, gash-washing, tall form, with T/S stopper).

PROCEDURE

1. Soak Whatman #1 filter paper in the silver nitrate solution and dry it. Cut circles 2.5 cm in diameter and insert one circular unit between the glass flanges of the paper holder (Figure 1C).
2. Place 5.0 ml of specimen (stomach content or blood) inside the jar (Figure 1A) and add 5.0 ml of water. Process 5.0 ml of each phosphorus reference solution in the same way.
3. Soak the glass wool with basic lead acetate

solution and dry it. Using forceps, pack the head of the tube (Figure 1B) with the impregnated glass wool.

4. Pass nitrogen through the jar (A) for a few seconds to eliminate any oxygen in the jar.
5. Put the tube (B) inside the jar (A) so that the lower end of the tube is below the diluted specimen.
6. Connect the paper holder (C) to the lower side arm of the tube (B) and place the jar (A) on top of a steam bath.
7. Connect nitrogen to the gas-input arm of the tube (B) and let it flow (150 bubbles/min) through the jar (A) for 30 min.
8. After 30 min remove the silver nitrate paper, which should show a dark gray stain if phosphorus is present. A low concentration gives a very faint stain.
9. Expose the paper to chlorine gas until the stain is completely decolorized.
10. Remove the excess chlorine from the paper by holding it in front of a stream of cold air flowing from the hair dryer.
11. Using a fine capillary tube, put a drop of ammonium molybdate solution on the area of the paper where the stain was seen. Wait 3 min.
12. Dry the paper by holding it in front of hot air from the hair dryer. Allow the paper to cool to room temperature.
13. Using a fine capillary tube, put a small drop of benzidine solution on the area of the paper where the stain was.
14. Expose the paper immediately to the fumes of ammonia.
15. Observe the spot for the appearance of a blue color.

CALCULATION

Compare the intensity of the blue color obtained from the specimen with the intensities obtained from the reference solutions.

INTERPRETATION (see p. 7)

The appearance of a blue color after the final step indicates the presence of phosphorus. Control stomach content gives a faint brownish-gray stain on the silver nitrate paper; no blue color is seen after final treatment of the paper upon exposure to ammonia fumes. If postmortem stomach content is old, it may give a very faint, transient blue color; this should not be considered an indication of the presence of phosphorus. Control blood samples tested by this method may give a very transient blue color due to a reaction of the natural constituents of blood.

A yellow-phosphorus dose of 50 mg or more is fatal.[2,3] In case of fatal phosphorus poisoning, either by yellow phosphorus or by zinc phosphide, the liver is the most appropriate organ to search for poison. This tissue can be analyzed in the same manner as the other biological samples.

ACCURACY AND PRECISION

The technique described can detect 20 μg of phosphorus in 100 ml of specimen.

INTERFERING SUBSTANCES

Arsine, zinc phosphide (rat poison), or phosphine liberated from putrified organs may interfere with this test. Arsine forms silver arsenide on the silver nitrate paper; silver arsenide, which is decolorized on exposure to chlorine gas, can be separated from silver phosphate by electrophoresis.[4] In the case of zinc phosphide poisoning, phosphine is liberated by nitrogen from zinc phosphide solution upon acidification and heating of the solution to 100°C. Phosphine liberation by nitrogen without acidification indicates yellow-phosphorus poisoning. To rule out the presence of zinc phosphide, add 10.0 ml of 0.5*N* sulfuric acid to the biological specimen, heat the jar to 100°C, then follow the procedure as described above. Phosphine liberated from putrified organs is difficult to interpret, since it may be due to bacterial reduction of phosphate and thus a false positive.

REFERENCES

1. **Curry, A. S.,** *Poison Detection in Human Organs,* 2nd ed., Charles C Thomas, Springfield, 1969, 137.
2. **Chernick, W. S.,** The ions: potassium, calcium, magnesium, fluoride, iodide, and others, in *Drill's Pharmacology in Medicine,* 3rd ed., DiPalma, J. R., Ed., McGraw-Hill, N.Y., 1965, 702.
3. **Dreisbach, R. H.,** *Poisoning: Diagnosis and Treatment,* 16th ed., Lange Medical Publications, Los Altos, Calif., 1969, 186.
4. **Curry, A. S., Rutter, E. R., and Lim, C. H.,** The detection of yellow phosphorus and phosphide in biological materials, *J. Pharm. Pharmacol.,* 10, 635, 1958.

POLYCHLORINATED BIPHENYLS (PCB)

PRINCIPLE

Polychlorinated biphenyls (PCB) can be extracted from a biological specimen with methylene chloride. After a clean-up procedure, the PCB can then be analyzed by electron-capture gas chromatography.

TYPE B PROCEDURE

Robert A. Maes

APPARATUS

1. Centrifuge bottles, conical, 250 ml
2. Centrifuge
3. Erlenmeyer flasks, 500 ml
4. Separatory funnels, 500 ml
5. Evaporator reduced pressure, rotary (Büchi)
6. Glass columns (35 cm × 6 mm i.d., without stopcock)
7. Syringes (Hamilton), 10 μl
8. Gas chromatograph (Varian Aerograph Model 1440), equipped with a nickel electron-capture detector, a 1 mV recorder (Varian Aerograph Model 25) with attached Disc integrator, and a glass column, 6′ × 1/8″ i.d., packed with 4% SE-30/6% QF-1 on Gas Chrom Q, 60 to 80 mesh, equipped with a Pyrex® injector insert proximal to the injection port which is silanized *in situ* with bistrimethylsilylacetamide. Condition the column for 24 hr at 230°C prior to its use.

Operating Conditions

Gas Flow Rate:
nitrogen (carrier gas) – 70 ml/min

Temperatures:
column – 200° C
injection port – 250° C
detector base – 250° C

REAGENTS

All chemicals should be analytical reagent grade.

1. Acetonitrile, Mallinckrodt Nanograde
2. Methylene chloride, Mallinckrodt Nanograde
3. Anhydrous sodium sulphate, Merck
4. Florisil® (Pennsylvania Glass Sand Corp., Pittsburgh). Activate by heating for 16 hr at 130°C.
5. PCB stock solution, 1 μg/ml
   Using *n*-hexane as the solvent, prepare stock solutions from either Aroclor 1254 or 1260 (Monsanto Chemical Company, U.S.A) or Phenoclor DP 6 (Prodelec, France).
6. PCB reference solutions
   Dilute each of the stock solutions with *n*-hexane to obtain the following concentrations: Aroclor 1254 or 1260, 0.01 and 0.05 μg/ml; Phenoclor DP 6, 0.1 and 0.5 μg/ml.

PROCEDURE

1. Transfer a 10-g sample of fecal matter or 10 ml of a 24-hr urine sample into a 250-ml centrifuge bottle.
2. Add approximately 25 ml of demineralized water and 150 ml of acetonitrile and shake for 1 min.
3. Centrifuge for 20 min at 1,500 rpm.
4. Decant the acetonitrile into a flask and discard.
5. Repeat the wash with 100 ml of acetonitrile, shake, centrifuge, decant, and discard the acetonitrile.
6. Measure the volume of the water layer, and transfer it to a 500-ml separatory funnel. Add an equal amount of methylene chloride.
7. Shake well and allow the mixture to settle for

15 min. Separate the lower methylene chloride layer. Save the aqueous layer.

8. Add 5 g of anhydrous sodium sulphate to the methylene chloride layer, and filter the dried methylene chloride through glass wool into a suitable container.
9. Reextract the aqueous layer (Step 8) with three more portions of methylene chloride, add each extract to the original methylene chloride extract. Evaporate the combined extracts to dryness in the Büchi evaporator under vacuum (30 mm Hg) in a bath at 50°C.
10. Dissolve the residue (Step 9) in 2 to 0.5 ml of *n*-hexane and pour the solution onto a column containing 2 g of Florisil® covered with 1 g of anhydrous sodium sulphate.
11. Elute any adsorbed PCB from the column with 7 ml of *n*-hexane.
12. Evaporate the *n*-hexane eluate to dryness in the Büchi evaporator and dissolve the residue in 0.5 ml of *n*-hexane.
13. Inject 5 μl of the *n*-hexane solution into the gas chromatograph, making sure that the operating conditions stated above are met.

CALCULATION

Identification is carried out by comparing the retention time of the sample's peaks with those of the reference peaks. Quantitative results are obtained by comparing the height of the most prominent peak in the sample with its analogue in the chromatogram of the reference solutions. Determine the concentration of PCB in the specimen by the following formula:

$$C_x = \frac{C_s \times H_x}{20 \times H_s}$$

where

C_x = concentration of PCB in the specimen;
C_s = concentration of the PCB in the reference solution;
H_x = peak height obtained from the specimen;
H_s = peak height from the reference solution.

INTERPRETATION (see p. 7)

The FDA has not yet established tolerance levels for PCB. It is suggested that 150 to 300 μg/day would be within the safe range as far as temporary dietary intake is concerned.

RECOVERY AND SENSITIVITY

Using the procedure above, the average recovery of PCB from samples of urine and fecal matter to which PCB has been added at a concentration of 0.1 μg/ml is 73%. Sensitivity for the determination is 0.001 μg/ml. Because of the change in the standing current of the electron-capture detector after prolonged use, reference samples must be analyzed with each injection.

INTERFERING SUBSTANCES

No significant gas-chromatographic response is observed from normal urine or fecal matter.

REFERENCES

Price, N. O., Young, R. W., and Dickinson, J. K., Pesticide residues and polychlorinated biphenyls levels in diets, urine and fecal matter of preadolescent girls (36347), *Proc. Soc. Exp. Biol. Med.,* 139, 1280, 1972.

Reynolds, L. M., Pesticide residue analyses in the presence of polychlorobiphenyls (PCB's), *Residue Rev.,* 34, 27, 1971.

Samuel, B. L., An improved screening method for chlorinated and thiophosphate organic insecticides in foods and feeds, *J. Assoc. Anal. Chem.,* 49, 346, 1966.

PRIMIDONE

PRINCIPLE

This procedure describes a method to rapidly determine the presence and concentration of primidone, diphenylhydantoin, and phenobarbital in biological fluids. The drugs are extracted from the sample with toluene. The toluene is then extracted with a methanolic solution of trimethylanilinium hydroxide (TMAH), which, upon injection into a gas chromatograph, produces the corresponding methylated derivatives of the anticonvulsants. The peaks produced are used for identification and quantitation of the drugs.

TYPE C PROCEDURE

Vijay Aggarwal, Michael McGee, and Irving Sunshine

APPARATUS

1. Culture tubes with Teflon® lined screw caps (Kimax #45066A)
2. Concentratubes®*
3. Vortex mixer (Scientific Industries Model IC-500J)
4. 10 μl syringe, Hamilton #701
5. 100 μl syringe, Hamilton #710
6. Gas chromatograph (Hewlett-Packard Model #7621) with dual flame ionization detectors, equipped with 6′ × 1/8″ i.d. stainless steel columns packed with 10% UCW-98 on 80/100 mesh Chromosorb W,HP, an integrator (Hewlett-Packard Model #3373) and a recorder (Hewlett-Packard Model #7127a)

Operating Conditions

Gas Flow Rates:
- helium – 30 ml/min
- hydrogen – 30 ml/min
- air – 400 ml/min

Temperatures:
- injection port – 260 °C
- detector – 290 °C
- oven – 235 °C

REAGENTS

All chemicals should be analytical reagent grade.

1. Phosphoric acid, 0.2*M*
   Dilute 1.15 ml of 85% H_3PO_4 to 100 ml with distilled water.
2. Trimethylanilinium hydroxide, (TMAH), 1.8*M*
   Mix 7.0 grams of trimethylphenyl ammonium iodide (Aldrich Chem. #13,914-9) with 10 ml of methanol contained in a 25 × 125 mm culture tube with Teflon®-lined screw cap. Add 3.6 g of silver oxide, cap, and shake for 2 min. Rotate on a mechanical rotator for 4 hr and centrifuge. The supernatant is decanted and stored at 20 °C. The solution is stable for at least 4 weeks.
3. Internal standard stock solution, 50 mg/dl
   Dissolve 50 mg of secobarbital in 100 ml of toluene.
4. Internal standard solution, 0.5 mg/dl
   Dilute 10.0 ml of the internal standard stock solution to 1000 ml with toluene.
5. Anticonvulsant stock solution, 50 mg/dl
   Transfer 50 mg each of primidone, phenobarbital, and diphenylhydantoin to a 100-ml volumetric flask. Add enough ethanol to dissolve the drugs and then dilute to 100 ml with

*Laboratory Research Co., P.O. Box 36509, Los Angeles, Calif. 90036.

Table 1

Drug	RT (min)	RRT*
N-Methyl-α-phenylbutyramide (EP)†	1.48	0.62
Secobarbital	2.39	1.00
Phenobarbital	3.82	1.60
Primidone	5.51	2.31
Diphenylhydantoin	9.60	4.01

* Retention time relative to secobarbital.
† Decomposition product of phenobarbital.

distilled water. The solution is stable for several months when stored at 4°C.

6. Anticonvulsant control solution, 2.0 mg/dl Dilute to 4.0 ml of the anticonvulsant stock solution to 100 ml with distilled water.
7. Anticonvulsant reference solution, 2.0 mg/dl Dilute 4.0 ml of the anticonvulsant stock solution to 100 ml with drug-free plasma or blood.

PROCEDURE

1. To 2.0 ml of sample (blood, plasma, urine, or reference solution) in a 16 X 100 mm screw-capped culture tube, add 1.0 ml of 0.2*M* phosphoric acid and 5.0 ml of the internal standard solution. Shake gently by hand for 2 min and centrifuge to separate phases.
2. Transfer approximately 4 ml of the toluene layer to a Concentratube®* using a Pasteur pipet. (Quantitative transfer is not necessary due to the internal standard in the toluene.) This extract may be stored several days without loss of accuracy.
3. While vortexing the Concentratube®, add 35 μl of the TMAH using a 100-μl syringe. Vortex for a total of 15 sec. Centrifuge the Concentratube® for 10 min to concentrate the TMAH in the tip of the tube.
4. With the chromatograph at 235°C, inject a 3-μl aliquot of the TMAH layer over a 10-sec interval. This slow injection is necessary as rapid injection of the TMAH solution will result in severe tailing of the solvent on some instruments. Figure 1 shows a chromatogram of a 2.0 mg/dl mixture of phenobarbital, primidone, and diphenylhydantoin. Table 1 lists the retention times of these compounds.

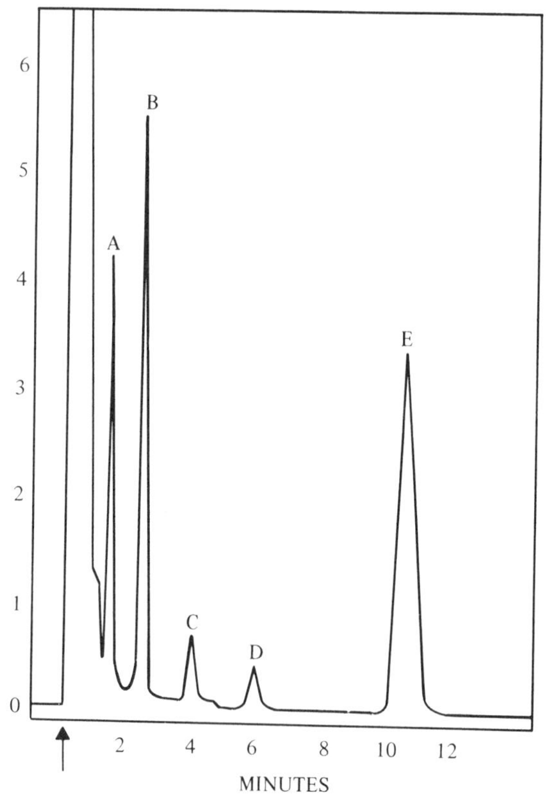

FIGURE 1. Chromatogram of a mixture of anticonvulants. (A) *N*-Methyl-α-phenylbutyramide (EP); (B) Secobarbital; (C) Phenobarbital; (D) Primidone; (E) Diphenylhydantoin. (From Osiewicz, R., Aggarwal, V., Young, R., and Sunshine, I., The quantitative analysis of phenobarbital with trimethylanilinium hydroxide, *J. Chromatogr.*, 88, 157, 1974. With permission.)

CALCULATION

The calculation of drug concentration may be done with either peak height or area data and the following formula:

*A test tube which contains approximately 20 ml and tapers to a sharp tip which contains approximately 10 μl.

$$C_U = C_s \times \frac{P_U}{I_U} \times \frac{I_s}{P_s}$$

where:

C_u = concentration of drug in sample;
C_s = concentration of drug in standard solution (2.0 mg/dl);
P_u = peak height or area of drug in sample;
I_u = peak height or area of secobarbital internal standard in the sample;
P_s = peak height or area of drug in the standard;
I_s = peak height or area of secobarbital internal standard in the standard.

INTERPRETATION (see p. 7)

Primidone is metabolized in man to phenobarbital and phenylethylmalonamide (PEMA). Thus, in cases where phenobarbital and primidone are administered concurrently, elevated levels of phenobarbital may be expected. Booker et al.[1] have reported that in well controlled epileptic patients, serum levels of primidone average 0.76 mg/dl. In the same study, phenobarbital levels averaged 4.4 mg/dl and dilantin levels averaged 1.2 mg/dl. Bailey and Jatlow[2] reported an apparent attempted primidone suicide in which blood levels of primidone reached 17.5 mg/dl and phenobarbital levels reached 2.5 mg/dl.

ACCURACY AND PRECISION

Peak area ratios of phenobarbital or Dilantin® to the internal standard are a linear function of concentration from 0.1 to 8.0 mg/dl. Peak area ratios of primidone to the internal standard are a linear function of concentration from 0.2 to at least 5.0 mg/dl. The coefficient of variation for replicate analyses of 1.0 mg/dl reference solutions is 3%.

INTERFERING SUBSTANCES

The peaks for phenobarbital, primidone, and dilantin are well resolved from common acidic drugs with the exception of glutethimide which has a retention time very close to that of phenobarbital. Osiewicz et al.[3] have shown, however, that the decomposition peak from phenobarbital (peak A in Figure 1) is a linear function of phenobarbital concentration and can thus be used to quantitate phenobarbital in the presence of glutethimide. Mephobarbital and phenobarbital yield the same derivatives and therefore cannot be differentiated by this method. The metabolism of primidone to PEMA does not interfere in the determination of primidone since PEMA is not extracted.

REFERENCES

1. **Booker, H. E., et al.**, A clinical study of serum primidone levels, *Epilepsia*, 11, 395, 1970.
2. **Bailey, D., and Jatlow, P.**, Chemical analysis of massive crystalluria following primidone overdose, *Am. J. Clin. Pathol.*, 58, 583, 1972.
3. **Osiewicz, R., Aggarwal, V., Young, R., and Sunshine, I.**, The quantitative analysis of phenobarbital with trimethylanilinium hydroxide, *J. Chromatogr.*, 88, 157, 1974.

GENERAL REFERENCES

Beam, R. E., Broad spectrum simultaneous GC assay of nonderivatized antiepileptic drugs, *Am. J. Med. Technol.*, 40, 211, 1974.

Booker, H. E., Primidone toxicity, in *Antiepileptic Drugs*, Woodbury, D. M., et al., Ed., Raven Press, N.Y., 1972.

Kuth, H., Pharmacodynamic and pharmacakinetic measurements of antiepileptic drugs, *Clin. Pharmacol. Ther.*, 16, 243, 1974.

Kupferberg, H. J., Quantitative estimation of diphenylhydantoin, primidone and phenobarbital in plasma by gas-liquid chromatography, *Clin. Chim. Acta*, 29, 283, 1970.

Solow, E. B., Metaxas, J. M., and Summers, T. R., Antiepileptic drugs: a current assessment of simultaneous determination of multiple drug therapy by gas liquid chromatography-on column methylation, *J. Chromatogr. Sci.*, 12, 256, 1974.

PROCAINE AMIDE HYDROCHLORIDE

PRINCIPLE

The drug is extracted from an alkalinized sample by an organic solvent. The extract may be concentrated and analyzed by gas chromatography (Procedure C) or it may be shaken with dilute acid which will remove the drug from the organic extract. The acid solution may be examined spectrophotometrically to identify the procaine amide (Procedure A).

TYPE A PROCEDURE

Frank E. Barnhardt

APPARATUS

1. pH paper (Hydrion) or pH meter
2. Extraction glassware
3. Graduate cylinders, 50 ml, glass-stoppered
4. Cuvettes, quartz or fused silica, 10-mm light path
5. Spectrophotometer, ratio-recording, with linear absorbance presentation

REAGENTS

All chemicals should be analytical reagent grade.

1. Sodium hydroxide, saturated aqueous solution, 19*M*
2. Procaine amide stock solution, 20.0 mg/100 cc
   Dissolve 231.5 mg of procaine amide hydrochloride in water and dilute to 1,000 ml.
3. Procaine amide control solution, 1.00 mg/100 ml
   Dilute 10.0 cc of procaine amide stock solution to 200 ml with water.
4. Dichloromethane/isopropyl alcohol 4:1 (v/v)
5. Sulfuric acid, 0.5*N*
   Dilute 14.0 ml of concentrated sulfuric to 1,000 ml with water.
6. Ammonium hydroxide, concentrated

PROCEDURE

1. To a separatory funnel, add 4 drops of saturated sodium hydroxide and 5.0 ml of sample (blood, control solution, and water as a blank). Test the mixture for alkalinity, using pH paper or a pH meter. Add more sodium hydroxide, if necessary, to obtain a pH of 10.
2. Extract each sample with 50 ml of dichloromethane/isopropyl alcohol (4:1) by shaking the mixture for 5 min. Allow the organic solvent and aqueous phases to separate completely.
3. With care, filter each solvent phase through Whatman #41 filter paper into a clean glass-stoppered graduate cylinder. Collect 40 ml.
4. Reextract the 40-ml aliquot with 5.0 ml of 0.5*N* sulfuric acid. Shake the cylinder for 5 min to insure complete extraction of the procaine amide from the solvent to the acid layer.
5. Allow the phases to separate and transfer the acid layer to a suitable test tube. Centrifuge and transfer 3.0 ml to a clean quartz or fused silica cuvette.
6. Determine the absorbance of the acidic phase from 190 to 390 nm. Use 0.5*N* sulfuric acid as the reference solution. This is the background curve.
7. To each cuvette add 0.5 ml of concentrated ammonium hydroxide, mix well, and let stand for 2 min. Determine the absorbance of the alkaline solution from 190 to 390 nm, using the processed water sample as the reference solution. Note the absorbance from 270 to 275 nm. This reflects the procaine amide level.

CALCULATION

$$\frac{A}{B} \times C_s = C_u$$

where

A = Difference in absorbance at 272 nm between the acid and alkaline curves for the unknown sample;
B = difference in absorbance at 272 nm between the acid and alkaline curve for the procaine amide control solution;
C_s = concentration of the procaine amide control solution in mg/100 cc;
C_u = concentration of procaine amide in the unknown blood in mg/100 cc.

INTERPRETATION (see p. 7)

The effective blood concentration following the therapeutic dose of 500 mg q.i.d. is 0.4 to 0.6 mg/100 ml. Concentrations above 0.7 mg/100 ml can produce adverse cardiovascular effects.

ACCURACY, PRECISION, AND SENSITIVITY

Data obtained using this procedure are comparable to those obtained by a commonly used colorimetric procedure (Table 1). This procedure is sensitive to 0.2μg/cc (0.02 mg/100 cc). The UV spectrum of procaine amide is shown in Figure 1. Drug interference can occur from those substances whose UV absorbance is similar to that of procaine amide.

Table 1

METHOD COMPARISON STUDY

	Colorimetric[1,2]	UV
1	0.70 mg/dl	0.66 mg/dl
2	0.90 mg/dl	0.92 mg/dl
3	0.19 mg/dl	0.14 mg/dl
4	0.86 mg/dl	0.64 mg/dl
5	0.05 mg/dl	0.02 mg/dl
6	1.10 mg/dl	1.20 mg/dl

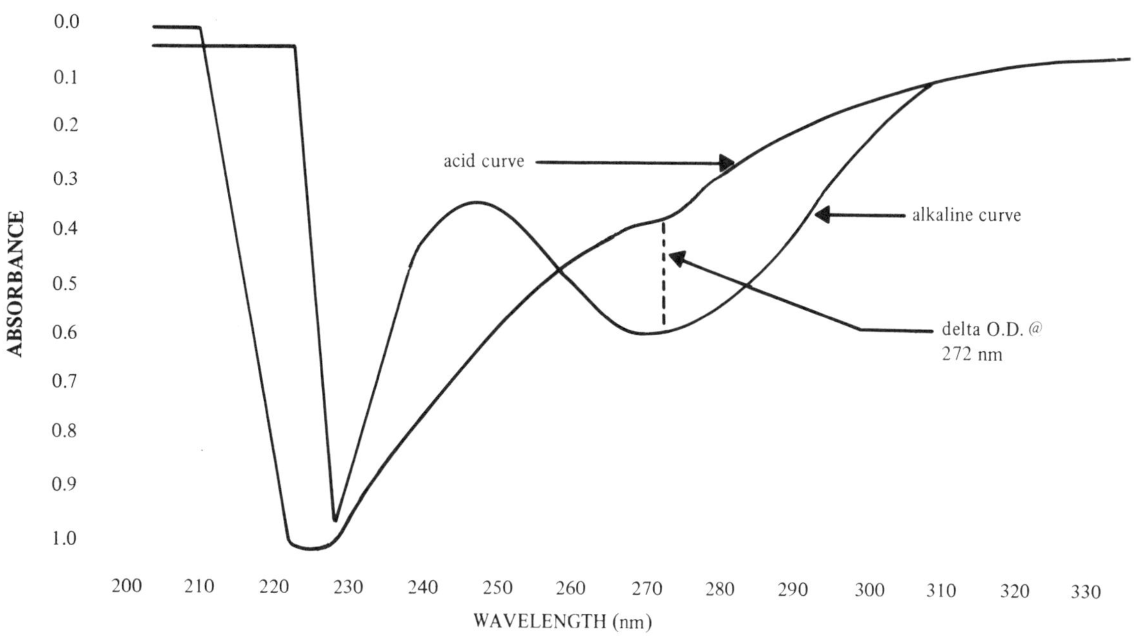

FIGURE 1. UV spectrum of procaine amide.

REFERENCES

1. **Mark, L. C., Kayden, H. J., Steele, J. M., et al.,** The physiological disposition and cardiac effects of procaine amide, *J. Pharmacol. Exp. Ther.*, 102, 5, 18, 1951.
2. **Koch-Weser, J., Klein, S. W., et al.,** Antiarrhythmic prophylaxis with procainamide in acute myocardial infarction, *N. Engl. J. Med.*, 281, 1253, 1969.

GENERAL REFERENCES*

Clarke, E. G. C., *Isolation and Identification of Drugs in Pharmaceuticals; Body Fluids and Postmortem Material,* Pharmaceutical Press, 1969, 512.

Hayes, A. H., Jr., Pharmacodynamic and pharmacokinetic measurements in cardiovascular-renal drugs, *Clin. Pharmacol. Ther.*, 16, 201, 1974.

TYPE C PROCEDURE[1]

John M. Meola

APPARATUS

1. 15-ml glass-stoppered tubes
2. 1 and 2 ml pipets
3. Small glass tubes, e.g., Kimble 75 × 2 mm
4. Centrifuge
5. Vortex mixer
6. Manifold connected to a supply of compressed air for evaporation
7. Gas chromatograph (Perkin-Elmer Model 900) with FID and Model 56 Recorder with a glass column 6′ × 0.08″ i.d. and 6′ × ¼″ o.d. packed with 0.2% OV-17 on Corning GLC 110 textured glass beads 100 to 200 mesh (The OV-17 liquid phase was stabilized by the addition of 0.2% Silanox.)

Operating Conditions

Gas Flow Rate:
nitrogen – 20 ml/min

Temperatures:
column – 250°C
injection port – 270°C
detector – 285°C

REAGENTS

All chemicals should be analytical reagent grade.

1. Norit®A, neutral charcoal†
2. Chloroform, Mallinckrodt® analytical grade
3. Bicarbonate, carbonate buffer, pH 11.0
   To a one-liter volumetric flask containing about 600 ml of distilled water, add 21.0 g of sodium carbonate (Na_2CO_3) and 420 mg of sodium bicarbonate. Mix well to dissolve, check the pH and adjust, if necessary, to 11.0 ± 0.1 with 2*N* NaOH or 2*N* HCl. Dilute to one liter with water and mix well. Store at 4°C.
4. Stock procaine amide solution, 100 mg/dl (as free base)
   Dissolve 28.75 mg procaine amide hydrochloride‡ in distilled water and dilute to 25 ml with water. When stored at 4°C this solution is stable for 6 weeks.
5. Procaine amide working standard, 0.5, 1.0, 1.5, and 2.0 mg/dl
   Dilute 0.5, 1.0, and 1.5 ml of procaine amide stock solution, respectively, to 100 ml with distilled water.
6. Librium®‡ stock solution for internal standard
   Transfer 10 mg of Librium® to a 25-ml volumetric flask containing 2 ml of 1*N* hydrochloric acid. Dilute to volume with distilled water. Store at 4°C.
7. Librium® working solution
   Transfer 5.0 ml of Librium® stock solution to a 100-ml volumetric flask and dilute to volume with distilled water.

*For an updated list of reference material, see General References, p. 319.
†Amend Drug and Chemical Co., Irvington, N.J. 07111.
‡E. R. Squibb and Sons, Inc., Princeton, N.J. 08540.
‡Hoffman-La Roche, Inc., Notley, N.J. 07110.

PROCEDURE[2,3]

1. Transfer 1 ml of serum and 1 ml of distilled water to a 15-ml glass-stoppered centrifuge tube. Add 1 ml of the internal standard Librium® working solution and 2 ml of carbonate-bicarbonate buffer. Add 5 mg of Norit® A neutral charcoal.
2. Standards are prepared by adding 1 ml of each working standard to 1 ml of drug-free serum or reconstituted serum (Hyland Normal) and proceeding as directed for serum samples under Step 1, except that the addition of 1 ml of distilled water is omitted.
3. Mix briefly on a Vortex mixer. Centrifuge at 2,000 × g for 4 min. Remove and discard the supernatant by aspiration.
4. Disperse charcoal over the wall of the tube using a Vortex mixer to insure maximum dispersion.
5. Add 2 ml of chloroform and extract the charcoal (shake tube contents vigorously).
6. Decant solvent into a small glass tube and evaporate it to dryness at room temperature using compressed air.
7. Dissolve the residue in 20 µl of chloroform and inject 1 µl into the gas chromatograph.
8. Measure the peak heights of the internal standard and procaine amide for both the serum samples and standards.
9. Determine the ratio of the peak height of the standard to that of the internal standard (S_r).
10. Determine the ratio of the peak height of the serum to that of internal standard (S_s).

CALCULATION

1. Plot the S_r values against their respective concentrations to form a standard curve.
2. Calculate the respective concentration of each serum sample by comparing S_s with the reference curve.

INTERPRETATION (see p. 7)

Plasma concentrations ranging from 5 to 10 µg/ml are considered optimal for procaine amide therapy.

SENSITIVITY AND PRECISION

The sensitivity for procaine amide is 5 µg/ml. The precision of the procedure was studied at 5 and 10 µg/ml. The CV at 5 µg/ml is 12% and at 10 µg/ml is 6%.

REFERENCES

1. **Atkinson, A. J.,** Rapid gas chromatographic measurement of plasma procainamide concentration, *Clin. Chem.*, 18, 643, 1972.
2. **Meola, J. and Vanko, M.,** A simple system for drug analysis, *Clin. Chem.*, 17, 556, 1971.
3. **Meola, J. and Vanko, M.,** The use of charcoal in the qualitative and quantitative analysis of drugs, *Clin. Chem.*, 18, 579, 1972.

GENERAL REFERENCES

Gly, G. O., et al., Plasma concentrations of procainamide and prevalence of exertional arrhythmias, *Ann. Int. Med.*, 80, 78, 1974.

Hayes, A. H., Jr., Pharmacodynamic and pharmacokinetic measurements in cardiovascular-renal drugs, *Clin. Pharmacol. Ther.*, 16, 201, 1974.

Koch-Weser, J. and Klein, S. W., Procainamide dosage schedules, plasma concentrations and clinical effects, *JAMA*, 215, 1454, 1971.

PROPOXYPHENE

PRINCIPLE

Acid refluxing of propoxyphene hydrolyzes the propionate ester linkage and subsequently dehydrates this intermediate. A conjugated product with a much higher absorptivity than propoxyphene is formed (Procedure A); this product lends itself to UV quantitation. Procedure B is a sensitive and specific UV spectrophotometric method for the determination of propoxyphene. The drug is extracted from acid-hydrolyzed tissue, and the UV spectrum is determined for the hydrolyzed product. Following UV irradiation, the UV spectrum is again determined. The spectrum thus produced is specific for propoxyphene. The absorbance difference at 255 nm between the irradiated and unirradiated solution is proportional to the propoxyphene concentration. The absorbance of the acid-hydrolyzed compound is about 30 times greater than that of propoxyphene, and irradiation increases the absorbance to about 80 times that of propoxyphene. In Procedure C propoxyphene is extracted from alkaline media into an organic solvent. In order to isolate the drug from neutral organic compounds and biological artifacts, it is back-extracted into dilute acid and then again into solvent. The final extract is concentrated and analyzed by gas chromatography, using a parallel standard as a reference for identification and quantitative calculation.

TYPE A PROCEDURE

Robert H. Cravey

APPARATUS

1. Separatory funnels, 500 ml
2. Graduated cylinders, 250 ml
3. Round-bottom flasks with standard taper ground-glass necks, 500 ml
4. Reflux condenser
5. Steam-distillation assembly
6. UV spectrophotometer

REAGENTS

All chemicals should be analytical reagent grade.

1. Propoxyphene hydrochloride stock solution, 20 mg/100 ml
   Dissolve 20 mg of propoxyphene hydrochloride in water and dilute to 100 ml.
2. Propoxyphene hydrochloride reference solution, 2 mg/100 ml
   Dilute 10.0 ml of the propoxyphene hydrochloride stock solution to 100 ml with water.
3. Sodium hydroxide, 5*N*
   Dissolve 200 g of sodium hydroxide in water and dilute to one liter.
4. Ether
5. Hydrochloric acid, 0.5*N*
   Dilute 10.0 ml of concentrated hydrochloric acid to 250 ml with water.
6. Hydrochloric acid, concentrated

PROCEDURE[1]

1. Place 10.0 ml of specimen (blood, serum, urine, or 10 g of homogenized tissue) in a 500-ml separatory funnel. Adjust the pH to 9.5 to 10 with 5*N* sodium hydroxide. Process 10.0 ml of the reference solution and 10.0 ml of water for a reagent blank in the same manner as the specimen.
2. Add 200 ml of ether and shake the mixture for 5 min. Remove and discard the aqueous layer.
3. Transfer the ether to a graduated cylinder by filtering it through Whatman #541 filter paper. Record the volume recovered.
4. Add 5.0 ml of 0.5*N* hydrochloric acid to the

ether and shake the mixture for 3 min. Allow the organic and aqueous phases to separate.

5. Place 4.0 ml of the aqueous phase in a 500-ml round-bottom flask with standard taper ground-glass neck. Add 6.0 ml of concentrated hydrochloric acid.
6. Attach the flask to a water-cooled reflux condenser and reflux the mixture for 20 min.
7. Allow the flask contents to cool, adjust the pH to 7.5 to 8.0, then steam-distill the mixture.
8. Determine the absorbance at 254 nm of the distillate which contains the propoxyphene reaction product. Use the distillate obtained by processing the water sample as the reference solution.
9. Compare the absorbance of the distillate obtained from the specimen with the absorbance obtained from the propoxyphene hydrochloride reference solution.

CALCULATION

Determine the propoxyphene concentration in the specimen by the following formula:

$$\frac{A_S}{A_R} \times C_R = C_S,$$

where

A_S = absorbance of the specimen at 254 nm;
A_R = absorbance of the reference solution at 254 mn;
C_R = propoxyphene hydrochloride concentration of the reference solution;
C_S = propoxyphene hydrochloride concentration of the specimen.

INTERPRETATION (see p. 7)

Plasma concentrations reach a maximum of 0.02 mg/dl in 1 hr following a 195-mg oral dose and 0.03 mg/dl in 30 min after a 50-mg intravenous dose.[2] Plasma concentrations reach a maximum of 0.03 mg/dl following the administration of 13 oral doses of 65 mg of the propoxyphene hydrochloride or 100 mg of the newer propoxyphene napsylate.[3] In fatal poisonings, concentrations of at least 0.2 mg/dl of blood and 3 ml/100 g of liver are attained. Where death has been attributed to propoxyphene, the blood levels have a range of 0.2 to 2.0 mg/dl, with the majority from 0.5 to 0.7 mg/dl. Liver concentrations have a range of 1.5 to 30 mg/100 g, with a majority from 5 to 13 mg/100 g. A high concentration in the liver might be indicative of chronic use of the drug.

ACCURACY AND PRECISION

The relationship between the concentration of propoxyphene and the absorbance of the reaction product is linear over the range from 0 to 50 μg/ml.

INTERFERING SUBSTANCES

No substance has been found that interferes with this method.

REFERENCES*

1. **Wallace, J. E., et al.,** A rapid and specific spectrophotometric method for determining propoxyphene, *J. Forensic Sci.*, 10, 179, 1965.
2. **Walen, R. L., Gruber, C. M., Kiplinger, G. F., and Scholz, N. E.,** Concentration of propoxyphene in human plasma following oral, intramuscular, and intravenous administration, *Toxicol. Appl. Pharmacol.*, 19, 480, 1971.
3. **Walen, R. L., Gruber, C. M., Kiplinger, G. F., and Scholz, N. E.,** Concentration of propoxyphene in human plasma following repeated oral doses, *Toxicol. Appl. Pharmacol.*, 19, 493, 1971.

GENERAL REFERENCES

Maxwell, S. B., personal communication, 1968.
McBay, A. J., Fatal Propoxyphene poisoning, *Bull. Int. Assoc. Forensic Toxicol.*, (Home Office Research Laboratory, Aldermaston, England), 3, 2, 1966.
Orange County, California, Coroner's Laboratory, Case #69-2494.

*For an updated list of reference material, see References, p. 327.

TYPE B PROCEDURE[1]

Arthur J. McBay

APPARATUS

1. Separatory funnels, 500 ml
2. Graduated cylinders, 250 and 10 ml
3. Glass funnels, small
4. Glass-stoppered Erlenmeyer flask, 500 ml
5. Filter paper, Whatman #1
6. Filter paper, Whatman #5
7. Recording UV spectrophotometer
8. UV light source, 257.3 nm
9. Water bath
10. Test tubes, 60 ml

REAGENTS

All chemicals should be analytical reagent grade.

1. Propoxyphene hydrochloride stock solution, 100 mg/dl
   Dissolve 100 mg of propoxyphene hydrochloride in water and dilute to 100 ml.
2. Propoxyphene hydrochloride working reference solutions, 10 and 1 mg/dl
   Dilute 10 ml of the stock solution to 100 ml. Dilute 10 ml of this solution to 100 ml (1 mg/100 ml).
3. Hydrochloric acid, concentrated
4. Sodium hydroxide, 50%
   Dissolve 50 g in water and dilute to 100 g with water.
5. Diethyl ether
6. Sodium sulfate, anhydrous

PROCEDURE

1. Place 10 ml of sample (blood, urine, gastric content, 10 g of homogenized tissue plus 10 ml of water, and working reference solutions) and 15 ml of concentrated hydrochloric acid in a 60-ml test tube. Heat the mixture in a boiling water bath for 20 min with occasional stirring.
2. Cool the test tube and transfer the contents to a 500-ml glass-stoppered Erlenmeyer flask. Add 15 ml of 50% sodium hydroxide solution.
3. After cooling the contents of the flask to room temperature, add 150 ml of ether and shake the mixture vigorously. Remove the ether layer and filter through dry Whatman #1 filter paper.
4. Shake the ether filtrate vigorously with 10 ml of water. Remove the water and discard. Filter the ether layer through dry Whatman #1 filter paper.
5. Add 5 ml of 0.2*N* hydrochloric acid to 100 ml of the filtrate and shake the mixture vigorously. Remove the aqueous layer and filter through water-washed Whatman #5 filter paper.
6. Determine the absorbance of the acid solution from 220 to 310 nm, using 0.2*N* hydrochloric acid as the reference solution. A broad peak at 255 nm could indicate the presence of propoxyphene. If the absorbance of the peak at 255 nm exceeds 0.3, dilute the solution with 0.2*N* hydrochloric acid so that the resulting solution has an absorbance of about 0.3.
7. Simultaneously irradiate each solution, the unknown and the working reference, for 5 min in quartz cuvettes placed a few millimeters from a 257.3 nm UV light. Determine the absorbances of the solutions from 220 to 310 nm, using 0.2*N* hydrochloric acid as the reference solution.
8. Compare the resulting UV absorption spectrum with that of a working reference solution. Acid-hydrolyzed UV irradiated propoxyphene has a sharp maximum at 255 nm with a shoulder at 247 nm and minor peaks at 277, 287, and 298 nm (Figure 1).

CALCULATION

Determine the propoxyphene concentration in the specimen by the following formula:

$$\frac{A_{S2} - A_{S1}}{A_{R2} - A_{R1}} \times C_R = C_S$$

where

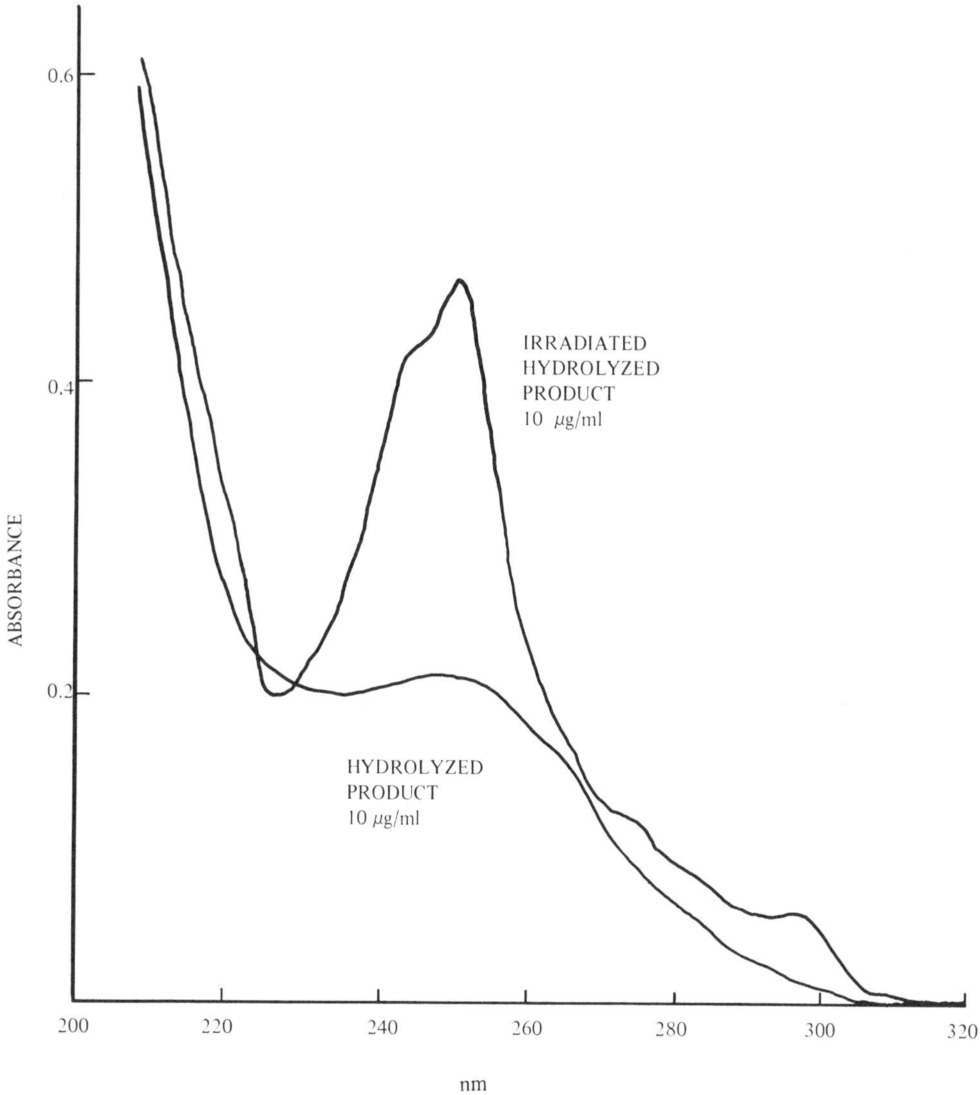

FIGURE 1. UV absorption spectra, the hydrolyzed product, and the irradiated hydrolyzed product of propoxyphene. (From McBay, A. J., Turk, R. F., Corbett, B. W., and Hudson, P., Determination of propoxyphene in biological materials, *J. Forensic Sci.*, 19(1), 84, 1974. With permission.)

A_{S1} = absorbance of specimen at 255 nm before irradiation;
A_{S2} = absorbance of specimen at 255 nm after irradiation;
A_{R1} = absorbance of working reference at 255 nm before irradiation;
A_{R2} = absorbance of working reference at 255 nm after irradiation;
C_R = propoxyphene concentration of the reference solution;
C_S = propoxyphene concentration of the specimen.

INTERPRETATION (see p. 7)

Plasma concentrations reach a maximum of 0.02 mg/dl in 1 hr following a 195-mg oral dose and 0.03 mg/dl in 30 min after a 50-mg intravenous dose.[2] Plasma concentrations reach a maximum of 0.03 mg/dl following the administration of 13 oral doses of 65 mg of the propoxyphene hydrochloride or 100 mg of the newer propoxyphene napsylate.[3] In fatal poisonings, concentrations of at least 0.2 mg/dl of blood and 3 ml/100 g of liver are attained. Where death has been attributed to propoxyphene, the blood levels have a range of 0.2 to 2.0 mg/dl, with the majority from 0.5 to 0.7 mg/dl. Liver concentrations have a range of 1.5 to 30 mg/100 g, with a majority from 5 to 13 mg/100 g. A high concentration in the liver might be indicative of chronic use of the drug.

INTERFERING SUBSTANCES

In order to establish which drugs might interfere with this method of propoxyphene determination, the compounds discussed hereafter were subjected to the hydrolysis and UV irradiation procedure. Ultraviolet spectra were determined for each of the compounds in acid solution after hydrolysis and UV irradiation of the hydrolyzed solution. Compounds showing no significant UV spectral changes included ephedrine, imipramine, meperidine, methaqualone, pentazocine, and phenylephrine. The following drugs had spectral changes which do not interefere with the quantitation of propoxyphene when their spectra are properly interpreted, as explained below.

Amitriptyline: Hydrolysis caused no spectral change. UV irradiation of the hydrolyzed solution causes a slight decrease in absorbance at 245 nm and a slight increase at 275 nm.

Chlordiazepoxide: Hydrolysis reduces the maxima at 250 and 312 nm. UV irradiation does not cause any further change.

Diazepam: Hydrolysis reduces the maxima at 245 and 288 nm to a shallow curve from 250 to 320 nm. UV irradiation does not cuase any further change.

Methadone: Hydrolysis does not change the normal absorbance spectrum; thus, propoxyphene and methadone are readily distinguishable by the comparison of the spectra of their hydrolysis products. UV irradiation of hydrolyzed methadone yields an increase in absorbance at 255 nm similar to that of propoxyphene. These spectra are also readily differentiated because methadone does not have a minimum before the peak at 255 nm, nor shoulders at 278, 287, and 298 nm. Instead, methadone has a broad peak extending from 280 through 300 nm.

REFERENCES

1. **McBay, A. J., Turk, R. F., Corbett, B. A., and Hudson, P.,** Determination of propoxyphene in biological materials, *J. Forensic Sci.*, 19, 81, 1974.
2. **Wolen, R. L., Gruber, C. M., Kiplinger, G. F., and Scholz, N. E.,** Concentration of propoxyphene in human plasma following oral, intramuscular, and intravenous administration, *Toxicol. Appl. Pharmacol.*, 19, 480, 1971.
3. **Wolen, R. L., Gruber, C. M., Kiplinger, G. F., and Scholz, N. E.,** Concentration of propoxyphene in human plasma following repeated oral doses, *Toxicol. Appl. Pharmacol.*, 19, 493, 1971.

GENERAL REFERENCES*

Cravey, R. H., Shaw, R. F., and Nakomura, G. R., Incidence of propoxyphene poisoning: A report of fatal cases, *J. Forensic Sci.*, 19, 72, 1974.

Evenson, M. A. and Koellner, S., Rapid method for quantitative determination of propoxyphene in serum by gas-liquid chromatography, *Clin. Chem.*, 19, 492, 1973.

Sturner, W. Q. and Garriott, S. C., Deaths involving propoxyphene, *JAMA*, 223, 1125, 1973.

Valentour, J. C., Monforte, J. R., and Sunshine, I., Fluorometric determination of propoxyphene, *Clin. Chem.*, 20, 275, 1974.

TYPE C PROCEDURE

Bryan S. Finkle

APPARATUS

1. Centrifuge tubes, ground-glass-stoppered, 15 ml
2. Separatory funnels, 30 ml
3. Beakers, 50 ml
4. Conical evaporating tubes, disposable, 2 ml (Cut Pasteur pipet to the desired lengths and seal the tips.)
5. Beakers, 10 ml
6. Gas chromatograph, fitted with a flame ionization detector and a U-shaped glass column, 2′ long, packed with 2.5% S.E. 30 on Chromosorb G, 80/100 mesh

*For an updated list of reference material, see References, p. 327.

Operating Conditions

Gas Flow Rate:
nitrogen (carrier gas) – 50 ml/min
Temperatures:
column – 210°C
injection port – 250°C
detector – 235°C

REAGENTS

All chemicals should be analytical reagent grade.

1. Propoxyphene stock solution, 100 μg/ml
Dissolve 111 mg of propoxyphene hydrochloride in water and dilute to one liter with water.
2. Propoxyphene reference solution, 5 μg/ml
Dilute 5.0 ml of the propoxyphene stock solution to 100 ml with water.
3. Parallel-standard solution, 250 μg/ml
Dissolve 25 mg of pyrroliphene hydrochloride (Eli Lilly Co.) in water and dilute to 100 ml.
4. Sodium bicarbonate, saturated aqueous solution
Saturate water with sodium bicarbonate. Prepare as needed.
5. *n*-Butyl chloride
6. Hydrochloric acid, concentrated
7. Hydrochloric acid, 0.2*N*
Dilute 5.0 ml of concentrated hydrochloric acid to 300 ml with water.
8. Sodium hydroxide, 6*N*
Dissolve 240 g of sodium hydroxide in water and dilute to one liter.
9. Chloroform, water-washed and dried over anhydrous sodium sulfate
10. Glass wool, acid-washed
11. Sodium sulfate, anhydrous

PROCEDURE

1. Transfer 1.0 ml of parallel-standard solution and 5.0 ml of whole blood or urine to a 15-ml ground-glass-stoppered centrifuge tube. Process a sample of propoxyphene reference solution concurrently and in the same manner as the specimen. If tissues are to be analyzed, prepare an aqueous homogenate, using 4.0 ml of water for each gram of tissue homogenized. Add 1.0 ml of parallel-standard solution to 5.0 ml of this homogenate and proceed as above.
2. Adjust the pH of each sample to above 6.0 by adding 10 drops of saturated sodium bicarbonate solution. Stopper the centrifuge tubes.
3. Extract each sample twice, using 5.0 ml of *n*-butyl chloride each time. Allow the phases to separate.
4. Pool the upper solvent layers obtained from the two extractions of each sample in a 30-ml separatory funnel.
5. Extract each of the pooled solvents twice, using 5.0 ml of 0.2*N* hydrochloric acid each time.
6. Pool the acid extracts in a second 30-ml separatory funnel and make it alkaline by adding approximately 0.5 ml of 6*N* sodium hydroxide.
7. Extract the alkaline solutions twice, using 10.0 ml of chloroform each time.
8. Filter each chloroform extract through anhydrous sodium sulfate supported on acid-washed glass wool in the neck of the funnel. Pool the filtered chloroform extracts of each sample in a 50-ml beaker.
9. Evaporate each pooled filtrate to approximately 1 ml, then transfer it to a disposable evaporating tube and continue the evaporation to about 50 μl. It is essential that the chloroform extract is not evaporated to less than 50 μl.
10. Inject approximately 1 μl of each concentrate into the gas chromatograph, making sure that the operating conditions stated above are met.
11. Note the retention times of the parallel standard and the specimen and compare them with the retention times obtained from the propoxyphene reference solution. The retention times should be approximately 2.5 and 5.7 min for propoxyphene and pyrroliphene, respectively.

Qualitative Confirmation

12. Transfer the residual gas-chromatographic solutions obtained from the propoxyphene reference solution and from the specimen to separate 10-ml beakers, using about 5 ml of concentrated hydrochloric acid to transfer each sample.

13. Heat the solutions for approximately 15 min in a steam bath.
14. Allow the solutions to cool, then make them alkaline with sodium hydroxide and extract them with chloroform.
15. Evaporate each chloroform extract to approximately 50 μl.
16. Inject 1 μl of each concentrate into the gas chromatograph, using the same operating conditions as in Step 10.
17. Note the disappearance of the propoxyphene peak and the appearance of a hydrolysis product at retention time 0.39 relative to propoxyphene. The pyrroliphene shows a hydrolysis product at retention time 0.63 relative to propoxyphene.

CALCULATION

1. Measure the peak heights of the parallel standard and propoxyphene for both the specimen and the reference solution.
2. Calculate the ratio of the peak height of propoxyphene to that of the peak height of parallel standard for each.
3. Calculate the concentration of propoxyphene in the blood or tissue by comparison of these ratios.

INTERPRETATION (see p. 7)

Plasma concentrations reach a maximum of 0.02 mg/dl in 1 hr following a 195-mg oral dose and 0.03 mg/dl in 30 min after a 50-mg intravenous dose.[1] Plasma concentrations reach a maximum of 0.03 mg/dl following the administration of 13 oral doses of 65 mg of the propoxyphene hydrochloride or 100 mg of the newer propoxyphene napsylate.[2] In fatal poisonings, concentrations of at least 0.2 mg/dl of blood and 3 ml/100 g of liver are attained. Where death has been attributed to propoxyphene, the blood levels have a range of 0.2 to 2.0 mg/dl, with the majority from 0.5 to 0.7 mg/dl. Liver concentrations have a range of 1.5 to 30 mg/100 g, with a majority from 5 to 13 mg/100 g. A high concentration in the liver might be indicative of chronic use of the drug.

ACCURACY AND PRECISION

Recovery of propoxyphene added to blood is 95% by this method. A concentration of 0.1 μg/ml blood can be detected with suitably adjusted gas-chromatographic conditions. The method is accurate within ±10% at values higher than 10 μg/ml and within ±20% at 5 μg/ml.

INTERFERING SUBSTANCES

On a 2′ gas-chromatography column, complete separation of all of the bases is impossible. The retention time of propoxyphene under the operating conditions given is not unique. Amitriptyline, doxepin, atropine, cocaine, mephenoxalone, and metaxalone are not completely separated from propoxyphene. Only propoxyphene, however, produces a hydrolysis product at retention time approximately 0.39 relative to propoxyphene.

Two metabolites almost always accompany the unchanged propoxyphene in liver and urine. Their retention times are 5.5 and 10 min. The minor metabolite cannot be separated from pyrroliphene. For this reason it is advisable to analyze urine and liver samples with and without the parallel standard in order to judge the degree of metabolite interference. It should be noted, however, that the typical three peak gas-chromatographic pattern of propoxyphene and its two metabolites adds considerable significance to the qualitative aspect of the analysis.

REFERENCES

1. **Wolen, R. L., Gruber, C. M., Kiplinger, G. F., and Scholz, N. E.,** Concentration of propoxyphene in human plasma following oral, intramuscular, and intravenous administration, *Toxicol. Appl. Pharmacol.*, 19, 480, 1971.
2. **Wolen, R. L., Gruber, C. M., Kiplinger, G. F., and Scholz, N. E.,** Concentration of propoxyphene in human plasma following repeated oral doses, *Toxicol. Appl. Pharmacol.* 19, 493, 1971.

GENERAL REFERENCES

Verebely, K. and Inturrisi, C. E., Disposition of propoxyphene and norpropoxyphene in man after a single oral dose, *Clin. Pharmacol. Ther.*, 15, 302, 1974.

Verebely, K. and Inturrisi, C. E., The simultaneous determination of propoxyphene and norpropoxyphene in human biofluids using gas-liquid chromatography, *J. Chromatogr.*, 75, 195, 1973.

Wolen, R. L. and Gruber, C. M., Determination of propoxyphene in human plasma by gas chromatography, *Anal. Chem.*, 40, 1243, 1968.

PROPRANOLOL

PRINCIPLE

Propranolol is first extracted into ether from alkaline solution and then reextracted into dilute acid. The acid extract is then made alkaline, extracted with ether, and then reextracted into dilute acid. The UV absorbance of this acid extract at 288.5 nm less that at 340 nm is the basis for the quantitative determination of propranolol.

TYPE B PROCEDURE

Richard F. Shaw

APPARATUS

1. UV recording spectrophotometer
2. Mechanical shaker
3. Serological pipets
4. Separatory funnels, 250 ml
5. Magnetic stirrer and stirrer bar
6. Centrifuge
7. Blender
8. Erlenmeyer flask, 2 l
9. Cuvettes, quartz or fused silica
10. Conical tubes, 12 ml
11. Microliter syringes, Hamilton, 5 μl
12. Thin-layer chromatography equipment: (a) Micropet, disposable; (b) glass plates (Brinkmann Silplate-F-22); (c) developing tanks; (d) Chromaflex Spray®, kantes)
13. Filter paper, Whatman #41
14. Screw-capped tubes, 13 × 100 mm
15. Gas chromatograph, fitted with flame ionization detector and a U-shaped glass column, 2′ × 4 mm i.d., packed with 2.5% SE-30 on 80/100 mesh Chromasorb G (AW-DMCS)[1]

Operating Conditions

Gas Flow Rate:
- nitrogen (carrier gas) – 40 ml/min

Temperatures:
- column* – 200°C
- injection port – 240°C
- detector – 220°C

REAGENTS

All chemicals should be analytical reagent grade.

1. Sodium hydroxide, saturated, 19*M*
2. Diethyl ether, anhydrous
3. Sulfuric acid, 0.5*N*
4. Ammonium hydroxide, concentrated
5. Chloroform:methanol, 1:1 (v/v)
6. Methyl alcohol
7. Hydrochloric acid, concentrated
8. TLC developing solutions, methanol: ammonium hydroxide, 100:1.5[2]
9. Platinum chloride, 5% in water (w/v)
10. Potassium iodide, 10% in water (w/v)
11. Iodoplatinate reagent
    Combine 5 ml of the platinum chloride solution with 45 ml of the potassium iodide solution and add 100 ml of water.
12. Propranolol stock solution, 1.0 mg/ml
    Dissolve 113.8 mg of propranolol hydrochloride in water and dilute to 100 ml.
13. Propranolol reference solution, 10 μg/ml
    Dilute 1 ml of the propranolol stock solution to 100 ml with water. The absorbance of this solution at 288.5 nm should be 0.220 with 1.0-cm light path cuvettes.
14. Codeine reference solution, 4 mg/ml
    Dissolve 567 mg of codeine phosphate (anhydrous salt) in 100 ml of chloroform and methanol (1:1).

*Adjust the column temperature so that codeine has a retention time of 3.8 ± 0.2 min.

SPECIMEN PREPARATION

1. To 10.0 ml of sample (blood, serum, 10.0-ml gastric content, 10.0-g homogenized tissue, and drug reference solution) and 10.0-ml water in a 500-ml Erlenmeyer flask containing a stirrer bar, add 200-ml ether. Mix the contents by placing the flask on a magnetic stirrer for 5 min.
2. Add 0.5 ml of saturated sodium hydroxide and allow the mixture to stir for an additional 5 min.
3. Allow the layers to separate. The ether layer is decanted into a 250-ml separatory funnel and washed with 25-ml H_2O. Discard the water and measure the ether volume (V_1).
4. Extract the ether two times, each time with 20.0 ml of 0.5*N* sulfuric acid. Pool the acid extracts in a clean 250-ml separatory funnel. Wash the acid extracted ether with 5.0 ml of water and add the water to the pooled acid extracts.
5. Adjust the acid solution to approximately pH 10 with saturated sodium hydroxide and extract with 200 ml of ether for 5 min on a mechanical shaker.
6. Allow the layers to separate. Discard the aqueous solution and wash the ether with 5.0-ml water. Discard the water and filter the ether through Whatman #41 filter paper into a 250-ml separatory funnel. Measure the ether volume (V_2).
7. Extract the measured ether with 5.0 ml of 0.5*N* sulfuric acid (V_3) for 5 min on a mechanical shaker.
8. Allow the layers to separate. Place 3.0 ml of the sulfuric acid solution into a 10-mm silica cell and determine the absorbance of the solution from 190 to 390 nm using a reference solution of 0.5*N* sulfuric acid (Figure 1). Propranolol will have inflexions at about 228 and 282 nm and maxima at 288.5, 305, and 319.5 nm.

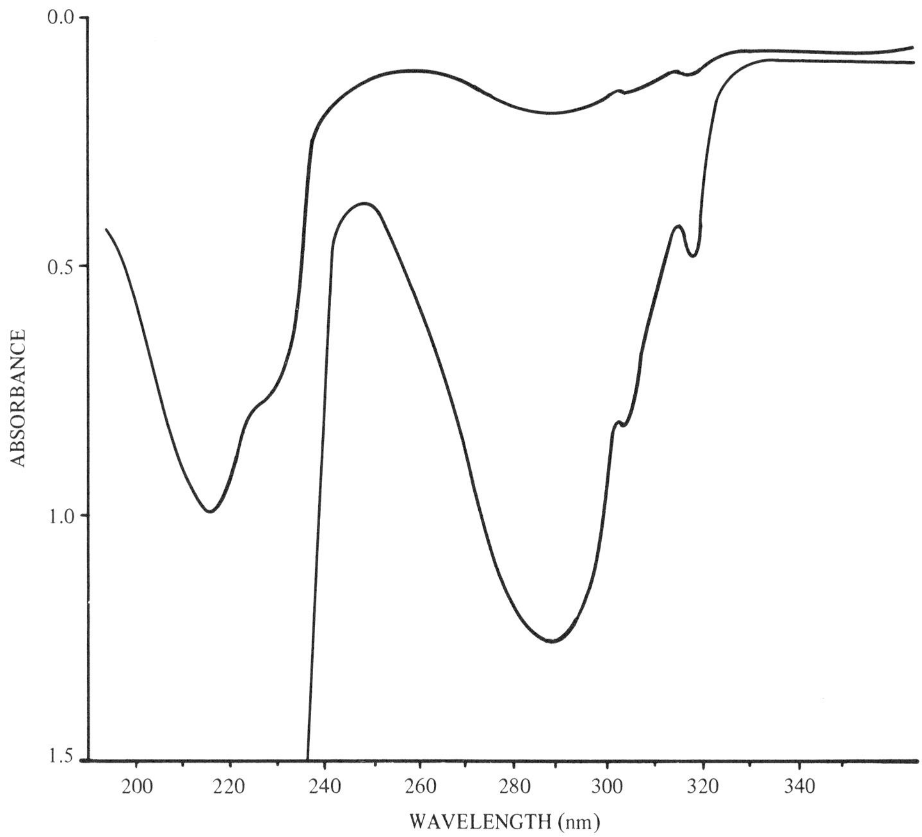

FIGURE 1. UV absorbance of propranolol in 0.5*N* H_2SO_4.

CALCULATION

Quantitation is based on the absorbance at 288.5 nm minus the absorbance at 340 nm. Use the following formula to calculate the propranolol concentration (mg/100 ml) in the specimen:

$$\frac{A_s}{A_r} \times C_r \times \frac{200}{V_1} \times \frac{200}{V_2} \times \frac{V_3}{S} \times \frac{100}{1000} = C_s$$

where

- A_s = absorbance of the sample at 288.5 nm minus the absorbance at 340 nm;
- A_r = absorbance of the propranolol reference solution at 288.5 nm minus the absorbance at 340 nm;
- C_r = concentration of the propranolol reference solution;
- V_1 = volume of solvent aliquot;
- V_2 = volume of solvent aliquot;
- V_3 = volume of 0.5*N* H_2SO_4 used to extract the final ether phase;
- S = sample volume;
- C_s = concentration of propranolol in the specimen.

CONFIRMATION

1. Transfer the solution in the cuvette to a 13 × 100 mm screw-capped tube. Make it alkaline by adding 0.5 ml of concentrated ammonium hydroxide and extract with 5.0 ml of ether. Evaporate the ether to dryness in a small conical tube.
2. Redissolve the residue in 20 μl of 1:1 methanol and chloroform and inject 1 to 2 μl into a gas chromatograph under the conditions listed above. Propranolol has a relative retention time of 0.51 relative to the codeine reference solution previously injected.
3. After the gas chromatography is complete, spot another aliquot of the solution of the residue on a thin-layer chromatography plate along with a propranolol standard. Develop the plate in methanol: ammonium hydroxide to approximately 10.0 cm above the point of application.
4. Remove the plates from the tank and allow them to dry 1 hr, preferably in a fume hood at room temperature.
5. Spray the plate lightly with concentrated hydrochloric acid and then with iodoplatinate reagent. Compare with the standard. Propranolol should have a R_f value of 0.53.

INTERPRETATION (see p. 7)

Plasma levels resulting from an oral dosage of 80 mg in a fasting state reached a maximum at 1½ to 2 and 2 to 4 hr when taken with a meal. In the fasting state the levels range from 36 to 212 ng/ml (five subjects). A plasma half-life of 3.2 hr was found after oral administration.[3] In a person whose death was probably due to propranolol and ethyl alcohol, the following concentrations of propranolol were found: blood, 0.99 mg/100 ml; liver, 26 mg/100 gm; and gastric contents, 56 mg. The blood contained 100 mg of ethyl alcohol/100 ml (w/v).[4]

SENSITIVITY

Recovery of propranolol added to blood is approximately 90%. The method will detect 0.1 mg of propranolol in 100 ml of blood.

INTERFERING SUBSTANCES

Other organic bases may interfere, especially if they have high UV absorbance in the region of propranolol's maximum absorption. The use of UV, GLC, and TLC should be adequate to confirm the specificity of the analysis.

REFERENCES

1. **Finkle, B. S., Cherry, E. J., and Taylor, D. M.,** A GLC based system for the detection of poisons, drugs, and human metabolites encountered in forensic toxicology, *J. Chromatogr. Sci.*, 9, 393, 1971.
2. **Sunshine, I.,** Use of thin-layer chromatography in the diagnosis of poisoning, *Am. J. Clin. Pathol.*, 40, 576, 1963.
3. **Shand, D. D. G., Nuckolls, E. M., and Oates, J. A.,** Plasma propranolol levels in adults with observations

in four children, *Clin. Pharmacol. Ther.*, 11, 112, 1970.

4. **Creason, R. L.,** Coroner's case file 337-72, San Diego County Coroner's Department, San Diego, California.

GENERAL REFERENCES

Coltart, D. J. and Shand, D. G., Plasma propranolol levels in the quantitative assessment of β-adrenergic blockade in man, *Br. Med. J.*, 3, 731, 1970.

Evans, G. H. and Shand, D. G., Disposition of propranolol: Drug accumulation and steady-state concentration during chronic oral administration in man, *Clin. Pharmacol. Ther.*, 14, 487, 1973.

Faulkner, S. L., et al., Time required for complete recovery from chronic propranolol therapy, *N. Engl. J. Med.*, 298, 607, 1973.

Lowenthal, D. T., Pharmacokinetics of oral propranolol in chronic renal disease, *Clin. Pharmacol. Ther.*, 16, 761, 1974.

PROTRIPTYLINE

PRINCIPLE

The drug may be extracted from an alkalinized sample by an organic solvent. Reextraction into dilute acid yields a solution whose protriptyline content can be assayed by spectrofluorometry.

TYPE C PROCEDURE

J. Grove

APPARATUS

1. Spectrofluorimeter (Aminoc-Bowman), equipped with an X-Y recorder
2. Centrifuge tubes, glass-stoppered, 30 ml
3. Multipurpose rotator (Model 150V)*

REAGENTS

All chemicals should be analytical reagent grade.

1. Sodium hydroxide, 1*N*
   Dissolve 40 g of sodium hydroxide in water and dilute to one liter.
2. Diethyl ether
3. Sulfuric acid, 0.1*N*
   Add 28 ml of concentrated sulfuric acid to water and dilute to one liter.
4. Protriptyline hydrochloride stock solution, 100 µg/ml
   Dissolve 50 mg of protriptyline hydrochloride in 0.1*N* sulfuric acid and dilute to 500 ml.
5. Proptriptyline hydrochloride reference solutions, 0.2, 0.5, and 1.0 µg/ml
   With 0.1*N* sulfuric acid, dilute 1.0 ml of the protriptyline stock solution to 500 ml, 5 to 1,000 ml, and 5 to 500 ml.

PROCEDURE

1. Be sure that the spectrofluorimeter is in operating order. Allow it to warm up for at least 15 min before making the determination. Adjust the dark current to zero reading.
2. To duplicate 1.0-ml plasma specimens in 30-ml glass-stoppered centrifuge tubes, add 2.0 ml of 1*N* sodium hydroxide and 25.0 ml of ether. Shake each mixture vigorously for 10 min then centrifuge the tubes. Process 1.0 ml of each reference solution and 1.0 ml of water for a reagent blank in the same manner as the specimen.
3. Pipet 20.0 ml of each ether layer into a clean tube and add 1.5 ml of 0.1*N* sulfuric acid. Rotate the tubes on the multipurpose rotator for 10 min then centrifuge them.
4. Carefully pipet each layer of sulfuric acid into a clean tube and determine its relative fluorescence at activation 300 nm and emission 375 nm, using sensitivity 30 and slit setting #1. Make these determinations promptly and try to complete them within 15 min.

CALCULATION

Use the following formula to calculate the protriptyline concentration in the specimen:

$$\frac{F_S}{F_R} \times C_R = C_S,$$

where

F_S = relative fluorescence of the specimen;
F_R = relative fluorescence of the reference solution;

*Scientific Industries, Inc., Springfield, Mass.

C_R = concentration of the reference solution used;

C_S = concentration of the specimen.

Note: Concentration-quenching occurs above 0.8 μg protriptyline/ml; hence, for more accurate analyses, "bracketing" is necessary. This involves determining the approximate concentration of the specimen and then using a reference solution within the same range for the calculation of its exact concentration. It is important to analyze the reference solutions every time a specimen is analyzed, because their relative fluorescence may vary considerably from day to day.

INTERPRETATION (see p. 7)

Patients receiving therapeutic doses after 3 weeks have plasma levels of 0.1 to 0.3 μg/ml.

ACCURACY AND PRECISION

Recovery of protriptyline added to plasma is 83%. Duplicate results agree within ± 5%.

REFERENCES

Greenblatt, D. J., Koch-Weser, J., and Shader, R. I., Multiple complications and death following protriptyline overdosage, *JAMA*, 229, 556, 1974.

Moody, J. P., Whyte, S. F., and Naylor, G. J., A simple method for the determination of protriptyline in plasma, *Clin. Chim. Acta.*, 43, 355, 1973.

PYRIMETHAMINE

PRINCIPLE

A concentrated organic solvent extract of an alkalinized sample is analyzed by gas chromatography.

TYPE C PROCEDURE

Leo Kazyak

APPARATUS

1. pH paper (Hydrion)
2. Graduated tubes or cylinders
3. Syringes (Hamilton), 10 μl
4. Gas chromatograph, equipped with a flame ionization detector, and a column packed with OV-17 liquid phase on silanized Chromosorb W (e.g., Gas Chrom Q or a comparable grade of support material)*

REAGENTS

All chemicals should be analytical reagent grade.

1. Potassium hydroxide, saturated aqueous solution
2. Pyrimethamine reference solution
   Dissolve 10 mg of pyrimethamine ($C_{12}H_{13}ClN_4$) in 10.0 ml of ethanol. When 1 μl of this reference solution is injected into the gas chromatograph, a peak of at least 30% of full-scale deflection should be detectable at an electrometer setting equivalent to 5×10^{-10} A ion current.
3. Chloroform
4. Hydrocarbon reference solution
   Dissolve 10 mg of *n*-tetracosane ($C_{24}H_{28}$) and 15 mg of *n*-octacosane ($C_{28}H_{32}$) in 20.0 ml of hexane. When 1 μl of this reference solution is injected into the gas chromatograph, it should produce a peak comparable in height and area to that of the pyrimethamine reference solution.

PROCEDURE

1. Add a drop of saturated potassium hydroxide to 5.0 ml of specimen (plasma or urine). Process 5.0 ml of pyrimethamine reference solution and 5.0 ml of water, or preferably pooled drug-free plasma or urine, for a reagent blank in the same manner as the specimen.
2. Test each sample for alkalinity with Hydrion pH paper. Add more potassium hydroxide if necessary.
3. Extract each sample with 30 ml of chloroform. Shake the extraction vessel for 5 min. Allow the solvent and aqueous phases to separate completely.
4. Carefully transfer 25 ml of each solvent phase to a clean graduated tube or cylinder. (Do not filter the solvent or add anhydrous sodium sulfate.) Measure the solvent volumes.
5. Reduce the volume of the solvent in each tube by evaporation. The concentrate may be transferred to a smaller tube with a constricted base to facilitate the withdrawing of aliquots with a Hamilton microliter syringe.
6. When the solvent has evaporated to 100 μl, add 10 μl of hydrocarbon reference solution to each solvent concentrate, then evaporate the mixture to 50 μl.
7. Inject a 5-μl aliquot of the solvent concentrate obtained from the specimen into the gas chromatograph. Column temperature and flow rate will depend on the particular column employed. Conditions should be such that the retention time for *n*-tetracosane ($C_{24}H_{28}$) is between 2.5 and 3.5 min. Under these condi-

*It is unnecessary to specify operating parameters because they place unnecessary limitations on the procedure, which can be based on retention index.

tions the retention time for pyrimethamine will be between 5.0 and 5.3 min.

8. Estimate the amount of drug in the aliquot injected by comparison of the *n*-octacosane peak area with the pyrimethamine peak.

CALCULATION

$$\frac{C_P}{V_S} \times V_P \times \frac{C}{S} \times \frac{V}{V_a} = C_S$$

where

C_p = concentration (μg/μl) of the pyrimethamine reference solution;
V_P = peak area ratio of pyrimethamine reference solution;
V_S = peak area ratio of the specimen;
C = solvent concentrate obtained in Step 6 (usually 50 μl);
V = initial volume of the solvent (Step 3);
V_a = volume of the solvent aliquot (Step 4);
S = volume of the specimen;
C_S = concentration (μg/ml) of pyrimethamine in the specimen.

Identification by retention index:

$$\left[\frac{\log S - \log C_{24}}{\log C_{28} - \log C_{24}}\right] \times 400 \quad + 2400 = I_R, \qquad (2)$$

where

log S = logarithm of the retention time of pyrimethamine;
log C_{24} = logarithm of the retention time of *n*-tetracosane ($C_{24}H_{28}$);
log C_{28} = logarithm of the retention time of *n*-octacosane ($C_{28}H_{32}$);
I_R = retention index for pyrimethamine (2630 ± 30).

INTERPRETATION (see p. 7)

Following therapeutic doses of pyrimethamine, plasma concentrations range from 0.05 to 0.15 mg/100 ml. However, plasma pyrimethamine concentrations as high as 0.40 mg/100 ml have been detected following a nonfatal overdose. Urine pyrimethamine concentrations range from 1.0 to 10.0 mg/100 ml.

ACCURACY AND PRECISION

Replicate determinations should vary no more than 2%. The retention index will not vary between injections, and day-to-day variations or those due to temperature change of the column should not exceed 2 to 3%. Recovery of the pyrimethamine will be better than 90%.

INTERFERING SUBSTANCES

Pentazocine, tetracaine, benactyzine, cocaine, dimethindine, and imipramine have retention indices in the same region as pyrimethamine.

QUINIDINE (or QUINIDINE)

PRINCIPLE

An organic base, quinine or its analogue, quinidine, can be extracted from an alkaline solution of the biological matrix. Reextraction of this extract into dilute acid produces a solution whose emission fluorescence spectrum (Procedure A), UV absorption spectrum (Procedure B), or retention time following gas chromatography (Procedure C) can be used to identify and quantitate either drug.

TYPE A PROCEDURE

Joseph Monforte

APPARATUS

1. Test tubes, screw-capped, 126 × 16 mm
2. Multipurpose rotator (Model 150 V)*
3. Centrifuge
4. Pasteur pipets
5. Spectrophotofluorometer (Perkin-Elmer Model MPF-2A)

REAGENTS

All chemicals should be analytical reagent grade.

1. Quinine sulfate stock solution, 100 mg/l
   Dissolve 100 mg of quinine sulfate in one liter of distilled water.
2. Quinine sulfate reference solution, 0.1 mg/100 ml
   Dilute 1.0 ml of the quinine sulfate stock solution to 100 ml with distilled water.
3. Buffer solution
   Dissolve 53.5 g of ammonium chloride in 950 ml of water. Add 10.0 ml of concentrated ammonium hydroxide and adjust the pH to 8.5 with ammonium hydroxide or hydrochloric acid.
4. Chloroform-isopropyl alcohol mixture, 3:1
   Mix 3 volumes of chloroform with 1 volume of isopropyl alcohol.
5. Sulfuric acid, 0.1*N*
   Dilute 2.8 ml of concentrated sulfuric acid to one liter with distilled water.

PROCEDURE

1. To 2.0 ml of sample (urine specimen, reference solution, and water for a reagent blank) in a screw-capped test tube, add 1.0 ml of buffer solution.
2. Add 4.0 ml of the chloroform-isopropyl alcohol mixture to each test tube and place the tubes on the rotator. Rotate the tubes for approximately 15 min.
3. Centrifuge the test tubes for 2 min at approximately 1,500 rpm.
4. Aspirate the upper (aqueous) layers. Decant each organic layer into a clean 15-ml screw-capped test tube.
5. Add 3.0 ml of 0.1*N* sulfuric acid to each chloroform extract, then cap the tubes and place them on the rotator. Rotate the test tubes for approximately 15 min.
6. Centrifuge the samples for 2 min at approximately 1,500 rpm.
7. Transfer each upper (aqueous) layer to a cuvette by means of a Pasteur pipet.
8. Excite the samples at 250 nm and record their emission spectra from approximately 400 to 460 nm. Observe their fluorescence at approximately 445 to 450 nm (Figure 1). In 0.1*N* sulfuric acid, quinine fluoresces at approximately 445 nm (uncorrected) as shown in Curve A.

Note: Quinine and morphine may be detected in the same urine sample by doubling the specimen

*Scientific Industries, Inc., Springfield, Mass.

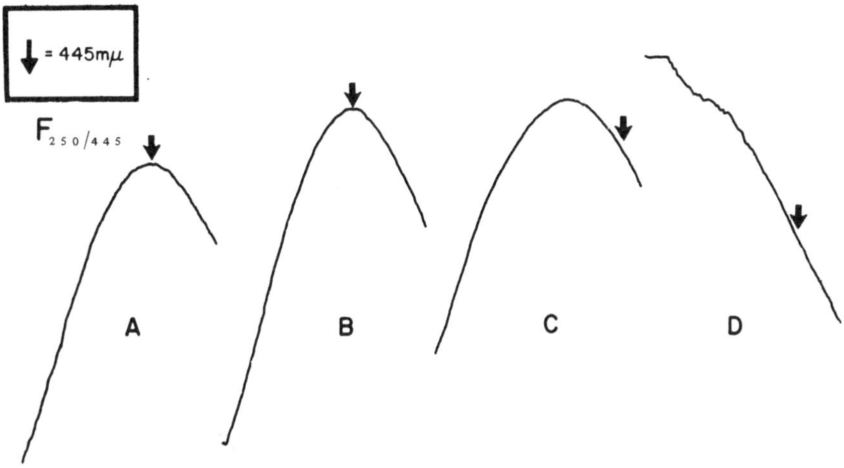

FIGURE 1. Fluorescence spectrum.

and reagent volumes and dividing the chloroform-isopropyl alcohol extract in half. The analysis for quinine is performed by completing Steps 5 to 8 above. The analysis for morphine is performed by completing Steps 4 to 10 in the morphine procedure.*

9. To confirm the fluorimetric data, add alkali to the sample and extract the alkaline solution with 2 ml of chloroform.
10. Centrifuge the solution, aspirate the aqueous phase, and concentrate the chloroform to about 50 μl.
11. To determine if quinine or quinidine is present, thin-layer chromatograph an aliquot of the organic extract on a silica gel G plate and develop the plate in cyclohexane, chloroform, and diethylamine (5:4:1). Quinine has an R_f of 0.07; quinidine is 0.15. They can be visualized by spraying the plate with dilute acid and observing the sprayed plate under 255-nm light.

INTERPRETATION (see p. 7)

Quinine is commonly associated with heroin in illicit drug preparations. Hence, a positive quinine test is often taken as an indication that heroin was used. If morphine is also present, this assumption is reasonable. If morphine is absent, the assumption is less valid, but not unreasonable, because the detection limit of quinine is lower than morphine's and quinine may constitute a large portion of the illicit heroin preparation. Quinine may, however, be found in over-the-counter medications and in tonic water, and these may be the source of the positive test.

INTERFERING SUBSTANCES

Pentazocine, morphine, percodan, meperidine, propoxyphene, chlorphentermine, methamphetamine, amphetamine, methaqualone, methapyrilene, and methadone do not interfere in the fluorometric procedure for quinine. Quinidine, the optical isomer of quinine, will give a positive fluorescence spectrum.

REFERENCES†

Härtel, G. and Korhonen, A., A TLC for the quantitative separation of quinidine and quinine metabolites from biological fluids and tissues, *J. Chromatogr.*, 37, 70, 1968.

Mulé, S. J. and Hushin, P. L., Semi-automated fluorometric assay for submicrogram quantities of morphine and quinine in human biological material, *Anal. Chem.*, 43, 708, 1971.

*See p. 268.

†For an updated list of reference material, see General References, p. 341.

TYPE B PROCEDURE

Leo Kazyak

APPARATUS

1. pH Paper (Hydrion)
2. Graduated tubes or cylinders
3. Cuvettes, quartz or fused silica
4. Spectrophotometer, preferably ratio-recording, with linear absorbance slidewire.

REAGENTS

All chemicals should be analytical reagent grade.

1. Potassium hydroxide, saturated aqueous solution
2. Quinine (or quinidine) stock solution, 1 mg/ml
   Dissolve 12 mg of quinine (mono-)hydrochloride, $C_{20}H_{24}N_2O_2 \cdot HCl \cdot 2H_2O$, (or 12 mg of quinidine sulfate, $(C_{20}H_{24}N_2O_2)_2 \cdot H_2SO_4 \cdot 2H_2O$) in water and dilute to 10 ml with water.
3. Quinine (or quinidine) reference solution, 10 μg/ml
   Dilute 1.0 ml of the quinine (or quinidine) stock solution to 100 ml with water. The absorbance of this solution at 250 nm should be 0.87.
4. Chloroform
5. Sulfuric acid, 0.5*N*
   Dissolve 7.0 ml of concentrated sulfuric acid in 300 to 400 ml of water, then dilute to 500 ml with water.

PROCEDURE

1. Add a drop of saturated potassium hydroxide to 5.0 ml of plasma or urine. Test the specimen for alkalinity with Hydrion pH paper. Add more potassium hydroxide, if necessary. Process 5.0 ml of reference solution and 5.0 ml of water for a reagent blank in the same manner as the specimen.
2. Extract each sample with 30 ml of chloroform. Shake the extraction vessel for at least 1 min. Allow the solvent and aqueous phases to separate completely.
3. Carefully transfer each solvent phase to a clean graduated tube or cylinder. Note the solvent volumes (V_a).
4. Reextract each solvent phase with 3.0 ml of 0.5*N* sulfuric acid. Shake the tubes or cylinders for at least 3 min to insure complete recovery of the quinine (or quinidine) from the solvent. Allow the phases to separate.
5. When the aqueous acidic phases have separated and cleared, aspirate them and transfer them to clean quartz or fused silica cuvettes.
6. Determine the absorbance of each solution from 400 to 240 nm, using the solution obtained from the processed water sample as the reference solution.
7. To confirm the fluorimetric data, add alkali to the sample and extract the alkaline solution with 2 ml of chloroform.
8. Centrifuge the solution, aspirate the aqueous phase, and concentrate the chloroform to about 50 μl.
9. To determine if quinine or quinidine is present, thin-layer chromatograph an aliquot of the organic extract on a silica gel G plate and develop the plate in cyclohexane, chloroform, and diethylamino (5:4:1). Quinine has an R_f value of 0.07; quinidine is 0.15. They can be visualized by spraying the plate with dilute acid and observing the sprayed plate under 255-nm light.

CALCULATION

1. Quantification is based on the absorbance at 250 nm; however, the ratio of the absorbance at 250 nm to that at 345 nm must not exceed 5.4 ± 0.1. If the ratio is greater than 5.5, the blank at 250 nm is significantly large and another aliquot of the specimen should be analyzed. If the first analysis depleted the sample, the following correction must be made:

$$A'_1 = A_1 - A_2$$

$$\frac{A'_1}{A_3} = 5.4 \pm 0.1,$$

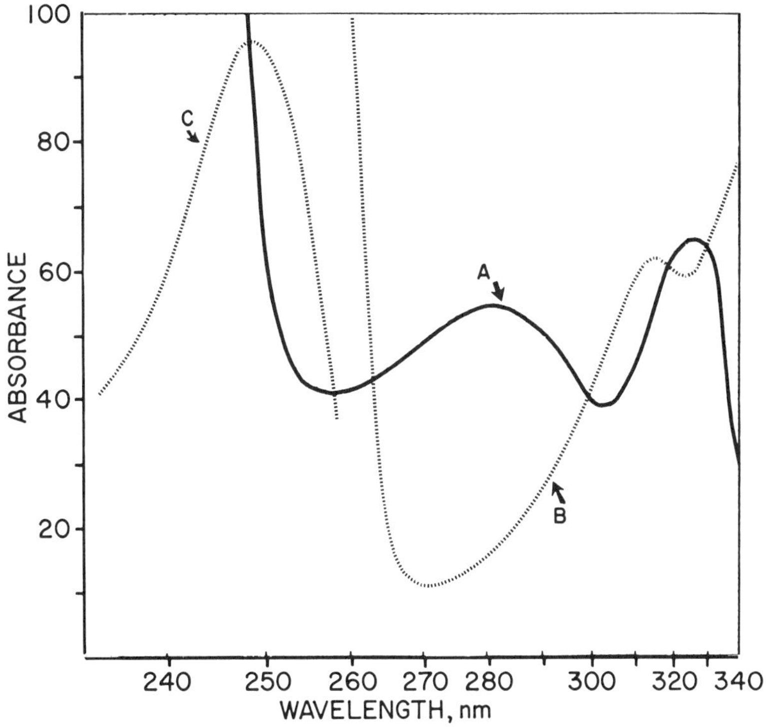

FIGURE 1. UV spectrum for quinine (or quinidine). A = 50 μg/ml base; B = 50 μg/ml acid; C = 10 μg/ml acid

where

A_1 = absorbance at 250 nm;
A_2 = absorbance at 275 nm;
A'_1 = corrected absorbance at 250 nm;
B = absorbance of the reagent blank;
A_3 = absorbance at 345 nm.

The relationship between concentration and absorbance is linear between 1.0 and 10.0 μg quinine (or quinidine)/ml solution.

2. Use the following formula to calculate the quinine (or quinidine) concentration in the specimen.

$$\frac{A_1 \text{ (or } A'_1)}{A_R} \times C_R \times \frac{V}{V_a} \times \frac{H}{S} = C_S,$$

where

A_R = absorbance of the reference solution;
C_R = concentration of the reference solution;
V = initial volume of the solvent;
V_a = volume of the solvent aliquot;
H = volume of 0.5*N* sulfuric acid used;
S = volume of the specimen;
C_S = quinine (or quinidine) concentration in the specimen.

INTERPRETATION (see p. 7)

Therapeutic plasma quinine (or quinidine) concentrations range from 3 to 5 μg/ml[1] depending on the size of the dose and the time elapsed between dose administration and specimen collection. Concentrations of 30 μg/ml are considered lethal.[2] After therapy, urine concentrations can range from 1.0 to 50.0 mg/100 ml. Patients receiving a daily dose of quinidine ranging from 100 to 2,000 mg (median 1,000 mg) achieved steady stage plasma quinidine concentration between 0.6 to 9.1 μg/ml (median 2.3 μg/ml). The plasma quinidine half-life ranged from 3.0 to 16.0 hr (median 7.0 hr). Although an appreciable quantity (10 to 15%) is excreted unchanged, hydroxyl metabolites have also been identified in urine.[3]

ACCURACY AND PRECISION

The UV absorption spectrum of quinine (or quinidine) is shown in Figure 1. Papaverine has a similar spectrum, with maximum absorbance occurring at 250 nm but with some absorbance at 345 nm also (maximum at 310 nm). Recovery of quinine (or quinidine) is 95 ± 2%.

INTERFERING SUBSTANCES

Besides papaverine, chloroquine and primaquine could interfere with this determination of quinine (or quinidine), although the therapeutic doses of these drugs are usually considerably less than those for quinine (or quinidine). The UV absorption spectrum will give an indication that interfering substances are present. Gas chromatography can then be utilized to confirm the analysis.

REFERENCES

1. **Sakalow, M. and Ball, E.,** Factors influencing conversion of chronic atrial fibrilation with special reference to serum quinidine concentration, *Circulation,* 14, 568, 1956.
2. **Halmos, P. B.,** Quinidine-induced syncope, *Br. Med. J.,* 2, 704, 1965.
3. **Goodman, L. S. and Gilman, A.,** The Pharmacological Basis of Therapeutics, 4th ed., MacMillan, N.Y., 1970, 717.

GENERAL REFERENCES*

Hartel, J. and Korhonen, A., Thin layer chromatography for the quantitative separation of quinidine and quinine metabolites from biological fluids, *J. Chromatogr.,* 37, 70, 1968.

Kessler, K. M., et al., Quinidine elimination in patients with congestive heart failure or poor renal function, *N. Engl. J. Med.,* 290, 706, 1974.

TYPE C PROCEDURE

K. K. Midha and C. Charette

APPARATUS

1. Centrifuge tubes, Teflon®-lined screw caps, 20 ml
2. Evaporating tubes, Teflon®-lined screw-caps, narrow bore base (tip 50 μl), total capacity, 10 ml
3. Rotating mixer
4. Oscillating mixer
5. Gas chromatograph (F/11 Perkin-Elmer), equipped with a flame ionization detector and a stainless steel column 4′ × 1/8″ o.d., packed with 5% OV-7 on Chromosorb W high performance, 80/100 mesh

   Operating Conditions

   Gas Flow Rates:
   - nitrogen (carrier gas) – 20/ml/min
   - Hydrogen and compressed air flow rates were adjusted to give maximum response.)

   Temperatures:
   - column – 270°C
   - injection port – 350°C
   - detector – 350°C

REAGENTS

All chemicals should be analytical reagent grade.

1. Stock quinidine and cinchonidine solution, 20 μg/ml
   Dissolve appropriate amounts of quinidine sulfate (J. T. Baker Laboratory Chemicals) and cinchonidine sulfate (Merck Chemical Co.) in distilled water to obtain the stock solutions.
2. Working standard quinidine solution, 0.2 to 12.0 μg/ml
   Dilute the quinidine stock solution to obtain the working solutions.
3. Working standard cinchonidine solution
   Dilute the stock solution to obtain 2 μg/ml.
4. Sodium hydroxide, 1.0*N*
5. Glass distilled benzene
6. Methanolic solution of trimethylanilinium hydroxide (TMAH), 0.2*M*

PROCEDURE

1. Place 1 ml of sample (plasma, whole blood, and working reference solution) in a centrifuge tube.

*For an updated list of reference material, see General References, p. 341.

2. Add 1 ml of distilled water, 1 ml of internal standard (≃ 2 μg of cinchonidine/ml), 1 ml of 1*N* NaOH, and 10 ml of benzene.
3. Extract the sample by shaking for 10 min at 19 rpm. Follow by centrifuging for 10 min at 2,500 rpm.
4. Transfer 9 ml of the organic layer into an evaporating tube. Evaporate at 75°C under a stream of dry nitrogen.
5. Add 25 μl of TMAH to the residue and mix, using an oscillating mixer.
6. Inject 2 μl into the gas chromatograph. Flash-heater methylated quinidine and cinchonidine gave retention times of 6.9 and 4.4 min, respectively.
7. Measure the peak heights of the methylated internal standard (cinchonidine) and methylated quinidine in the unknown specimen and the reference (known concentrations).
8. Calculate the ratio of the peak height of methylated quinidine to that of the peak height of internal standard for each chromatogram.

CALCULATION

Calculate the concentration of quinidine in the blood or plasma by comparison of the sample's peak height to that of the reference solution's.

INTERPRETATION (see p. 7)

Therapeutic plasma quinine (or quinidine) concentrations range from 3 to 5 μg/ml,[1] depending on the size of the dose and the time elapsed between dose administration and specimen collection. Concentrations of 30 μg/ml are considered lethal.[2] After therapy, urine concentrations can range from 1 to 500 μg/ml. Patients receiving a daily dose of quinidine ranging from 100 to 2,000 mg (median 1,000 mg) achieved steady stage plasma quinidine concentration between 0.6 to 9.1 μg/ml (median 2.3 μg/ml). The plasma quinidine half-life ranged from 3.0 to 16.0 hr (median 7.0 hr). Although an appreciable quantity (10 to 15%) is excreted unchanged, hydroxyl metabolites have also been identified in urine.[3]

ACCURACY AND PRECISION

1. The overall recoveries of quinidine and cinchonidine from plasma are 98.27 ± 3.61% and 81.63 ± 2.84%, respectively.
2. Concentrations as low as 0.20 μg/ml can be determined with a coefficient of variation of 10%.

INTERFERING SUBSTANCES

The metabolites of quinidine (i.e., 2-hydroxyquinidine and monohydroxyquinidine) do not interfere in the assay as they have retention times of 12.1 and 10.6 min, respectively, on flash-heater methylation.

REFERENCES

1. **Sokolow, M. and Ball, E.,** Factors influencing conversion of chronic atrial fibrilation with special reference to serum quinidine concentration, *Circulation,* 14, 568, 1956.
2. **Halmos, P. B.,** Quinidine-induced syncope, *Br. Med. J.,* 2, 704, 1965.
3. **Goodman, L. S. and Gilman, A.,** *The Pharmacological Basis of Therapeutics,* 4th ed., MacMillan, N.Y., 1970, 717.

GENERAL REFERENCES

Hall, A. P., Czerwinski, W., Madonia, E. C., and Evenson, K. L., Human plasma and urine quinine levels following tablets, capsules and intravenous infusion, *Clin. Pharmacol. Ther.,* 14, 580, 1973.

Midha, K. K. and Charette, C., GLC determination of quinidine from plasma, *J. Pharm. Sci.,* 63, 1245, 1974.

Winek, C., et al., Quinine fatality – case report, *Clin. Toxicol.,* 7, 129, 1974.

SALICYLATE

PRINCIPLE

In the presence of ferric salts, salicylates produce a violet color whose absorbance is a function of the salicylate concentration (Procedure A). A more elegant, reliable, and specific test requires the extraction of the salicylate from the acidified biological specimen, and the reextraction of the salicylate into alkali. The ultraviolet absorption spectrum of the alkali solution can then be used to qualitatively identify and quantitatively determine any salicylate present in the solution (Procedure B).

TYPE A PROCEDURE

Irving Sunshine

APPARATUS

1. Centrifuge tubes, 15 ml
2. Centrifuge
3. Photometer, photoelectric, with a 540-nm filter

REAGENTS

All chemicals should be analytical reagent grade.

1. Hydrochloric acid, 1*N*
   Dilute 8.0 ml of concentrated hydrochloric acid to 100 ml with water.
2. Trinder's reagent[1]
   Transfer 4 g of ferric nitrate ($Fe(NO_3)_3 \cdot 9H_2O$) and 4 g of mercuric chloride to a 100-ml volumetric flask. Add 12.0 ml of 1*N* hydrochloric acid. Dissolve the salts, dilute the solution to 100 ml with water, then filter it. Store the reagent at room temperature.
3. Salicylic acid stock solution, 200 mg/dl
   Transfer 232 mg of sodium salicylate to a 100-ml volumetric flask. Dissolve the salt with water, then dilute the solution to 100 ml. Add a few drops of chloroform as a preservative, then store the solution in a refrigerator. Discard the solution after 6 months.
4. Salicylic acid reference solution, 20 mg/dl
   Dilute 10.0 ml of the salicylic acid stock solution to 100 ml with water. Add a few drops of chloroform as a preservative, then store the solution in a refrigerator. Discard the solution after 6 months.
5. Phosphoric acid, 85%

PROCEDURE

1. To 15-ml centrifuge tubes containing 5.0 ml of water and 0.5 ml of sample (blood or urine specimen, reference solution, and water for a reagent blank), add 5.0 ml of Trinder's reagent. If a urine specimen is used, prepare a urine blank by processing a second 0.5-ml aliquot of urine, adding 0.5 ml of 85% phosphoric acid and only 4.5 ml of Trinder's reagent.
2. Mix the contents of each tube well, allow the samples to stand for 5 min, then centrifuge them.
3. Using the processed water sample as the reference solution, determine the absorbance of each solution at 540 nm. The resulting absorbances are stable for 1 hr.

CALCULATION

Determine the salicylate concentration (mg/100 ml) in the specimen by the following formula:

$$\frac{A_S}{A_R} \times 20 = C_S,$$

where

A_S = absorbance of the blood specimen at 540 nm; if a urine specimen was analyzed, A_S is the difference in absorbance between the test sample and the urine blank;
A_R = absorbance of the reference solution at 540 nm;
C_S = salicylate concentration of the specimen.

If the salicylate concentration of any specimen is determined to be higher than 40 mg/100 ml, perform a second analysis on the specimen after diluting it so that the ensuing concentration is below 40 mg/100 ml.

INTERPRETATION (see p. 7)

Sodium salicylate and aspirin are both easily absorbed, some from the stomach, but more generally from the upper GI tract. Maximum salicylate concentration usually occurs 2 hr after ingestion.[2] The common adult therapeutic dose of 600 mg aspirin yields a serum concentration of about 5 mg/100 ml.[3] Doses of 100 mg sodium salicylate/kg body weight usually produce serum concentrations of 20 to 30 mg/100 ml. At this concentration the first overt sign of toxicity, tinnitus, may be noticed. If higher concentrations are found, increased toxic reactions occur. Following an initial respiratory alkalosis, metabolic acidosis may occur at a plasma salicylate concentration between 50 and 70 mg/100 ml. Patients with these or higher serum salicylate concentrations require considerable supportive therapy.

Chemical analyses of serum or urine for their salicylate concentration can be valuable aids to corroborate whether or not a patient is intoxicated and can help predict the clinical course of a salicylate-intoxicated patient. Precise quantitation of salicylate concentration (within ±1 mg/100 ml) is not essential for this purpose, and the procedure described above is more than adequate.

ACCURACY AND PRECISION

The results obtained by this procedure are accurate within ±5%.

INTERFERING SUBSTANCES

Urine specimens should be boiled before they are analyzed. This will remove any diacetic acid, which, if present, would interfere. Phenothiazine drugs, if present, would also interfere.

REFERENCES

1. **Trinder, P.,** Rapid determination of salicylates in biological materials, *Biochem. J.*, 57, 301, 1954.
2. **Done, A. K.,** Salicylate intoxication: Significance of measurements of salicylate in blood in cases of acute congestion, *Pediatrics*, 26, 800, 1960.
3. **Leonards, J. R.,** The influence of solubility on the rate of gastrointestinal absorption of aspirin, *Clin. Pharmacol. Ther.*, 5, 476, 1963.

TYPE B PROCEDURE[1]

Louis A. Williams

APPARATUS

1. Culture tubes with Teflon®-lined screw caps, 25 × 150 mm (Kimble Cat. No. 45066-A)
2. UV spectrophotometer, preferably ratio-recording

REAGENTS

All chemicals should be analytical reagent grade.

1. Chloroform, washed
   Fill a 2 liter volumetric flask to the base of the neck with chloroform. Add sodium hydroxide solution to the mark and stir the flask contents for 5 min on a mixer. Aspirate the top layer. Add water to the mark, mix for 5 min, then aspirate the water. Add 1*N* hydrochloric acid to the mark, mix for 5 min, then aspirate the acid. Wash three times with water in the same manner. Filter the reagent into a dark bottle.
2. Sodium hydroxide, 2.5*N*
   Dissolve 10 g of sodium hydroxide in water and dilute to 100 ml.
3. Hydrochloric acid, 1*N*
   Dilute 8.0 ml of concentrated hydrochloric acid to 100 ml with water.

4. Salicylate stock solution, 100 mg/dl
   Dissolve 117 mg of sodium salicylate in water and dilute to 100 ml.
5. Salicylate reference solution, 20 mg/dl
   Dilute 20.0 ml of the salicylate stock solution to 100 ml with water.
6. Phosphate buffer, 0.1*M*, pH 7.4
   Dissolve 11.419 g of anhydrous sodium phosphate, dibasic (Na_2HPO_4), 2.668 g of anhydrous potassium phosphate, monobasic (KH_2PO_4), in water and dilute to one liter. Check the pH of the solution and adjust as needed.
7. Hydrochloric acid, 6*N*
   Mix equal volumes of concentrated hydrochloric acid and water.
8. Sodium hydroxide, 1*N*
   Dissolve 4 g of sodium hydroxide in water and dilute to 100 ml.
9. Sodium hydroxide, 0.45*N*
   Dilute 90 ml of 1*N* sodium hydroxide to 200 ml with water or dissolve 18 g of sodium hydroxide in water and dilute to one liter with water. Adjust this solution as described in Step 10.
10. Ammonium chloride, 16 g/dl
    Dissolve 16 g of ammonium chloride in water and dilute to 100 ml. Adjust this solution so that 0.5 ml added to 3.0 ml of 0.45*N* sodium hydroxide produces a solution with a pH of 10.5 ± 0.1. Dilute one solution or the other, if necessary, to insure that the mixture will have this pH.

PROCEDURE

1. Add 30 ml of chloroform to each of two 25 X 150 mm screw-capped culture tubes.
2. Add 1.0 ml of specimen to one tube and 1.0 ml of reference solution to the second. If the presence of barbiturates is suspected, treat the samples as noted under Interfering Substances.*
3. Add 1.0 ml of 6*N* hydrochloric acid to each tube. Stopper the tubes and mix the contents vigorously for 1 min. Allow the tubes to stand for 1 min.
4. Remove the aqueous layers by aspiration. Filter the chloroform layers through Whatman #1 filter paper into clean, dry tubes.
5. Add 8.0 ml of 0.45*N* sodium hydroxide to each tube. Cap the tubes and mix the contents vigorously for 1 min. Allow the layers to separate.
6. Remove the lower (organic) layers by aspiration. Pour each sodium hydroxide layer into a centrifuge tube and centrifuge it for 5 min at 2,000 rpm.
7. Pipet duplicate 3.0-ml aliquots of each supernatant into 16 X 100 mm test tubes.
8. To one tube of each set add 0.5 ml of the ammonium chloride solution. Add 0.5 ml of 0.45*N* sodium hydroxide to the other. Mix the contents of each tube.
9. Pour each mixture into a 1-cm silica cuvette.
10. Record the differential spectra from 340 to 220 nm, placing the cuvette with the ammonium chloride on the reference side and the other cuvette on the sample side. Use one of the following three techniques to obtain the differential spectra. Techniques A and B are for recording spectrophotometers, and C is for a manual spectrophotometer. (A) Turn the 100% control knob of the instrument to manually displace the zero absorbance setting to 0.3 absorbance at 340 nm. This method can be used for such instruments as the Beckman DK, the Hitachi 124, and the Beckman DB, on which the instrument's original 100% control 250-K potentiometer has been replaced with a 1-M potentiometer. (B) For recording spectrophotometers not able to perform as described above, use a variable aperture on the reference beam, such as the Beckman variable beam attenuator (Part #104185 or #104186), or a fine mesh screen. (C) If a manual spectrophotometer is used, set the instrument to read 0.3 absorbance at 340 nm. With the cuvette containing ammonium chloride in place, determine the absorbance of the specimen at 340, 325, 320, 318, 315, 300, 290, 285, 283, 280, 270, 260, 255, 250, 246, 242, 235, and 225 nm, resetting the instrument at each wavelength to the initial setting, 0.3 absorbance. Plot the results obtained. Salicylates have a positive peak at 318 nm, a negative peak at 283 nm, and a second positive peak at 246 nm.

*See p. 346.

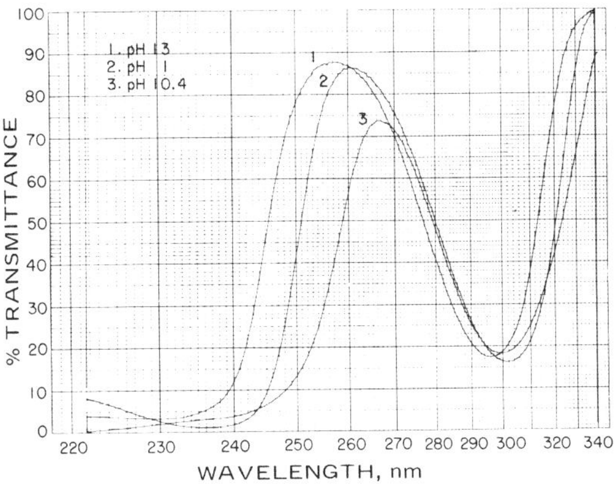

FIGURE 1. Percent transmission of salicylate solutions at various pH's. (Reproduced with permission of C. V. Mosby Co., St. Louis, Missouri, from Williams, L. A., Linn, R. A., and Zak, B., Differential ultraviolet spectrophotometric determination of serum salicylates, *J. Lab. Clin. Med.*, 53, 156–162, 1959.)

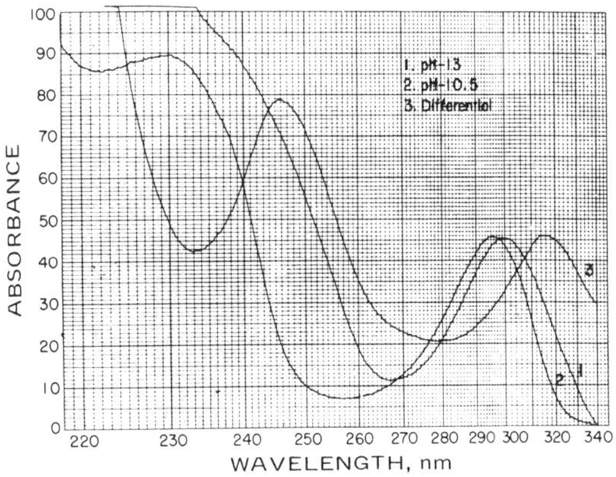

FIGURE 2. Absorbance spectra of salicylate at pH 13 and pH 10.5, and the resultant differential spectrum. (Reproduced with permission of C. V. Mosby Co., St. Louis, Missouri, from Williams, L. A., Linn, R. A., and Zak, B., Differential ultraviolet spectrophotometric determination of serum salicylates, *J. Lab. Clin. Med.*, 53, 156–162, 1959.)

CALCULATION

Figure 1 shows the UV shifts of salicylate at various pH's. Figure 2 shows the absorbance spectra at pH 13,[1] pH 10.5,[2] and the differential spectrum obtained by placing an equal concentration of salicylate in both the reference and sample compartments at the two pH's and recording the resultant spectrum after displacing the zero absorbance to 0.3. The positive peak at 318 nm can be used to calculate concentrations from 0 to 50 mg/100 ml, while the most sensitive peak, 246 nm, is used for concentrations from 0 to 20 mg/100 ml. For salicylate concentrations over 50 mg/100 ml, the negative peak at 283 nm is used. If a series of reference solutions of different concentrations is analyzed, as shown in Figure 3 where the respective concentrations for Curves A to F are 4, 8, 15, 20, 40, and 55 mg/100 ml, linear curves are obtained when the absorbance of the reference solutions are plotted against their respective concentrations. For calculation, therefore, a reference solution must be carried through the entire procedure and the absorbance peak chosen must be in the proper range. The following formula can then be used to determine the salicylate concentration in the specimen:

$$\frac{A_x}{A_R} \times 20 = \text{mg}/100\ \text{ml},$$

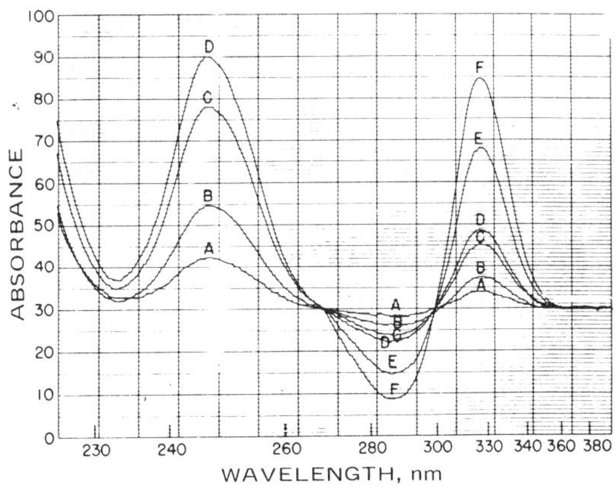

FIGURE 3. Differential spectra of various concentrations of salicylate. (Reproduced with permission of C. V. Mosby Co., St Louis, Missouri, from Williams, L. A., Linn, R. A., and Zak, B., Differential ultraviolet spectrophotometric determination of serum salicylates, *J. Lab. Clin. Med.*, 53, 156–162, 1959.)

where

A_x = absorbance of the specimen;
A_R = absorbance of the reference solution.

INTERPRETATION (see p. 7)

Sodium salicylate and aspirin are both easily absorbed, some from the stomach, but more generally, from the upper GI tract. Maximum salicylate concentration usually occurs 2 hr after ingestion. The common adult therapeutic dose of 600 mg aspirin yields a serum concentration of about 5 mg/100 ml.[3] Doses of 100 mg sodium salicylate/kg body weight usually produce serum concentrations of 20 to 30 mg/100 ml. At this concentration the first overt sign of toxicity, tinnitus, may be noticed. If higher concentrations are found, increased toxic reactions occur. Following an initial respiratory alkalosis, metabolic acidosis may occur at a plasma salicylate concentration between 50 and 70 mg/100 ml. Patients with these or higher serum salicylate concentrations require considerable supportive therapy.

Chemical analyses of serum or urine for their salicylate concentration can be valuable aids to corroborate whether or not a patient is intoxicated and can help predict the clinical course of a salicylate-intoxicated patient. Precise quantitation of salicylate concentration (within ±1 mg/100 ml) is not essential for this purpose, and the procedure described above is more than adequate.

ACCURACY AND PRECISION

The coefficient of variation for salicylate is ±6%. Recovery from samples of known concentrations is 93%.

INTERFERING SUBSTANCES

The low pH used for salicylate extraction will also cause extraction of barbiturates if they are present. Figure 4 shows the differential spectra of salicylate (Curve A), barbiturate (Curve B), and a mixture of salicylate and barbiturate (Curve C).

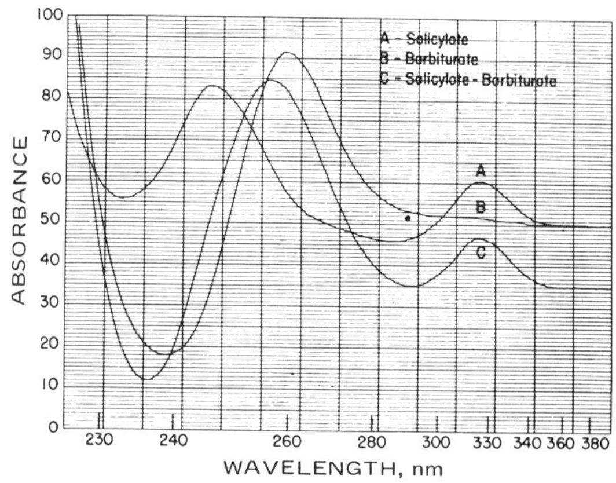

FIGURE 4. Differential spectra of salicylate, barbiturate, and a mixture of both. (Reproduced with permission of C. V. Mosby Co., St. Louis, Missouri, from Williams, L. A., Linn, R. A., and Zak, B., Differential ultraviolet spectrophotometric determination of serum salicylates, *J. Lab. Clin. Med.*, 53, 156–162, 1959.)

The 318-nm peak of salicylate is undistorted, whereas the other peaks are changed. If the specimen is extracted first with chloroform at pH 7.4, the barbiturates will be extracted and can be subsequently determined. The aqueous phase is then made acid and the extraction of salicylates is then accomplished.

REFERENCES

1. **Williams, L. A., Linn, R. A., and Zak, B.,** Differential ultraviolet spectrophotometric determination of serum salicylates, *J. Lab. Clin. Med.*, 53, 156, 1959.
2. **Done, A. K.,** Salicylate intoxication: Significance of measurements of salicylate in blood and cases of acute congestion, *Pediatrics,* 26, 800, 1960.
3. **Leonards, J. R.,** The influence of solubility on the rate of gastrointestinal absorption of aspirin, *Clin. Pharmacol. Ther.*, 5, 476, 1963.

SELENIUM

PRINCIPLE

Copper, zinc, and selenium can be complexed in urine with sodium diethyldithiocarbamate. The zinc and copper complexes are extractable from alkaline medium into methylisobutylketone; thus, they may be extracted first, leaving the selenium complex to be extracted under acid conditions into the solvent. The concentration of the metalloid then can be determined by atomic absorption spectrophotometry.

TYPE C PROCEDURE

Robert A. Maes

APPARATUS

1. Centrifuge
2. Centrifuge tubes, 50 ml
3. Mechanical shaker
4. pH meter
5. Separatory funnels, 100 ml
6. Pipets, volumetric, 1 and 10 ml
7. Flasks, volumetric, one liter and 100 ml
8. Spectrophotometer, atomic absorption (Varian Techtron Model 5 A.A.), equipped with a selenium hollow cathode lamp, a Boling three-slot acetylene air burner, and one 10 in. strip-chart with a 1 to 50 mV span (A selenium electrodeless discharge lamp (EDL) may be more desirable for some laboratories.)

   Operating Conditions

   Gas Flow Rates:
   acetylene – 2.2 l/min
   air – 6.8 l/min
   Adjust the fuel and oxidant flows to obtain a lean, blue flame when aspirating MIBK.
   Wavelength: 196.1 nm
   Selenium Lamp Current: 10 mA
   Range: UV
   Slit Width: 300 μ
   Aspiration: 4 to 6 ml/min
   Curve Correction: 0
   Warm-up Time: 15 min
   Chart Speed: 1 in./min

REAGENTS

All chemicals should be analytical reagent grade. All water used in this procedure must be deionized and then distilled in an all-glass still.

1. Sodium diethyldithiocarbamate (NaDEDC), 1 g/dl
   Dissolve 1 g in 10 ml of water and dilute to 100 ml with water. Prepare this reagent fresh each day.
2. Hydrochloric acid, concentrated (35%)
3. Hydrochloric acid, 4*N*
   Dilute 344 ml of concentrated (35%) hydrochloric acid to one liter with water.
4. Hydrochloric acid, 0.1*N*
   Dilute 8.6 ml of concentrated (35%) hydrochloric acid to one liter with water.
5. Hydrochloric acid, 1.2*N*
   Dilute 10 ml of concentrated hydrochloric acid to 100 ml with water.
6. Nitric acid, concentrated
7. Sodium hydroxide, 4*N*
   Dissolve 160 g of sodium hydroxide in one liter of water.
8. Sodium hydroxide, 0.1*N*
   Dissolve 4 g of sodium hydroxide in one liter of water.
9. Methylisobutylketone (MIBK), Fisher Scientific Co.
10. Selenium stock solution, 1,000 μg/ml
    Dissolve 1.000 g of selenium metal in a minimum volume of concentrated nitric acid.

Evaporate the solution to dryness, add 2 ml of water, and evaporate to dryness 2 or 3 additional times. Dissolve the residue after the third washing in 1.2*N* hydrochloric acid, and dilute to one liter with 1.2*N* hydrochloric acid.

11. Selenium reference solutions, 5, 10, 15, and 20 μg/ml
    Transfer 0.5, 1.0, 1.5, and 2.0 ml of the selenium stock solution to 100-ml volumetric flasks, then dilute each to the calibration marks with water.

PROCEDURE

1. Transfer 30 ml of sample (urines and each of the reference solutions) to duplicate 50-ml centrifuge tubes.
2. Add 4*N* sodium hydroxide drop by drop to each sample, constantly mixing, until the pH reaches approximately 12. Monitor the additions with a pH meter. Adjust the pH to 12.0 by dropwise addition of 0.1*N* sodium hydroxide.
3. Add 1.0 ml of the NaDEDC solution to each sample and mix.
4. Add 10.0 ml of MIBK, shake for 3 min, and centrifuge for 5 min at 3,000 rpm.
5. Transfer the MIBK in the centrifuge tubes to a 100-ml separatory funnel and allow the layers to separate. Place the aqueous phase in a 100-ml separatory funnel. Discard the MIBK (contains Cu and Zn).
6. To the separatory funnel containing the aqueous phase (Step 5), add 4*N* hydrochloric acid drop by drop, constantly mixing, until the pH reaches approximately 4.0. Monitor this with a pH meter. Adjust the pH to 4.5 by dropwise addition of 0.1*N* hydrochloric acid.
7. Add 1.0 ml of the NaDEDC solution and mix.
8. Add 10.0 ml of MIBK, shake for 3 min, and allow the layers to separate.
9. Collect the organic layer in a small stoppered test tube, avoiding the transfer of any aqueous phase.
10. Aspirate the MIBK extract into the burner of the atomic absorption spectrometer and record the absorbance of the samples.
11. Measure the heights of the absorbance peaks.
12. Determine the selenium concentration in the urine sample by comparing the heights of the absorbance peaks of the extracts with those of the reference samples analyzed in the same way.

INTERPRETATION (see p. 7)

According to Sterner and Lidfeldt,[1] the normal concentration of selenium in a 24-hr urine ranges from 0 to 0.15 μg/ml. Lemley,[2] however, considers a concentration of 0.04 μg/ml to be an indication of selenium poisoning. Intoxications,[3] as well as the possibility of selenium being teratogenic,[4] are discussed in literature.

SENSITIVITY AND PRECISION

In urine determinations, precision is within 3% in the normal range for selenium. The precision is increased if higher concentrations are present. The limit of detection is 1.2 μg of selenium/liter.

INTERFERING SUBSTANCES

No other element interferes with the determination of selenium in urine by this atomic absorption procedure.

REFERENCES

1. **Sterner, J. H. and Lidfeldt, V.,** Selenium content of "normal" urine, *J. Pharmacol. Exp. Ther.,* 73, 205, 1941.
2. **Lemley, R. E.,** Selenium poisoning in the human. A preliminary case report, *Lancet,* 60, 528, 1940.
3. **Carter, R. F.,** Acute selenium poisoning, *Med. J. Aust.,* 1, 525, 1968.
4. **Robertson, D. S. F.,** Selenium – a possible teratogen? *Lancet,* 1, 518, 1970.

STRYCHNINE

PRINCIPLE

Strychnine can be extracted from an alkaline solution of the sample. An aliquot of this concentrated extract, when exposed to Mandelin's reagent, yields a very characteristic series of color changes. Another aliquot, when chromatographed on thin-layer plates, can be used to identify strychnine by its R_f values (Procedure A). If the organic extract is reextracted into acid, the UV absorption spectrum of the acid solution can be used to identify strychnine (Procedure B).

TYPE A PROCEDURE

Joseph Monforte

APPARATUS

1. Separatory funnels, 250 ml
2. Evaporating dishes
3. Pasteur pipets
4. Microscope slides, glass
5. Micropipets (diSPo*)
6. Thin-layer chromatography (TLC) equipment: (a) glass plates coated with silica gel G-F; (b) scriber for chromatographic plates†; (c) developing tanks; (d) spray bottle
7. UV lamp, 250 nm radiation

REAGENTS

All chemicals should be analytical reagent grade.

1. Strychnine reference solution, 100 mg of strychnine/dl
   Dissolve 122 mg of strychnine hydrochloride ($C_{21}H_{22}N_2O_2 \cdot HCl \cdot 2H_2O$) in ethanol and dilute to 100 ml with ethanol.
2. Sodium hydroxide, 6*N*
   With stirring, add 60 g of sodium hydroxide to 200 ml of distilled water. Dilute to 250 ml with distilled water.
3. Sulfuric acid, 0.1*N*
   Add 2.8 ml of concentrated sulfuric acid to approximately 500 ml of distilled water. Dilute to one liter with distilled water.
4. Mandelin's reagent
   Dissolve 50 mg of ammonium vandate in 50 ml of concentrated sulfuric acid.
5. Chloroform
6. Developing solutions
   Solution 1, chloroform-methanol, 80:20 – Mix 80 ml of chloroform with 20 ml of methanol. Solution 2, methanol-ammonia, 100:1.5 – Mix 100 ml of methanol with 1.5 ml of concentrated ammonium hydroxide.

PROCEDURE

1. Adjust the pH of the specimen (blood, urine, gastric wash, or bile) to approximately 10 with 6*N* sodium hydroxide. If the specimen is stomach content or a solid, triturate it first with 0.1*N* sulfuric acid, then adjust the pH to approximately 10 with 6*N* sodium hydroxide. Process comparable samples of strychnine reference solution and of water for a reagent blank in the same manner as the specimen.
2. Extract each sample with chloroform, using a solvent-to-sample ratio of at least 4:1. Allow the mixtures to stand until the layers have separated. Centrifuge, if necessary.
3. Aspirate the aqueous layers. Filter each chloroform layer into an evaporating dish.
4. Evaporate the chloroform to dryness in a fume hood.
5. Dissolve each residue in 200 μl of chloroform.
6. Place a 10-μl aliquot of each dissolved residue on a glass microscope slide. Allow the solvent to evaporate. Add one drop of Mandelin's

*Available from Scientific Products Co., Evanston, Ill.
†CRC Press, Inc., 18901 Cranwood Parkway, Cleveland, Ohio 44128, Cat. No. 8705/975.

reagent to both the specimen and the reference samples. Note the color changes of the specimen and of the reference material.
7. Scribe two TLC glass plates so that 18 samples can be processed simultaneously.
8. Apply 25-μl aliquots of each chloroform solution (Step 5) to each of the two plates.
9. Develop one plate in Solution 1 and the other in Solution 2. Allow the plates to air-dry.
10. Observe the plates under a 250-nm light, then spray each with Mandelin's reagent.

INTERPRETATION (see p. 7)

Upon addition of Mandelin's reagent (as in Step 6), a color change from blue to violet to red-orange occurs if strychnine is present. This sequence of color changes is relatively specific for strychnine. It is also observed when the TLC plate containing strychnine is sprayed with Mandelin's reagent. Strychnine has a R_f of 0.29 in developing Solution 1 and a R_f of 0.15 in developing Solution 2.

REFERENCE

Sidney, K., *Handbook of Emergency Toxicology,* 2nd ed., Charles C Thomas, Springfield, Ill., 1961, 79.

TYPE B PROCEDURE

Joseph Monforte

APPARATUS

1. Separatory funnels, 250 ml
2. Filter paper (Whatman #1)
3. Graduated cylinders, 100 ml
4. Centrifuge
5. UV spectrophotometer, equipped with microcells

REAGENTS

All chemicals should be analytical reagent grade.

1. Strychnine stock solution, 100 mg of strychnine/dl
   Dissolve 122 mg of strychnine hydrochloride ($C_{21}H_{22}N_2O_2 \cdot HCl \cdot 2H_2O$) in 100 ml of distilled water.
2. Strychnine reference solutions
   Dilute appropriate quantities of the strychnine stock solution to obtain strychnine concentrations of 1.0, 0.5, and 0.1 mg/dl.
3. Ammonium hydroxide, 3*N*
   Dilute 20.0 ml of concentrated ammonium hydroxide to 100 ml with distilled water.
4. Chloroform
5. Sulfuric acid, 0.1*N*
   Add 1.8 ml of concentrated sulfuric acid to approximately 500 ml of distilled water, then dilute to one liter.

PROCEDURE

1. To 10.0 ml of specimen (blood or urine) in a 250-ml separatory funnel, add 0.5 ml of the ammonium hydroxide solution. Process 10.0 ml of each reference solution and 10.0 ml of water for a reagent blank simultaneously and in the same manner as the specimen.
2. Extract each sample with 125 ml of chloroform.
3. Filter the chloroform through Whatman #1 filter paper. Collect 100 ml of the filtrate in a graduated cylinder.
4. Transfer 50.0 ml of the chloroform filtrate into a clean 250-ml separatory funnel. Add 2.0 ml of 0.1*N* sulfuric acid and shake the mixture for approximately 2 min. Allow the layers to separate.
5. Discard the chloroform. Add the second 50.0-ml portion of the chloroform filtrate, and extract it with the same 0.1*N* sulfuric acid used in the first extraction.

6. Discard the chloroform. Centrifuge the acid remaining in the separatory funnel.
7. Transfer the sulfuric acid layer to a microcell. Determine its UV absorbance from 340 to 230 nm, using the sulfuric acid obtained from the processed water sample as the reference solution.

CALCULATION

If specimen and reference solutions are treated identically, the strychnine content in the specimen may be determined as follows:

$$C_X = \frac{A_X}{A_R} \times C_R,$$

where

C_X = strychnine concentration of the specimen;

A_x = absorbance of the specimen at 286 nm;

A_R = absorbance of the aqueous reference solution at 286 nm;

C_R = strychnine concentration of the reference solution.

INTERPRETATION (see p. 7)

Strychnine is not a normal component of biological specimens. Its presence is an indication that an exogenous chemical agent has been ingested. Should the UV data indicate that strychnine may have been involved, the acid obtained in Step 6 should be treated as described in the Type A Procedure for strychnine* to corroborate that strychnine was the agent whose UV data were recorded.

ACCURACY AND PRECISION

Recoveries of strychnine added to water are approximately 70%.

*See p. 349.

"SULFA" COMPOUNDS

PRINCIPLE

A simple color test is available for urine specimens (Procedure A). Quantitation is possible by diazotizing and coupling the aromatic amine and then determining the absorbance of the resulting solution (Procedure B).

TYPE A PROCEDURE

Irving Sunshine

REAGENTS

All chemicals should be analytical reagent grade.

1. Hydrochloric acid, concentrated

PROCEDURE

1. Streak some urine on a piece of newspaper.
2. Cover this streak with concentrated hydrochloric acid.

INTERPRETATION (see p. 7)

An orange color indicates that a "sulfa" drug may be present. To quantitate and confirm this, use Procedure B.

SENSITIVITY

The test is sensitive to 2 μg of drug.

TYPE B PROCEDURE

Irving Sunshine

REAGENTS

All chemicals should be analytical reagent grade.

1. Drug reference solution, 8 mg/dl
   Dissolve 20 mg of the "sulfa" drug under investigation in water and dilute to 250 ml.
2. Trichloroacetic acid, 15 g/dl
   Dissolve 15 g of trichloroacetic acid in water and dilute to 100 ml.
3. Sodium nitrite, 10 g/dl
   Dissolve 10 g of sodium nitrite in water and dilute to 100 ml. Store this solution in a refrigerator. Before use, dilute this reagent 1:100 with water.
4. Ammonium sulfamate, 0.5 g/dl
   Dissolve 0.5 g of ammonium sulfamate in water and dilute to 100 ml.
5. N-(1-naphthyl)-ethylenediamine dihydrochloride, 0.1 g/dl
   Dissolve 0.1 g of N-(1-naphthyl)-ethylenediamine dihydrochloride in water and dilute to 100 ml. Store this solution at 4°C.
6. Hydrochloric acid, 4*N*
   Add 100 ml of water to 50 ml of concentrated hydrochloric acid.

PROCEDURE

Direct-Reacting Sulfonamide (Free "Sulfa" Drugs)

1. Dilute 0.50 ml of sample (blood or urine specimen, reference solution, and water for a reagent blank) with water to 20 ml. Slowly add 5.0 ml of trichloroacetic acid and mix. Allow the mixtures to stand for 10 min, then filter them.
2. Transfer 5.0 ml of each clean filtrate to a test tube.
3. Add 0.5 ml of the sodium nitrite solution to each tube and mix. Allow the samples to stand for 6 min.
4. Add 0.5 ml of the ammonium sulfamate solution and mix. Allow the samples to stand for 2 min.
5. Add 0.5 ml of the N-(1-naphthyl)-ethylenediamine dihydrochloride solution and mix. Allow the samples to stand for 15 min in the dark.
6. Determine the absorbance of each sample at 550 nm, using the solution obtained by processing the water sample as the reference solution.

Total Sulfonamide (Free plus N_4-Acetylated "Sulfa" Drugs)

1. Transfer 5.0 ml of each filtrate obtained in Step 1 (above) to a test tube. Add 0.5 ml of 4*N* hydrochloric acid, then heat the mixtures for 1 hr in a 100°C water bath.
2. Cool, adjust the volumes to the original level, then proceed as above, beginning with Step 2.

CALCULATION

Determine the drug concentration (mg/100 ml) in the specimen by using the following formula:

$$\frac{A_U}{A_R} \times 8 = \text{mg/100 ml},$$

where

A_U = absorbance of the specimen at 550 nm;
A_R = absorbance of the reference solution at 550 nm.

INTERPRETATION (see p. 7)

Following ingestion of 2 g of sulfisoxazole, a concentration of 9 to 10 mg/100 ml of blood may be expected. Excretion of 70 ti 80% of an oral dose can be expected within 24 hr after ingestion. The major urinary product (70%) is unchanged sulfisoxazole. The remainder is the N_4-acetylated compound and a glucuronide. (Similar data are available for other "sulfa" drugs.[1])

INTERFERING SUBSTANCES

The reaction is not specific for "sulfa" drugs. Any compound with a free aromatic amine or one that is easily hydrolyzed to a free amine will interfere.

REFERENCE

1. **Kananen, G.**, in *Handbook of Analytical Toxicology*, Sunshine, I., Ed., Chemical Rubber Co., Cleveland, 1970, 374.

SULFONYLUREAS

PRINCIPLE

Several commonly used sulfonylureas (tolbutamide, chlorpropamide, and tolazamide), with the following general structure, are separated from the biological matrix by extraction into toluene.

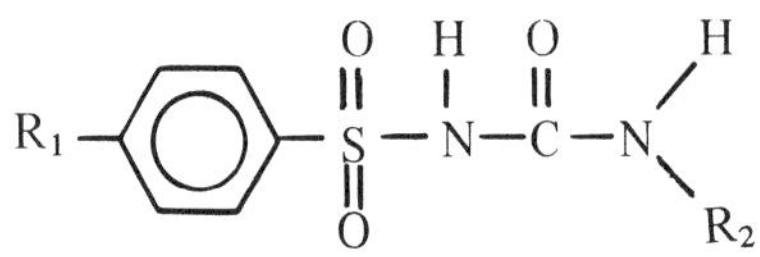

The toluene is then reextracted into a methanolic solution of trimethylanilinium (TMAH). When injected into a gas chromatograph, the TMAH extracts of these drugs fragment to give products of the following structure:

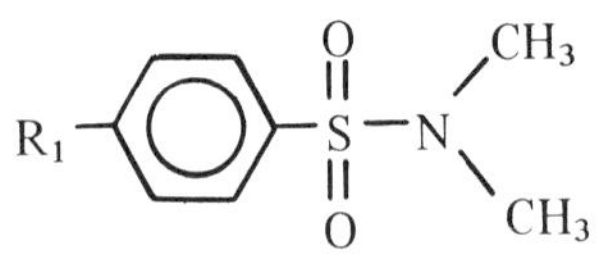

The gas chromatographic peaks from these products are then used to determine the identity and concentration of sulfonylurea in the original sample.

TYPE C PROCEDURE

Vijay Aggarwal and Irving Sunshine

APPARATUS

1. Test tubes, 10 ml with Teflon®-lined screw caps
2. Concentratubes®*
3. Pasteur pipets
4. 50-μl syringe (Hamilton #705-N)
5. 10-μl syringe (Hamilton #701-N)
6. Vortex (Vortex Genie #58223)
7. Centrifuge
8. Gas chromatograph, fitted with flame ionizations detectors and a coiled stainless steel column 6′ × 1/8″ i.d., packed with 10% UCW 98 on Chromsorb W-HP 80/100 mesh (A stainless steel injection port liner packed with silanized glass wool is used in the injection port.)

Operating Conditions

Gas Flow Rates:
- air – 240 ml/min
- hydrogen – 25 ml/min
- helium – 30 ml/min

Temperatures:
- column – 180°C
- injection port – 260°C
- detector – 290°C

*Test tubes, 20 ml, which taper to a small tip which holds about 10 μl. Available from Laboratory Research Co., P.O. Box 36409, Los Angeles, California 90035.

REAGENTS

All chemicals should be analytical reagent grade.

1. Trimethylanilinium hydroxide (TMAH)
   Add 7.0 g of trimethylphenylammonium iodide (Aldrich # 13,914-9) to 10 ml of methanol contained in a culture tube with a Teflon®-lined screw cap. Add 3.6 g of silver oxide and shake for 2 min. Rotate the tube on a mechanical rotator for 2 hr, centrifuge, and decant the supernatant into a brown glass bottle. The molarity of the resulting solution should be 2.0 ± 0.1. It is stable for at least one month when stored at 4°C.
2. Stock internal standard solution, 100 mg/ml
   Dissolve 500 mg of aprobarbital in toluene and dilute to 500 ml with toluene.
3. Working internal standard solution, 10 mg/100 ml
   Dilute 10 mg of the stock internal standard solution to 100 ml with toluene.
4. H_3PO_4
   Dilute 1.15 ml of 85% H_3PO_4 to 100 ml with distilled water.
5. Stock sulfonylurea standard solution
   Dissolve 25 mg of the drug (e.g., tolbutamide, chlorpropamide, or tolazamide) in 50 ml of distilled water.
6. Working sulfonylurea reference solutions
   Dilute these stock solutions with fresh drug, free plasma, urine, or distilled water, depending on the type of samples to be analyzed, to give concentrations in the range expected in the samples. At least two reference solutions (e.g., 2.0 and 5.0 mg/100 ml) should be processed with each group of samples.

PROCEDURE

1. To 3.0 ml of plasma sample and appropriate standards, each contained in a 10-ml culture tube, add 1.0 ml of the H_3PO_4 solution, and 5.0 ml of the internal standard solution. If urine or aqueous samples and standards are to be analyzed, substitute 1 ml of a one mol/l acetate buffer (pH 5.2) for the 1 ml of H_3PO_4.
2. Shake the capped tubes for 2 min and then centrifuge them to separate the phases. Transfer 4 ml of the toluene layer to a Concentratube®.
3. Vortex the Concentratube®. While vortexing, slowly add 20 μl of the TMAH solution with a 50-μl syringe. Continue vortexing for 25 sec, and then centrifuge the tubes for 5 min.
4. Withdraw 3 μl of the TMAH (lower) phase with a 10-μl syringe and inject this aliquot into the gas chromatograph over a 10-sec interval. This slow injection is necessary on several types of gas chromatographs to avoid severe tailing of the solvent which results when normal injection speeds are used.

CALCULATIONS

The concentration of sulfonylurea can be calculated from either peak height or peak area data and the following formula:

$$C_i = C_s \times \frac{P_i}{A_i} \times \frac{A_s}{P_s},$$

where

- C_i = concentration of sulfonylurea in the sample;
- C_s = concentration of sulfonylurea in the standard;
- P_i = peak height or area of drug in the sample;
- A_i = peak height or area of aprobarbital in the sample;
- P_s = peak height or area of drug in the standard;
- A_s = peak height or area of aprobarbital in the standard.

INTERPRETATION (see p. 7)

Sheldon et al.[1] reported that well-controlled diabetic patients have average serum concentrations of 7.1 mg of tolbutamide/100 ml and 7.7 mg/100 ml of chlorpropamide. Dowell and Imrie[2] reported a fatal chlorpropamide poisoning in a nondiabetic where plasma chlorpropamide was 70 mg/100 ml.

PRECISION

The ratio of the peak area of the drug fragment to peak area of aprobarbital is a linear function of drug concentration from 0.05 to 10.0 mg/100 ml for chlorpropamide, tolbutamide and tolazamide. Over this concentration range the average coefficient of variation is 3.1%. The minimum detectable amount is 0.03 mg/100 ml.

INTERFERING SUBSTANCES

Table 1 lists the retention times of the sulfonylurea fragments produced in this procedure. Both tolbutamide and tolazamide fragment in the injection port of the gas chromatograph to yield the same product and thus their retention times in this system are identical. Since the most common need for sulfonylurea determinations is for monitoring of diabetic's blood sulfonylurea level where the identity of the agent is known, the identity of the drug is not a major problem.

Barbiturates are extracted by this procedure; using the gas chromatographic conditions described above, the sulfonylurea fragments are resolved from them (Table 1). In cases where the patient is known to be free of barbiturates, the total time for analysis of a sample may be shortened by raising the gas chromatograph oven temperature to 200°C.

REFERENCES

1. **Sheldon, J., et al.,** Serum concentration and urinary excretion of oral sulfonylurea compounds, *Diabetes,* 14(6), 362, 1965.
2. **Dowell, R. C. and Imrie, A. H.,** Chlorpropamide poisoning in nondiabetics, *Scott. Med. J.,* 17, 305, 1972.

Table 1

RETENTION TIMES OF TMAH DERIVATIVES OF SUBSTANCES CO-EXTRACTED WITH SULFONYLUREAS

	Retention times at 180°C (min)
Amobarbital	6.81
Pentobarbital	7.68
Tolbutamide fragment	7.80
Tolazamide fragment	7.80
Chlorpropamide fragment	8.23
Secobarbital	8.86
Phenobarbital	12.92

GENERAL REFERENCES

Aggarwal, V. and Sunshine, I., Determination of sulfonylureas and metabolites by pyrolysis gas chromatography, *Clin. Chem.,* 20(2), 200, 1974.

Forrest, J. H., Chlorpropramide overdosage, *Clin. Toxicol.,* 7, 19, 1974.

Martin, S. B. and Rowland, M., Determination of tolbutamide and chlorpropramide in biological fluids, *J. Pharm. Pharmacol.,* 25, 186, 1973.

Taylor, J. A., Pharmacokinetics and biotransformation of chlorpropramide in man, *Clin. Pharmacol. Ther.,* 13, 710, 1972.

THALLIUM

PRINCIPLE

The organic matter in the sample is removed by wet oxidative digestion. The thallium in the resulting solution is oxidized to thallic ions by bromine. In Procedure A the stabilized tetrabromothallate anion formed reacts with the cation of the basic dye, methyl violet, to form a nonionized benzene-extractable blue complex. In Procedure B an iodometric redox reaction is used to quantitate the thallium present. This redox procedure is not feasible if bismuth, chromium, or copper salts are present. If this is so, the digest is treated with sulfur dioxide to reduce all thallium present to the thallous ion which is then precipitated as the bromide and determined gravimetrically. In Procedure C the thallic bromide is extracted into diethyl ether, and the ether is evaporated to dryness. The residue is dissolved in dilute acid and aspirated into the flame of an atomic absorption spectrometer. The absorption of light at 277 nm is proportional to the concentration of thallium in the sample.

TYPE A PROCEDURE

Fredric Rieders

APPARATUS

1. Centrifuge tubes borosilicate, conical, 10 ml

REAGENTS

All chemicals should be analytical reagent grade.

1. Thallium stock solution, 10 mg/100 ml
   Dissolve 123.5 mg of anhydrous thallous sulfate in distilled water and dilute to one liter.
2. Thallium reference solution, 1 μg/ml
   Dilute 1.0 ml of the thallium stock solution to 100 ml with distilled water.
3. Nitric acid, 3*N*
   Dilute 20.0 ml of concentrated nitric acid to 100 ml with distilled water.
4. Hydrochloric acid, concentrated
5. Bromine water
   Place 40 ml of distilled water and approximately 5 ml of bromine into a 60-ml ground-glass-stoppered dropping bottle of clear borosilicate glass and shake. Store the solution in a refrigerator when not in use. Some undissolved bromine should remain in the bottle.
6. Sulfosalicylic acid, 20 g/100 ml
   Dissolve 10 g of sulfosalicylic acid (Eastman 676) in approximately 30.0 ml of distilled water. Dilute this solution to 50.0 ml with distilled water and store it in a polyethylene-stoppered amber glass bottle. The reagent is stable indefinitely.
7. Methyl violet, 200 mg/100 ml
   Dissolve 200 mg of methyl violet (Eastman 1309) in distilled water. Dilute this solution to 100 ml with distilled water. Stored in a ground-glass-stoppered clear bottle, this reagent is stable indefinitely.
8. Benzene

SPECIMEN REQUIREMENTS

Specimens and containers must be free of detergent residues. Wash all glassware with the dilute nitric acid, rinse with distilled water, drain, then dry in an oven.

Urine

Use as received unless contamination by detergent is suspected. If so, add 2.0 ml of concentrated nitric acid to 2.0 ml of urine, gently heat the mixture just to dryness, then dissolve the residue in 1.0 ml of distilled water.

Gastric Content

Centrifuge the specimen for 15 min at 6,000 rpm. Use 1.0 ml of the clear aqueous portion, usually from the middle layer between the fat on top and the debris at the bottom of the centrifuge tube.

PROCEDURE

1. Place 1.0 ml of specimen (urine, aqueous phase of centrifuged gastric content, or neutralized digest of other biologic material) in a 10-ml conical borosilicate centrifuge tube. Into similar tubes place 1.0 ml of distilled water containing 1 ml of the thallium reference solution (to be processed as a reference control) and 1.0 ml of water to serve as reagent blank.
2. Add 0.05 ml (1 drop) of the concentrated hydrochloric acid and 0.3 ml (6 drops) of the bromine water to each tube. Shake the mixtures, then allow them to stand for 1 min.
3. Add 0.3 ml (6 drops) of the sulfosalicylic acid solution to each tube. Shake the mixtures, then allow them to stand for 3 min to effect complete removal of excess bromine.
4. Add 1.0 ml of benzene to each tube. Stopper the tubes, shake them vigorously for about 20 sec, then allow the benzene layers to separate. A blue, green, or orange color could be due to interfering medicines, medication dyes, or food dyes; other procedures for the detection of thallium should then be used. If the benzene is colorless, proceed with Step 5.
5. Add 0.1 ml (2 drops) of the aqueous methyl violet solution to each sample. Stopper the tubes, then shake them vigorously for about 30 sec.
6. Centrifuge the tubes for approximately 5 min at 3,000 rpm.
7. Examine the supernatant benzene layers against a white, well-illuminated background for the presence of a blue color.
8. If the benzene appears to contain a blue dye, filter it through a small pledget of packed glass wool, then examine the filtrate for the presence of a blue color.
9. Compare the solution obtained from the specimen with those obtained from the reference sample and from the reagent blank.

INTERPRETATION (see p. 7)

If the benzene is colorless, the specimen did not contain a toxicologically significant amount of thallium. A positive test result may be obtained on urine as long as 3 weeks after ingestion of a single, moderately toxic dose of thallium sulfate.

SENSITIVITY

The detection limit for thallium in urine by this method is approximately 0.15 μg of thallium.

INTERFERING SUBSTANCES

Color formation is inhibited by the presence of 1.0 mg of nitrite, sulfite, sulfide, thiosulfate, or thiocyanate. False positives may be obtained if an alkylaryl sulfonate detergent, 20 μg or more of mercury, 200 μg of iodide, or vanadium is present, or if the pH of the final solution is greater than 4.

REFERENCE

Rieders, F., Possibilities and limitations of chemical exclusion screening for some common poisons, *Ann. N.Y. Acad. Sci.,* 111, 591, 1964.

TYPE B PROCEDURE

William J. Wilson, Jr.

APPARATUS

1. Volumetric flasks, 500 ml and one liter
2. Pregl filter tubes
3. Erlenmeyer flasks, 125 ml
4. Microburettes, 10 ml
5. Beakers
6. Kjeldahl flasks, 300 to 500 ml
7. Glass beads
8. Filter paper
9. Measuring cylinders, various sizes
10. Spot plates

REAGENTS

All chemicals should be analytical reagent grade.

1. Hydriodic acid, 5.51*N*
2. Hydriodic acid, 1*N*
   Dilute 9.1 ml of 5.51*N* hydriodic acid to 50 ml with distilled water.
3. Acetone
4. Sulfuric acid, concentrated
5. Bromine water
   Wash a ¼-in. layer of bromine, contained in a glass-stoppered brown bottle, three times with distilled water by decantation. Add distilled water equivalent to 10 volumes of the bromine used. Protect the solution from light.
6. Phenol, 5 g/100 ml
   Dissolve 5 g of white phenol crystals in 100 ml of water.
7. Potassium iodide
8. Starch-potassium iodide-phenol indicator
   Triturate 0.5 g of soluble starch with 5.0 ml of water, then add it, with stirring, to 50 ml of boiling water. Add 0.5 g of potassium iodide. When the solution has cooled, add 2.5 ml of the phenol solution.
9. Chloroform
10. Sodium thiosulfate solution, 0.01*N*
    Boil a volume of distilled water for 10 min. Cool it to room temperature. While cooling, protect the water from air and carbon dioxide. Dissolve 2.5 g of sodium thiosulfate pentahydrate in the specially prepared water. Add 0.1 ml of chloroform to prevent bacterial growth and decomposition, then dilute the solution to one liter with the boiled water.
11. Thallous sulfate stock solution, 1 mg/ml
    Dissolve 0.6174 g of pure dry thallous sulfate in distilled water and dilute to exactly 500 ml. Check the concentration by addition of hydriodic acid to a proper aliquot. Filter the precipitate with a Pregl filter tube. Wash the precipitate first with 1*N* hydriodic acid, then with acetone. Dry it for 1 hr at 80 to 100°C while passing filtered air through the tube. Weigh it as thallous iodide. Calculate the thallium content, using the factor 0.6169. Recovery is 98.8%. Do not use bromine, since thallous bromide is appreciably soluble in water.
12. Thallous sulfate reference solutions
    Pipet 1.0, 2.0, 3.0, 4.0, 5.0, and 10.0 ml of the thallous sulfate stock solution into a series of 125-ml Erlenmeyer flasks. Add 40 ml of water and 1 drop of concentrated sulfuric acid to each flask. Add bromine water, drop by drop, until a persistent yellow color is obtained. Wait 3 to 5 min, then add 1.0 ml of the phenol solution to remove excess bromine. Wait 3 to 5 min, then add 0.5 g of potassium iodide. Agitate the solutions until the potassium iodide dissolves, cover the flasks with watch glasses, then let them stand for 10 min. Add 1.0 ml of starch-potassium iodide-phenol indicator, then titrate with 0.01*N* sodium thiosulfate solution, using microburettes, until the color just disappears. One ml of 0.01*N* sodium thiosulfate solution is equivalent to 1.06 mg of thallium. Calculate the exact equivalence of the sodium thiosulfate solution.
13. Nitric acid, concentrated
14. Perchloric acid, concentrated (72%)
15. Hydrogen peroxide, 30% (Superoxol®)
16. Sodium phosphate, dibasic, dodecahydrate ($Na_2HPO_4 \cdot 12H_2O$)
17. Phosphoric acid, concentrated (85%)
18. Cinchonine solution
    Dissolve 1 g of cinchonine by heating it in 100

ml of water containing a little nitric acid. Add 2 g of potassium iodide when the solution has cooled to room temperature.

19. Potassium hydroxide, 5*N*
    Dissolve 28.1 g of potassium hydroxide in 100 ml of water.
20. Potassium bromide
21. Hypobromite solution, alkaline
    To 8.0 ml of bromine water add 2.0 ml of 5*N* potassium hydroxide and 2 g of potassium bromide. Prepare fresh as needed.
22. Sulfosalicylic acid, 20 g/100 ml
    Dissolve 20 g of sulfosalicylic acid in 100 ml of water.
23. Diphenylcarbazide, saturated ethanol solution
    Dissolve an excess of diphenylcarbazide in hot ethanol, cool, then use the supernatant liquid.
24. Alizarin blue, saturated pyridine solution
25. Acetic anhydride
26. Sulfur dioxide
27. Hydrobromic acid, 8.89*N*
28. Hydrobromic acid, 5.5*N*
    Dilute 62 ml of 8.89*N* hydrobromic acid to 100 ml with distilled water.
29. Hydrobromic acid, 1*N*
    Dilute 11.3 ml of 8.89*N* hydrobromic acid to 100 ml with distilled water.
30. Hydrochloric acid, concentrated

PROCEDURE, VOLUMETRIC[1]

1. Place the specimen (50 to 100 g of minced tissue, 50 to 100 ml of blood, or one liter of urine concentrated to about 80 ml on a steam bath) in a large beaker. Add 100 to 150 ml of concentrated nitric acid and 5 to 7 ml of concentrated sulfuric acid, depending on the amount of specimen. Process appropriate reference samples and a reagent blank concomitantly in the same manner.
2. Heat the mixture very cautiously to prevent foaming. If foaming occurs, lower the heat until it subsides. Continue the digestion with increased heat until the mixture becomes a homogeneous solution.
3. Transfer the solution quantitatively with small increments of concentrated nitric acid to a Kjeldahl flask and dilute it to about 100 ml with concentrated nitric acid. Allow the solution to cool.
4. After making sure that the solution is cool, add several glass beads. Slowly and *carefully* add 3 to 4 ml of concentrated (72%) perchloric acid, then continue heating at the highest possible temperature. Avoid charring by adding small increments of 30% hydrogen peroxide and, if necessary, concentrated nitric acid.
5. When all the organic matter has been destroyed, continue heating until dense white sulfur trioxide fumes evolve.
6. Cool the flask, add 20 ml of water, then heat the flask again until sulfur trioxide fumes appear.
7. Repeat this wash step twice.
8. Cool the flask to ambient temperature, then add 10.0 ml of distilled water. Allow the flask to stand for several hours, preferably overnight, stirring occasionally.
9. Filter the flask contents into a 25-ml graduated cylinder. Wash the flask and filter paper with distilled water, adding the washings to the cylinder, then dilute the filtrate to 20 ml.
10. Remove an aliquot of 3 drops to test for the presence of interfering substances. If interfering cations are present, the gravimetric thallium bromide procedure of Gettler and Weiss[2] should be used. If not, proceed as described below.
11. To the clear digest (Step 9) add 150 ml of water, 10 g of dibasic sodium phosphate (dodecahydrate), and 20 ml of concentrated (85%) phosphoric acid. This buffers the solution and eliminates iron interference.
12. Add bromine water to slight excess (yellow color), oxidizing any Tl^{+1} to Tl^{+3}. Allow the solution to stand for 5 min.
13. Add 2.0 ml of the phenol solution to remove any excess bromine. Wait several minutes.
14. Add 0.5 g of potassium iodide, then allow the solution to stand for 10 min.
15. Add 2.0 ml of starch-potassium iodide-phenol indicator.
16. Using a microburette, titrate the mixture with 0.01*N* sodium thiosulfate solution to the disappearance of the blue color. The titer for a reagent blank on 50 g of thallium-free tissue usually is 0.11 ± 0.03 ml of 0.01*N* sodium thiosulfate solution. If the titer for the specimen is very close to this amount, no thallium is present.

CALCULATION

The average loss of thallium due to wet digestion is about 10%. One ml of 0.01*N* sodium thiosulfate solution is equivalent to 1.06 mg of thallium; therefore,

$$T = (\text{ml of } Na_2S_2O_3 \text{ solution} - 0.11) \times \frac{1.06}{0.9} \times f,$$

where

T = milligrams of thallium in the weighed specimen;
f = correction factor for $Na_2S_2O_3$ solution if it is not 0.01*N*.

INTERFERING SUBSTANCES

Bismuth, chromium, and copper give positive results in the above procedure, and it must be determined whether these cations are present.

1. Bismuth
   Impregnate filter paper with cinchonine solution. Add 1 drop of the dilute digest. If Bi^{+3} is present, it will give an orange-red precipitate of the double iodide. If the solution (digest) contains bismuth, mercury, lead and copper, four rings will be formed as follows:[3] (a) an orange ring due to bismuth; (b) a white central ring due to mercury; (c) a yellow ring due to lead iodide; (d) a brown ring of iodine, released by cupric ions. The width of these zones will vary according to the concentrations of these metals. The limit for identification of bismuth is 0.14 μg; in the presence of copper, lead, and mercury it is 10 μg.
2. Chromium[4]
   To 1 drop of neutral or weakly acid digest on a spot plate, add 1 or 2 drops of alkaline hypobromite solution. Wait 1 min, then add 1 drop of concentrated sulfuric acid, 1 or 2 drops of the sulfosalicylic acid solution, and 1 drop of saturated alcoholic diphenylcarbazide solution. A violet color appears, whose intensity indicates the amount of chromium present. The limit for identification of chromium is 0.25 μg.
3. Copper[5]
   Place 1 drop of alizarin blue solution in each of two depressions on a spot plate. Add 1 drop of the acid digest to one depression and a copper-free water blank to the other. An intense blue color results in both. Add 1 or 2 drops of acetic anhydride to both solutions. The blank will become honey-yellow, whereas the copper-bearing solution will have a blue-violet precipitate. The limit for identification of copper is 0.04 μg.

If the tests for bismuth, copper, or chromium yield positive results, the gravimetric procedure of Gettler and Weiss,[2] described below, should be substituted for Steps 11 through 16 of the volumetric procedure.

PROCEDURE, GRAVIMETRIC[2]

1. Pass sulfur dioxide through the solution obtained in Step 9 of the volumetric procedure until it is saturated. This prevents the oxidation of T^{+1} to T^{+3} by bromide, which may form when hydrogen bromide is added in the next step.
2. While sulfur dioxide is still bubbling through the liquid, add 1.0 ml of 5.5*N* hydrobromic acid drop by drop. A white flocculent precipitate of thallous bromide forms in a few minutes.
3. Filter the solution by means of a previously weighed Pregl filter tube, using an inverted syphon and suction.
4. Wash the centrifuge tube, syphon, and precipitate successively with 2.0 ml of 1*N* hydrobromic acid saturated with sulfur dioxide, followed by acetone.
5. Plug the filter tube with a stopper that has been fitted with a glass tube packed with cotton.
6. Connect the tube to a suction pump and heat it to 80 to 90°C while pumping air through it.
7. Cool the tube to ambient temperature, wipe it with a chamois cloth, then weight it as thallous bromide.

CALCULATION

Calculate the thallium concentration in tissue (mg/100 g) as follows:

$$\frac{P \times 0.7189^{*} \times 100}{8} = mg/100\ g,$$

where

P = weight (mg) of the precipitate plus correction factor for the solubility of thallous bromide, which is 0.4 mg of TlBr/15 ml of solution;

S = weight (g) or volume (ml) of the original material.

INTERFERING SUBSTANCES

Test the solution obtained in Step 9 of the volumetric procedure for the presence of silver by adding 2 or 3 drops of concentrated hydrochloric acid. If no precipitate is formed, no silver is present. If a precipitate forms, place the solution in a water bath for 30 min, then remove the precipitated silver chloride by filtration. Proceed with the precipitation of thallous bromide, as described above, from the clear filtrate. Although silver bromide is less soluble than silver chloride, silver bromide will not precipitate from a solution free of silver chloride.

INTERPRETATION (see p. 7)

The volumetric procedure is sensitive to amounts of thallium ranging from 10 to 30 μg. For the gravimetric procedure at least 100 μg of thallium should be present; enough material must be used, therefore, to insure this amount. A minimum of 50 g is recommended for tissue specimens. Urinary excretion, in the nonfatal poisoning, may vary from 30 μg/liter to several milligrams.[6] It is also necessary to use a 24-hr specimen, since the urine excretion may be erratic. Blood is not recommended for the thallium determination, because it has a high iron content and low thallium concentration (10 μg/100 ml). With very few exceptions, fatal urinary thallium concentrations range from 0.5 to 10 mg.[7-9] In two fatal cases the total respective urine concentrations were 5.5 and 6.2 mg/24-hr urine specimen. Fatal tissue concentrations range from 4 to 5 mg of thallium/100 g of liver or kidney; kidney tissue generally shows a higher concentration than liver.

*Gravimetric factor: $\frac{Tl}{Tl\,Br} = \frac{204.37}{284.28} = 0.7198.$

SENSITIVITY

The sensitivity of the volumetric procedure ranges from 10 to 30 μg.[10] For the gravimetric method it is recommended to have at least 100 μg of thallium present, although smaller quantities can be detected.

REFERENCES

1. **Gettler, A. O. and Weiss, L.,** Thallium poisoning II: The quantitative determination of thallium in biologic material, *Am. J. Clin. Pathol.,* 13, 368, 1943.
2. **Gettler, A. O. and Weiss, L.,** Thallium poisoning II: The quantitative determination of thallium in biologic material, *Am. J. Clin. Pathol.,* 13, 375, 1943.
3. **Feigl, F.,** *Spot Test in Inorganic Analysis,* Elsevier, Amsterdam, 1958, 76.
4. **Feigl, F.,** *Spot Test in Inorganic Analysis,* Elsevier, Amsterdam, 1958, 168.
5. **Feigl, F.,** *Spot Test in Inorganic Analysis,* Elsevier, Amsterdam, 1958, 92.
6. **Curry, A. S.,** *Poison Detection in Human Organs,* 2nd ed., Charles C Thomas, Springfield, 1969, 249.
7. **Gettler, A. O. and Weiss, L.,** Thallium poisoning: Clinical toxicology of thallium, *Am. J. Clin. Pathol.,* 13, 422, 1943.
8. **Prick, J. J. G., Smitt, W. G. S., and Miller, L.,** *Thallium Poisoning,* Elsevier, Amsterdam, 1955, 122.
9. **Hausman, R. and Wilson, W. J., Jr.,** Thallotoxicosis – a social menace, *J. Forensic Sci.,* 9, 92, 1964.
10. **Gettler, A. O. and Weiss, L.,** Thallium poisoning II: The quantitative determination of thallium in biologic material, *Am. J. Clin. Pathol.,* 13, 374, 1943.

TYPE C PROCEDURE

F. William Sunderman, Jr.

APPARATUS

1. Erlenmeyer flasks, 125 ml
2. Beads (Pyrex®)
3. Hot plate
4. Centrifuge tubes, glass-stoppered, 50 ml
5. Pasteur pipets
6. Beakers (Pyrex®), 100 ml
7. Volumetric flasks, 25 ml
8. Homogenizer, Teflon® glass, motor-driven
9. Spectrometer, atomic absorption (Perkin-Elmer Model 303), fitted with a thallium hollow cathode lamp and a Boling burner

REAGENTS

All chemicals should be analytical reagent grade.

1. Thallium stock solution, 10 mg/100 ml
   Dissolve 123.5 mg of anhydrous thallous sulfate in distilled water and dilute to one liter.
2. Thallium reference solutions
   Dilute appropriate volumes of the thallium stock solution with water to obtain thallium concentrations of 12.5, 25, 50, and 100 μg/ml of solution.
3. Nitric acid, concentrated (70%)
4. Sulfuric acid, concentrated (sp gr 1.84)
5. Perchloric acid, 35%
6. Hydrochloric acid, concentrated (39%)
7. Bromine water, saturated aqueous solution
8. Diethyl ether, peroxide-free

PROCEDURE

Preparation of Specimens

Urine

1. To duplicate sets of six 125-ml Erlenmeyer flasks transfer, respectively, 50 ml of urine, 50 ml of distilled water for reagent blanks, and 1 ml of each thallium reference solution added to 50 ml of distilled water.
2. Add 6 ml of 70% nitric acid and 2 ml of concentrated sulfuric acid to each sample, then insert 3 Pyrex® beads into each flask.
3. Heat the flasks on a hot plate in a fume hood until the contents have boiled down to approximately 4 ml and charring has occurred in the urine samples. Allow the flasks to cool to room temperature.
4. Add 6 ml of 70% nitric acid and 0.2 ml of 35% perchloric acid, then reheat the flasks until the urine samples become yellow and finally colorless. Allow the flasks to cool. (If the solutions fail to become colorless, additional 0.2-ml volumes of perchloric acid may be added. Be certain to cool the flasks to room temperature before adding any perchloric acid.)
5. Add 5 ml of distilled water to each sample.
6. Transfer the flask contents to 50-ml glass-stoppered centrifuge tubes, using three 4-ml rinses of concentrated (39%) hydrochloric acid.
7. Add 2 ml of bromine water to each centrifuge tube, then cool the samples in an ice bath.
8. Extract the thallic bromide with four 20-ml volumes of peroxide-free diethyl ether. After each extraction, remove the ether layers with Pasteur pipets. Combine each set of four extracts obtained from one sample in a 100-ml Pyrex® beaker.
9. Evaporate each of the combined ether extracts to dryness on a steam bath in a fume hood.
10. Dissolve the residues in 3 ml of concentrated sulfuric acid and 0.2 ml of 35% perchloric acid. Be sure the solution is at room temperature before adding the perchloric acid.
11. Heat the beakers on the hot plate until dense white fumes of sulfur trioxide appear. Continue to heat them for 3 min longer, then allow them to cool.
12. Transfer the contents of each beaker to a 25-ml volumetric flask, using three 5-ml rinses of distilled water.
13. Dilute the contents of the volumetric flasks to 25 ml with distilled water. The samples are now ready for measurements by atomic absorption spectrometry.

Feces

1. Transfer duplicate 1-g specimens of feces and 50 ml of distilled water to each of two 125-ml Erlenmeyer flasks. Mix the contents thoroughly with a glass rod.
2. Digest and extract the samples in the same manner as the urine specimens.

Tissues

1. Homogenize duplicate 1-g specimen of tissues (wet weight) with 10 ml of distilled water, using a motor-driven Teflon® glass homogenizer.
2. Transfer each of the homogenates to a 125-ml Erlenmeyer flask, using four 10-ml washings of distilled water.
3. Digest and extract the samples in the same manner as the urine specimens.

Serum or Blood

1. Transfer duplicate 5-ml specimens of serum or blood to each of two 125-ml Erlenmeyer flasks and dilute them to 50 ml with distilled water.
2. Digest and extract the samples in the same manner as the urine specimens.

Adjustment of the Atomic Absorption Spectrometer

1. Adjust the atomic absorption spectrometer to the following operating conditions:

Air pressure: 25 psi
Air flow: 9 meter units
Acetylene pressure: 10.5 psi
Acetylene flow: 8.5 meter units
Sample aspiration rate: 5 ml/min
Lamp current: 12 mA
Absorption wavelength: 277.0 nm
Entrance slit: 4 μ
Scale expansion: 5 X
Meter response: position 3

2. Set the potentiometer knob at 0% absorption.
3. While water is aspirated into the burner, set the null meter at the null point by means of the background-adjustment knob.
4. Verify the stability of the burner and of the optical and electronic systems by monitoring the null meter for several minutes while water is continuously aspirated into the burner.

Measurement of Atomic Absorption

1. Aspirate the blank, reference, and unknown samples into the flame.
2. Determine the percentage of absorption of each sample by adjusting the null meter to the null point, using the potentiometer knob.

CALCULATION

1. Convert the measurements of percent absorption (%A) into absorbance units (A) by the equation:

$$A = 2 \log_{10}(100 - \%A)$$

2. Determine the amount of thallium in the specimen by comparing its absorbance with that of a suitable reference sample. For determinations on a large number of specimens, a standard curve can be prepared by plotting the absorbances of the reference solutions against their respective thallium concentrations.

INTERPRETATION (see p. 7)

As reported by Savory et al.,[1] thallium is normally not detectable in biological materials from healthy subjects. The reported levels of sensitivity are sufficient for clinical management of thallotoxicosis.[2]

ACCURACY, PRECISION, AND SENSITIVITY

The coefficients of variation of duplicate analyses of thallium are 6.9% for urine specimens containing 10 to 30 μg of thallium/100 ml, and 3.5% for urine specimens containing 90 to 150 μg of thallium/100 ml. The mean recoveries of thallium added to urine, serum, liver, or feces range from 95 to 107%. Measurements of thallium by atomic absorption spectrometry correlate closely with analyses by a coulometric procedure.[3] The limit of sensitivity (A = 0.01) for the detection of thallium in urine is 3.5 μg in a 50-ml specimen or 7 μg/100 ml. The limit of sensitivity (A = 0.01) for the detection of thallium in urine is 3.5 μg in a 5-ml specimen or 70 μg/100 ml.

INTERFERING SUBSTANCES

Despite careful search, no other element interferes with the determination of thallium in biological materials by the atomic absorption technique.[1]

REFERENCES

1. **Savory, J., Roszel, N. O., Mushak, P., and Sunderman, F. W., Jr.,** Measurements of thallium in biologic materials by atomic-absorption spectrometry, *Am. J. Clin. Pathol.*, 50, 505, 1968.
2. **Sunderman, F. W., Jr.,** Diethyldithiocarbamate therapy of thallotoxicosis, *Am. J. Med. Sci.*, 253, 209, 1967.
3. **Christian, G. D. and Purdy, W. C.,** Coulometric determination of thallium in blood and urine, *Am. J. Clin. Pathol.*, 46, 185, 1966.

GENERAL REFERENCES

Gettler, A. O. and Weiss, L., Thallium poisoning: Clinical toxicology of thallium, *Am. J. Pathol.*, 13, 422, 1943.

Gettler, A. O. and Weiss, L., Thallium poisoning II: The quantitative determination of thallium in biologic material, *Am. J. Clin. Pathol.*, 13, 374, 1943.

Hausman, R. and Wilson, W. J., Jr., Thallotoxicosis – a social menace, *J. Forensic Sci.*, 9, 72, 1964.

Prick, J. J. G., Smitt, W. G. S., and Miller, L., *Thallium Poisoning*, Elsevier, Amsterdam, 1955, 122.

THEOPHYLLINE

PRINCIPLE

Theophylline is extracted from serum or saliva with an organic solvent. This may be reextracted into a pH 9.0 buffer, and the theophylline then is identified and quantitated from the UV absorption spectrum of this alkaline solution (Procedure A). Another approach is to evaporate the original organic extract to dryness and then dissolve the residue in toluene. The toluene is extracted with ammonium hydroxide to remove the theophylline. The ammonium hydroxide is evaporated, and the *N*-butyl derivative of theophylline is prepared by reaction with butyl iodide in *N,N*-dimethylacetamide. This derivative is quantitated relative to the internal standard by gas chromatography. Theobromine and phenobarbital are well-separated from theophylline and can also be determined by this method (Procedure C).

TYPE A PROCEDURE

Jocelyn M. Hicks

APPARATUS

1. Separatory funnels, 60 ml
2. Graduated cylinders, glass-stoppered, 25 ml
3. Filter paper (Whatman #41)
4. Volumetric flask, 100 ml
5. Volumetric flask, 1,000 ml
6. Serological pipets, 5 ml
7. Volumetric pipets, 2 ml
8. Pasteur pipets, disposable
9. Mettler balance, type H15
10. pH meter
11. Recording spectrophotometer (UV)
12. Quartz cuvettes, 1-cm light path

REAGENTS

All chemicals should be analytical reagent grade.

1. Chloroform
2. Bicarbonate/carbonate buffer (pH 9.0)
   (A) 0.1*M* sodium carbonate (Na_2CO_3)
   Place 10.6 g of sodium carbonate in a 1,000-ml volumetric flask and dilute to volume with deionized water.
   (B) 0.1*M* sodium bicarbonate ($NaHCO_3$)
   Place 8.4 g of sodium bicarbonate in 1,000-ml volumetric flask and dilute to volume with deionized water. Add 110 ml of the sodium carbonate solution to 890 ml of the sodium bicarbonate solution. Check the pH and adjust if necessary. Store the buffer in a dark polyethylene bottle at room temperature. It is stable for several months.
3. Stock standard theophylline, 100 mg/dl (theophylline anhydrous, Merck)
   Place 100 mg of theophylline in a 100-ml volumetric flask, and dilute to volume with deionized water. Store this standard in a brown glass container at 4°C. It is stable for several months.
4. Working standard, 2 mg/dl
   Place 2 ml of the stock standard in a 100-ml volumetric flask and dilute to volume with deionized water. This solution should be made fresh on the day of the analysis.
5. Theophylline control solution, 1.5 mg/dl
   Transfer 1.5 ml of the theophylline stock solution to a 100-ml volumetric flask and dilute to volume with pooled theophylline free serum.

PROCEDURE

1. Transfer 2.5 ml of the sample, (serum, working standard, and control solution) to a 60-ml separatory funnel containing 25 ml of chloroform.
2. Shake for at least 3 min, and allow the layers to separate.
3. Filter the chloroform layer (bottom layer)

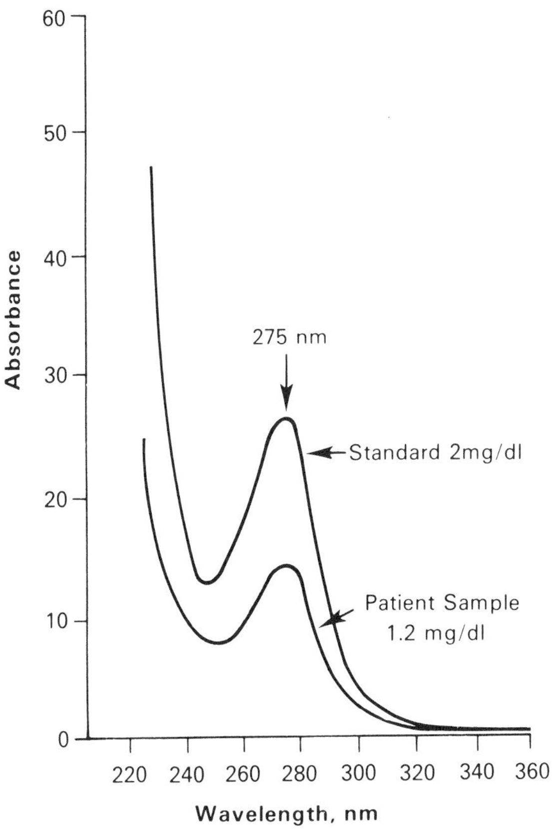

FIGURE 1. UV absorbance of theophylline.

through a double thickness of Whatman #41 filter paper into a 25-ml glass-stoppered graduated cylinder.

4. Collect 20 ml of the chloroform extract. Add 2.5 ml of the pH 9.0 bicarbonate/carbonate buffer.
5. Stopper the cylinder, shake for at least 3 min, and allow the layers to separate.
6. Pipet at least 2 ml of the buffer (top layer) into a quartz cuvette.
7. Determine the UV absorption spectrum (Figure 1) of each sample (working standard, control and unknown solutions) from 360 to 230 nm using the pH 9.0 buffer as the reference solution. (The readings are taken at 280 nm, although maximum absorbance is at 275 nm.)
8. Record the absorbance at 280 nm.

CALCULATION

$$\frac{A_T}{A_R} \times 2 = \text{mg/dl theophylline}$$

where

A_T = the absorbance at 280 nm of the sample being tested

A_R = the absorbance at 280 nm of 2.0 mg/dl standard theophylline solution

INTERPRETATION (see p. 7)

Theophylline compounds, particularly aminophylline, play an important role in the management of bronchial and cardiac asthma. They act by dilating the bronchi. Theophylline is also a myocardial stimulant and a diuretic.

Optimum therapeutic serum concentrations of theophylline range from 8 to 20 μg/ml. Concentrations below 5 μg/ml usually do not produce maximum therapeutic benefits, while those greater than 20 μg/ml are often associated with signs of toxicity. Administration of aminophylline (theophylline ethylenediamine) to children with asthma at a dose of 8.1 mg/kg results in serum concentrations of theophylline averaging 13 and 9 μg/ml at 2 and 4 hr, respectively.

PRECISION

At the 2 mg/dl level the coefficient of variation is 6%. This was determined by analyzing the same specimen (approximately 2 mg/dl) 41 times.

INTERFERING SUBSTANCES

Interference from other xanthine compounds should be avoided by placing the patient on a diet free of coffee, tea, chocolate, or cocoa at least 16 hr before a specimen is drawn for theophylline analysis. The analysis is performed at pH 9.0 to avoid interference from barbiturates, which would interfere at higher pHs.

REFERENCES*

Schack, J. A. and Waxler, S. H., An ultraviolet spectrophotometric method for the determination of theophylline and theobromine in blood and tissues, *J. Pharmacol. Exp. Ther.*, 97, 283, 1949.

Weinberger, M. M. and Bronsky, E. A., Evaluation of oral bronchodilation therapy in asthmatic children, *J. Pediatr.*, 84, 421, 1973.

ACKNOWLEDGMENTS

My thanks to Ms. Aida Gutierrez and Ms. Brenda Worthy for technical assistance.

TYPE C PROCEDURE

George F. Johnson, Walter A. Dechtiaruk, and Harvey M. Solomon

APPARATUS

1. Eppendorf pipets, 50, 100, 200, and 1,000 μl
2. Repipets®, 10 and 5 ml
3. Microsyringes, 250 and 10 μl
4. Culture tubes, screw-capped, 16 × 125 mm with caps, Teflon®-lined
5. Concentratubes®,[†] 18 × 114 mm with polyethylene caps (nipple tubes)
6. Pasteur pipets
7. Centrifuge
8. Water bath
9. Vortex mixer
10. Eberbach shaker
11. Nitrogen evaporator Model 10, N-EVAP, Organomation Assoc.
12. Gas chromatograph equipped with a flame ionization detector, a 1 mV recorder and a glass column 4′ × 2 mm i.d., packed with 3% SP 2250 on 100/120 mesh Supelcoport

   Operating Conditions

   Gas Flow Rate:
   nitrogen – 40 ml/min
   Temperatures:
   column – programmed from 160 to 240°C at 8°C/min
   injection port – 250°C
   detector – 300°C

REAGENTS

All chemical should be analytical reagent grade.

1. Theophylline stock solution, 100 μg/ml
   Dissolve 10 mg of theophylline[‡] in ethanol and dilute to 100 ml with ethanol
2. Theophylline working standard solutions, 5, 10, 15, and 20 μg/ml
   To 16 × 125 mm screw-capped culture tubes add 50, 100, 150, and 200 μl of the theophylline stock solution and evaporate each solution to dryness under nitrogen. Add 1 ml of normal serum to each residue.
3. Alphenal stock solution, 100 μg/ml
   Dissolve 10 mg of alphenal[‡‡] in ethanol and dilute to 100 ml with ethanol.
4. Internal standard – alphenal in methylene chloride, 5 μg/10 ml
   To a tube add 5 ml of alphenal stock solution and evaporate this solution to dryness under nitrogen using a water bath. Dissolve the residue in methylene chloride and dilute to 1,000 ml.
5. Methanol
6. Sodium chloride
7. Phosphate buffer, 1*M*, pH 6.8
   (a) Prepare 1*M* K_2HPO_4. Dissolve 87.1 g of K_2HPO_4 in 500 ml of distilled water. (b) Prepare 1*M* KH_2PO_4. Dissolve 68.0 g of

*For an updated list of reference material, see References, p. 370.
[†]Laboratory Research Co., P.O. Box 36509, Los Angeles, California.
[‡]Sigma Chemical Co., St. Louis, Mo.
[‡‡]Gane's Chemical Co., Carlstadt, N.J.

KH_2PO_4 in 500 ml of distilled water. (c) Using a pH meter, adjust the K_2HPO_4 with KH_2PO_4 to a pH of 6.8

8. Ammonium hydroxide, 0.5*M*
   Dilute 3.4 ml of concentrated NH_4OH to 100 ml with distilled water
9. Toluene, chromatoquality (Matheson, Coleman, and Bell)
10. *N,N*,-Dimethylacetamide, spectrophotometric grade, Aldrich Chemical Co.
11. Iodobutane, 99%, Aldrich Chemical Co.
12. Tetramethylammonium hydroxide (TMH)
    Dilute the 24% in methanol solution (obtainable from Matheson, Coleman and Bell) 1:10 (V:V) with methanol. Store at 4°C.

PROCEDURE

1. Transfer 1.0 ml of sample (serum and each working standard solution), 1 ml of phosphate buffer, 2 g of sodium chloride, and 10 ml of the internal standard to a 16 × 125 mm screw-capped culture tube. Mix well after each addition.
2. Shake for 10 min in the Eberbach shaker at 250 oscillations/min.
3. Centrifuge at 2,000 rpm for 10 min.
4. Remove the aqueous phase by aspiration. If any emulsion forms, stir the tube with a glass rod to break up the emulsion, centrifuge, and aspirate any aqueous phase.
5. Using a Pasteur pipet, transfer the methylene chloride to a nipple tube and evaporate the solution to dryness under nitrogen in a water bath at 40°C.
6. Wash the walls of the nipple tube with 100 μl of 0.5*M* NH_4OH to dissolve the residue and mix the tube on a vortex for 30 sec.
7. Add 5 ml of toluene and shake the tube in the Eberbach shaker for 10 min.
8. Centrifuge at 2,000 rpm for 5 min.
9. Remove the toluene layer by aspiration. Evaporate the aqueous phase to dryness under nitrogen in a water bath at 55°C.
10. Mix 50 μl of the diluted TMH with 400 μl of *N,N*-dimethylacetamide and add 20 μl of this solution to the dried residue. Mix on a vortex for 5 sec. Add 10 μl of iodobutane and mix on a vortex for 5 sec. Allow the tube to stand for 10 min.
11. Centrifuge for 1 min at 2,000 rpm and inject 2 μl of the supernate into the gas chromatograph.
12. Measure the peak heights of the internal standard and the theophylline from the theophylline standard solutions and each specimen.
13. Calculate the ratio of the peak height due to the theophylline to that of the one due to alphenal.

CALCULATION

1. Construct a standard curve of the peak height of the theophylline standards against the concentration of theophylline (μg/ml) in the standards.
2. Determine the concentration of theophylline in the specimen from the standard curve.

INTERPRETATION (see p. 7)

Theophylline compounds, particularly aminophylline, play an important role in the management of bronchial and cardiac asthma. They act by dilating the bronchi. Theophylline is also a myocardial stimulant and a diuretic.

Optimum therapeutic serum concentrations of theophylline range from 8 to 20 μg/ml. Concentrations below 5 μg/ml usually do not produce maximum therapeutic benefits, while those greater than 20 μg/ml are often associated with signs of toxicity. Administration of aminophylline (theophylline ethylenediamine) to children with asthma at a dose of 8.1 mg/kg results in serum concentrations of theophylline averaging 13 and 9 μg/ml at 2 and 4 hr, respectively.

ACCURACY AND PRECISION

Recovery of theophylline from serum ranged from 91 to 109%. The limit of sensitivity of the procedure is 1 μg of theophylline/ml of serum. The coefficient of variation of the assay at 15 μg/ml is 8% between runs.

INTERFERING SUBSTANCES

Theobromine and phenobarbital are well separated from theophylline in this assay and can be quantitated if so desired.

REFERENCES

Greeley, R. H., New approach to derivatization and gas chromatographic analysis of barbiturates, *Clin. Chem.,* 20, 192, 1974.

Kowblansky, M., Scheinthal, B. M., Cravello, G. D., and Chafetz, L., Specific gas chromatographic determination of xanthines and barbiturates by flash-heater N-butylation, *J. Chromatogr.,* 76, 467, 1973.

Koysooko, R., Ellis, E. F., and Levy, G., Relationship between theophylline concentration in plasma and saliva of man, *Clin. Pharmacol. Ther.,* 15, 454, 1974.

Levy, G., Ellis, E. F., and Koysooko, R., Indirect plasma-theophylline monitoring in asthmatic children by determination of theophylline concentration in saliva, *Pediatrics,* 53, 873, 1974.

Mitenko, P. A. and Ogilvie, R. I., Rapidly achieved plasma concentration plateaus, with observations on theophylline kinetics, *Clin. Pharmacol. Ther.,* 13, 329, 1972.

Shah, V. P. and Riegelman, S., GLC determination of theophylline in biological fluids, *J. Pharm. Sci.,* 63, 1283, 1974.

Weinberger, M. M. and Bronsky, E. A., Evaluation of oral bronchodilator therapy in asthmatic children, *J. Pediatr.,* 84, 421, 1974.

THIAMPHENICOL

PRINCIPLE

Thiamphenicol can be extracted with ethyl acetate. After concentration of the extract, the trimethylsilyl derivative of the drug can be determined by electron-capture gas chromatography using chloramphenicol as the internal standard.

TYPE C PROCEDURE

Robert A. Maes

APPARATUS

1. Graduated test tubes, conical (Kontes 41055)
2. A vacuum desiccator
3. Culture tubes with Teflon®-lined screw caps, 15 × 100 mm and 16 × 126 mm
4. Centrifuge
5. Volumetric pipets, 2 ml
6. Syringe (Hamilton 701-N), 10 μl
7. Gas chromatograph (Varian Aerograph Model 1440), equipped with a ^{63}Ni electron-capture detector, a 1 mV recorder (Varian Aerograph model 25) with attached Disc integrator and a glass column, 75 × 0.4 cm i.d., packed with 3% OV-17 on Gas Chrom Q, 60 to 80 mesh (Condition the column for 24 hr at 230°C prior to use.)

Operating Conditions

Gas Flow Rate:
- nitrogen (carrier gas)—50 ml/min

Temperatures:
- column – 215°C
- injection port – 240°C
- detector base – 240°C

REAGENTS

All chemicals should be analytical reagent grade.

1. Ethyl acetate
2. Anhydrous sodium sulfate
3. Tri-Sil/BSA® reagent*
4. Internal standard, 100 mg/dl
   Dissolve 100 mg of chloramphenicol in 100 ml of ethyl acetate
5. Thiamphenicol reference solution, 0.5 mg/dl
   Dissolve 250 mg of thiamphenicol in 500 ml of the internal standard. Aliquots of 0.2, 0.6, 1.0, and 1.4 μl of this solution are equivalent to 1, 3, 5, and 7 μg of thiamphenicol, respectively.

PROCEDURE

1. Add 10.0 ml of ethyl acetate to 2.0 ml of sample (blood, serum, plasma and reference solutions) in screw-capped test tubes.
2. Shake vigorously for 5 min.
3. Transfer the ethyl acetate to a clean screw-capped tube.
4. Add approximately 1 g of sodium sulfate, mix well, and centrifuge the tubes for 3 min at 1,500 rpm.
5. Pipet 2.0 ml of the ethyl acetate extract into a graduated conical test tube.
6. Add 25 μl of internal standard.
7. Evaporate the organic solvent in a vacuum desiccator.
8. Add 0.2 ml of trimethylsilyl reagent and leave at room temperature for 15 min.
9. Evaporate the solution to dryness in a vacuum desiccator.
10. Dissolve the residue in 25 μl of pyridine.
11. Inject 2 μl of this solution into the gas chromatograph. The retention times under the conditions stated above are approximately 5.5

*Tri-Sil/BSA® (= *N,O*-bis-TMS-acetamide), Formula "P" – Pierce Chemical Co., P.O. Box 117, Rockford, Ill. 61105.

min for thiamphenicol and approximately 1.3 min for the internal standard.

CALCULATION

Calculate the thiamphenicol concentration (μg/ml) in the specimen by the following formula:

$$C_X = \frac{C_S \times H_X \times I_S}{H_S \times I_X},$$

where

C_X = concentration of thiamphenicol in the specimen;
C_S = concentration of thiamphenicol in the reference solution;
H_X = peak height of thiamphenicol in the specimen;
H_S = peak height of thiamphenicol in the reference solution;
I_X = peak height of the internal standard in the specimen;
I_S = peak height of the internal standard in the reference solution.

INTERPRETATION (see p. 7)

Blood levels at 1 hr after administration of a single dose of 500 mg of thiamphenicol by oral, intramuscular, and intravenous routes were 2.8, 5.7, and 5.1 μg/ml, respectively. Detectable levels of the antibiotic are still present in the blood 24 hr after intravenous administration of a therapeutic dose.

SENSITIVITY AND PRECISION

Sensitivity for the determination is 0.01 μg/ml. Because of the change in the standing current of the electron-capture detector after prolonged use, reference samples must be analyzed with each injection. The average recovery of thiamphenicol from samples of plasma containing 0.01 g/liter is 97 ± 3%.

INTERFERING SUBSTANCES

No significant gas-chromatographic response is observed from normal blood constituents that might be extracted.

REFERENCE

Aoyama, T. and Iguchi, S., Determination of thiamphenicol in biological fluids by gas chromatography, *J. Chromatogr.*, 43, 253, 1969.

THIOPENTAL

PRINCIPLE

Thiopental is extracted into petroleum ether containing isoamyl alcohol and reextracted into dilute alkali. The UV absorption spectrum of the alkaline extract is used to identify and quantitate any thiopental in the sample.

TYPE B PROCEDURE

Gerald Kananen

APPARATUS

1. Pasteur pipets
2. Bottles, glass-stoppered, 60 ml, or separatory funnels, 100 ml
3. UV spectrophotometer, recording

REAGENTS

All chemicals should be analytical reagent grade.

1. Thiopental stock solution, 50 mg/dl
   Dissolve 50.0 mg of thiopental with water in a volumetric flask and dilute to 100 ml. If the free acid is used, add a trace of alkali to help dissolve the solid, add 50.0 ml of water, then acidify the solution and dilute it to 100.0 ml with water. Prepare fresh solution each week and store it at 4°C.
2. Thiopental reference solution, 2 mg/dl
   Dilute 1.0 ml of the stock solution to 25.0 ml with water. Prepare a fresh solution each time it is required.
3. Sodium dihydrogen phosphate, 1.5*M*
   Dissolve 208.5 g of the monohydrate salt in water and dilute to one liter. Store the solution in a polyethylene bottle.
4. Petroleum ether
5. Sodium hydroxide, 0.4*N*
   Dissolve 18 g of sodium hydroxide in water and dilute to one liter. Store the solution in a polyethylene bottle.
6. Petroleum ether-isoamyl alcohol mixture
   Dilute 15.0 ml of isoamyl alcohol to one liter with petroleum ether. Extract an aliquot of each freshly mixed batch with 0.45*N* sodium hydroxide and compare the absorbance of this alkaline solution with that of 0.45*N* sodium hydroxide. It should have no significant absorbance between 240 and 300 nm. If there is, wash the mixture with dilute alkali, dilute acid, and water.
7. Sodium chloride
8. Sodium hydroxide, 2.5*N*
   Dissolve 100 g of sodium hydroxide in water and dilute to one liter. Store the solution in a polyethylene bottle.
9. Sulfuric acid, concentrated

PROCEDURE

1. Pipet 2.0 ml of each sample (plasma or urine specimen, reference solution, and water for a reagent blank), 2.0 ml of 1.5*M* sodium dihydrogen phosphate, and 30.0 ml of the petroleum ether-isoamyl alcohol mixture into a 60-ml glass-stoppered bottle or separatory funnel. To all samples other than plasma, add 0.5 g of sodium chloride. Shake the containers for 10 min.
2. Centrifuge the samples, then transfer 25.0 ml of each organic phase to a clean 60-ml bottle.
3. Add 15.0 ml of 1.5*M* sodium dihydrogen phosphate to the organic extracts. Shake the containers for 2 min.
4. Centrifuge the solutions, then transfer 20.0 ml of each organic phase to a 60-ml glass-stoppered bottle containing 5.0 ml of 2.5*N* sodium hydroxide. Shake the bottles for 2 min.
5. Centrifuge the solutions, then transfer 3.0 ml of each aqueous phase to a cuvette.
6. Determine the absorbances at 305 nm, A_A, using the extract obtained from the reagent

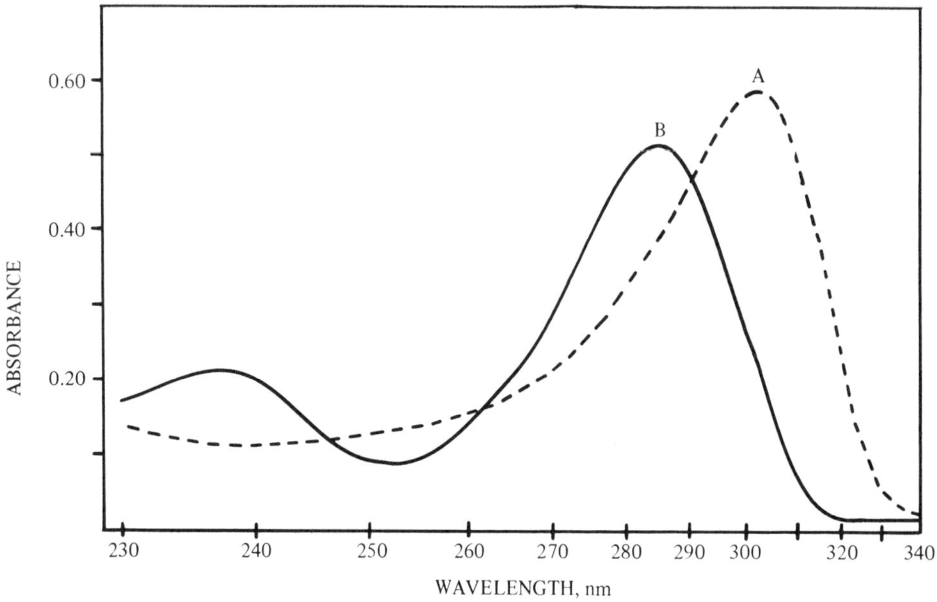

FIGURE 1. Absorption curves for thiopental. A = 0.45*N* NaOH; B = dilute acid.

blank as the reference solution (see Figure 1, Curve A).

7. Add 1 or 2 drops of concentrated sulfuric acid to each cuvette. Mix thoroughly.
8. Determine the absorbances at 305 nm, A_B (see Figure 1, Curve B).

CALCULATION

Determine the thiopental concentration in the specimen by the following formula:

$$\frac{(A_A - A_B)\text{ specimen}}{(A_A - A_B)\text{ reference}} \times C_R = C_S,$$

where

A_A = absorbance at 305 nm in basic solution;
A_B = absorbance at 305 nm in acid solution;
C_R = concentration of the reference solution;
C_S = concentration of the specimen.

A typical $(A_A - A_B)$ value obtained after analyzing 2.0 ml of a solution containing 2.0 mg of Pentothal®/100 ml is 310.

INTERPRETATION (see p. 7)

Patients receiving 0.4 g of thiopental intravenousl: had plasma concentrations decreasing from 0.' mg/100 ml at 15 min to 0.3 mg/100 ml at 1½ hr

PRECISION

A precision of 96 ± 3% can be achieved with this method.

INTERFERING SUBSTANCES

The double-extraction procedure precludes most interfering substances. A large quantity of salicylate, if present, may have significant absorbance at 340 nm.

REFERENCE

Brodie, B. et al., The fate of thiopental in man and a method for its estimation in biological material, *J. Pharmacol. Exp. Ther.*, 98, 85, 1950.

THIORIDAZINE

PRINCIPLE

Thioridizine produces an unusual color when treated with ferric chloride and sulfuric acid (Procedure A). It is extracted from the biological sample into heptane, then it is reextracted into acid, and oxidized to produce a fluorophore whose fluorescent properties can be used to determine the thioridazine concentration (Procedure B).

TYPE A PROCEDURE

Irving Sunshine

REAGENTS

All chemicals should be analytical reagent grade.

1. Ferric chloride, 5 g/100 ml
   Dissolve 5 g of ferric chloride in 100 ml of water.
2. Sulfuric acid, 10*N*
   Dilute 30 ml of concentrated sulfuric acid to 100 ml with water.
3. Color reagent
   Add 1 ml of the ferric chloride solution to a 50-ml volumetric flask, then dilute to the mark with 10*N* sulfuric acid.

PROCEDURE

1. Add 1 ml of urine to 1 ml of the color reagent.
2. Note the color change that appears in the first 15 sec after mixing the two substances.

INTERPRETATION (see p. 7)

A pink or blue color indicates that thioridazine may be present. This *must* be confirmed by other, more definitive tests. The absence of a color indicates that thioridazine is not present.

INTERFERING SUBSTANCES

Phenothiazine compounds may give similar color reactions.

REFERENCE *

Forrest, I. S., Forrest, F. M., and Mason, A. S., A rapid urine color test for thioridazine, *Am. J. Psychiatry,* 116, 928, 1960.

TYPE B PROCEDURE

Joseph Monforte

APPARATUS

1. Volumetric pipets, 3, 4, and 5 ml
2. Graduated pipets, 10 ml
3. Test tubes, screw-capped, 15 × 100 mm and 16 × 126 mm
4. Multipurpose rotator (Model 150V)[†]
5. Centrifuge
6. Temp-Blok®[‡]
7. Spectrophotofluorometer (Perkin-Elmer Model MPF-2A)

*For an updated list of reference material, see References, p. 377.
†Scientific Industries, Inc., Springfield, Mass.
‡Labline Instruments, Inc., Melrose Park, Ill.,

REAGENTS

All chemicals should be analytical reagent grade.

1. Thioridazine stock solution, 100 mg/100 ml
   Dissolve 110 mg of thioridazine hydrochloride in water and dilute to 100 ml with water.
2. Thioridazine reference solutions
   Dilute appropriate quantities of the stock solution with distilled water to obtain thioridazine concentrations of 0.1, 0.5, and 4.0 mg/100 ml solution. Duplicate this dilution, substituting 8.7*M* acetic acid for the distilled water.
3. Acetic acid, 8.7*M*
   Dilute 50.0 ml of glacial acetic acid to 100 ml with water.
4. Ammonium hydroxide, 3*N*
   Dilute 20.0 ml of concentrated ammonium hydroxide to 100 ml with distilled water.
5. *n*-Heptane-isoamyl alcohol mixture
   Dilute 17.0 ml of isoamyl alcohol to one liter with *n*-heptane.
6. Hydrogen peroxide, 30%

PROCEDURE

1. Add 1.0 ml of 3*N* ammonium hydroxide to 4.0 ml of sample (blood or urine specimen, aqueous reference solutions, and water for a reagent blank) in screw-capped test tubes.
2. Add 10.0 ml of the *n*-heptane-isoamyl alcohol mixture to each tube.
3. Place the tubes on the rotator and allow them to rotate for approximately 45 min.
4. Centrifuge the tubes for approximately 2 min at 1,500 rpm.
5. Transfer 8.0 ml of each upper (organic) layer to a clean screw-capped tube. Add 4.0 ml of 8.7*M* acetic acid to each tube.
6. Place the tubes on the rotator and allow them to rotate for approximately 45 min.
7. Centrifuge the tubes for approximately 2 min at 1,500 rpm.
8. Transfer 3.0 ml of each lower (aqueous acetic acid) layer to a clean test tube. If recovery of thioridazine is to be determined, place 3.0 ml of the 8.7*M* acetic acid thioridazine reference solutions in test tubes.
9. Add 0.2 ml of 30% hydrogen peroxide to each test tube.
10. Heat the test tubes for 15 min at 100°C in the Temp-Blok®.
11. Cool the samples to room temperature, then record their fluorescence spectra (see Figure 1). Excite the samples at 352 nm and record the emission spectra from 400 to 480 nm. Record the fluorescence at 430 nm.

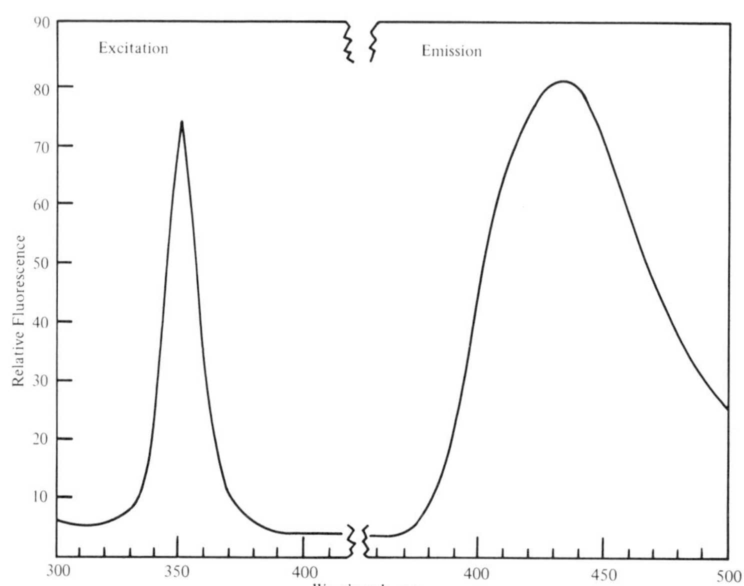

FIGURE 1. Relative fluorescence of thioridazine.

CALCULATION

1. The fluorometric response of thioridazine varies linearly with thioridazine concentration within the range from 0.1 to 1.0 mg/100 ml.
2. Determine the thioridazine concentration (mg/100 ml) in the specimen by using the following formula:

$$C_X = \frac{10 \times (F_X - F_C) \times C_R}{8 \times F_R},$$

where

C_X = thioridazine concentration of the specimen;
C_R = thioridazine concentration of the reference solution in 8.7*M* acetic acid;
F_X = fluorescence of the specimen;
F_C = fluorescence of the reagent blank;
F_R = fluorescence of the reference solution in 8.7*M* acetic acid;
10/8 = dilution factor.

INTERPRETATION (see p. 7)

Patients whose blood contained from 0.2 to 1.2 mg thioridazine/100 ml have survived.

ACCURACY AND PRECISION

Recoveries of thioridazine added to blood, urine, and water are 65 to 70% for blood and 85 to 95% for urine and aqueous reference solutions.

INTERFERING SUBSTANCES

This procedure is a variant of one designed to the quantitative determination of phenothiazines. It is not specific for thioridazine. The fluorophores resulting from a variety of phenothiazine sulfoxides undergo excitation and emission at wavelengths near that of thioridazine.

REFERENCES

Joubert, P. H. and Olivier, J. A., Fatal suicide ingestion of thioridazine, *Clin. Toxicol.*, 7, 133, 1974.

Martensson, E. and Roos, B. E., Serum levels of thioridazine in psychiatric patients and healthy volunteers, *Eur. J. Clin. Pharmacol.*, 6, 181, 1973.

Ragland, J. B. and Kinross-Wright, V. J., Spectrofluorometric measurement of phenothiazines, *Anal. Chem.*, 36, 1356, 1964.

Ragland, J. B., Kinross-Wright, V. J., and Ragland, R. S., Determination of phenothiazines in biological samples, *Anal. Biochem.*, 12, 60, 1965.

Tompsett, S. L., The spectrofluorometric determination of phenothiazine drugs in blood serum, *Acta Pharmacol. Toxicol.*, 26, 298, 1968.

West, N. R., et al., Assay procedures for thioridazine, trifluoperazine and their sulfoxides and determination of urinary excretion of these compounds in mental patients, *J. Pharm. Sci.*, 63, 417, 1974.

VOLATILE COMPOUNDS (TOLUENE, XYLENE, AND BENZENE)

PRINCIPLE

The solvents, if present, are extracted into carbon tetrachloride and reacted with Marquis reagent to form a characteristic colored complex.

TYPE A PROCEDURE

Sidney Kaye

APPARATUS

1. Centrifuge

REAGENTS

All chemicals should be analytical reagent grade.

1. Hydrochloric acid, 0.1*N*
2. Carbon tetrachloride
3. Marquis reagent
   Just prior to use, add 0.1 ml of formaldehyde to 10 ml of sulfuric acid.

PROCEDURE

1. Mix 35 ml of 0.1*N* hydrochloric acid and 5 ml of blood. Gently shake and extract with 5 ml of carbon tetrachloride.
2. Separate the lower carbon tetrachloride layer and centrifuge.
3. Add 5 ml of the Marquis reagent and mix.
4. Compare the resulting red color with standards fixed at 0, 5, 10, 20, and 30 ppm.

INTERPRETATION (see p. 7)

This test is positive and may be used as a screening for xylene, toluene, and benzene.

REFERENCES

Collon, W. D. and Winek, C. L., Detection of glue constituents in fatalities due to "glue sniffing," *Clin. Toxicol.,* 3(1), 125, 1970.

Gerarde, H., Toxicologic studies on hydrocarbons, Part VI. A colorimetric method for the determination of kerosene in blood, *Clin. Chem.,* 6, 327, 1960.

Kaye, S., *Emergency Toxicology,* 3rd ed., Charles C Thomas, Springfield, Ill., 1970.

TYPE C PROCEDURE

The volatile compounds of glue, such as benzene, toluene, and xylene, are separated from blood or tissue homogenate directly on the gas-chromatographic column and detected using a flame ionization detector. The high volatility of these compounds permits the gas chromatograph to be operated at a relatively low temperature. The nonvolatile and high boiling components of the biological matrix are left behind in the injection port. This insures long column life and requires only occasional cleaning of the injection chamber. For details of the gas-chromatographic analysis, see screening method for volatile substances (p. 407).

WARFARIN

PRINCIPLE

In Procedure B warfarin may be extracted from plasma into acetone. The native fluoresence of the extracted warfarin and some of its metabolites can then be measured before and after quenching with acid. The difference in fluoresence is a measure of warfarin concentration. In Procedure C the warfarin is extracted from alkaline solution and the warfarin in the concentrated extracts is separated from the biological coextracted material by thin-layer chromatography. The warfarin on the TLC chromatogram is eluted and assayed by GLC.

TYPE B PROCEDURE

Method of Corn and Berberich[1]

Peter I. Jatlow

APPARATUS

1. Centrifuge tubes, conical, 12 ml
2. Centrifuge
3. Fluorometer, excitation, 340 nm; emission, 400 nm

REAGENTS

All chemicals should be analytical reagent grade.

1. Acetone
2. HCl, 0.1*N*
   Dilute 0.8 ml of concentrated HCl to 100 ml with water.
3. Stock warfarin standard, 1 mg/ml
   Dissolve 25 mg of warfarin (Sigma) in methanol and dilute to 25 ml with methanol. Store at −20°C.
4. Working warfarin standard, 5 and 10 μg/ml
   Add 5 and 10 μl of the stock standard to 1 ml of warfarin-free plasma. Prepare each time an analysis is to be done.
5. Negative control, warfarin-free plasma

PROCEDURE

All blood samples should contain heparin or citrate as anticoagulants.

1. To 4 ml of acetone in a centrifuge tube, add 0.2 ml of sample (plasma, both standards, negative control, and water which serves as a reagent blank).
2. Mix thoroughly.
3. Centrifuge and decant into a glass fluoresence cuvette.
4. Measure fluoresence (F_1), setting the reagent blank to zero and the high standard to the upper end of the scale.
5. Add 0.05 ml of 0.1*N* HCl to each cuvette. Mix and measure the fluoresence (F_2).

CALCULATION

$$\frac{Cs}{F_1 - F_2)s} \times (F_1 - F_2)\mu = C\mu$$

where

Cs	=	concentration of plasma standard (μg/ml)
Cμ	=	concentration of unknown (μg/ml)
$(F_1 - F_2)s$	=	fluoresence of plasma standard
$(F_1 - F_2)\mu$	=	fluoresence of unknown

INTERPRETATION (see p. 7)

Patients receiving anticoagulant therapy will usually have warfarin concentrations between 2 to

8 μg/ml; however, there is no consistent correlation between warfarin concentration and prothrombin time. Blood warfarin concentrations achieved during optimal therapy will vary widely, because an individual response to warfarin, which inhibits synthesis of Vitamin K dependent clotting factors, varies. Prothrombin time, and not warfarin concentration, should be used to monitor therapy. In cases of bleeding, a prothrombin time should be used to categorize the type and determine the severity of a hemorrhagin diathesis. This fluormetric procedure is suitable for establishing that warfarin ingestion has occurred.

INTERFERING SUBSTANCES

This procedure will measure some warfarin metabolites as well as the parent drug. Some of these metabolites, which may be present in plasma in low concentrations, are active. The method is, therefore, not specific for unchanged warfarin. The concentrations determined by this procedure are slightly higher than those obtained by spectrophotometry. More specific methods that separate warfarin from its metabolites have been described by Lewis et al.,[2] who used thin-layer chromatography, and Vesell,[3] who employed liquid chromatography.

Acidification does not quench the small variable fluoresence found in warfarin-free plasma. $F_1 - F_2$ should be zero for the negative plasma control. This method is not suitable for measurement of warfarin in urine. Urine has considerable endogenous fluorescence as well as a greater proportion of warfarin metabolites, some of which are measured by this procedure.

REFERENCES

1. **Corn, M. and Berberich, R.,** Rapid fluorometric assay for plasma warfarin, *Clin. Chem.,* 13, 126, 1967.
2. **Lewis, R. J., Ilnicki, L. P., and Carlstrom, M.,** The assay of warfarin in plasma or stool, *Biochem. Med.,* 4, 376, 1970.
3. **Vesell, R. J. and Shively, C. A.,** Liquid chromatographic assay of warfarin: Similarity of warfarin half lives in human subjects, *Science,* 184, 466, 1974.

GENERAL REFERENCE*

O'Reilly, R. A., Aggeler, P. M., and Hoag, M. S., Studies on the coumadin anticoagulant drugs: the assay of warfarin, and its biologic application, *Thromb. Diath. Haemorrh.,* 8, 82, 1962.

TYPE C PROCEDURE

D. G. Kaiser and R. S. Martin

APPARATUS

1. Centrifuge tubes, 15 ml, with ground glass joints
2. Vortex mixer (Model K-500, Scientific Industries) or its equivalent
3. Reciprocating shaker, two-speed (Eberbach), or its equivalent
4. Centrifuge
5. Chromatography plates, 250-μm thin layers of silica gel F_{254}
6. UV lamp, short wavelength, 254 nm
7. Water bath, temperature controlled (60°C)
8. Gas chromatograph (Micro-Tek MT-220 or its equivalent) equipped with a ^{63}Ni electron-capture detector and U-shaped glass columns, 0.61 m × 3 mm i.d., packed with 1% OV-17 on 80 to 100 mesh Gas Chrom Q

Operating Conditions

Gas Flow Rates:
  nitrogen (carrier gas) – 75 ml/min
  nitrogen (purge gas) – 30 ml/min
Temperatures:
  column – 240°C
  injection port – 275°C
  detector – 285°C

Electron-Capture Detector: 14.5 V (DC mode)

*For an updated list of reference material, see General References, p. 383.

Precondition newly prepared columns at 275°C for 1 hr without carrier gas flow and for 16 hr with a carrier gas flow of 10 ml/min.

REAGENTS

All chemicals should be analytical reagent grade unless otherwise indicated. All organic solvents (Burdick and Jackson) should be redistilled in glass unless otherwise stated.

1. Acetone
2. Ethylene chloride
3. Hexane
4. Methanol
5. Sodium hydroxide, 0.01*N*
   Dissolve 4 g of sodium hydroxide in water and dilute to one liter. Dilute 100 ml of this stock solution to 1,000 ml with water.
6. Warfarin stock solution, 100 μg/ml
   Dissolve 10 mg of warfarin [3-α-acetonyl-benzyl)-4-hydroxycoumarin] (S. B. Penick) in 0.01*N* sodium hydroxide and dilute to 100 ml with 0.01*N* sodium hydroxide.
7. Warfarin reference solutions
   Respectively dilute 0.2, 0.4, 0.8, 1.2, 1.6, and 2.0 ml of the warfarin stock solution to 100 ml with 0.01*N* sodium hydroxide.
8. Internal standard stock solution, 10 mg/100 ml
   Dissolve 10 mg of 3-(α-acetonyl-*p*-chloro-benzyl)-4-hydroxycoumarin (Aldrich) in acetone and dilute to 100 ml with acetone.
9. Internal standard working solution, 20 μg/ml
   Dilute 5 ml of the internal standard stock solution to 25 ml with acetone.
10. Pentafluorobenzyl bromide stock solution, 0.1 ml/100 ml
    (Caution – Pentafluorobenzyl bromide (Pierce) is a lachrymator. Prepare all stock solutions in a well-ventilated hood.) Dilute 0.1 ml of pentafluorobenzyl bromide to 100 ml with acetone.
11. Sulfuric acid, 3*N*
    Dilute 8 ml of concentrated sulfuric acid (sp gr = 1.84) to 100 ml with water.
12. Potassium carbonate, anhydrous
13. Developing solution, acetone-ethylene chloride mixture, 10:90
    Mix 10 volumes of acetone with 90 volumes of ethylene chloride. Prepare this mixture just prior to use.
14. Control plasma
    Human plasma known to be free of warfarin is satisfactory.

PROCEDURE

1. Pipet 0.1-ml aliquots of the internal standard working solution into a series of 15-ml glass-stoppered centrifuge tubes and evaporate them to dryness with a gentle stream of nitrogen gas or air.
2. For each specimen to be analyzed add 0.5 ml of 0.01*N* sodium hydroxide and 1 ml of the plasma specimen* to one of the tubes prepared in Step 1. Mix well. In addition, pipet 0.5-ml aliquots of the warfarin reference solutions into successive centrifuge tubes containing the evaporated internal standard. Include 0.5 ml of 0.01*N* sodium hydroxide in another tube to serve as a reagent blank. Add 1 ml of the control plasma to each of the centrifuge tubes and mix well.
3. To each tube add 0.5 ml of 3*N* sulfuric acid and 10 ml of ethylene chloride. Shake all of the tubes in the horizontal position for 10 min. Centrifuge the tubes for 10 min at 2,000 rpm and discard the aqueous layer.
4. Transfer an 8-ml aliquot of the ethylene chloride layer to a fresh glass-stoppered centrifuge tube and evaporate to dryness. Wash down the walls of the centrifuge tube with 1 ml of ethylene chloride and evaporate to dryness.
5. Dissolve the residue in 100 μl of ethylene chloride. Spot all of each sample, including the reference solutions and control solution, on silica gel F_{254} thin-layer plates. Using the acetone-ethylene chloride mixture, develop each plate for a distance of 165 mm. Remove the plates from the tank and air-dry all chromatograms thoroughly at room temperature (24°C). Visualize the zones by irradiation with a 254-nm UV lamp.
6. Scrape the zones corresponding to warfarin (R_f = 0.40) into separate glass-stoppered centrifuge tubes. Add 2 ml of methanol to

*If the concentrations of warfarin in plasma are anticipated to be greater than 5 μg/ml, an appropriately smaller aliquot of the original specimen should be analyzed.

each tube, shake for 10 min in a horizontal position, and centrifuge for 10 min at 2,000 rpm. Transfer 1 ml of the methanol layer to a fresh glass-stoppered centrifuge tube and evaporate to dryness.

7. Add 25 mg of anhydrous potassium carbonate and 0.5 ml of the pentafluorobenzyl bromide stock solution to each centrifuge tube. Stopper tightly and heat in a water bath at 60°C for 1 hr. Evaporate to dryness.
8. Add 1 ml of water and 2 ml of hexane, shake for 10 min, and allow the phases to separate. Inject a 1-μl aliquot of the hexane layer into the chromatograph for analysis. The retention times for the pentafluorobenzyl derivatives of warfarin and the internal standard are approximately 3.6 and 6.1 min, respectively.
9. Determine the ratio of the peak heights of the warfarin and the internal standard pentafluorobenzyl derivatives.

CALCULATION

To obtain a calibration curve, plot the peak height ratios for the known concentrations of warfarin in plasma against their warfarin concentrations. Concentrations of warfarin in plasma specimens are analyzed along with the reference solutions and then determined directly from the calibration curve. In the absence of adequate amounts of control plasma or internal standard for preparation of a standard curve, warfarin concentrations can be estimated by comparing the peak height ratios obtained from the plasma specimens with those obtained from appropriate dilutions of the warfarin pentafluorobenzyl derivative.

INTERPRETATION (see p. 7)

Concentrations of 0.4 to 1.0 μg of warfarin/ml of plasma are achieved 2 to 6 hr after a single oral dose of 7.5 mg of warfarin. Substantial amounts of intact drug (0.2 to 0.4 μg/ml) are found in peripheral circulation at 24 hr post-drug administration. The relationship between circulating drug concentrations and prothrombin times in humans has been demonstrated.[1] Depending upon intersubject variability,[2-7] the therapeutic range (prothrombin complex activity <35% of normal) is reached soon after plasma warfarin concentrations of 2 μg/ml are attained.[8] Plasma warfarin concentrations in excess of 10 μg/ml may be associated with (a) a loading dose, (b) impaired metabolism and/or clearance of the drug, or (c) surreptitious drug ingestion.

ACCURACY AND PRECISION

The lower limit of assay detection sensitivity for warfarin in human plasma is 0.02 μg/ml. Recoveries (±S.D.) of warfarin (98.8 ± 10.9%) and the internal standard (95.6 ± 3.7%) from plasma are essentially quantitative over the concentration range of 0.1 to 2.0 μg/ml. The method is capable of measuring warfarin concentrations of 0.25 to 1.0 μg/ml of plasma with a coefficient of variation of 9%.

INTERFERING SUBSTANCES

The specificity of the method is as good as any gas-liquid chromatographic procedure, coupled with selective extraction, thin-layer chromatography, derivative formation, and selective detection. Compounds which potentially could interfere must (a) extract into ethylene chloride at acidic pH, (b) have a TLC mobility approximately the same as warfarin (R_f = 0.35 to 0.45), (c) form a pentafluorobenzyl derivative, and (d) have a retention time approximately the same as warfarin (R_t = 3.0 to 4.5 min). No interferences from control plasma have been observed.

REFERENCES

1. **O'Reilly, R. A., Aggeler, P. M., Hoag, M. S., and Leong, L.,** Studies on the coumarin anticoagulant drugs: the assay of warfarin and its biological application, *Thromb. Diath. Haemorrh.,* 8, 82, 1962.
2. **O'Reilly, R. A. and Aggeler, P. M.,** Studies on coumarin anti-coagulant drugs: initiation of warfarin therapy without a loading dose, *Circulation,* 38, 169, 1968.
3. **Nagashima, R., O'Reilly, R. A., and Levy, G.,** Kinetics of pharmacologic effects in man: the anticoagulant action of warfarin, *Clin. Pharmacol. Ther.,* 10, 22, 1969.
4. **Breckenridge, A. and Orme, M.,** Kinetics of warfarin absorption in man, *Clin. Pharmacol. Ther.,* 14, 955, 1973.
5. **Levy, G., O'Reilly, R. A., and Wingard, L. B., Jr.,** Relationship between the kinetics of the anticoagu-

lant effects of racemic warfarin and its individual enantiomers in man, *Res. Comm. Chem. Pathol. Pharmacol.*, 7, 359, 1974.

6. **Breckenridge, A., Orme, M., Wesseling, H., Lewis, R. J., and Gibbons, R.,** Pharmacokinetics and pharmacodynamics of the enantiomers of warfarin in man, *Clin. Pharmacol. Ther.*, 15, 424, 1974.
7. **O'Reilly, R. A.,** Studies on the optical enantiomers of warfarin in man, *Clin. Pharmacol. Ther.*, 16, 348, 1974.
8. **O'Reilly, R. A., Aggeler, P. M., and Leong, L. S.,** Studies on the coumarin anticoagulant drugs: the pharmacodynamics of warfarin in man, *J. Clin. Invest.*, 42, 1542, 1963.

GENERAL REFERENCES

Hewick, D. S., and McEwen, J., Analysis of warfarin and metabolites in plasma, *J. Pharm. Pharmacol.*, 25, 458, 1973.

Kaiser, D. G. and Martin, R. S., GLC determination of warfarin in human plasma, *J. Pharm. Sci.*, 63, 1579, 1974.

Midha, K. K., McGilveray, I. J., and Cooper, J. K., GLC determination of plasma levels of warfarin, *J. Pharm. Sci.*, 63(11), 1725, 1974.

O'Reilly, R. A., Sahud, M. A., and Robinson, A. J., Studies on the interaction of warfarin and clofibrate in man, *Thromb. Diath. Haemorrh.*, 27, 309, 1972.

ZINC

PRINCIPLE

Zinc may be determined by atomic absorption spectrophotometry by aspiration of diluted samples of biological fluids.

TYPE C PROCEDURE

Kurt M. Dubowski

APPARATUS

1. Spectrophotometer, atomic absorption (Model 153),* single channel, equipped with a zinc hollow cathode lamp (#62811), a Boling three slot acetylene-air burner, 11 cm long, with the top 6 mm below the optical axis, and a 10-in. strip chart recorder with a 50-mV span
2. Recorder, potentiometric, 10 in. (Model 194)†

REAGENTS

All chemicals should be Ultra Pure‡ or analytical reagent grade. Use ion-free water, chemically clean plastic disposable containers, and pipets rinsed in ion-free water.

1. Control substances
   To prepare a serum control or a urine control, pool the respective specimens, clarify them as needed by centrifugation and filtration, then add aliquots of the zinc stock solution (see below) to obtain the desired concentrations. Establish the zinc concentrations by replicate analyses as outlined below.
2. Zinc stock solution, 100 mg/liter
   Dissolve 1.00000 g of zinc in a minimal volume of concentrated hydrochloric acid. When solution is complete, dilute to one liter with ion-free water and mix well. Dilute 100 ml of this solution to one liter with ion-free water.
3. Sodium solution, 2.8 meq Na^+/ml
   Dissolve 164 g of sodium chloride in ion-free water and dilute to one liter.
4. Potassium solution, 4 meq K^+/ml
   Dissolve 300 g of potassium chloride in ion-free water and dilute to one liter.
5. Phosphorus solution, 30 mg P/ml
   Dissolve 132 g of potassium phosphate in ion-free water and dilute to one liter.
6. Zinc reference solutions, serum standards
   Dilute 5.0, 15.0, and 25.0 ml of the zinc stock solution to one liter with ion-free water. Before diluting, add to each aliquot of the zinc stock solution 50 ml of sodium solution, 1.0 ml of potassium solution, and 1.0 ml of phosphorus solution. Each of the resulting zinc reference solutions will then contain 140 meq of Na^+, 5 meq of K^+, and 30 mg (or 1.74 meq) of phosphorus/liter. Include one solution containing all the reagents except the zinc stock solution as a control specimen.
7. Zinc reference solutions, urine standards
   Dilute 1.0, 5.0, 10.0, 15.0, and 20.0 ml of the zinc stock solution to one liter with ion-free water. Before diluting, add to each aliquot of the zinc stock solution 6.0 ml of sodium solution, 5.0 ml of potassium solution, and 20.0 ml of phosphorus solution. Each of the resulting zinc reference solutions will then contain 80 meq of Na^+, 40 meq of K^+, and 600 mg of phosphorus/liter. Include one solution containing all the reagents except the zinc stock solution as a control specimen.

PROCEDURE

1. Prepare serum specimens, control serum, and serum standards by adding 5 volumes of

*Instrumentation Laboratory, Inc., Lexington, Mass. 02173.
†Honeywell, Inc., Fort Washington, Pa. 19034.
‡Manufactured by E. Merck Co., Darmstadt, West Germany; available from Brinkmann Instruments, Inc., Westbury, N.Y.

ion-free water to 1 volume of each of the above. Urine specimens, control urine, and urine standards require no dilution and may be used directly.

2. Adjust the operating parameters of the atomic absorption spectrophotometer as recommended by the manufacturer. For the unit suggested above (I/L Model 153), the conditions are as follows:

   Wavelength: 213.8 nm (zinc line)
   Zinc Lamp Current: 9 mA
   Slit Width: 320 μ
   Flame: very slightly fuel-rich (yellow tinge)
   Air Pressure:
   - nebulizer – 40 psig supply, finely regulated and passed through a drying column to insure that all water is removed
   - auxiliary – 6 psig dial setting

   Acetylene Pressure: 15 psig supply, regulated to 4 psig
   Aspiration: 4 to 6 ml/min
   Curve Correction: none
   Instrument Range: 0.5
   Warm-up Time: 15 min
   Chart Speed: 1 in./min

3. Adjust the digital readout of the atomic absorption spectrophotometer and the recorder response to zero while aspirating water, then adjust the recorder response to 90% of full scale while aspirating the highest standard of interest.
4. Establish calibration by aspirating each reference solution for 15 sec, interspersing a 15-sec aspiration of ion-free water between successive reference solutions. At a sampling rate of 5 ml/min, 1.25 ml of sample is required.
5. Aspirate each unknown sample for 15 sec, interspersing a 15-sec aspiration of ion-free water between successive samples. Every fifth sample should be followed by a control specimen. If a large series of samples is processed, the set of reference solutions (interspersed with ion-free water) and the corresponding controls are analyzed after every 30 samples. With automatic sampling (e.g., with an AutoAnalyzer Sampler II), employ a sampling rate of 120 samples/hr and a sampling-rinse ratio of 1:1.
6. Clean the burner and the aspirator after 30 protein-containing samples have been analyzed.

CALCULATION

1. Plot the recorder response peak heights of the reference solutions against their respective concentrations on rectilinear graph paper, and draw a best-fit straight line through these points and the origin.
2. Obtain the zinc concentrations of the control specimens and test samples from the observed recorder response peak heights and the standard curve.

INTERPRETATION (see p. 7)

Normal zinc concentrations range from 750 to 1,500 μg/liter of serum or plasma, with a mean of 1,050 μg; whole blood normally contains 4,000 to 12,000 μg/liter, with a mean of 5,450 μg.[1-4] It has been reported[5] that the serum zinc concentration exceeds that of plasma by 15%. Normal urinary zinc excretion in adult subjects usually ranges from 150 to 1,250 μg/24 hr, with a mean of 650 μg.

High zinc concentrations in the human body are toxic, though zinc toxicity is relatively infrequent compared to that of other trace elements such as copper, lead, and mercury. The normal human dietary zinc intake is approximately 10 to 15 mg/day. Excess zinc intake usually occurs through increased dietary sources, direct skin contact with zinc salts, or inhalation of zinc oxide fumes. The resulting zinc intoxication is often termed "metal fume fever." The maximum U.S. Occupational Standard (TWA) value for zinc oxide fumes in air is 5 mg/cubic meter.[6]

ACCURACY AND PRECISION

Replicate analyses of a pooled urine specimen with a mean zinc concentration of 370 μg/liter yielded a standard deviation of 15 μg/liter, and replicate analyses of a pooled urine specimen with a mean zinc concentration of 1,100 μg/liter yielded a standard deviation of 14 μg/liter. Replicate

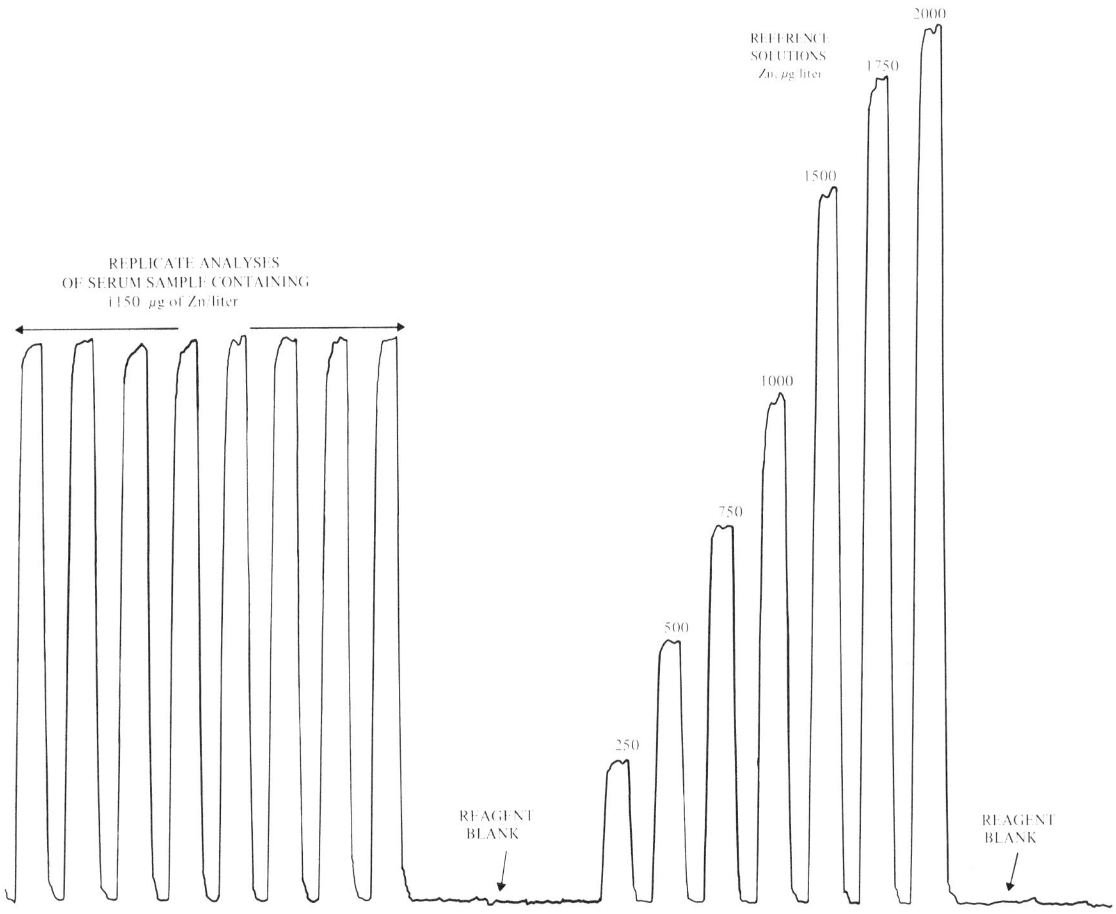

FIGURE 1. Atomic absorption spectrophotometric analysis of zinc: recorder responses to reference solutions to replicate analyses of a pooled serum sample.

analyses of a pooled serum specimen with a mean zinc concentration of 1,240 μg/liter yielded a standard deviation of 59 μg/liter. Mean recovery of 750 μg of zinc added to one liter of pooled serum was 101.3%. The limit of detection was 2.8 μg of zinc/liter.

INTERFERING SUBSTANCES

Zinc is present in trace quantities in many reagents, in water, and on most glass surfaces. It is, therefore, advisable to reduce the number and quantity of reagents employed in zinc analysis to a minimum, to employ only ion-free water, and to use chemically clean plastic containers rather than glassware whenever possible. Containers can be freed of zinc traces by washing with detergent and rinsing thoroughly, followed by immersion for 1 to 2 hr in 1% (w/v) disodium ethylenediaminetetraacetate and copious rinsing with ion-free water. Syringes, needles, and containers used in collecting blood specimens for zinc analysis must be checked for absence of zinc contamination. To further minimize sample contamination with zinc, simple water dilution of proteinaceous specimens, such as plasma, before atomic absorption measurement is preferable to treatment with trichloroacetic acid or other deproteinizing agents. Addition of dextran or other colloids to the reference solutions, as advised by Hackley et al.[5] and by Parker et al.,[7] produced no detectable differences in analytical results when sample aspiration rates and burner and flame conditions were optimized and standardized. Suppression of up to 15% of the apparent zinc content by inorganic compounds present in biological samples has been reported.[8] The reference solutions, therefore, contain concentrations of sodium, potassium, and phosphate equivalent to the average normal values in serum or urine.

REFERENCES

1. **Malström, G.,** Determination of zinc in biological materials, in *Methods of Biochemical Analysis,* Vol. 3, Glick, D., Ed., Interscience, N.Y., 1956, 327.
2. **Vallee, B. L.,** Biochemistry, physiology, and pathology of zinc, *Physiol. Rev.,* 39, 443, 1959.
3. **Prasad, A. S.,** *Zinc Metabolism,* Charles C Thomas, Springfield, Ill., 1966.
4. **Mikac-Dević, D.,** Methodology of zinc determinations and the role of zinc in biological processes, in *Advances in Clinical Chemistry,* Vol. 13, Bodansky, O., and Stewart, C. P., Eds., Academic Press, N.Y., 1970, 271.
5. **Hackley, B. M., Smith, J. C., and Halstead, J. A.,** A simplified method for plasma zinc determination by atomic-absorption spectrophotometry, *Clin. Chem.,* 14, 1, 1968.
6. Toxic Substances List – 1974 ed., Hen Publication No. (NIOSH) 74-134, Christensen, H. E. and Luginbyhi, T. T., Ed., National Institute for Occupational Safety and Health, June 1974, 817.
7. **Parker, M. M., Humoller, F. L., and Mahler, D. J.,** Determination of copper and zinc in biological material, *Clin. Chem.,* 13, 40, 1967.
8. **Dawson, J. B. and Walker, B. G.,** Direct determination of zinc in whole blood, plasma and urine by atomic-absorption spectroscopy, *Clin. Chim. Acta,* 26, 465, 1969.

GENERAL REFERENCE

Carter, P., Spectrophotometric submicrogram serum zinc assay application for the routine service laboratory, *Clin. Chim. Acta,* 52, 277, 1974.

Section II

Screening Procedures

ASIDE TO THE ANALYST

Once help is requested, the analyst must decide which analytical procedure should be followed. This decision will depend on the request that accompanies the specimen. If the request is for determination of a specific substance, Section I of the manual provides suitable directions.

A word of caution is in order, however. A positive result is self-explanatory. A negative result poses the question whether the substance selected for the analysis was the relevant one. Eyewitnesses are notoriously unreliable, and often the containers or products found at the scene or on the victim are not the causative agents. Yet, they may have been the basis for the original request to analyze for a particular substance. If the decision was based on this type of evidence and the test for the substance allegedly involved is negative, either another agent may be involved or the patient's condition may be caused by some process that does not involve a chemical agent. The attending physician must be apprised of the analyst's negative findings, and together they must decide what other analyses, if any, are in order. If further analyses are indicated, two alternatives present themselves – one, a pragmatic approach based on the art of toxicology and the other based on the science of this subject.

Pragmatic Approach

The artful approach says that common substances are frequently involved and uncommon substances are infrequently involved; therefore, chances of getting a positive result are high if the analyst tests for substances that are most frequently involved. Of course, the current local pattern of drug use must be known – pesticides are a reasonable probability in Dade County, Florida or in a rural, agricultural area, whereas in urban New York or Los Angeles sedatives would be the primary suspects. Coupled with this knowledge of local usage must be experience with the signs and symptoms of poisoning. These could indicate that certain agents are more likely to be involved than others; nausea, vomiting and diarrhea may suggest that poisoning is due to heavy metals and not to sedatives; pinpoint pupils suggest opiates or methanol, and so on. The attending physician should be involved in the decision concerning the substance most likely to be involved.

The artful approach leads to analyses for many specific substances, and Section I of the manual provides the necessary procedures. The number of procedures that can be attempted depends on the size and type of specimen. The volume of urine and/or stomach content available is usually larger than the volume of available blood; hence, they are the specimens of choice for a qualitative analysis. Blood samples should be reserved for confirmation and quantitative analysis. Another reason for preferring urine for the first probe is that many substances, particularly the organic bases, are present in such low concentration in blood that they might not be found unless they were the specific target of the analysis.

In the absence of any guidelines, common experience indicates that the first determination should be for ethanol and the next for central nervous system depressants. These substances account for a majority of acute poisonings in adults. Thereafter all options concerning the identity of the offending agent are open and subject to local ground rules.

Systematic Approach

Most systematic toxicological analyses can be divided into several unit operations – separation of the toxic agent from its biological matrix, isolation of the agent and/or its metabolites, identification of the isolated material, and quantitative estimation.

For organic substances separation techniques usually involve distillation, solvent extraction, or adsorption techniques. Distillation effectively separates many volatile organic toxins and is used effectively. It is simple, inexpensive, and reliable. Unfortunately, not too many substances can be detected by this procedure; therefore, toxicologists do not use it extensively.

Solvent extraction, with or without previous precipitation of proteins, is the procedure most commonly used for the separation of organic poisons. If blood or tissues are to be analyzed, protein precipitation by one of many common methods may be used prior to the extraction step. Urine is usually extracted without any previous treatment. The choice of the extracting solvent is difficult. Many good reasons can be given for preferring one over another. In the final analysis, because of a dearth of objective information, the decision is usually a subjective one, based on the analyst's experience and prejudices. By performing the extractions at different pH's, the organic toxins can be separated into strong acids, weak acids, neutrals, weak bases, strong bases, and amphoteric compounds.

Adsorption techniques have been used in recent years as a separation procedure. In vogue is a nonionic resin XAD-2 and activated charcoal. Either batch or column techniques are used. The pH of the sample may or may not be adjusted to some preferable value. In the batch approach the sample is then put in contact with the adsorbent and the matrix is poured off; alternatively, it is passed through an adsorbent packed column. The adsorbent is first washed and then the drug is desorbed with a suitable solvent (eluant). This separation procedure is a very efficient, economic method, particularly if a large number of samples must be processed. Many laboratories faced with the problem of analyzing many urine samples for drugs of abuse prefer this approach.

Isolation of the drug from concomitantly extracted "normal" materials is usually carried out by chromatography. Paper was originally preferred, but in the last decade this technique has yielded to thin-layer films. Both of these methods are yielding to gas chromatography. Many factors will govern the method of choice – expense, experience, ease with instruments, and personnel available, to mention but a few.

Identification is a difficult problem. Criteria satisfactory to one analyst may be wholly inadequate to another. One spot on a chromatogram or a GC peak may be considered sufficient data for positive identification by some, but not by others. The use to which the result is to be put should help govern the criteria used. In a clinical situation a "yes" or "no" answer may be satisfactory if it is obtained quickly; in medicolegal situations very exact identifications are essential. To obtain these exact identifications, other physical parameters, such as infrared absorption or mass spectrum, may be required.

Quantitative analysis is a relatively simple problem once the identity of the substance(s) in question has been ascertained. In most laboratories the quantitative procedure that is selected depends on the equipment available. Spectrophotometry still commands a respectable position. Usually the UV absorption spectrum is involved, but several very respectable procedures utilize the visible region of the spectrum because suitable colored derivatives of the compounds involved are easily prepared. Fluorimetry is also a useful technique, yielding some specificity and, usually, significantly improved sensitivity.

Although most chemists recognize the value of spectrophotometric procedures and utilize them, the trend toward gas chromatography is very apparent and for good reasons. Generally speaking, the gas-chromatographic procedure is more sensitive and specific than the spectrophotometric analogue. In many instances the spectrophotometric procedure will measure the parent drug as well as its metabolites. This is most undesirable because the resulting number is a relatively unreliable index for the physician, since it reflects the total amount of drug and metabolite present (i.e., active and inactive components).

Hence, there is inherent difficulty in interpreting the value reported. In gas chromatography, the active parent drug usually can be resolved from the inactive metabolites, and the value reported can be just that of the active components. In those instances where the drug and its metabolite are active (e.g., imipramine and desipramine), both can be reported. It is true that many clinical laboratories are currently not equipped with gas chromatographs and tend to resist obtaining them because, allegedly, they are too complex, too troublesome, and require superior personnel to use the instruments effectively. This just is not so. Those concerned have to recognize that gas chromatography is here to stay and will be a commonplace tool in most laboratories before long.

Having said all this, where does it lead? One point of this section is systematic analysis, and this has to be spelled out in detail. The problem in doing this is that there is no one optimal procedure that is ideal for every laboratory. Each must select an approach that is best suited to the available equipment, the skills of the personnel involved, and the time and specificity requirements of the client served. To this end, the section that follows will present alternative pathways and leave the choice to each individual. Whichever technique is chosen, with use it will become simpler to perform and in time both performance and results will improve. There is no substitute for experience.

OUTLINE OF ALTERNATIVE TECHNIQUES FOR SYSTEMATIC ANALYSIS

A. Nonseparation (direct) techniques – may be performed directly on the available specimens without any prior manipulation
   1. Spot tests – addition of specific reagents to aliquots of urine, stomach content, emesis, or a protein-free filtrate of blood to determine if a substance is present
   2. Heavy metals
   3. Immunoassays – amphetamine (p. 22), barbiturates (p. 34), benzoylecgonine (p. 387), digitoxin (p. 124), digoxin (p. 127), diphenylhydantoin and phenobarbital (p. 132), methadone (p. 231), morphine (p. 267)
   4. Gas chromatography – head space or direct injection of an aliquot of urine or blood on the column (organic volatile substances)

B. Indirect techniques – require prior preparation of samples for identification and quantitation
   1. Distillation – direct or microdiffusion (see Section I for details) (The gas-chromatographic procedure listed under Item 4 is the optimal method for the systematic detection of volatile substances.)
   2. Solvent extraction
      a. followed by TLC (sedative screen)
      b. followed by UV spectrophotometry (sedative screen)
      c. followed by GC (sedative screen)
      d. followed by TLC (organic bases)
      e. followed by GC (organic bases)
   3. Adsorption
      a. XAD-2 resin
      b. charcoal

SPOT TESTS

Aliquots of the urine, gastric content, or emesis fluid are distributed into each of several test tubes or into several wells in a spot plate. Each of the test reagents is added to an aliquot and any color changes are noted. If the spot test reagent produces a reaction, the inference is that the substance in question may be present. This must be confirmed by using one of the other procedures for the substance in question. These confirmatory procedures are described in Section I. In some tests a protein-free filtrate of blood is required. Usually, 10% trichloracetic acid is used to precipitate the proteins. Details are presented in Section I. Substances and page citations follow: acetaminophen (p. 13), borate (p. 51), bromide (p. 54), cholinesterase (p. 86), cyanide (p. 113), diquat (p. 137), ethchlorvynol (p. 155), imipramine (p. 192), methanol (p. 236), paraquat (p. 294), phenothiazines (p. 301), salicylate (p. 342), "sulfa" drugs (p. 352), thioridazine (p. 375), volatiles (p. 378).

HEAVY METALS

Sidney Kaye

The following procedure is designed so that rapid detection and estimation of several heavy-metal cations may be made. Several of these tests are specific and sensitive to 10 μg. The procedure is based on the fact that deposition on copper provides a simple means for rapid separation, detection, and estimation of mercury, bismuth, antimony, and arsenic from a biological matrix. Because selenium, tellurium, and sulfur may interfere with this test, they have been included in this scheme.

APPARATUS

1. Gutzeit apparatus
2. Filter paper (Whatman #40)

REAGENTS

All chemicals should be analytical reagent grade.

1. Copper strip, 5 × 10 mm, or a spiral of #20 copper wire wound tightly around a glass rod ten times
2. Nitric acid, 2.25*N*
   Dilute 15 ml of concentrated nitric acid to 100 ml with water.
3. Hydrochloric acid, concentrated
4. Hydrochloric acid, 1.2*N*
   Dilute 10 ml of concentrated hydrochloric acid to 100 ml with water.
5. Cuprous iodide suspension
   Dissolve 5 g of copper sulfate and 3 g of ferrous sulfate in 10 ml of water. Add 7 g of potassium iodide in 50 ml of water while stirring. Filter and wash the precipitate with water. Transfer the precipitated cuprous iodide to a brown bottle, keeping it in the form of a suspension with the aid of a little water. This suspension is quite stable.
6. Sodium sulfite, 5 g/100 ml
   Dissolve 5 g of sodium sulfite in water and dilute to 100 ml.
7. Quinine-potassium iodide reagent
   Dissolve 1 g of quinine sulfate in 100 ml of water containing 0.5 ml of concentrated nitric acid. Add 2 g of potassium iodide and allow it to dissolve. This reagent is stable if kept in a brown bottle.
8. Potassium cyanide, 10 g/100 ml
   Dissolve 10 g of potassium cyanide in water and dilute to 100 ml.
9. Ethanol, 95%
10. Silver nitrate, 5 g/100 ml
    Dissolve 5 g of silver nitrate in 95% ethanol. Dilute this solution to 100 ml with 95% ethanol.
11. Cadmium acetate reagent, 2-5 g/100 ml
    Dissolve 2.5 g of cadmium acetate in 20 ml of glacial acetic acid. Dilute this solution to 100 ml with distilled water.
12. Lead acetate, 2 g/100 ml
    Dissolve 2 g of lead acetate in water and dilute to 100 ml.
13. Mercuric bromide, 5 g/100 ml
    Dissolve 5 g of mercuric bromide in 95% ethanol. Dilute this solution to 100 ml with 95% ethanol.
14. Stannous chloride, 40 g/100 ml
    Dissolve 40 g of stannous chloride in 100 ml of water. If solution is incomplete, add a minimum of hydrochloric acid, drop by drop, until the solution is clear.
15. Potassium iodide, 20 g/100 ml
    Dissolve 20 g of potassium iodide in 100 ml of water.
16. Sulfuric acid, 3.6*N*
    Dilute 10.0 ml of concentrated sulfuric acid to 100 ml with water.

PROCEDURE

1. Clean the copper strip or spiral with 2.25*N* nitric acid. Discard the acid.
2. Wash the copper first with ethanol, then with ether. Discard the washings.
3. Place the strip or spiral in a 50-ml Erlenmeyer flask containing 4 ml of concentrated hydrochloric acid.

4. Add 20 ml of urine or stomach content, or 10 g of tissue macerated with 10 ml of water.
5. Heat the contents of the flask and let it boil gently for approximately 1 hr. Maintain the original volume by adding 1.2*N* hydrochloric acid.
6. After 1 hr remove the spiral. Wash it with water, then examine it. (A large amount of mercury or bismuth may require a longer heating period.) A silvery coating indicates that mercury may be present. Dark discoloration indicates that antimony, arsenic, bismuth, selenium, sulfur, or tellurium (or any combination of these substances) may be present.
7. Identification procedures should be carried out even in the absence of a visible deposit. The suggested confirmation tests will detect amounts smaller than visual inspection of the copper spiral can.

IDENTIFICATION AND ESTIMATION

Mercury

Mercury may be readily identified by a simple test described by Gettler.[1]

1. Place a small piece of filter paper on a watch glass, then place 2 drops of a suspension of cuprous iodide on the filter paper.
2. Place the coated copper spiral on the spot of cuprous iodide, cover it with a watch glass, then allow it to stand for approximately 1 hr. A rose to salmon-pink color, due to the formation of cuprous mercuric iodide, develops if 0.020 mg or more of mercury is present.
3. Make a set of cuprous mercuric iodide reference stains, using solutions containing from 0.020 to 0.20 mg of mercury and processed in the same manner as the specimen.
4. Estimate the quantity of mercury in the specimen by comparing the stain obtained from it with the reference stains. The test is specific for mercury. If a more accurate quantitative determination is desired, use another procedure.*
5. After completing the analysis for mercury, wash the original coated copper spiral so that it is free from any adhering cuprous iodide and transfer it to a small test tube.

Bismuth[2]

A bismuth deposit on copper may be quantitatively dissolved with 2.25*N* nitric acid. Other deposited metals will neither dissolve nor interfere with the subsequent test for bismuth described below. This test is sensitive to 0.010 mg of bismuth.

1. Add to the washed copper spiral 1 ml of the sodium sulfite solution and 1 ml of 2.25*N* nitric acid.
2. Agitate the copper spiral in this mixture until the deposited bismuth dissolves. If the deposit of bismuth is not too large, 5 min is usually sufficient.
3. Carefully remove the copper spiral from the test tube with the aid of a wooden applicator. Wash it with water and retain it for subsequent testing.
4. To the solution remaining in the test tube add 1 ml of distilled water and 1 ml of the quinine-potasssium iodide reagent.
5. Shake the resulting suspension of quinine-bismuth-iodide, and compare its color and turbidity with those of suspensions obtained from solutions containing known amounts of bismuth, prepared as described in Step 6.
6. Into each of 6 small test tubes, introduce 1 ml of the sodium sulfite solution and 1 ml of 2.25*N* nitric acid. Add to each tube, respectively, 0, 0.010, 0.020, 0.040, 0.070, and 0.100 mg of bismuth. Dilute the contents of each tube to 3 ml with distilled water, then add 1 ml of the quinine-potassium iodide reagent. Shake the tubes for comparison of color and turbidity. The color of the reagent blank is slightly yellow, but clear; 0.010 mg of bismuth produces a slight turbidity and a faint orange color; 0.020 mg yields greater turbidity and a more distinct orange color. With higher concentrations, turbidity and color progressively increase.
7. Estimate the bismuth content in the specimen after evaluating the results. The turbidity resulting from "pure" reference samples is approximately 25% greater than that of the

*See Mercury, Type B Procedure (dithizone method), p. 225, and Mercury, Type C Procedure (atomic absorption spectroscopy), p. 227.

test sample, the loss being due to deposition. Use of a correction factor of 4/3 gives a reliable estimate of the bismuth content in the specimen. This method is specific for bismuth under the conditions of the test. Addition of sodium sulfite inhibits any reaction of dissolved copper with the iodide. If a more accurate determination of bismuth is required, once its presence has been established by the foregoing technique, a more precise procedure should be employed.*

Antimony

If the deposit on the copper reagent has a purplish sheen, the presence of antimony is sugested. In any case, the following procedure should be employed.

1. Wash the copper spiral from which the bismuth has been dissolved (Step 3 of the bismuth determination) and place it in a small test tube.
2. Add 0.5 ml of the potassium cyanide solution and shake the tube gently for 5 min. A deposit, due partially or totally to the presence of arsenic, selenium, tellurium, or sulfur, will be dissolved by this treatment, whereas an antimony deposit will be unaffected.
3. Remove the copper spiral from the solution and wash it with a little water. Preserve the solution for the detection of arsenic, selenium, tellurium, and sulfur (see below). Proceed immediately with the test for antimony, because on standing 1 hr or more antimony becomes passive and is difficult to determine. The modified Gutzeit method described by Kaye,[3] which is sensitive to 0.010 mg of antimony, is recommended for a more accurate analysis.
4. Compare the antimony deposit on the copper spiral with that obtained from known quantities of antimony. This allows a fair estimate of the quantity of antimony present.
5. Place the copper spiral in the Gutzeit flask, then impregnate the disc of filter paper in the Gutzeit apparatus with the silver nitrate solution. If antimony is present, it is converted in the Gutzeit apparatus into stibine, which stains the silver nitrate paper light-gray to black. The intensity of the stain is proportional to the quantity of stibine produced. (For details on the generation of stibine in the Gutzeit apparatus, refer to the arsenic determination, Step 5 of the next procedure.)
6. Determine the quantity of antimony present in the specimen by comparing the stain on the paper disc with a series of reference stains, prepared in a similar manner from known quantities of antimony ranging from 0.01 to 0.10 mg. The reference stains are stable if stored in the dark.
7. Arsenic and antimony act similarly in the Gutzeit test. However, if arsenic was previously present on the copper spiral, it was dissolved and removed by the potassium cyanide solution in Step 2. To confirm that the stain is due to antimony, expose it to hydrochloric acid fumes. If it is due to antimony, the stain fades; if it is due to arsenic, the stain remains unchanged.

Arsenic, Selenium, Tellurium, and Sulfur

The potassium cyanide solution previously preserved (Step 3 of the antimony determination) is now tested for arsenic, selenium, tellurium, and sulfur. Under ideal conditions, the darkening will take place with as little as 0.050 mg of these elements, but the conditions as described in this test are not ideal for the quantitative deposition of selenium and tellurium. In the presence of 4 ml of concentrated hydrochloric acid, most of the volatile hydrides of selenium, tellurium, and sulfur are lost during the procedure. If 0.25 ml of concentrated hydrochloric acid is added, these elements may be semiquantitatively deposited on the copper. If a large quantity (0.2 mg or more) of these elements is present, however, the copper spiral would darken in spite of the excess of acid. In the event that the spiral is tarnished and it is known (or has already been determined by the preceding procedures) that arsenic, bismuth, and antimony are absent, it would be of some importance to know whether the deposit is due to sulfur from decomposed biologic material, sulfur-containing administered drugs, or selenium or tellurium. If one is specifically interested in the identification and estimation of selenium and tellurium, deposition on the copper spiral should be repeated on 20

*See p. 48.

g of the original material after adding 0.25 ml of concentrated hydrochloric acid.

1. To the 0.5 ml of potassium cyanide solution previously preserved, introduce, as a catalyst, the washed copper spiral from which the antimony has been removed.
2. Add 4 drops of ethanol and 5 drops of the cadmium acetate reagent. Shake the mixture, then let the tube rest for 5 min. An orange precipitate indicates selenium, a black precipitate (tellurium), and a yellow precipitate (sulfur). These three elements cannot be detected in the presence of one another, but may be detected in the presence of mercury, antimony, bismuth, or arsenic. The precipitates resulting from this test are distinctive and specific; none of the other metals that deposit on the copper spiral interferes with the test. The cadmium acetate test, although sensitive to 0.050 mg in each case, does not give positive results with pure solutions of these elements. The deposition on copper and the solution of the deposit in the cyanide reagent are integral parts of the test.
3. To estimate the approximate quantity of selenium or tellurium present, prepare a series of reference solutions containing 0.025 to 0.100 mg of these cations in 20 ml of water containing 0.25 ml of concentrated hydrochloric acid. Deposit these known quantities of selenium or tellurium, as the case may be, on a series of copper spirals as previously described. Dissolve the deposit in 0.5 ml of the potassium cyanide solution, then add 4 drops of 95% ethanol and 5 drops of the cadmium acetate reagent to the solution. Shake this mixture, then allow it to stand for 5 min. By comparing the precipitated suspension obtained from the biologic specimen with suspensions obtained from a series of reference samples, a fair estimate of the quantity present can be made.
4. Arsenic, although dissolved by the cyanide solution together with the selenium and tellurium, does not give any visible reaction with the cadmium acetate reagent. If the copper spiral was tarnished and the cyanide solution of the deposit yielded a negative cadmium acetate test, there is strong indication that arsenic was originally present. To confirm the presence of arsenic, acidify the cyanide solution of the deposit with 3.6*N* sulfuric acid, and subject it to the modified Gutzeit test as described by Kaye.[3] This procedure serves only as a qualitative method for the detection of arsenic in the presence of potassium cyanide.
5. For a quantitative estimation, take another 20-ml sample of tissue homogenate or body fluid and allow all of the arsenic to deposit on a fresh copper spiral. Place the coated copper spiral in the modified Gutzeit apparatus.[3] Place a cotton pledget into the small drying tube supported by the flask and moisten it with lead acetate solution. Impregnate a disc of filter paper for 3 min with the mercuric bromide solution. Blot the disc dry. Insert the impregnated filter paper between the flanges attached above the drying tube, then clamp the flanges together with a rubber band. Charge the apparatus with a few small pieces of arsenic-free mossy zinc, 2 drops of the stannous chloride solution, 2 drops of the potassium iodide solution, and 15 ml of 3.6*N* sulfuric acid. The hydrogen thus liberated reacts with the deposited arsenic and forms arsine (AsH_3). Allow the generation of arsine to proceed for 1 hr. Do not allow the gas to generate too rapidly; if generation is too rapid, cool the apparatus in an ice bath to decelerate the process. As the arsine rises, any hydrogen sulfide impurity is removed by passage through the cotton moistened with lead acetate. Arsine turns the mercuric bromide paper to colors ranging from clear canary-yellow to orange-brown. The intensity of the yellow color is a very sensitive indicator and is directly proportional to the arsine liberated.

REFERENCES

1. **Gettler, A. O.,** Simple tests for mercury in body fluids and tissues, *Am. J. Clin. Pathol.* (Tech. Suppl.), 7, 13, 1937.
2. **Kaye, S. and Castillo, J. C.,** A rapid and specific method for the estimation of bismuth in urine, *Am. J. Clin. Pathol.* (Tech. Suppl.), 14, 81, 1944.
3. **Kaye, S.,** Simple procedure for the detection of arsenic body fluids, *Am. J. Clin. Pathol.,* 14, 36, 1944.

IMMUNOASSAYS*

Irving Sunshine

Immunoassay of drugs is based on classical immunochemical procedures and utilizes an antigen-antibody reaction as an analytical tool. An antigen is any substance capable of eliciting an immune response when injected into a host animal. Generally, the best antigens are high molecular weight proteins, polysaccharides, or lipoproteins. Low molecular weight compounds, such as steroids and drugs, will usually not elicit an immune response. If these compounds are coupled to a large carrier protein or polysaccharide, they then can be antigens. Antibodies are immunoglobins that are formed in an animal as part of its immune response to an antigenic stimulus. The antibodies thus formed have a highly specific ability to react with the antigen that stimulated their formation. Thus, these can serve as detectors for the drug in the antigen in a suitable analytical system.

The first step in the production of drug-specific antibodies is the coupling of the drug to a suitable carrier protein. This preparation requires significant laboratory skill. Many synthetic pathways can be used. These include the use of diazonium salts for primary aromatic amines and phenols, carbodiimide for carboxylic acids, and dihalodinitrobenzenes or diisocyanates for aliphatic amines. This synthesis of the antigen is very critical because the specificity of the antibody is dependent on the results. In several instances alternative pathways may be used, and the resulting antigens will be different and have properties which will affect the sensitivity and specificity of the resulting antibody.

Having synthesized and purified the antigen, the antibody is formed by injecting a mixture of the antigen and Freund's adjuvant (a suitable carrier vehicle) into an animal (usually a rabbit, but goats, sheep, and horses have been used when larger volumes of antisera are required). Some animals are preferable to others because, among other reasons, they have a better ability to recognize the antigen as a foreign body and thus generate a better antiserum. The site and frequency of injection vary with each preparation. Usually the animal is bled 3 to 6 months after the initial injection. The resulting serum is then checked for its sensitivity and specificity for the antigen. The titer is determined by measuring the ability of varying dilutions of the antiserum to react with a given small amount of antigen. The specificity is determined by detecting to what extent chemically similar substances react as does the antigen. Once a suitable antiserum has been prepared, the probability is great that the animal involved will continue to produce it for a reasonable subsequent period; thus, some animals literally become worth their weight in gold. To produce significant amounts of antibodies one may repeat this experiment with other animals of the same or different species. There is no guarantee, however, that each animal will produce identical antibodies; continual vigilance is required if a desired titer and specificity is required. Once a suitable antiserum is obtained, it can be stored frozen at -80 to $-20°C$ or it can be lyophilized and stored at -20 to $4°C$. Once thawed or reconstituted, it is undesirable to refreeze or relyophilize the unused material; hence, small aliquots are preferred for storage. Most laboratories prefer to purchase commercially available immunoassay kits rather than try to prepare their own.

*Abridged from Sunshine, I., Immunoassay of drugs, in *The Poisoned Patient: The Role of the Laboratory*, CIBA Foundation Symposium 26, Elsevier, Amsterdam, 1974, 193. With permission.

All immunoassays are based on a similar principle – the competitive displacement of the labeled drug from the antibody complex by unlabeled drug in the sample. The concentration of the drug in the sample can then be determined by measuring the amount of the displaced labeled drug or alternately, by measuring the amount of labeled drug still bound to the antibody. In some immunoassays this involves a separation of the free and bound drug forms; this is usually accomplished easily by standard techniques. In other procedures this separation step is not required, and the resulting procedure then requires fewer manipulations.

Several immunoassay systems have been developed. Only two have been generally accepted for clinical use and they will be the only ones described herein. The Enzyme Multiplied Immunoassay Technique (EMIT) uses the enzyme lysozyme as the label attached to the drug in question. This enzyme catalyzes the hydrolysis of the mucopolysaccharide component of the cell walls of certain bacteria. When the antibody binds the drug attached to the enzyme, the enzyme is rendered inactive. In the presence of drug in the sample the enzyme is released; the hydrolysis takes place and can be measured. There is no need to separate the components of the reaction because a negative sample will not displace the enzyme label; hence, no activity will ensue. If the drug in question is present in the sample, the enzyme is released and its activity, and hence the drug concentration, can be determined by measuring the rate of clearing of the suspension of the cell walls (the decrease in absorbance) as the enzyme hydrolyzes them into small soluble pieces. This involves three measurements: the initial and subsequent optical density and the time between these measurements. Instrumentation is available to perform this automatically as part of the semiautomated EMIT system. This determination requires 1 min to complete and is simple to perform. Its primary advantages are its speed and its relatively moderate instrument cost – approximately \$6,000 to \$8,000. Of course, the cost of the antiserum is significant – \$0.50 to \$0.60 a test; but when prompt results are required, this system is the one that can provide the necessary results.

Another advantage of the EMIT system is its applicability to many drugs (morphine, amphetamine, barbiturate, cocaine, and methadone). Thus, this system can be very valuable in clinical situations which require rapid analyses to aid in the diagnosis of poisoning due to drugs of abuse. Recent advances have led to a new EMIT system for phenobarbital and diphenylhydantoin analyses. Should this prove to be adequate, the potential value of this new modification is high, particularly for neurologists.

An additional deterring factor of the EMIT system over those usually present for most immunoassays is that natural lysozyme does exist in some samples, and this may be a source of false positive results. Of course, one can easily check for this interference by adding the urine sample to the bacteria suspension and noting if any activity results. This is inexpensive since it does not require any antibody to obtain a result. Details of the EMIT procedure are given on the following page.

ENZYME MULTIPLIED IMMUNOASSAY TECHNIQUE (EMIT)

Beverly Lorenzo

APPARATUS

1. Disposable auto-analyzer sample cups, conical, 2 ml
2. Spectrophotometer with flow-through cuvette and constant temperature control (Gifford 300-N or Bausch and Lamb Spectronic 100) with a timer/printer/calculator
3. Micro sampler/dilutor

REAGENTS*

1. Antibody solution (Reagent A)
2. Antigen-lysozyme solution (Reagent B)
3. *tris*-Maleate buffer, pH 6.0, 0.25*M*
4. Bacterial cell wall suspension, 75 mg of M. luteus in 100 ml of 0.25*M* *tris*-maleate pH 6.0 buffer
5. Urine controls of known concentration and a "normal" urine or urine pool from "normal" drug-free individuals

PROCEDURE

The technique for the assay of morphine and other drugs by EMIT was described by Rubenstein et al.[1] The following procedure is similar to that suggested by the Syva Corp.

1. Into the 2-ml conical sample cups dispense 0.5 ml of the bacterial cell wall suspension. (Be sure to resuspend the bacteria before each use.)
2. Using the automatic sampler/dilutor, add to the suspension in the sample cup in order: (a) 0.05 ml of the urine sample or standard plus 0.25 ml of the *tris*-maleate buffer; (b) 0.05 ml of the antibody solution (Reagent A) plus 0.25 ml of the buffer; (c) 0.05 ml of the antigen-lysozyme solution (Reagent B) plus 0.25 ml of the buffer.
3. Immediately draw the reaction mixture into the temperature-controlled (37°C) flow-through cuvette of a spectrophotometer adjusted to read the absorbance at 436 nm. Set the timer/printer/calculator to record the absorbance after 10 sec to allow for temperature equilibration and again at 50 sec after the cuvette is filled. Calculate the decrease in absorbance over the 40-sec span.
4. Determine the concentration of the drug in the sample by comparing the decrease in absorbance with a standard curve. Even a negative sample will give some decrease in absorbance; therefore, a positive sample must have a greater decrease than that of the lowest detectable level of the drug to which the antibody is specific. All positive samples should have an exogenous lysozyme check to eliminate possible false positives. To check for this, reanalyze the sample as in the procedure substituting 0.05 ml of the buffer for both the antibody and antigen-lysozyme solutions (Reagents A and B). Subtract this decrease from the original decrease, and if this answer is still greater than that of the lowest detectable level, the sample is indeed positive. The reagents for this procedure are available commercially for morphine, methadone, amphetamine, barbiturates, and benzoyleconine, the metabolite of cocaine. The sensitivity of the technique for each of the drugs is:

	μg/ml
Morphine	0.5
Methadone	0.5
Amphetamine	1.0
Barbiturate	1.0
Benzoylecgonine	1.0

*All the reagents are available from the Syva Corp., Porter Drive, Palo Alto, Cal. 94304.

A similar procedure based on glucose-6-phosphate dehydrogenase has been developed for phenobarbital and diphenylhydantoin. An important innovation here is the application to serum or plasma. The previously described EMIT procedures were only applicable to urine. Details for these assays follow.

APPARATUS

1. Disposable auto-analyzer sample cups, conical, 2 ml
2. Spectrophotometer with flow-through cuvette and constant temperature control (Gifford 300-N or Bausch and Lomb Spectronic 100) with a timer/printer/calculator
3. Micro sampler/dilutor

REAGENTS*

1. Antibody-glucose-6-phosphate and nicotinamide-adenine dinucleotide antibody-substrate solution (Reagent A)
2. Antigen-glucose-6-phosphate dehydrogenase solution (Reagent B)
3. *tris*-Hydrochloride, pH 7.9 buffer with surfactant, 0.055*M*
4. Sera controls of known concentrations and a "normal" serum or sera pool from "normal" drug-free individuals

PROCEDURE

1. Using the automatic sampler/dilutor, add 0.05 ml of the serum sample or standard plus 0.25 ml of the *tris*-hydrochloride buffer to a 2-ml conical sample cup. Let it equilibrate for 1 min.
2. Aspirate 0.05 ml of the above diluted sample plus 0.25 ml of the buffer into each of three clean 2-ml conical sample cups. Let them equilibrate for 1 min.
3. To one of the doubly diluted samples add, in order: (a) 0.05 ml of the antibody-substrate solution (Reagent A) plus 0.25 ml of the buffer; (b) 0.05 ml of the antigen-glucose-6-phosphate dihydrogenase solution (Reagent B) plus 0.25 ml of the buffer.
4. Immediately draw the reaction mixture into the temperature-controlled (30°C) flow-through cuvette of a spectrophotometer adjusted to read the absorbance at 340 nm. Set the timer/printer/calculator to record the absorbance at 15 sec to allow the temperature to equilibrate and again at 80 sec. After the cuvette is filled calculate the increase in absorbance over the 65-sec span. From this increase subtract the increase of a "normal" serum determined at the beginning of the set of samples.
5. Take another of the doubly diluted samples from Step 2 and repeat Steps 3 and 4. If the difference from this sample agrees within 6 absorbance units with the first difference, determine the concentration of the drug in the sample by comparing the averaged difference with a standard curve. If, however, the two differences do not agree within 6 absorbance units, then take the third doubly diluted sample from Step 2 and repeat Steps 3 and 4. The sensitivity limit of this procedure is:

Diphenylhydantoin	0.25 μg/ml
Phenobarbital	0.5 μg/ml

Another immunoassay, which has become very popular and has been applied to many different substances (rather than only drugs of abuse), is radioimmunoassay (RIA). In this technique the antigen is labeled with a suitable radioactive isotope. Many can be used, but most frequently the isotope is either I^{125}, H^3, or ^{14}C. The usual antigen-antibody reaction is performed, and either the bound or the displaced radioactive drug in the resulting mixture is separated and measured. Usually the latter is involved, and the measuring device used depends on the label. Products of I^{125} are measured in a gamma counter, while the H^3 compounds require a scintillation counter. Of course, the I^{125} can also be counted in a scintillation counter, but this imposes additional cost and effort that

*All the reagents are available from the Syva Corp., Porter Drive, Palo Alto, Cal. 94304.

are seldom warranted. The inherent advantage of the RIA technique is that, since the radioactivity-labeled drug has a high specific radioactivity, its concentration can be determined with a high degree of sensitivity and precision. Standard curves are obtained by plotting counts per minute against concentration. Usually, these have a limited linear portion, and above these concentrations, unless the sample is diluted, all one can determine is that the reaction is positive. One attribute of RIA over most of the EMIT assays is that it is applicable to serum and thus opens a whole new horizon, which up until now could not be attained by the other procedure.

The general objections to immunoassays also prevail for this procedure, with a few additional ones. Since radioactive substances are involved, additional precautions and safety measures, all reasonable and easily met, are required. Shelf life may be a problem also, particularly for I^{125} compounds. The time for one determination is relatively long (40 min), but when many are done concomitantly, as they can be, the time per sample decreases significantly. The procedural details for the RIA technique are given below.

RADIOIMMUNOASSAY (RIA)

Beverly Lorenzo

Radioimmunoassay of morphine was first described by Spector and Parker.[2] The technique was applied to other classifications of drugs. The following procedure is a generalized one, modifying that suggested by the manufacturer.

APPARATUS

1. Disposable culture tubes, 10 × 75 mm
2. Semiautomatic pipets (Eppendorf pipets, Schwartz/Mann Biopettes) or glass transfer pipets (Lang-Levy). (Because this procedure involves both low concentrations and small volumes, carry-over, accuracy, and reproducibility of measurements are critical.)
3. Vortex mixer
4. Centrifuge
5. Gamma scintillation counter for I^{125} or liquid scintillation spectrometer for tritium

REAGENTS

1. Antibody reagent*
2. Radioactivity-labeled antigen reagent* (the radioactively-labeled drug to which the antibody is specific)
3. Positive urine control
   Use urine containing the appropriate concentration for the lowest detectable level of the drug to which the antibody is specific.
4. "Normal" urine control
   Use urine or a urine pool from "normal" drug-free individuals.
5. Saturated solution or ammonium sulfate

PROCEDURE

1. In a 10 × 75 mm test tube mix 0.1 ml of urine sample or standard and 0.4 ml of the combined antibody and radioactively-labeled antigen mixture. (Always analyze a positive and "normal" urine control in duplicate with each set of samples.) Wait 1 hr to approach equilibrium.
2. Add 0.5 ml of the saturated $(NH_4)_2\ SO_4$ solution to precipitate the antibody and antibody-antigen complex. Mix and wait 5 to 10 min to ensure that precipitation is complete. Centrifuge for 10 to 20 min at 1,000 to 1,500 × g.
3. Place 0.5 ml of the clear supernatant into either a counting vial for the gamma scintillation counter when using I^{125} or a scintillation vial containing 12 ml of Bray's solution for the

*These reagents are available from Roche Diagnostics, Nutley, N.J. 07110.

liquid scintillation spectrometer when using tritium. **Note**: Be extremely cautious to avoid drawing any precipitate into the supernatant. Measure the amount of radioactivity by the appropriate method.

4. Determine the amount of drug present by use of a standard curve. If the drug concentration in a sample is found to be greater than the positive urine control and if quantitative results are desired, the sample should be diluted (to yield a final concentration lower than the positive control, but discernable from the "normal" control urine) and reanalyzed. The reagents for this procedure are available commercially for morphine, barbiturates, amphetamine, and methadone. The stated sensitivities for these substances are:

Morphine	40	ng/ml
Methadone	100	ng/ml
Barbiturates	100	ng/ml
Amphetamine	0.1	μg/ml

Having mentioned some of the advantages and disadvantages of immunoassays, one of its major faults deserves particular attention.[3] The greatest defect is specificity, or lack thereof (Table 1). Very few antisera exist that are specific for one compound, although some have been prepared with very high specificity when cost was no object.[4] Hence, there is great need to confirm all positive results by some other procedure if specificity is important. If one does not care whether morphine, codeine, or another related opiate-like drug is the cause of a positive opiate reaction, the need for confirmation is minimal. If resolving the problem of what specific substance is present is important, because a job may be in jeopardy or a parolee incarcerated, or any one of several other vital situations, *then confirmation is essential.*[5]

Immunotechniques are sensitive and relatively specific, can be performed easily and rapidly by personnel with modest scientific training, and most of them provide objective results. These attributes are designed to suit those laboratories burdened with ongoing demands for the analysis of a large number of samples to be analyzed for a given substance, particularly when a large number of the specimens to be analyzed are predictably negative (Screening Techniques). This ability to satisfy a service need for many samples highlights the advantage of these techniques. Many other elegant procedures satisfy similar needs for one or more of the attributes listed, but few combine them all, as do the immunoassays.

REFERENCES

1. **Rubenstein, K., Schneider, R., and Ullman, E.,** Homogeneous enzyme immunoassay, *Biochem. Biophys. Res. Commun.*, 47, 846, 1972.
2. **Spector, S. and Parker, C. W.,** Morphine radioimmunoassays, *Science*, 168, 1374, 1970.
3. **Mulé, S. J., Bastos, M. L., and Jukofsky, D.,** Evaluation of immunoassay methods for detection, in urine, or drugs subject to abuse, *Clin. Chem.*, 20, 243, 1974.
4. **Gross, S. J., et al.,** Critical antigenic determinants for production of antibody to distinguish morphine from heroin, codeine and dextromorphan, *Immunochem.*, 11, 8, 1974.
5. **Foltz, R. and Clark, P.,** Quantitative analysis of morphine in urine by gas chromatography – chemical ionization mass spectrophotometry, *Clin. Chem.*, 20, 465, 1974.

GENERAL REFERENCES

Adler, F. and Liu, C. T., Detection of morphine by hemagglutination inhibition, *J. Immunol.*, 106, 1684, 1971.

Adler, F., Liu, C. T., and Catlin, D., Methodology and application of a hemagglutination inhibition test for the detection of morphine, *Clin. Immunol. and Immunopathol.*, 1, 53, 1972.

Bastiani, R., Phillips, R., Schneider, R., and Ullman, E., Homogeneous immunochemical drug assays, *Am. J. Med. Technol.*, 39, 211, 1973.

Bidanset, J. H., Drug analysis by immunoassays, *J. Chromatogr. Sci.*, 12, 4, 1974.

Catlin, D., Cleeland, R., and Grunberg, E., A sensitive and rapid radioimmunoassay for morphine and immunologically related substances in urine and serum, *Clin. Chem.*, 19, 216, 1973.

Cravey, R. H. and Jain, N. C., Current status of blood alcohol methods, *J. Chromatogr. Sci.*, 12, 209, 1974.

Dubowski, K., Free radical assay technique for drugs, *Ann. Clin. Lab. Sci.*, 1, 199, 1971.

Mulé, S. and Hushin, P. L., Semiautomated fluorometric assay for submicrogram quantities of morphine and quinine in human biological material, *Anal. Chem.*, 43, 708, 1971.

Mulé, S. J., Sunshine, I., Braude, M., and Willette, R. E., *Immunoassay for Drugs Subject to Abuse*, CRC Press, Cleveland, 1974.

Skelly, D. S., Brown, L. P., and Besch, P. K., Radioimmunoassay, *Clin. Chem.*, 19, 146, 1973.

Table 1

CROSS-REACTIVITY OF COMPOUNDS* IN URINE WITH VARIOUS IMMUNOASSAYS

Methadone			*d*-Amphetamine			Barbiturate		
Compound	$\mu g/ml$	RR‡	Compound	$\mu g/ml$	RR‡	Compound	$\mu g/ml$	RR‡
Methadone	1.0	1.00	*d*-Amphetamine	1.0	1.00	Secobarbital	1.0	1.00
Morphine	NR‡	–	Phenethylamine	3.1	0.32	Phenobarbital	2.0	0.50
Meperidine	1,000	0.001	Phenylpropanolamine	5.0	0.20	Pentobarbital	1.1	0.90
2-Ethylidene-1,5-dimethyl-3,3-diphenylpyrrolidine	NR	–	Methamphetamine (Methedrine®)	0.9	1.08	Amobarbital	1.8	0.55
2-Ethyl-5-methyl-3,3-diphenyl-1-pyrroline	NR	–	Methylphenidate (Ritalin®)	50.0	0.02	Thiopental	0.7	1.42
d-Propoxyphene (Darvon®)	NR	–	Phenmetrazine (Preludin®)	0.95	1.05	Glutethimide (Doriden®)	50	0.02
			Ephedrine	4.5	0.22			
			Mephentermine (Wyamine®)	1.6	0.62			
			Phentermine	1.6	0.62			
			Propylhexedrine	20	0.05			
			Phenylethylamine	5	0.20			
			Benzphetamine	3	0.33			
			Cyclopentamine	3	0.33			
			Nylidrin	3.7	0.27			
			Isoxsuprine	5.0	0.20			
			Methoxyphenamine	3.0	0.33			
			Phenformin	5.5	0.18			
			p-Hydroxyamphetamine	80.0	0.01			

* All values ($\mu g/ml$) for each compound are equivalent to 1 $\mu g/ml$ of the assay drug.
** This EMIT assay is for benzoylecgonine, a metabolite of cocaine.
† RIA for morphine and the EMIT for opiates.
‡ RR, relative reactivity, is the ratio obtained by dividing 1 $\mu g/ml$ by the concentration ($\mu g/ml$) of the cross-reacting drug.
‡ NR, no reaction at concentrations of 500 to 1,000 g/ml.

Table 1 (continued)

CROSS-REACTIVITY OF COMPOUNDS* IN URINE WITH VARIOUS IMMUNOASSAYS

Cocaine**

Compound	μg/ml	RR[‡]
Benzoylecgonine	1.0	1.000
Ecgonine	9.5	0.105
Ecgonine	380	0.003
Ecgonine methylester	460	0.002
Cocaine	460	0.002
Homatropine	NR	–
Scopolamine	NR	–
Morphine	NR	–
Methadone	NR	–
Secobarbital	NR	–

Morphine[†]

Compound	RIA μg/ml	RIA RR[‡]	EMIT μg/ml	EMIT RR[‡]
Normorphine	41.6	0.02	44.4	0.02
Codeine	0.76	1.32	0.78	1.28
Diacetylmorphine (heroin)	1.0	1.00	2.4	0.42
N-Allylnormorphine (nalorphine)	10.0	0.10	15.8	0.05
N-Allyl-7,8-dihydro-14-hydroxy normorphinone (Naloxone®)	290.0	0.00	NR	–
Dihydromorphinone (Dilaudid®)	1.2	0.83	2.6	0.38
Apomorphine	350.0	0.00	NR	–
Dihydromorphine	1.5	0.68	1.8	0.55
Morphine glucuronide	–	–	2.6	0.38
1,3-Hydroxy-*N*-methylmorphinan (levorphanol)	2.0	0.50	6.2	0.16
d-3-Methoxy-*N*-methylmorphinan (dextromethorphan)	878.0	0.00	268.0	0.00
2-Ethylidene-1,5-dimethyl-3,3-diphenylpyrrolidine (methadone metabolite)	–	–	NR	–
2-Ethyl-5-methyl-3,3-diphenyl-1-pyrroline (methadone metabolite)	–	–	1,000	0.00
Methadone	1,780.0	0.00	NR	–
d-Propoxyphene (Darvon®)	680.0	0.00	NR	–
Cyclazocine	380.0	0.00	NR	–

ORGANIC VOLATILE SUBSTANCES

Kurt M. Dubowski

Volatile substances can be separated from biological liquids after injection onto packed gas-chromatographic columns or in a closed vessel or by controlled temperature diffusion from the liquid phase into the air above the sample (head space). The separated volatile component may be identified by its gas-chromatographic retention time and quantitated by means of the gas chromatograph detector response.

APPARATUS

1. Septum vials, 15 ml, screw-capped with butyl rubber stoppers
2. Water bath (e.g., Lauda-Brinkmann Model K-4) with ±0.01 to 0.05°C regulation
3. Tuberculin syringe, plastic, 1 ml with a 25-gauge 1 ½-in. needle
4. Chaney adaptor
5. Gas chromatograph, equipped with a flame ionization detector (e.g., Varian Model 1860), a stainless steel (or glass) column, 6′ × 1/8″ i.d., packed with Porapak S (80 to 100 mesh), and a suitable potentiometric recorder (1 mV full-scale sensitivity and 250-mm chart width). An electronic or recorder-coupled mechanical integrator is very desirable. If liquid samples are to be injected, the injection port is fitted with a removable glass liner. Operating conditions and electrometer settings of the chromatograph should be adjusted so that injection of 2 μl of 200 mg/dl of ethanol produces a full-scale recorder response with a retention time of approximately 2 min. A recorder chart speed of 5 mm/min is used if peak heights are employed for quantitation; higher chart speeds can be used if peak areas are measured. (Other column packings may be used for the analysis of volatile substances. Table 1 provides reference data relative to these other materials.)

Operating Conditions

(Typical operating conditions are shown for a Varian Model 1860-3 gas chromatograph.)

Gases:	Inlet pressure	Flow rate
He, NH_2	55 psig	45 ml/min
H_2	20 psig	45 ml/min
air	15 psig	330 ml/min

Temperatures:
column – 165°C
injection port – 175°C
detector – 225°C

Recorder:
chart speed – 5 mm/min

REAGENTS

All chemicals should be analytical reagent grade.

1. Mixed volatiles reference solutions
   Using absolute ethanol and chromatographically pure absolute acetone, isopropanol, and methanol, prepare the following low concentration and high concentration solutions.

	Low concentration	High concentration
Acetone	50 mg/dl	100 mg/dl
Ethanol	100 mg/dl	200 mg/dl
Isopropanol	50 mg/dl	100 mg/dl
Methanol	50 mg/dl	100 mg/dl

   In sealed glass containers, at 4°C, these reference solutions are stable for at least 6 months.
2. Diluent internal standard solution
   Dissolve 12 g of Triton® X-100 in water, add 1.80 g (= 2.2 g/ml at 20°C) of acetonitrile, and dilute to one liter.

Table 1

ABSOLUTE RETENTION TIMES FOR ETHANOL USING THE GAS-CHROMATOGRAPHIC CONDITIONS DESCRIBED BELOW

Packing	Temperature, °C	Absolute retention time for ethanol (min)
1. 0.5% Carbowax K-600 and 3.8% Hallcomid 18 on Teflon® 6HC 40 to 60 mesh	100	0.24
2. 0.5% Carbowax K-600 and 3.8% Hallcomid 18 on Teflon® 6HC 40 to 60 mesh*	50	1.8
3. 0.4% Carbowax 1500 on Carbopak A	80	1.47
4. Porapak Q, 80 to 100 mesh	155	1.60
5. Chromosorb 102, 100 to 120 mesh	155	2.16
6. 15% Carbowax 1500 on Celite 525 80 to 100 mesh	80	2.58
7. Porapak S, 80 to 100 mesh	155	2.51
8. 30% Carbowax 20M* on Chromosorb W, AW, 60 to 80 mesh	130	2.12

* 6′ × 1/4″ o.d. column, rather than the 6′ × 1/8″ size used for the other supports.

PROCEDURE

Head Space Analysis Procedure

1. Into a 15-ml screw-capped septum vial with a butyl rubber septum stopper, place 1.0 g of sodium chloride and 1 ml of well-mixed whole blood (or other liquid sample). Close the vial and mix well by rotation and lateral shaking (swirling).
2. Prepare vials (following the procedure in Step 1) containing 1 ml of low concentration and 1 ml of high concentration mixed volatiles reference solution, respectively. When the specimens supplied for analysis have limited volume, the same procedure is followed with 0.2 g of sodium chloride and 0.1 ml of specimen.
3. Place all vials into a water bath maintained at 38 ± 0.05°C and allow the vials (immersed to just below the screw caps) to equilibrate for 45 min.
4. Using a plastic 1-ml tuberculin syringe fitted with a volume-limiting Chaney adaptor and a 25-gauge 1½-in. needle preheated to 38°C withdraw a fixed volume (approximately 0.25 ml) of the head space vapor (after repeated pumping to obtain an equilibrated sample aliquot), and immediately inject it into the gas chromatograph. (For gas chromatographs equipped with a heated gas-sampling valve and a 0.25-ml sample loop, a larger head space sample can be withdrawn from a septum vial and transferred to the gas-sampling valve.) Thoroughly purge the syringe and needle by rapid repetitive intake and expulsion of room air.
5. Record each chromatogram for 5 min.
6. It is convenient and advisable to sample and chromatograph the head space vapors in the following sequence: low concentration reference solution, unknown specimen(s), and high concentration reference solution. The reference solutions (or at least one reference solution) should be analyzed completely in parallel with every unknown specimen (or repeated with every ten unknown specimens). The same syringe is used for all unknown and reference specimens.

Table 2

RELATIVE RETENTION TIMES OF VOLATILE SUBSTANCES

Relative retention time*	Compound	Relative retention time*	Compound
0.19	Petroleum ether	1.22	Benzene
0.20	Acetaldehyde	1.24	Isopropanol
0.21	*n*-Pentane	1.32	Methyl cyclohexane
0.25	Diethyl ether	1.39	Allyl ether
0.36	Propionaldehyde	1.40	Butanol, tertiary
0.38	Methylacetate	1.63	*N*-Propyl acetate
0.40	Acetone	1.64	Chloroform
0.40	Carbon disulfide	1.69	Allyl acetate
0.41	Acrolein	1.72	1-Chloro-3-methyl butane
0.44	*n*-Hexane	1.80	Trichlorethanol
0.44	Methyl iodide	1.81	1,4-Dioxane
0.47	Isopropyl ether	1.84	Ethylene dichloride
0.57	Diethylamine	2.10	Trichlorethylene
0.60	Methanol	2.40	*n*-Octane
0.65	Acetonitrile	2.50	*n*-Propanol
0.69	Methylene chloride	2.63	2,3-Dichloropropane
0.71	Ethyl acetate	2.75	Methyl isobutyl ketone
0.72	Cyclohexane	3.04	Butanol, secondary
0.78	Tetrahydrofuran	3.15	Toluene
0.80	Acrylonitrile	3.45	Paraldehyde
0.84	Butanone	4.00	*n*-Butylacetate
0.98	*n*-Heptane	4.68	Isobutanol
0.98	1,1,1-Trichloroethane	5.95	*n*-Nonane
1.00	Ethanol	6.08	Pyridine
1.01	Carbon tetrachloride	6.60	*n*-Butanol
1.14	Propionitrile	7.57	Xylene

* Relative to ethanol, whose absolute retention time is 1.9 ± 0.1 min on a 6′ × 1/4″ o.d. column packed with 5% Carbowax K-600 and 3% Halcomid 18 on 60 to 80 mesh Teflon® 6HC.

Note: The retention time is measured from the blip resulting from the pressure drop in the column at the moment of injection.

7. For analyses of critical importance, repeat Steps 4, 5, and 6 after allowing the vials to equilibrate for at least 20 min after the prior head space vapor withdrawal.
8. Identify ethanol or any other volatile in the unknown specimen, if present, by its retention time in comparison with the reference solutions. For the system described, the volatile substances appear in the following order: methanol, ethanol, acetone, and isopropanol. Typical retention times are shown in Table 3. R_f data for other volatiles are given in Table 2.
9. If any volatile substance is present in the unknown specimen, its concentration in the original blood (or other) specimen is determined with the following formula:

$$\frac{P_A}{P_R} \times C_R = C_A$$

where

P_A = peak area of the volatile substance in question in the unknown specimen;
P_R = peak area of the volatile substance in question in the reference specimen;
C_R = reference concentration of the volatile in question in a reference solution;
C_A = concentration of the volatile in question in the unknown sample (mg/dl).

Direct Injection Procedure

1. With a fully quantitative technique, add ex-

Table 3

TYPICAL RELATIVE RETENTION TIMES*
OF VOLATILE SUBSTANCES

(ON PORAPAK S COLUMN)

Compound	RR_+*
Acetone	1.44
Acetonitrile	1.23
Ethanol	1.00
Isopropanol	1.80
Methanol	0.48

* Retention times relative to that of ethanol, whose absolute retention time for this analytical system is 2.0 min.

actly equal volumes of the well-mixed whole blood (or other liquid sample) and the diluent internal standard solution to a suitable container, and mix thoroughly. (Glass-stoppered microcentrifuge tubes are convenient for this purpose; use of a high precision manual or mechanical sampler/diluter is helpful when many specimens are to be analyzed.)

2. Mix exactly equal volumes of low concentration and high concentration mixed volatiles reference solution, respectively, and diluent internal standard solution.
3. Centrifuge all mixtures briefly in closed containers, if necessary, to obtain a perfectly clear mixture free of debris, blood cell ghosts, etc.
4. Using a suitable gas-chromatographic syringe, inject 2 μl of each unknown and reference specimen, prepared as per Step 1 or 2 above, into the gas chromatograph. Immediately after each injection separate the syringe plunger and barrel, and thoroughly clean and dry them.
5. Record each chromatogram for 5 min.
6. It is convenient and advisable to sample and chromatograph low concentration reference solution, unknown specimen(s), and high concentration reference solution, in that sequence. The reference solutions (or at least one reference solution) should be analyzed completely in parallel with every unknown specimen (or repeated with every ten unknown specimens). Different syringes can be used to inject the several specimens.
7. For analyses of critical importance, repeat Steps 4, 5, and 6.
8. Identify the volatile in question in the unknown specimen, if present, by its retention time in comparison with the simultaneously analyzed reference solutions. For the system described, the volatile substances appear in the following order: methanol, ethanol, acetonitrile, acetone, and isopropanol. Typical retention times are shown in Table 3.
9. If a volatile substance is present in the unknown specimen, its concentration in the original blood (or other specimen) is determined with the following formula:

$$\frac{S_E/S_R}{K_E/K_R} \times C_R = C_E$$

where

S_E = peak area of the volatile in question in unknown sample and diluent internal standard mixture;

S_R = peak area of acetonitrile in unknown sample and diluent internal standard mixture;

K_E = peak area of the volatile in question in reference sample and diluent internal standard mixture;

K_R = peak area of acetonitrile in reference sample and diluent internal standard mixture;

C_R = reference sample concentration of the volatile in question;

C_E = concentration of the volatile in question in the unknown sample (mg/dl).

ACCURACY AND PRECISION

When peak area measurements are used to calculate sample ethanol concentrations, the standard deviation and coefficient of variation (= relative standard deviation) of replicate analyses for the procedures described above are as follows for specimens with a mean ethanol concentration of 100 mg/dl:

	Head space analysis	Direct injection
Standard deviation	± 2.80 mg/dl	2.8%
Coefficient of variation	± 2.18 mg/dl	2.2%

When peak height measurements are used to calculate sample ethanol concentrations, the standard deviation and coefficient of variation of replicate analyses are somewhat greater than listed above unless the procedure is fully optimized with respect to sample size, peak slope, chart speed, and other gas-chromatographic analysis conditions.

DETECTABLE SUBSTANCES

Commonly occurring volatile substances are shown in Table 3. These compounds can be readily separated from each other and identified by their relative retention time according to the procedure outlined. In critically important analyses, it is good and recommended practice to confirm the tentative identifications based on a single set of gas-chromatographic conditions by additional methods, which can include reanalysis of the prepared sample by gas-chromatographic means with a different column and other conditions. If an internal standard with a retention time different than that of acetonitrile is desired, *n*-propanol, *tert*-butanol, and dioxane, among others, are suitable compounds.

REFERENCES

Baker, R. N., et al., Toxic volatiles in alcoholic coma, *Bull. Los Angeles County Neurol. Soc.,* 33, 140, 1968.

Wallace, J. E. and Dahl, E. V., Rapid vapor phase method for determining ethanol in blood and urine by gas chromatography, *Am. J. Clin. Pathol.,* 46, 152, 1966.

TLC FOR WEAK ACIDS, NEUTRALS, AND WEAK BASES

Irving Sunshine

APPARATUS

1. Bottles, ground-glass-stoppered, 60 ml, or separatory funnels
2. Beakers, 50 ml
3. Evaporating tubes, disposable, 2 ml (Cut Pasteur pipets to the desired lengths and seal the tips.)
4. Thin-layer chromatography (TLC) equipment: (a) micropipets; (b) glass plates, coated with silica gel G; (c) developing tanks; (d) spray bottles
5. UV light source, 254-nm radiation

REAGENTS

All chemicals should be analytical reagent grade.

1. Chloroform
2. Sodium hydroxide, 0.45*N*
   Dissolve 18 g of sodium hydroxide in water and dilute to one liter with water.
3. Ethanol-chloroform mixture, 1:1
   Mix equal volumes of ethanol and chloroform.
4. Hydrochloric acid, 6*N*
   Dilute concentrated hydrochloric acid with an equal volume of water.
5. Thin-layer chromatography (TLC) developing systems
   (a) Chloroform-acetone, 9:1 (S-1) – Mix 9 volumes of chloroform with 1 volume of acetone; (b) Isopropyl ether (S-2); (c) Mix 85 ml of ethyl acetate with 10 ml of methanol and 5 ml of concentrated ammonium hydroxide (S-3).
6. Stock drug solutions, 1 mg/ml
   Dissolve 10 mg of each drug in methanol and dilute to 10 ml with methanol. Solutions of the following drugs should be prepared: (1) secobarbital, (2) amobarbital, (3) phenobarbital, (4) meprobamate, (5) chlordiazepoxide, (6) diazepam, and (7) glutethimide.
7. Working drug solutions
   Dilute 1 ml of Solutions 1, 2, and 4 and 1 ml of Solutions 3, 5, 6, and 7 to 50 ml with methanol.
8. Thin-layer chromatography (TLC) detection reagents
   (a) Mercuric sulfate, 1 g/100 ml – Suspend, with mixing, 5 g of mercuric oxide in 100 ml of water. Add, while mixing, 20 ml of concentrated sulfuric acid. Cool the suspension, then dilute it to 250 ml with water; (b) Furfural, freshly redistilled furfural, stored in a dark bottle at 4°C – This chemical has a shelf life of approximately 1 month; (c) Hydrochloric acid, concentrated; (d) Potassium permanganate, 100 mg/100 ml – Dissolve 100 mg of potassium permanganate in water and dilute to 100 ml with water.

PROCEDURE

1. Acidify 3 ml of blood or 10 ml of urine and extract with 50 ml of chloroform in a 60-ml ground-glass-stoppered bottle or in a suitable separatory funnel. Allow the phases to separate.
2. Filter the chloroform phase through filter paper.
3. Collect the chloroform filtrate.
4. Evaporate the filtrate to dryness. Use low heat and an air stream. Remove the sample from the heat source as soon as it is dry.
5. Dissolve the residue in 20 μl of the 1:1 ethanol-chloroform mixture.
6. Apply 10-μl aliquots of the dissolved residue (Step 5) to a TLC plate coated with silica gel G. Spot aliquots from a suitable number of reference drug solutions on each plate to serve as reference points.
7. Develop one plate in the chloroform-acetone developing system and the other in isopropyl ether. After they are developed (i.e., after the solvent fronts have moved 10 to 12 cm beyond the application points), remove the plates from the developing jars and air-dry them. Inspect each plate under the UV lamp. Note the results. Spray each plate with the potassium permanganate, mercuric sulfate, furfural, and concentrated hydrochloric acid, in that order. Tentatively identify any spots that appear by

Table 1

R_f VALUES OF ACIDIC AND NEUTRAL DRUGS

	$R_f \times 100$		
Compound	S-1	S-2	S-3
Amobarbital	62	78	75
Butabarbital	57	76	73
Carisoprodol	34	16	–
Chlordiazepoxide	84	35	88
Diazepam	64	22	98
Diphenylhydantoin	33	33	75
Glutethimide	80	49	99
Hexobarbital	78	58	67
Meprobamate	5	4	75
Pentobarbital	62	79	75
Phenobarbital	45	65	46
Secobarbital	72	87	75

comparison with spots obtained by applying reference solutions to the same plates (Table 1).

INTERPRETATION (see p. 7)

One swallow does not indicate spring is here, and just as surely, one spot on a thin-layer chromatogram does not indicate a particular drug is present. The spot at a particular R_f with particular reactions to given spray reagents is a necessary condition for proof of identity, but *it is not sufficient for positive proof*. All drugs presumed to be present as a result of a spot on a chromatograph should be confirmed by other tests. Thin-layer chromatography using other developing solvents is one procedure that can be considered. If this is done, care in the selection of the other solvents is essential. The second solvent may produce a series of spots that have different R_f values; if they are in the same sequence as those obtainable from the use of the original solvent, no further element of proof has been added. Only when the other developing solvent produces a different order of R_f value does this become another confirmatory datum. Whenever the quantum of proof must be high, the TLC data must be confirmed by another method using different physical properties of the substance.

UV SPECTROPHOTOMETRY FOR SEDATIVE DRUGS FREQUENTLY INVOLVED IN OVERDOSE EMERGENCIES

Peter I. Jatlow

The sedative drugs, which are usually involved in poisoning episodes and develop measurable concentrations in blood, are chemically weak organic acids, neutrals, or weak organic bases. This procedure, in conjunction with rapid tests for blood salicylate and alcohol, and urine screening tests for phenothiazines, imipramine and ethchlorvynol, constitutes a fairly comprehensive rapid procedure for the testing of those drugs most frequently involved in cases of coma of unknown origin.

APPARATUS

1. Separatory funnels, 60 ml
2. Centrifuge tubes, round-bottomed, 50 ml
3. Filter paper, Whatman #1
4. UV spectrophotometer, recording
5. Quartz cuvettes, 10-mm light path, 2-ml capacity
6. Centrifuge
7. pH Meter
8. Graduate cylinders, 50 ml

REAGENTS

All chemicals should be analytical reagent grade.

1. Stock drug standards, 1 mg/ml in methanol*
   Dissolve 10 mg of each drug separately in methanol and dilute each to 10 ml. Store at −20°C.
2. Working serum standards, 1 mg/100 ml
   Add 50 μl of stock to 5 ml of serum. Use a separate aliquot of serum for each drug.† Methanol stock (1 ml) can be added to 100 ml of serum, and 5-ml aliquots can be stored at −20°C. Individual aliquots are thawed and used as needed.
3. Chloroform
   Extract a 25-ml aliquot of chloroform solvent successively with 5 ml of 0.45*N* NaOH and 0.5*N* HCl, and determine the UV absorption spectrum of each, using NaOH and HCl as the reference solutions, respectively. If the absorbance is greater than 0.02, between 235 and 310 nm, wash all the chloroform successively with 0.45*N* NaOH, 0.5*N* HCl, and water until neutral. Check the washed chloroform as directed above until the absorbance of the extracts is below 0.02. Store in a dark glass bottle. Spectrograde chloroform may contain less UV absorbing material and, if cost is not a deterrent, may prove more acceptable than the analytical reagent.
4. Sodium hydroxide, 5*N*
   Dissolve 100 g of sodium hydroxide in water and dilute to 500 ml with water.
5. Sodium hydroxide, 0.45*N*
   Dilute 90 ml of 5*N* NaOH to 1,000 ml with water.
6. Hydrochloric acid, 1*N*
   Add 42 ml of 12*N* (concentrated) HCl to water and dilute to 500 ml.
7. Hydrochloric acid, 0.5*N*
   Add 21 ml of 12*N* (concentrated) HCl to water and dilute to 500 ml.
8. Hexane, spectrograde or redistilled
9. Ethanol, 80%
10. NH_4Cl, 10.7 g/100 ml
    Dissolve 10.7 g of ammonium chloride in water and dilute the mixture to 100 ml with water.
11. Potassium hydroxide, 5*N*
    Dissolve 31 g of 85% KOH pellets in water and dilute to 100 ml.
12. Phosphate buffer, pH 7.4, 0.5*M*
    Dissolve 35.3 g of Na_2HPO_4 in water and dilute to 500 ml. Dissolve 34 g of KH_2PO_4 in

*If the sodium salts of the barbiturates are used, their concentration should be 1.1 mg/ml to correspond to 1 mg/ml of the free acid. Use 1.1 mg/ml of chlordiazepoxide HCl and methaqualone HCl. Diazepam, oxazepam, and glutethimide are used as the free bases and acid, respectively.

†Chlordiazepoxide, glutethimide, and *one* of the barbiturates can be combined in a single stock methanol standard and added together to one serum standard.

water and dilute to 500 ml. To 500 ml of Na_2HPO_4, add KH_2PO_4 until the pH of the mixture measures 7.4 with a pH meter. About 110 to 115 ml of the KH_2PO_4 will be required.

PROCEDURE (see Flow Chart)

1. Place 3 ml of serum (sample or serum standard), 2 ml of phosphate buffer, and 30 ml of chloroform into a separatory funnel and extract gently for about 5 min.
2. Filter the chloroform (lower) layer into a graduate cylinder. Place 25 ml into a 50-ml centrifuge tube. Discard the extracted serum.
3. Add 5 ml of 0.45*N* NaOH, and shake for about 3 to 5 min. Centrifuge for about 5 min.
4. Remove the entire NaOH (upper) layer with a Pasteur pipet and prepare two 2-ml aliquots, A and B. Save the chloroform for Step 9.
5. Add 0.5 ml of 0.45*N* NaOH to aliquot A (pH 13) and 0.5 ml of the 10.7% NH_4Cl to aliquot B (pH 10).
6. Place aliquot B (pH 10) in the reference cuvette and aliquot A (pH 13) in the sample cuvette. Set the recorder pen zero at 0.3 to 0.5 absorbance units and determine the UV absorption spectra.
7. A characteristic biomodal absorption spectrum indicates a barbiturate may be present (Figure 1A). The barbiturate concentration may be calculated from the absolute difference in the absorbance at 260 and 240 nm (maximum and minimum).
8. If the characteristic biomodal barbiturate spectrum is not obtained in Step 7, the contents of the reference cuvette B should be replaced with 0.45*N* NaOH, and the UV absorption spectrum of A determined again. If other UV absorbing weakly acidic drugs are present, their typical spectra will be obtained.
9. Add 0.5*N* HCl to the chloroform remaining in the centrifuge tube (Step 4 above). Shake for 3 to 5 min and centrifuge. Save the chloroform for Step 11.
10. Remove the entire HCl fraction and separate into two 2.0-ml aliquots, A and B. Add 0.5 ml of 0.5*N* HCl to A and, using 0.5*N* HCl in the reference cuvette, determine its UV absorption spectrum. If the result is positive, add 0.5 ml of 5*N* NaOH to B and to the 0.5*N* HCl reference solution. Determine the UV absorption spectrum of the alkalinized solution. Chlordiazepoxide is the most common drug in this fraction (Figure 1B). Calculate the concentration from the absorbance at the major acid peak (247 nm for chlordiazepoxide). If this step is positive, wash the remaining chloroform (Step 9) with an additional 10 ml of 0.5*N* HCl, discarding the HCl. This prevents carry-over of drug from interfering in the test for diazepam and related drugs (Step 13 below).
11. Refilter the chloroform (Step 9 above) and evaporate the filtrate to dryness.
12. Dissolve the residue in 5 ml of hexane. Proceed directly to Step 16 (glutethimide analysis) if the determination of diazepam, oxazepam, chlorazepate (as nordiazepam), or methaqualone is not required (Figures 1C and 1D).
13. Extract the hexane with 4 ml of 1*N* HCl. Centrifuge and remove the entire HCl (lower) layer. Save the hexane for Step 16.
14. Determine the UV absorption of the aqueous phase (Step 13), using 1*N* HCl in the reference cell.
15. Diazepam (Figure 2A), oxazepam, methaqualone (Figure 2B), and caffeine (Figures 2C and D) are the drugs usually found in this fraction. Subtract the absorbance at 260 nm from that at 240 nm to determine the concentration of diazepam or oxazepam. Identify, but do not quantify, methaqualone because metabolites as well as the unchanged drug are extracted by chloroform.[1] The quantitation of methaqualone requires a separate analysis.
16. Add 5 ml of 80% ethanol to the remaining hexane, (Step 12 or 13 above), and shake for 1 to 2 min.
17. Prepare a blank consisting of 2 ml of 80% ethanol and 0.1 ml of 5*N* KOH.
18. Remove the ethanol (Step 16). Add 0.1 ml of 5*N* KOH to a 2-ml aliquot of the 80% ethanol, and note the time. Determine the UV absorption spectrum using as a reference solution the *prepared* blank (Step 17).
19. Note the absorbance at 235 nm at 2 and 10 min. Calculate the concentration from the absorbance *decrease* at 235 nm during this 8-min interval. Figure 1D shows the spectrum obtained if glutethimide is present.

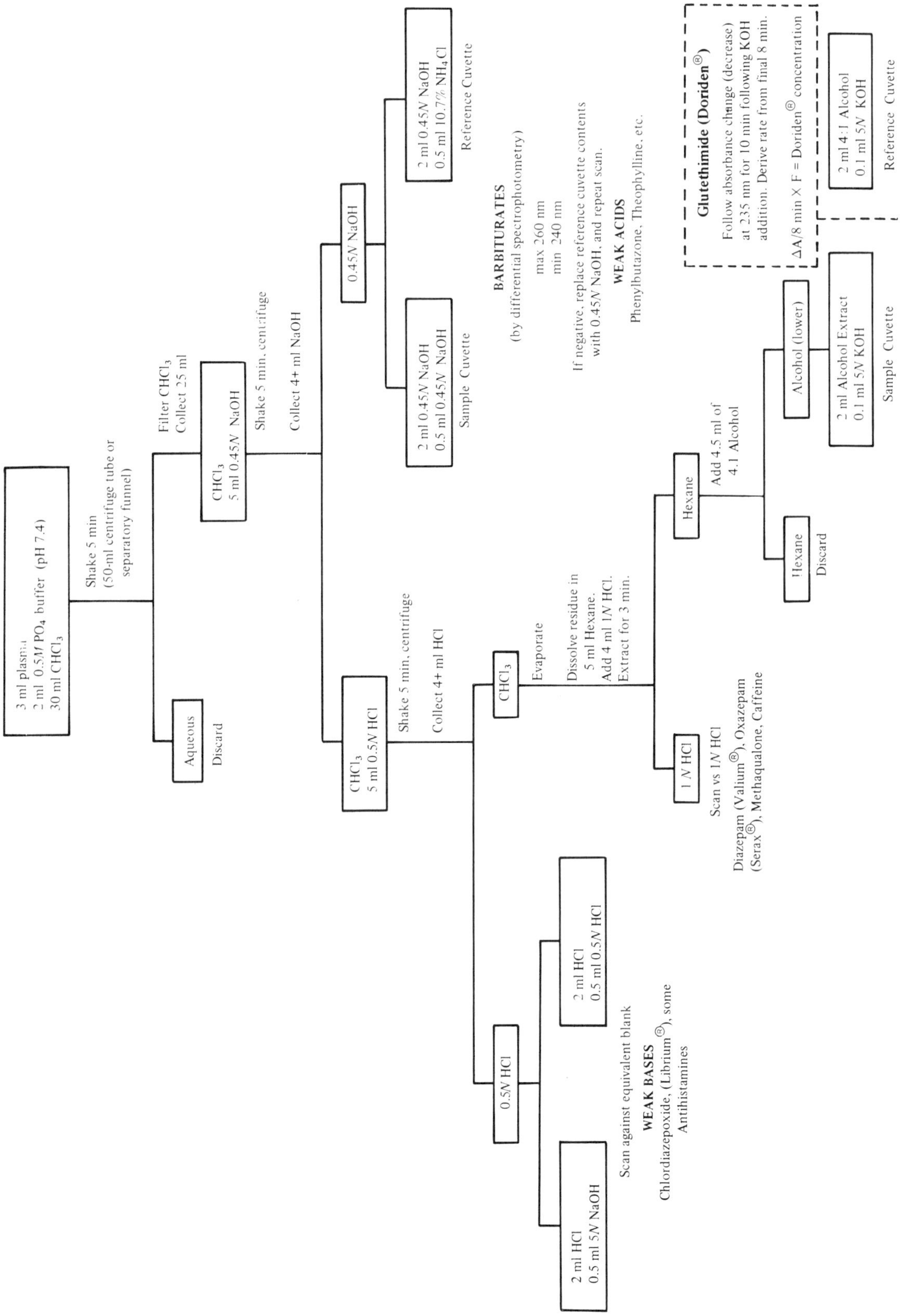

Flow chart for UV procedure for sedative drugs.

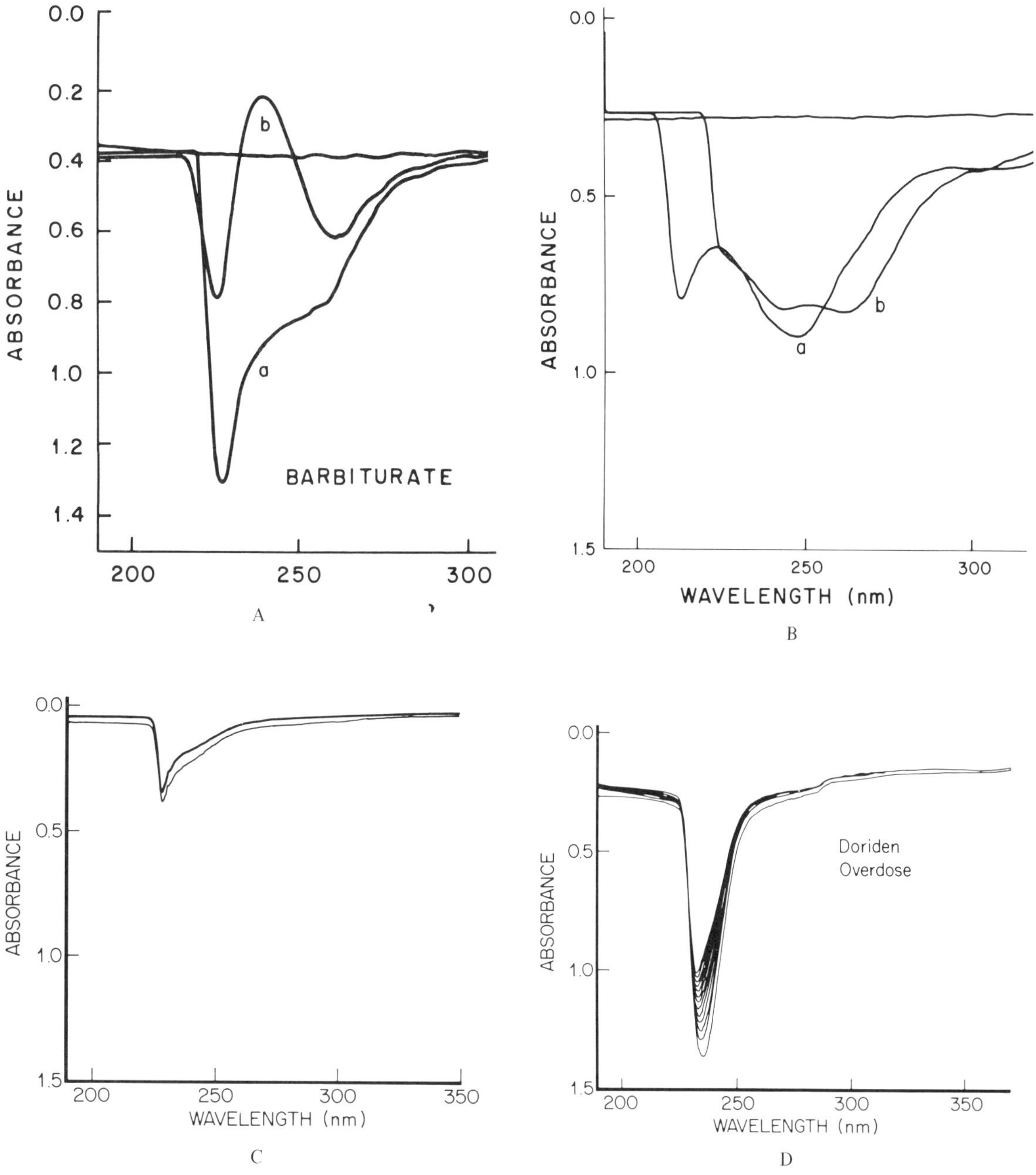

FIGURE 1. (A) Barbiturate overdose (phenobarbital). Curve a is conventional spectrum at pH 13, using 0.45*N* NaOH as blank. Curve b is differential spectrum. Use absorbance difference between minimum and maximum of differential spectrum to calculate concentration; (B) Chlordiazepoxide (Librium®) overdose. Curve a in 0.5*N* HCl. Curve b in 0.6*N* NaOH; (C) Negative glutethimide (Doriden®) (in alcoholic KOH). Note that a peak is present at 235 nm, but there is no decrease in absorbance when followed for 10 min with repeated scans; (D) Glutethimide (Doriden®) overdose (in alcoholic KOH). Note that absorbance at 235 nm decreases when followed for 10 min with repeated scans.

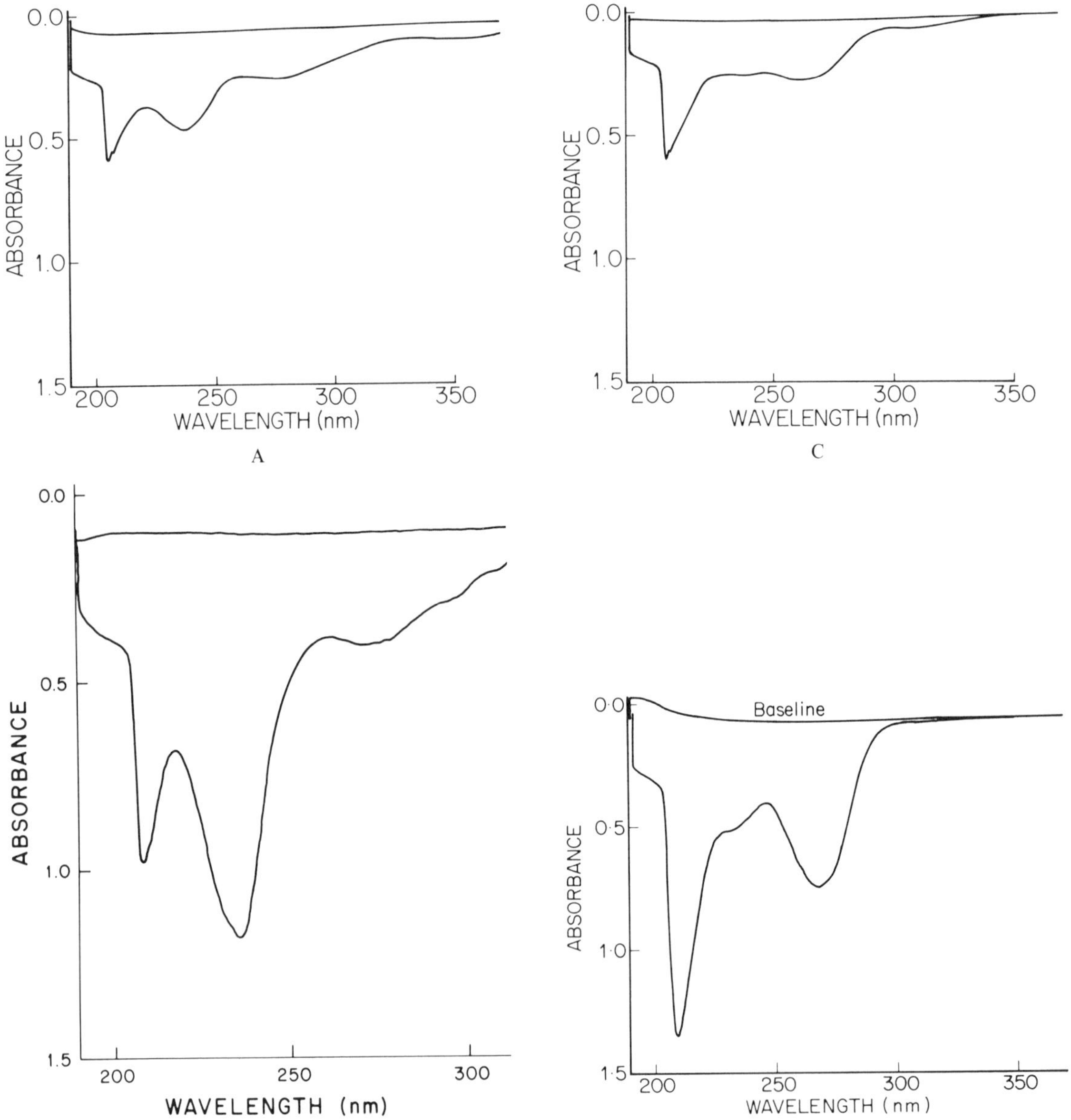

FIGURE 2. (A) Diazepam (Valium®) overdose (spectrum in 1*N* HCl). Oxazepam (Serax®) and metabolite of chlorazepate (Transxene®) have same spectra; (B) Methaqualone (Quaalude®) overdose (in 1*N* HCl). Methaqualone metabolites have same spectrum; (C) Caffeine (moderate) (in 1*N*HCl). Note spectrum is relatively flat between 240 to 260 nm and permits determination of diazepam and recognition of methaqualone; (D) Caffeine (very high). This would obscure diazepam and methaqualone, if present. Other methods must be used.

CALCULATION

$$C_u = \frac{C_s}{A_s} \times A_u$$

C_s = concentration of drug in the serum standard

A_s* = absorbance of serum standard at the indicated wavelengths

A_u* = absorbance of unknown at the indicated wavelengths

C_u = concentration of unknown

*For barbiturate A = 260 nm (maximum) to 240 nm (minimum). For chlordiazepoxide determine A at 247 nm. For glutethimide determine ΔA at 235 nm for 8 min. For diazepam and oxazepam A = 260 to 240 nm.

Table 1

SUMMARY OF DATA OBTAINED FROM SEDATIVE SCREENS

Drug	Fraction	Major acid peak (nm)	Minor acid peak (nm)	Major basic peak (nm)	Calculation*
Barbiturate	0.45*N* NaOH (differential scan)	–	–	260 max 240 min	A260–A240
Theophylline and other weak acids	0.45*N* NaOH (direct scan)	–	–	274 †	A274 (base)
Chlordiazepoxide	0.5*N* HCl	247	305	362	A247 (acid)
Methapyrilene	0.5*N* HCl	239	315	241	A241 (acid)
Diazepam	1*N* HCl	240	285	–	A240–A260
Oxazepam	1*N* HCl	240	285	–	A240–A260
Caffeine	1*N* HCl	–	275	‡	
Methaqualone	1*N* HCl	235	265	–	‡
Glutethimide	Ethanol-KOH	–	–	235	Δ A235 (8 min)

* See Calculation.
† Depends upon drug present.
‡ See Interfering Substances.

Supplemented serum standards should be carried through the entire procedure. For emergency work it may be more practical to use a factor ($\frac{C_S}{A_S}$) derived previously from different extracted serum standards containing each drug, if the calibration of the spectrophotometer and procedure is checked monthly. If the specific barbiturate is unknown, it is satisfactory for emergency work to calculate the concentration using any single barbiturate standard. The extinction coefficients of the common barbiturates differ by less than 15%. *Each analyst should become familiar with the UV absorption spectra of the various drugs discussed on his instrument before attempting routine analyses.* The absorption peaks of drugs extracted from biological specimens are not always as sharply defined as those obtained from pure drugs (Table 1). Some minor peaks may be broad at low concentration. The analyst should allow a tolerance of about ±2 nm in identifying absorption peaks.

INTERPRETATION (see p. 7)

See individual drugs.

SENSITIVITY

With the exception of phenobarbital, UV methods are not suitable for determination of therapeutic levels of the above drugs (i.e., less than 0.1 mg/100 ml of barbiturates and 0.2 mg/100 ml of the other drugs).

INTERFERING SUBSTANCES

In contrast to thin-layer and gas chromatography, UV procedures are not specific, nor do they resolve mixtures. For example, a mixture of diazepam and methaqualone (rare) will not be resolved by this procedure; however, the occurrence of a combination of drugs in the same step is rare. Interference or drug combinations may distort spectra, but will not cause false positives. Unrecognized spectra should be compared with a published collection of spectra.[2]

The barbiturate procedure is specific for the 5-5′ disubstituted class of barbiturates, but will not differentiate between the long and short acting drugs, identical concentrations of which have different clinical significance. For example, concentrations of short acting barbiturates (secobarbital and pentobarbital) greater than 2 mg/100 ml are associated with serious coma. On the other hand, concentrations of phenobarbital greater than 10 mg/100 ml are usually required to produce a similar clinical picture. Salicylate would interfere if it were extracted. Because it has a pKa of 2.97, however, it is not extracted by this procedure.

UV absorbing basic drugs, such as the phenothiazines and tricyclic antidepressants, do not achieve "measurable" blood levels, nor are they extracted from serum at pH 7.4. The various benzodiazepines, diazepam, oxazepam, and nordiazepam (the major metabolite of clorazepate), all have similar spectra and cannot be differentiated by this procedure. Fluorazepam does not reach sufficiently high blood levels to be detected by UV spectrophotometry. Caffeine is a common interference in the 1*N* HCl, and the analyst should be intimately familiar with its spectrum at low and high concentrations (Figures 2C and D). At moderate concentrations its spectrum is essentially flat between 240 and 260 nm, and it will not distort the location of the primary peak of diazepam or methaqualone. Caffeine will broaden the secondary peak of these drugs, but will not significantly affect the value of A240 to A260. High levels of caffeine (uncommon), void the 1*N* HCl step, and more specific assays for diazepam and methaqualone should be performed. A high concentration of caffeine does not affect the subsequent glutethimide step.[3] In such cases proceed with Step 16 (glutethimide).

Normal serum will show a peak at about 235 nm in Step 18 (Figure 1C). Evidence of hydrolysis (decreasing absorbance) (Figure 1D) indicates the presence of glutethimide. This procedure also measures some glutethimide metabolites; therefore, results from this UV procedure may be higher than those obtained with gas-chromatographic procedures. Methaqualone can be identified, but should not be quantified, by this procedure because UV absorbing metabolites with similar spectra are extracted by the chloroform. Use a supplementary procedure to quantify methaqualone.

REFERENCES

1. **Bailey, D. and Jatlow, P.,** Methaqualone overdose: analytical methodology, and the significance of serum drug concentrations, *Clin. Chem.*, 19, 615, 1973.
2. **Sunshine, I.,** *Handbook of Analytical Toxicology*, Chemical Rubber Co., Cleveland, 1969.
3. **Sunshine, I., Maes, R., and Faracci, R.,** Determination of glutethimide (Doriden) and its metabolites in biological specimens, *Clin. Chem.*, 14, 595, 1968.

GENERAL REFERENCES

Dauphinais, L. R. and McComb, R., A specific procedure for serum glutethimide (Doriden) determination, *Am. J. Clin. Pathol.*, 44, 440, 1965.

Goldbaum, L. R., Determination of glutethimide in biological fluids, *Anal. Chem.*, 32, 81, 1960.

Goldbaum, L. R., Williams, M. A., and Kopanyi, R., Analytical determination of barbiturates, *Anal. Chem.*, 24, 1600, 1952.

Jatlow, P., Ultraviolet spectrophotometric analysis of barbiturates: Evaluation of potential interferences, *Am. J. Clin. Pathol.*, 59, 167, 1973.

Jatlow, P., Ultraviolet spectrophotometric measurement of chlordiazepoxide in plasma, *Clin. Chem.*, 18, 516, 1972.

Sunshine, I., Barbiturates, in *Standard Methods*, Vol. 3, Seligson, D., Ed., Academic Press, N.Y., 1961, 46.

GC FOR SEDATIVE DRUGS

Jerry Thoma and Paul Bondo

This procedure provides for the identification and quantitative analysis of the barbiturates, glutethimide, meprobamate, methyprylon, the benzodiazepines, methaqualone, and propoxyphene as the free drugs in serum. The drugs are extracted into diethyl ether using a single step direct extraction. Two internal standards, barbital and 5-(*p*-methylphenyl)-5-phenylhydantoin, are contained in a pH 6.4 phosphate buffer. Confirmation of the barbiturates, glutethimide, and methyprylon is performed by redrying the original extract and redissolving in 0.2*M* methanolic solution of trimethylanilinium hydroxide (TMAH). The methylated derivatives are formed on-column. Meprobamate is decomposed by the TMAH, yielding a product which is useful for confirmation of this drug. Confirmation of propoxyphene, methaqualone, and the benzodiazepines is done by thin-layer chromatography.

APPARATUS

1. Screw-capped culture tubes, 20 × 150 mm
2. Centrifuge tubes, conical, 15 ml
3. Polyethylene hollow stoppers, size 00
4. Gas chromatograph, dual column with a 1 mV 10-in. recorder, equipped with two flame ionization detectors, temperature programming, and glass columns, 6′ × 2 mm i.d. (¼″ o.d.), one packed with 3% OV-17 on 100/120 mesh Gas Chrom Q and the other with 3% OV-1 on 100/120 mesh Gas Chrom Q. Before using the columns for the first time disconnect them from the detectors, and condition the columns at 300°C for 12 hr with no carrier gas flow and then for 12 hr with carrier gas flowing. Immediately prior to each use some OV-17 columns may require preconditioning with 2 to 5 μl of the serum extract to be chromatographed. Inject the serum extract with the column temperature at about 260°C and allow about 5 min for all of the components to be eluted before setting Program I. An optimally prepared column will not require such preconditioning before each use.

   Operating Conditions

   Gas Flow Rate:
      nitrogen (carrier gas) – 10 to 20 ml/min
   Temperatures:
      injection port – 280°C
      detector – 280°C
   Program I:
      Initial temperature – 165°C
      program rate – 32°C/min
      final temperature – 280°C
      hold at 280° for – 5 min
   Program II:
      initial temperature – 135°C
      program rate – 20°C/min
      final temperature – 250°C
      hold at 250° for – 5 min

REAGENTS

All chemicals should be analytical reagent grade. All drugs should be reference standard grade.

1. Drug stock standard solutions, 100 mg/dl
   Dissolve an amount of drug equivalent to 100 mg of the free acid or base in methanol in a 100-ml volumetric flask and dilute to volume with methanol. Store each solution in a glass bottle with Teflon®-lined cap at -10°C. These solutions are stable for at least 1 year.
2. Drug working standard
   Add the quantities of each stock standard indicated in Table 1 to a 100-ml volumetric flask. Place the flask in a warm water bath and, with the aid of vacuum or a stream of nitrogen, evaporate the methanol to about 2 ml and dilute to volume with water. Store in a glass bottle at 4°C. This is stable for at least 6 months.
3. Sodium phosphate, dibasic (Na_2HPO_4), 1.15*M*
   Dry anhydrous or hydrated Na_2HPO_4 in a 120°C oven for at least 2 hr. (The hydrates are converted to the anhydrous form at tempera-

Table 1

DIRECTIONS FOR PREPARATION OF THE DRUG WORKING STANDARD AND THE WORKING INTERNAL STANDARD

Compound	Concentration	Stock standard added, ml	Relative retention time,* min
	Working Standard		
Methyprylon	0.7	0.7	0.22
Butabarbital	0.7	0.7	0.65
Amobarbital	0.7	0.7	0.77
Pentobarbital	0.7	0.7	0.90
Secobarbital	0.7	0.7	1.10
Meprobamate	0.7	0.7	1.48
Glutethimide	0.4	0.4	1.60
Phenobarbital	0.7	0.7	2.14
Propoxyphene	0.4	0.4	2.34
Methaqualone	0.4	0.4	2.84
Oxazepam	0.7	0.7	3.22
Diazepam	0.4	0.4	3.66
Chlordiazepoxide	0.7	0.7	4.17
Flurazepam	0.7	0.7	4.84
	Working Internal Standard		
Barbital	1.0	1.0	
5-(*p*-Methylphenyl)-5-phenylhydantoin	1.0	1.0	

* All retention times are relative to barbital.

tures above 95°C.) Store in a desiccator. Dissolve 4.73 g of the dried Na_2HPO_4 in water in a 500-ml volumetric flask. Dilute to volume with water. Store at 4°C.

4. Potassium phosphate, monobasic (KH_2PO_4), 1.15*M*
   Dissolve 4.54 g of KH_2PO_4 in water in a 500-ml volumetric flask. Dilute to volume with water. Store at 4°C.
5. Phosphate buffer, pH 6.4
   Mix 80 ml of 1.15*M* KH_2PO_4 with 30 ml of 1.15*M* Na_2HPO_4. If reagents 3, 4, and 5 are prepared properly, the pH will be 6.4 ± 0.1. It is preferable that the pH be 6.4 ± 0.1. If pH adjustment is necessary, add reagent 4 to lower the pH and reagent 3 to raise the pH.
6. Working internal standard
   Add the quantities of stock standards indicated in Table 1 to a 100-ml volumetric flask. Dilute to volume with pH 6.4 phosphate buffer.
7. Serum control, 0.5 mg/dl
   Dilute 500 μl of the stock standard to 100 ml with drug-free serum. Transfer 2-ml aliquots to 2-ml Vacutainers® and store at −10°C.
8. Diethyl ether, USP
9. Sodium sulfate, anhydrous
10. Trimethylanilinium hydroxide* (TMAH), 0.2*M* in methanol

*Pierce Chemical Co., Rockford, Ill. 61105.

PROCEDURE

1. Into suitably labeled 20 × 150 mm culture tubes, pipet 1.0 ml of the working internal standard and 1.0 ml of the sample (working standard, patient serum, and control serum).
2. Add 10 ml of diethyl ether to each tube, stopper with a polyethylene hollow stopper, and vortex for 30 sec.
3. Use a Pasteur pipet to transfer the ether layer to a clean 20 × 150 mm culture tube. Add 2.5 g of anhydrous sodium sulfate to the ether and mix on a Vortex mixer.

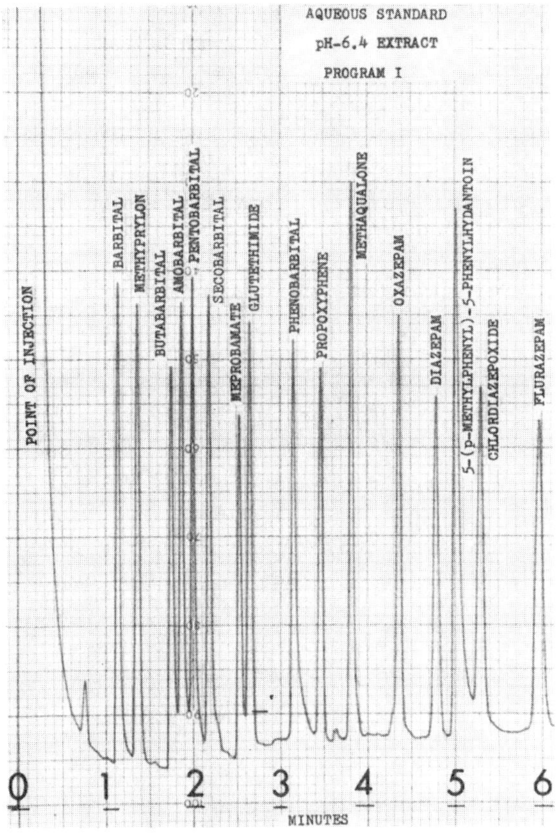

FIGURE 1. Chromatogram of underivatized drugs obtained by processing the working standard as outlined in Steps 1 to 6 of the Procedure (Program I).

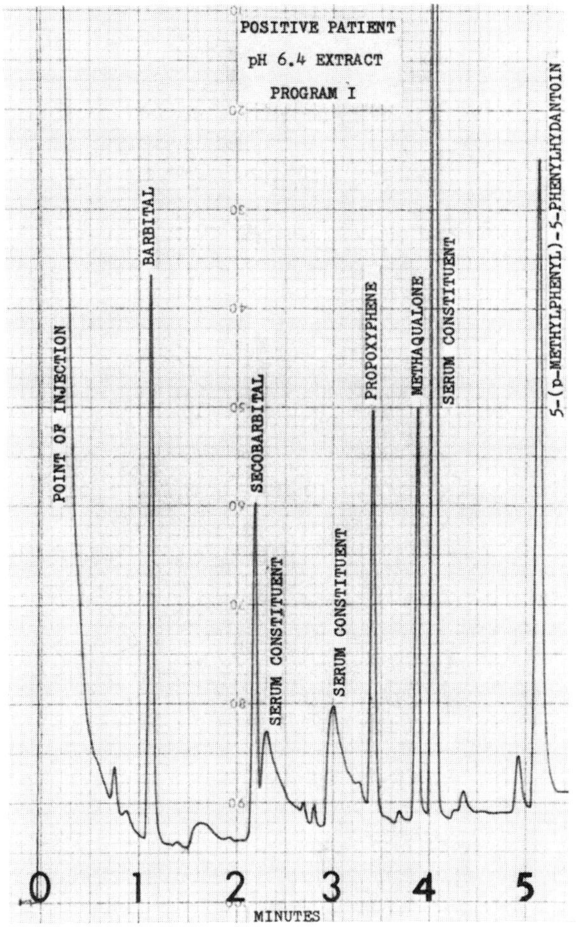

FIGURE 2. Chromatogram of patient serum containing 0.3 mg/dl of secobarbital and 0.3 mg/dl of methaqualone (Program I).

4. Decant the ether into 15-ml conical tubes, and evaporate to dryness under a stream of nitrogen in a 40°C water bath.
5. Dissolve each dried extract in 50 μl of chloroform, taking care to rinse the walls of the tube. Mix on a Vortex mixer.
6. Inject 2 μl of each chloroform solution into the OV-17 column using Program I (Figures 1 and 2).
7. Compare the retention times of any peaks in the unknown to those in the standard.
8. If peaks are present in the unknown with the same retention times as those in the standard, evaporate the extracts from Step 5 to dryness and add 50 μl of TMAH. Mix on a Vortex mixer.
9. Inject into the OV-1 column using Program II, and compare the retention times of the peaks obtained from the sample with those for the standard (Figure 3).

NOTES

1. The drug 5-(*p*-methylphenyl)-5-phenylhydantoin serves as the internal standard for diphenylhydantoin, which was determined in our laboratory by a procedure similar to that presented here. For this analysis the benzodiazepines are left out of the working standard and primidone and diphenylhydantoin are added. The working internal standard is made up in 0.2*M* HCl, as a cleaner extract results. In the pH 6.4 extract the second internal standard serves as an excellent time marker from which relative retention times may be determined for those drugs appearing late in the program.

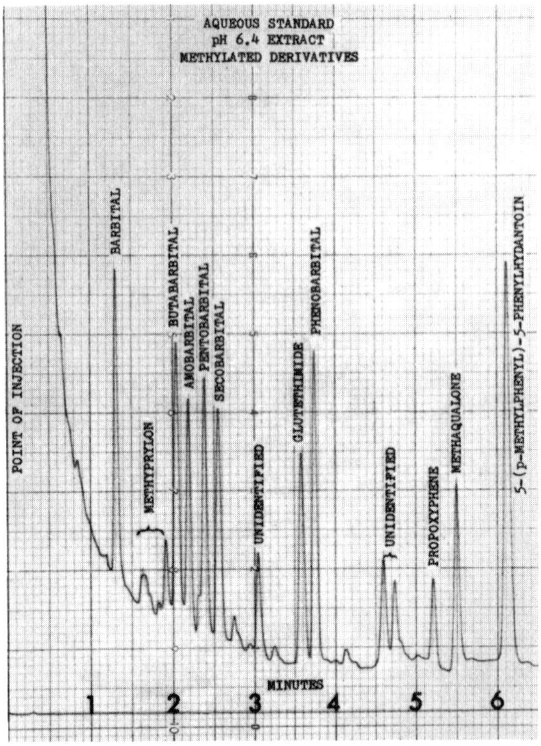

FIGURE 3. Chromatogram of TMAH derivatives of the drugs obtained by processing the working standard as outlined in Steps 8 to 9 of the Procedure (Program II).

2. Megadon® (nitrazepam) is also extracted by this method; however, it is not well-resolved from chlordiazepoxide. It is readily separated from chlordiazepoxide using the standard methods of thin-layer chromatography.
3. Barbital is somewhat volatile and care must be taken in evaporating the extracts to dryness. Aprobarbital and diallylbarbital are less volatile and can also serve as internal standards.

CALCULATION

Calculate C_u, the concentration of each drug in the unknown, by using the following equation:

$$C_u = \frac{C_s \times R_s}{Ru}$$

where

R_s = the ratio of the peak height of drug in the standard extract to that of the internal standard in the standard extract;

R_u = the ratio of the peak height of drug in the test extract to that of the internal standard in the test extract;

C_s = concentration of the drug in the drug working standard;

C_u = concentration of the drug in the patient's serum.

Barbital is the internal standard for all drugs.

ACCURACY AND PRECISION

Table 2 lists the precision data for the serum control prepared in our laboratory. These results were obtained over a period of 3 months by three different analysts. This data was obtained using a working internal standard in a 0.2*N* HCl solution. If the pH 6.4 working internal standard described in Reagents (Step 6) is used, the recovery from serum relative to aqueous may be different.

Table 2

ACCURACY AND PRECISION DATA

Drug	N	$\overline{X}$	S.D.
Secobarbital	50	0.5	0.04
Glutethimide	50	0.4	0.04
Phenobarbital	57	0.5	0.06
Methaqualone	55	0.4	0.04
Diphenylhydantoin	57	0.5	0.03

INTERFERING SUBSTANCES

On properly prepared columns no interferences have been found which give false positives, both as the underivatized drug in Program I and as the TMAH derivative in Program II. In over 1,000 determinations by this method, fewer than 1% have had interfering peaks on Program I. Salicylamide interferes with the barbital peak on Program I, but such interference is readily apparent because the heptobarbital/barbital peak-height ratio will be shifted.

POINTERS ON GAS CHROMATOGRAPHY

GC methods pose many problems for less experienced toxicologists. The described conditions, the column packages, and their supports vary significantly. Is one advised to have a multitude of columns and interchange them to satisfy the demand for a given procedure? Surely this would lead to inefficiency and ineffective work. Not many laboratories will have sufficient chromatographs to ensure availability of the described columns, nor is this desirable. One should install and become familiar with a few columns and modify the procedures to suit the available instrumentation. Since gas chromatography is still a relatively new technique for many, some "pointers" may be helpful. The following material is provided for the reader's guidance.

A good column should provide sharp nontailing peaks, while a poor column may produce broad tailing peaks which make detection difficult and have a very adverse effect on detection limits. Quantitation by any method becomes less precise, while quantitation by peak height is rendered all but impossible. Figures 4 and 5 are chromatograms of the same drug mixture chromatographed on identical column packings run in the same instrument under identical conditions. The marked differences in column performance they illustrate can be caused by improper packing, conditioning, or maintenance of a

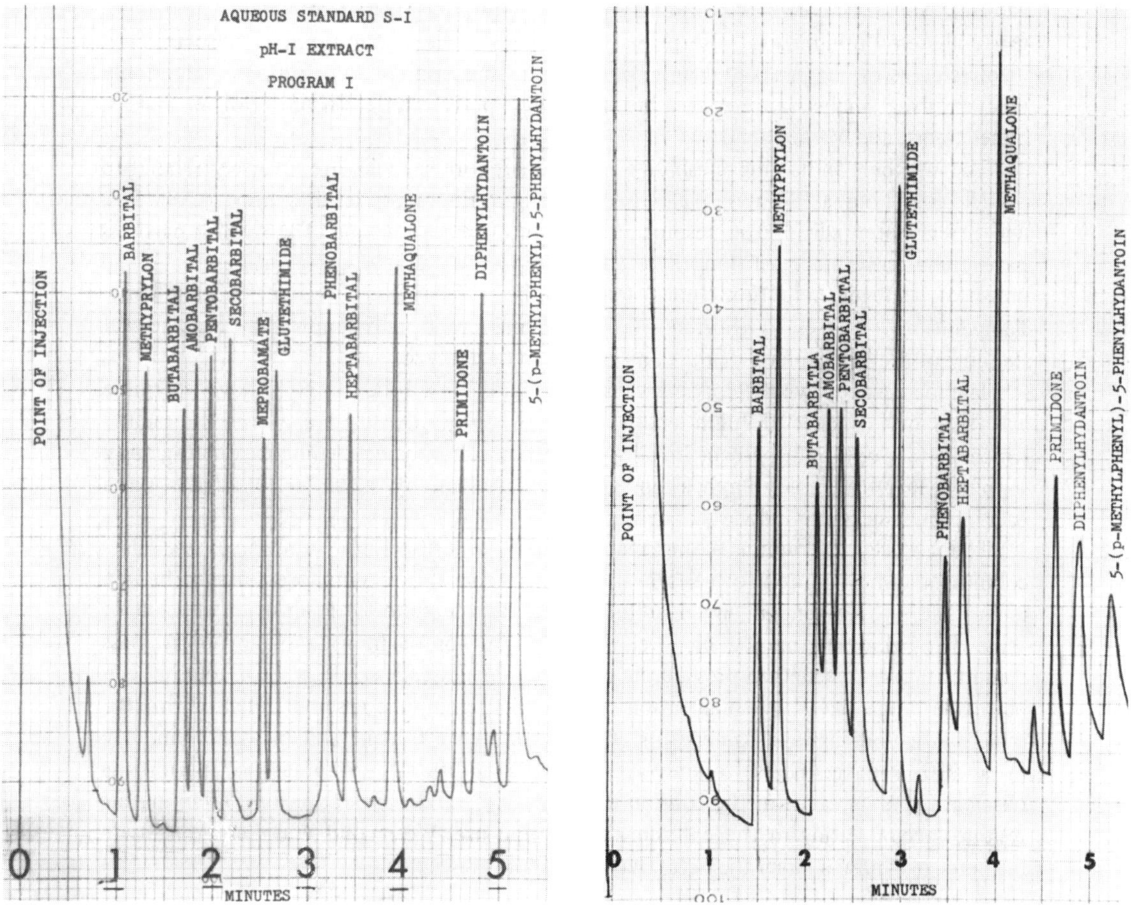

FIGURES 4 and 5. Comparison of two analyses on two different columns containing the same packing and analyzed in the same chromatograph under identical conditions.

column. In addition, there are many other circumstances related to the type of material injected on the column that can change the column used to obtain Figure 4 to one that produced Figure 5.

Each gas chromatography procedure in this manual lists the type of column packing used by the author. This does not mean that the analysis cannot be performed without this particular packing; other satisfactory phases may produce equally good results. Tables classifying various liquid phases according to their general selectivities are explained in chromatography supply catalogues, such as those of Varian, Applied Science, or Supelco (Table 3). Liquid phases listed as having similar selectivities can generally be substituted for one another. Consideration must also be given to the lower and upper temperature limits of each stationary phase. If the available column has characteristics similar to the one recommended in the procedure for an anticipated analysis, try it.

Among the liquid phases frequently used for analysis of nonvolatiles are OV-17, OV-1, Dexil 300, and SE-30. The OV-1 and SE-30 possess similar selectivities or polarities and will, therefore, give comparable separations with similar retention times. The OV-17, classified as having a higher selectivity or polarity than the OV-1, may resolve some drugs better than the OV-1, but will generally give longer retention times.[1,2] For GLC analysis of volatiles, liquid phases such as Carbowax® or Halcomid® are commonly used. Alternatively, volatiles are frequently analyzed by gas-solid-chromatography (GSC), employing Porapak® or Carbopack® as the stationary phase.

Solid supports marketed under various brand names may also be substituted for one another. Supports used for drug analyses are chemically treated to render them more inert, thereby minimizing adsorption of drugs on the columns. Such adsorption is manifested as tailing peaks and possibly peaks of smaller area. Some supports commonly used in drug analyses are Gas Chrom Q, high-performance Chromosorb W and G, Supelcoport, and Varaport 30.

The numbers indicating mesh size of solid support particles are inversely related to particle size. Thus, a 120 mesh packing, consisting of finer particles, has more surface area and offers potentially better resolution than an 80 mesh packing. The smaller particles have the disadvantage of longer retention times for similar temperatures and head pressures. Longer retention times tend to be accompanied by peak broadening. Temperature increases to shorten retention times are usually limited by the thermal stability of the liquid phase or the components to be analyzed.

The percent by weight loading of liquid phase on a solid support may determine analytical performance. Column length and solid support density are two of the factors which dictate optimum percent loading. In any case, companies selling chromatography supplies generally employ applications chemists, available by telephone for advice on the packings best suited to individual needs.

The choice of column tubing material may be critical for some analyses. Glass columns may be required for certain drugs which tend to be decomposed or adsorbed by metal columns. In general, metal columns may be adequate for analysis of drugs at or somewhat below the microgram level. For analyses approaching nanogram levels, glass columns may be needed to provide the required inertness. If necessary, glass columns can be made more inert by silanization. Allow the column to stand filled with 10% dimethyldichlorosilane in toluene for 20 min, rinse with toluene and methanol, and dry in a 110°C oven. Glass columns provide the additional advantages of permitting observation of air gaps in the column during packing and observation of contaminating residues accumulating in the column head during use. We recommend a column inside diameter of 2 mm; a larger diameter may give poorer resolution.

Packing, Conditioning, and Maintenance

The manner in which a column is packed is critical to column performance. We recommend that the analyst purchase solid supports precoated with liquid phase, unless he is experienced in the coating procedures. The user can successfully pack his own columns, and the following suggestions may prove helpful. Plug one end of the column with silanized glass wool and apply a vacuum to this end. Add the packing material through the other end from a reservoir, such as a funnel attached to the column. Use an electric engraver/vibrator to gently vibrate the column, always working from the plugged end of the column toward the reservoir end. The packing material must be firmly packed to achieve the best resolution; however, care must be used in vibrating solid supports, such as Gas Chrom Q, which are quite fragile and easily crumbled by rough vibration. Crumbling of a silanized solid support exposes unsilanized areas of the support which can cause adsorption of polar compounds, resulting in peak tailing and decreased sensitivity. For packings which are difficult to transfer into the column, dry nitrogen pressure may be applied to the packing reservoir.

The silanized surface of the solid support and the inner walls of a glass column are subject to attack by moisture. For this reason, some packing materials (such as the silicone phases) should be stored in a desiccator. The interior of a packed column should be protected from atmospheric moisture by a low flow rate (20 ml/min) of dry carrier gas or by sealing the ends of the column. Those who feel they cannot adequately pack a column need not despair. Reputable vendors are very willing to sell well-prepared columns of almost any type, and even experienced chromatographers use them.

Column conditioning is essential to proper column performance. The conditioning process elutes volatile components of the liquid phase which might otherwise undergo constant slow elution (bleed), adding to the background or causing a rising baseline during temperature programing. In general, conditioning involves heating the column 1 to 12 hr at a low carrier gas flow rate (20 ml/min) to about 20°C above the highest temperature to be used in analyses. The exit end of the column must be disconnected from the detector during conditioning to prevent contamination of the detector. Conditioning is adequate when the baseline does not rise during temperature programing.

Even the most optimally functioning column requires regular maintenance if it is to continue working efficiently during months of injections of extracts of biological specimens. On chromatographs equipped with injection port liners, tarry residues from biological extracts build up in the liner and can adsorb some compounds to be analyzed. These liners are easily and quickly changed and should be replaced whenever significant deposits become visible. The glass wool in the entrance end of the column should be replaced periodically, as tarry residues also accumulate here imparting a brown or gray color.

An obvious but frequently overlooked maintenance item is the septum. Lack of resistance to the needle or a hissing sound upon injection are clues that septum replacement is due. Among the problems which can be caused by a leaking septum are broad solvent fronts, broad peaks, tailing peaks, increased retention times, and decreased sensitivity.

The carrier gas pressure on the head of the column should never be released suddenly when removing septum caps, disconnecting the carrier gas tank, or disconnecting the entrance end of the column. Prior to such maintenance procedures the carrier gas pressure should be bled down slowly, usually by closing the supply valve and allowing the gas to bleed through the column. A sudden release of pressure causes the packing to be thrown violently toward the column head, disturbing the packing bed and crushing solid support particles.

After weeks of use columns may begin to show peak tailing and decreased sensitivity for certain drugs. Some packings, such as the silicones, are sometimes restored by injecting silating compounds marketed for column treatment (e.g., Silyl-8)*. For some drugs, columns may show decreased sensitivity during the first few injections each day, apparently because of adsorbing column sites which must be filled. The column can be preconditioned by injecting a concentrated solution of the drugs to be chromatographed. Injection of an extract of biological specimen is often even more effective in preconditioning the column.

General Precautions

Of the many things that can cause a good column to go bad, the least subtle is simply heating the column above the maximum recommended temperature for extended periods of time. Although these maximums are approximate, it can be said that above these temperatures either the column will not perform properly or the column bleed will be such that it will interfere with the response of the detector.

With silicone phases and, quite possibly, other liquid phases, moisture injected into the column at high temperatures can be extremely detrimental. Complicating matters is the fact that easily chromatographed compounds, such as glutethemide or methaqualone, may appear quite normal, whereas phenobarbital will appear broad and tailing. This is quite evident in Figure 4 and 5.

Two other common liquid phase demons are anhydrides and iodine. Acetic anhydride can be very useful for on-column acetylation of amines and alcohols, but the same column cannot be used for the barbiturates (as free acid) or diphenylhydantoin. Iodine carried over into a chloroform extract of a TLC spot produces the same result. Columns subjected to such use may still be quite adequate for the analysis of less sensitive drugs and should not be discarded without due consideration.

A similar situation occurs if one attempts to use the same column for analysis of both acidic and basic drugs. Chances are good that under these conditions the performance will be hindered for both groups. Columns should be set aside for use with one group only, and it may be necessary to be even more discriminating than simply using different columns for acidic and basic compounds.

For analyses where temperature programing is necessary, consideration must be given to the type of ferrules used to install the column, particularly when glass columns are employed. High temperatures (in excess of 250°C) and rapid programing rates tend to exacerbate ferrule problems. Many ferrules tend to expand and flow as the temperature increases and contract as the temperature falls, resulting in carrier gas leaks. The advent of graphite ferrules has certainly alleviated this problem for most chromatographers. For lower temperature work (below 200°C) Teflon® ferrules are quite adequate and are generally much cheaper.

REFERENCES

McReynolds, W. O., Characterization of some liquid phases, *J. Chromatogr. Sci.*, 8, 230, 1970.

Supena, W. R. and Rose, L. P., The use of Rohrschneider Constants for classification of GLC columns, *J. Chromatogr. Sci.*, 8, 214, 1970.

*Pierce Chemical Co., Rockford, Ill. 61105.

The reference compounds 1 through 7 in Table 3 were analyzed by GC on the phases listed. The values shown are differences in Kovats Index units between the reference compound run on squalane and on the other phases listed. The last entry shows the actual elution point (in Kovats Index units) for the reference compound on squalane (i.e., benzene elutes at a KI of 653). On phase 121 benzene elutes 690 index units later than on squalane. Thus, benzene elutes at a Kovats Index of 1343 from a column packing coated with phase 121. The value of Σ should be treated as a general selectivity guide. The higher the value, the more selective overall is the phase. A 30 unit difference in the value of Σ is almost insignificant. Similarly, a difference of 20 units in Δ1 is also not very significant.

1. If phase #8 (Σ is 217) will not effect a separation, then do not expect to be able to do it on phases #1 to 15. You would do best to look at phases numbered between 20 and 60 with Σ values of 474 to 1426.

2. If phase #50 will not do a separation, then try phase #104 or phase #12.

Remember, the higher the Σ value, the greater is the general selectivity of the phase.

Table 3

PHASE SELECTIVITY DATA

Phase reference number	Phase name	Δ1 Values: Benzene	1-Butanol	2-Pentanone	Nitropropane	Pyridine	2-Methyl-2-pentanol	2-Octyne	Σ_1^5
1	Squalane	0	0	0	0	0	0	0	0
2	Nujol®	9	5	2	6	11	2	2	33
3	Apiezon® M	31	22	15	30	40	12	10	138
4	Apiezon® L	32	22	15	32	42	13	11	143
5	SF 96	12	53	42	61	37	31	21	205
6	Apiezon® J	38	36	27	49	57	23	15	207
7	Apiezon® N	38	40	28	52	58	25	15	216
8	SE 30	15	53	44	64	41	31	22	217
9	OV-1	16	55	44	65	42	32	23	222
10	M and B silicone oil	14	57	46	67	43	33	22	227
11	DC 200 (12,500 cSt)	16	57	45	66	43	33	23	227
12	OV-101	17	57	45	67	43	33	23	229
13	DC-410	18	57	47	68	44	34	24	234
14	Versilube F-50	19	57	48	69	47	36	23	240
15	DC 11	17	86	48	69	56	36	23	276

(From Supena, W. R. and Rose, L. R., *J. Chromatogr. Sci.*, 8, 214, 1970. With permission.)

Table 3 (Continued)

PHASE SELECTIVITY TABLE

Phase reference number	Phase name	Δ1 Values							
		Benzene	1-Butanol	2-Pentanone	Nitropropane	Pyridine	2-Methyl-2-pentanol	2-Octyne	Σ_1^5
16	SE 52	32	72	65	98	67	44	36	334
17	SE 54	33	72	66	99	67	46	36	337
18	DC 560	32	72	70	100	68	49	35	342
19	OV-3	44	86	81	124	88	55	46	423
20	Dexsil 300	47	80	103	148	96	55	–	474
21	Fluorolube HG 1200	51	68	114	144	118	68	53	495
22	Kel F wax	55	67	114	143	116	73	57	495
23	Apiezon® H	59	86	81	151	129	46	23	506
24	OV-7	69	113	111	171	128	77	66	592
25	DC 550	74	116	117	178	135	81	72	620
26	Di(2-ethylhexyl) sebacate	72	168	108	180	125	132	49	653
27	Diisodecyl adipate	71	171	113	185	128	134	52	668
28	Octyl decyl adipate	79	179	119	193	134	141	57	704
29	Dilauryl phthalate	79	158	120	192	158	120	52	707
30	Bis(2-ethylhexyl) tetrachlorophthalate	112	150	123	168	181	110	–	734
31	Diisodecyl phthalate	84	173	137	218	155	133	59	767
32	Dinonyl phthalate	83	183	147	231	159	141	65	803
33	DC 710	107	149	153	228	190	107	98	827
34	Dioctyl phthalate	92	186	150	236	167	143	66	831
35	POLY-I 110	115	194	122	204	202	152	55	837
36	Hallcomid® M-18	79	268	130	222	146	202	48	845
37	Diisooctyl phthalate (not available)	94	193	154	243	174	149	69	858
38	OV-17	119	158	162	243	202	112	105	884
39	UCON® LB-550-X	118	271	158	243	206	177	91	996
40	Span® 80	97	266	170	216	268	207	66	1017
41	Castorwax®	108	265	175	229	246	202	73	1023
42	POLY-A 103	115	331	149	263	214	221	62	1072
43	OV-22	160	188	191	283	253	133	132	1075

Table 3 (Continued)

PHASE SELECTIVITY TABLE

Phase reference number	Phase name	Δ1 Values							
		Benzene	1-Butanol	2-Pentanone	Nitropropane	Pyridine	2-Methyl-2-pentanol	2-Octyne	Σ_1^5
44	Polypropylene glycol	128	294	173	264	226	196	98	1085
45	Trimer acid	94	271	163	182	378	234	57	1088
46	POLY-A 101A	115	357	151	262	214	233	64	1099
47	Amine 220	117	380	181	293	133	274	–	1104
48	UCON® LB-1715	132	297	180	275	235	201	100	1119
49	Acetyl tributyl citrate	135	268	202	314	233	214	102	1152
50	Didecyl phthalate	136	255	213	320	235	201	101	1159
51	OV-25	178	204	208	305	280	144	147	1175
52	Polyphenyl ether OS-124 (5 rings)	176	227	224	306	283	177	135	1216
53	Tributyl citrate	135	286	213	324	262	226	102	1220
54	Polyphenyl ether OS-138 (6 rings)	182	233	228	313	293	181	136	1249
55	POLY-A 135	163	389	168	340	269	282	–	1329
56	Neopentyl glycol sebacate (HI-EFF-3CP®)	172	327	225	344	326	257	109	1394
57	Squalene	152	341	238	329	344	248	101	1404
58	UCON® 50-HB-280X	177	362	227	351	302	252	130	1419
59	Tricresyl phosphate	176	321	250	374	299	242	131	1420
60	Sucrose acetate isobutyrate	172	330	251	378	295	264	128	1426
61	QF-1	144	233	355	463	305	203	53	1500
62	OV-210	146	238	358	468	310	206	56	1520
63	Ethofat® 60/25	191	382	244	380	333	277	131	1530
64	Igepal CO-630	192	381	253	382	344	277	136	1552
65	DC LSX-3-0295	152	241	366	479	319	208	55	1557
66	Tergitol® NPX	197	386	258	389	351	281	39	1581
67	UCON® 50-HB-2000	202	394	253	392	341	277	147	1582
68	Emulphor® ON-870	202	395	251	395	344	282	140	1587
69	Triton® X-100	203	399	268	402	362	290	145	1634
70	UCON® 50-HB-5100	214	418	278	421	375	301	155	1706

Table 3 (Continued)

PHASE SELECTIVITY TABLE

Phase reference number	Phase name	Δ1 Values							
		Benzene	1-Butanol	2-Pentanone	Nitropropane	Pyridine	2-Methyl-2-pentanol	2-Octyne	Σ_1^5
71	Siponate® DS-10	99	569	320	344	388	466	61	1720
72	Tween® 80	227	430	283	438	396	310	–	1747
73	XE 60	204	381	340	493	367	289	120	1785
74	OV-225	228	369	338	492	386	282	150	1813
75	Neopentyl glycol adipate (HI-EFF-3AP®)	232	421	311	461	424	335	156	1849
76	UCON® 75-H-90000	255	452	299	470	406	321	180	1882
77	Igepal CO 880	259	461	311	482	426	334	180	1939
78	Triton® X-305	262	467	314	488	430	336	183	1961
79	HI-EFF-8BP®	271	444	330	498	463	346	175	2006
80	Quadrol®	214	571	357	472	489	431	142	2103
81	Neopentyl glycol succinate (HI-EFF-3BP®)	272	469	366	539	474	371	184	2120
82	Igepal CO 990	298	508	345	540	475	366	205	2166
83	EGSP-Z	308	474	399	548	549	373	220	2278
84	Carbowax® 20M	322	536	368	572	510	387	221	2308
85	Carbowax® 20M (TPA)	321	537	367	573	520	387	220	2318
86	Epon® 1001	284	489	406	539	601	378	207	2319
87	Carbowax® 6000	322	540	369	577	512	390	222	2320
88	Carbowax® 4000	325	551	375	582	520	399	224	2353
89	Silicone ASI 50-phenyl-50-cyanopropyl*	319	495	446	637	531	379	216	2428
90	Ethylene glycol isophthalate (HI-EFF-2EP®)	326	508	425	607	561	400	213	2427
91	XF-1150	308	520	470	669	528	401	174	2495
92	Carbowax® 1000	347	607	418	626	589	449	240	2587
93	Ethylene glycol adipate (HI-EFF-2AP®)	372	576	453	655	617	462	250	2673
94	Butane-1,4-diol succinate (HI-EFF-4BP®)	369	591	457	661	629	476	243	2707
95	Phenyldiethanolamine succinate (HI-EFF-10BP®)	386	555	472	674	654	437	242	2741
96	Reoplex® 400	364	619	449	647	671	482	245	2750
97	LAC-1-R-296®	377	601	458	663	655	477	253	2754
98	Diethylene glycol adipate (HI-EFF-1AP®)	378	603	460	665	658	479	254	2764
99	Carbowax® 1540	371	639	453	666	641	479	255	2770
100	LAC-2-R-466®	387	616	471	679	667	489	257	2820

Table 3 (Continued)

PHASE SELECTIVITY TABLE

Phase reference number	Phase name	Δ1 Values							
		Benzene	1-Butanol	2-Pentanone	Nitropropane	Pyridine	2-Methyl-2-pentanol	2-Octyne	Σ_1^5
101	EGSS-Y	391	597	493	693	661	469	261	2835
102	Hyprose® SP-80	336	742	492	639	727	565	227	2936
103	EGSP-A	397	629	519	727	700	496	278	2972
104	Silicone APOLAR-7CP (formerly SILAR-7CP)	440	638	605	844	673	492	268	3200
105	ECNSS-M	421	690	581	803	732	548	259	3227
106	ECNSS-S	438	659	566	820	722	530	286	3205
107	Diglycerol	371	826	560	676	854	608	141	3287
108	EGSS-X	484	710	585	831	778	566	316	3388
109	Ethylene glycol phthalate (HI-EFF-2GP®)	453	697	602	816	872	560	306	3410
110	Silicone APOLAR-9CP (formerly SILAR-9CP)	489	725	631	913	778	566	292	3536
111	Diethylene glycol succinate (HI-EFF-1BP®)	499	751	593	840	860	595	323	3543
112	LAC-3-R-728®	502	755	597	849	852	599	329	3555
113	Silicone APOLAR-10C (formerly SILAR-10C)	523	757	659	942	801	584	298	3682
114	THEED	463	942	626	801	893	746	269	3725
115	Tetracyanoethylated pentaerythritol	526	782	677	920	837	621	333	3742
116	Ethylene glycol succinate (HI-EFF-2BP®)	537	787	643	903	889	633	348	3759
117	1,2,3,4,5,6-Hexakis (CYCLO-N)	567	825	713	978	901	620	–	3984
118	1,2,3-Tris(2-cyanoethoxy)propane	593	857	752	1028	915	672	375	4145
119	1,2,3,4-Tetrakis (CYANO-B)	617	860	773	1048	941	685	–	4239
120	Cyanoethylsucrose	647	919	797	1043	976	713	388	4382
121	N,N-Bis(2-cyanoethyl)formamide	690	991	853	1110	1000	773	371	4644
NA	Absolute Δ1 values for squalane	653	590	627	652	699	690	841	NA

TLC OF BASIC ORGANIC DRUGS

Milton L. Bastos, Gerald E. Kananen, Joseph R. Monforte, and Irving Sunshine

APPARATUS

1. Test tubes, screw-capped, 125 × 16 mm
2. Mixer (Vortex Jr*)
3. Centrifuge
4. Pasteur pipets
5. Capillary tubes, sealed
6. Capillary pipets
7. Thin-layer chromatography (TLC) equipment: (a) scriber for chromatographic plates†; (b) glass plates, coated with silica gel G (*nach* Stahl‡); (c) developing tanks; (d) spray bottles
8. UV lamps, 350- and 254-nm radiation

REAGENTS

All chemicals should be analytical reagent grade.

1. Ethanol, 95%
2. Potassium carbonate, anhydrous
3. Ether
4. Buffer solution, pH 8.5
   Dissolve 53.5 g of ammonium chloride in 950 ml of water. Add 18 ml of concentrated ammonium hydroxide. Adjust the pH to 8.5 by adding either ammonium hydroxide or hydrochloric acid. Check the pH before using a previously prepared solution.
5. Acetic acid, 3.5*N*
   Dilute 20 ml of glacial acetic acid to 100 ml with water.
6. Drug reference solutions, 10 mg/10 ml
   Dissolve 10 mg of suitable pharmaceutical-quality salts in 10 ml of ethanol. For salts with limited solubility in ethanol, add a few drops of dilute acid to ensure solution.
7. Developing solutions
   System 1 (S-1), chloroform-methanol, 90:10 – To 90 ml of chloroform add 10 ml of methanol. System 2 (S-2), methanol-ammonia, 100:1.5 – To 100 ml of methanol add 1.5 ml of aqua ammonia (28% NH_3 in water). System 3 (S-3), isopropyl ether-ethanol, 80:20 – To 80 ml of isopropyl ether add 20 ml of ethanol. System 4 (S-4), ethyl acetate methanol-ammonia, 170:20:10 – Mix 170 ml of ethyl acetate with 20 ml of methanol and 10 ml of concentrated ammonium hydroxide. System 5 (S-5), benzene/dioxane/diethylamine/absolute ethanol, 50:40:5:5 (v/v) – Mix 50 ml of benzene, 40 ml of dioxane, 5 ml of diethylamine, and 5 ml of absolute ethanol.
8. Ninhydrin®-acetone spray reagent
   Dissolve 0.4 g of Ninhydrin® in acetone. Dilute the solution to 100 ml with acetone. Prepare this reagent fresh just prior to use.
9. Potassium iodoplatinate spray reagent
   Dissolve 1 g of platinum chloride in 100 ml of water containing 10 g of potassium iodide. Dilute this mixture to 500 ml with water.
10. Nitric acid, concentrated
11. Mercuric sulfate spray reagent
    Suspend, with mixing, 5 g of mercuric oxide in 100 ml of water. Add, while stirring, 20 ml of concentrated sulfuric acid. Cool the suspension, then dilute it to 250 ml with water.
12. Furfural
    Freshly redistill furfural, and store in a dark bottle under refrigeration. This reagent has a shelf life of approximately 1 month. If it blackens, it may be redistilled and reused.
13. Ninhydrin®-acid spray reagent
    Dissolve 0.3 g of Ninhydrin® in 100 ml of isopropyl alcohol and 1 ml of glacial acetic acid.
14. Hydrochloric acid, concentrated
15. Hydrochloric acid, 1*N*
    Dilute 8.0 ml of concentrated hydrochloric acid to 100 ml with water.
16. Sodium nitrite spray reagent
    Dissolve 5 g of sodium nitrite in water and dilute to 100 ml.
17. *p*-Nitroaniline (PNA) spray reagent
    Dissolve 2.5 g of PNA in 250 ml of 1*N* hydrochloric acid. Dilute the solution to 500 ml with ethanol. Just before use add 2 ml of the sodium nitrite solution to 10 ml of PNA.

*Scientific Instruments, Inc., Springfield, Mass.
†CRC Press, Inc., 18901 Cranwood Parkway, Cleveland, Ohio 44128.
‡Available from Brinkmann Instruments, Inc., Westbury, N. Y. A Desaga apparatus may be used to apply the coatings; alternatively, commercially available coated plates may be purchased.

Cool this mixture to approximately 5°C by placing it in a refrigerator for 10 min. Use this reagent only when cold.

18. Sodium hydroxide spray reagent, 0.125*N*
    Dissolve 50 g of sodium hydroxide in 100 ml of water. Dilute 10 ml of this solution to 100 ml with 95% ethanol just before use.
19. Hydrochloric acid, 6*N*
    Mix equal volumes of hydrochloric acid and water.
20. Alkali mixture
    Mix 30 g of anhydrous potassium carbonate with 20 g of anhydrous sodium bicarbonate.
21. Chloroform-isopropanol mixture, 3:1
    To 30.0 ml of chloroform add 10.0 ml of isopropanol. Prepare this reagent just prior to use.

PROCEDURE

Separation of Drugs from Urine

1. To 1.0 ml of ethanol in a screw-capped test tube, add 10 ml of urine and mix. Incline the tube so that it is not in a vertical position. Add anhydrous potassium carbonate until the solution is saturated (about 12 g). Cap the tube, then immediately mix its contents by inversion.
2. Agitate the tube with a Vortex Jr mixer for 20 sec. Because the process is exothermic, the tube must be securely capped.
3. Place the tube in an upright position. After 5 min a creamy dark-brown suspension should float to the surface.
4. Centrifuge the tube for 3 min. Usually, 0.8 to 0.9 ml of ethanol separates from the aqueous phase. If a smaller amount separates, add more potassium carbonate, recap the tube, mix, and recentrifuge.
5. Using a rubber bulb, aspirate the highly colored ethanol concentrate into a Pasteur pipet, rejecting any aqueous phase by squeezing the bulb. Some urines form a film of protein between the water and ethanol phases. If this film is present, use the tip of the Pasteur pipet to push the film against the wall of the test tube before transferring the ethanol into the pipet.
6. Transfer the ethanol concentrate to a 10-ml test tube. If the volume is less than 0.8 ml, add several drops of ethanol to the original tube to wash the protein layer. Add this wash solution to the ethanol concentrate in the test tube.
7. Add 5 ml of ether and 1.0 ml of buffer to the ethanol concentrate. Agitate the mixture thoroughly with a Vortex mixer, then allow it to stand until two layers are formed. The (upper) ether-ethanol layer should be clear. If it is not, agitate the mixture again with a Vortex mixer.
8. Transfer the (upper) ethanol-ether layer, which contains any basic organic drugs, to a second test tube. Save this for subsequent testing. The (lower) ethanol-buffer mixture contains the water-soluble fraction, which includes any morphine glucuronides that may be present. Save this for the morphine detection procedure described below.
9. Add a drop of dilute acetic acid to the ether-ethanol layer (Step 8 of the separation procedure), then place the test tube in a water bath at 50°C in a hood. To help prevent bumping during the evaporation (Step 2), insert a sealed capillary tube into the test tube.
10. Evaporate the ether-ethanol mixture to dryness. Blowing air over the surface of the tubes facilitates evaporation.
11. Dissolve the residue in 50 μl of ethanol. Shake the tube vigorously to insure complete solution of the residue.
12. Using a capillary pipet, transfer 10- to 15-μl aliquots of this solution from the test tube to each of two chromatographic plates, previously scribed so that 20 columns are formed. Save the test tubes and the capillaries, which usually contain sufficient material for another plate, should another chromatogram be required.
13. Apply aliquots of suitable drug reference solutions to each plate. The number used depends on the circumstances, but at least one primary amine (amphetamine), one secondary amine (methamphetamine), and one tertiary amine (morphine) should be included on each plate.
14. Develop one plate in System 1 and the other in System 2.
15. After the developing solution on each plate has ascended 10 to 12 cm above the application points, remove the plates from the developing tanks and air-dry them.
16. Heat the plate that was developed in System 2

for 5 min at 90°C. Do not heat the other plate.*

Identification Procedures

Every colored spot that forms should be recorded after each spray operation.

System 1

1. Expose the chromatogram to 350-and 254-nm radiation. Observe any absorption or fluorescence.
2. Spray the plate with the Ninhydrin®-acetone reagent. Expose it to 350-nm radiation for 10 min or until the background becomes slightly pink.
3. Spray the plate with the potassium iodoplatinate reagent, then air-dry it.
4. Gently overspray the plate with concentrated hydrochloric acid.
5. Spray the plate again with the potassium iodoplatinate reagent. Observation of the color intensity of the drug reference spots serves as a guide to the amount of spray required. Air-dry the plate.
6. Overspray the plate with concentrated nitric acid, then dry it in an oven.
7. Spray the plate with mercuric sulfate.
8. Overspray the plate with furfural and concentrated hydrochloric acid.

System 2

1. Spray the plate with acid Ninhydrin,® then place it for 5 min in an oven at 90°C. Allow it to cool to room temperature. Note any color that forms.
2. Spray the plate with the potassium iodoplatinate reagent.
3. Overspray the plate with concentrated hydrochloric acid, then air-dry it.
4. Spray the plate lightly with PNA reagent. A black background should appear promptly; if it does not, this indicates that the PNA reagent was not diazotized. In that case, allow the mixture of PNA and sodium nitrite to react at 5°C for 5 to 10 min more, then respray the plate. The background should now become black. Avoid wetting the plate; should this happen, air-dry the plate until the background turns gray.
5. Spray the plate with the sodium hydroxide reagent until the dark background disappears or until the amphetamine reference spot becomes red.

Morphine Determination

If morphine is suspected, the ethanol-buffer layer (Step 8 of the separation procedure) must be analyzed. Morphine may not be detected on the two chromatograms of the ether-ethanol extract because most of the morphine is excreted as the glucuronide. The glucuronide, being a highly polar compound, remains in the ethanol-buffer solution if it is present. Hence, the ethanol-buffer must be hydrolyzed to release the morphine.

1. Add 0.5 ml of 6*N* hydrochloric acid to the ethanol-buffer solution, then heat the mixture in a water bath for 1 hr at 100°C.
2. After cooling, neutralize the acid by slowly adding the alkali mixture until there is no further effervescence. This should bring the pH of the solution to 8.8 ± 0.3.
3. Extract the neutralized solution with 10 ml of the chloroform-isopropanol mixture. Allow the solvent to separate from the aqueous phase.
4. Evaporate the solvent to dryness
5. Dissolve the residue in 50 μl of ethanol. Shake the tube vigorously to insure complete solution of the residue.
6. Spot the dissolved residue on a chromatography plate and develop it in System 4. This system is preferred because it separates morphine and codeine.
7. Spray the developed plate successively with iodoplatinate and concentrated hydrochloric acid.

INTERPRETATION (see p. 7)

The sensitivity and R_f value of each drug in each developing solution are given in Tables 1,2, and 3.

*Spots with R_f values of 0.80 or greater when developed in System 1 can be better identified in System 3, which uses a mixture of isopropyl ether and ethanol as the developing solution. The tubes containing aliquots of samples with high R_f values should be separated from those previously saved; aliquots of each of these should be applied to a third plate coated with silica gel G and developed in the isopropyl ether-ethanol system. When developed and dried, this plate should be sprayed in the same sequence as that developed in System 1.

Table 1

PRIMARY AMINES REACTING WITH NINHYDRIN®-ACETONE (NA) AND WITH *p*-NITROANILINE (PNA)

Number	Compound	Minimum amount detected, μg		$R_f \times 100$				
		NA	PNA	S-1	S-2	S-3	S-4	S-5
1	Amphetamine	3	1	26	45	10	78	57
2	Betazole	50	–	05	36	00	–	–
3	Chlorphentermine	50	–	44	50	–	–	64
4	Metaraminol	20	1	08	51	02	–	–
5	Methoxamine	2	1	14	48	07	–	26
6	Naphazoline*	10	5	10	10	00	–	–
7	Phenylpropanolamine	2	1	15	55	09	60	35
8	Tranylcypromine	5	2	76	73	25	–	93
9	Tuaminoheptane	3	1	14	29	09	–	–

*Fluorescence.

Table 2

SECONDARY AMINES REACTING WITH NINHYDRIN®-ACID

Number	Compound	Minimum amount detected, μg	$R_f \times 100$				
			S-1	S-2	S-3	S-4	S-5
10	Butethamine*	10 (UV)†	49	70	23	–	–
11	Cyclopentamine	10 (UV)	20	21	05	–	–
12	Desipramine	3 (UV)	28	33	06	–	66
13	Ephedrine	3	10	30	07	00	40
14	Isocarboxazid‡	6 (UV)	91	77	88	–	88
15	Isonicotinylhydrazine	4 (UV)	22	65	09	–	–
16	Mephentermine	15	21	28	15	–	66
17	Methamphetamine	5	21	37	07	00	–
18	Methoxyphenylamine	3	15	33	07	–	–
19	Methylphenidate	6 (UV)	79	76	19	92	90
20	Nialamid‡	6 (UV)	30	75	14	–	20
21	Nortriptyline	2	48	38	13	75	67
22	Phenothiazine	3 (UV)	97	81	94	–	–
23	Phenylephrine	10	05	38	06	00	30
24	Phenylpropylmethylamine	1	23	34	05	–	35
25	Pipradol‡	5	69	75	26	–	88
26	Propitocaine	10 (UV)	20	79	60	–	–
27	Propylhexedrine	6	14	23	05	–	–

*Also detected in the primary aromatic amine group.
†UV denotes UV absorption after application of Ninhydrin®-acid and heat.
‡Fluorescence.

Table 3 (Continued)

TERTIARY AMINES REACTING WITH IODOPLATINATE*

Number	Compound	Minimum amount detected, μg	$R_f \times 100$ S-1	S-2	S-3	S-4	S-5
28	Adiphenine	1	90	70	55	–	–
29	Aminophenylline	5	95	67	41	–	–
30	Aminopyrine	5	87	79	42	–	–
31	Amitriptyline	1	55	56	14	98	90
32	Atropine	5	18	24	00	43	31
33	Benactyzine	5	87	75	52	–	89
34	Benzonatate	10	94	74	–	–	–
35	Benzphetamine	1	98	81	63	–	–
36	Brompheniramine	1	30	–	07	–	74
37	Bupivacaine	5	95	80	46	–	–
38	Caffeine	1	89	73	24	80	65
39	Carbetapentane	20	44	49	08	–	–
40	Chlordiazepoxide	1	85	78	91	88	52
41	Chlorpheniramine	1	37	42	07	88	87
42	Cinchocaine	1	78	78	11	–	–
43	Cinchonine	1	31	55	09	–	–
44	Cocaine	10	80	74	14	98	92
45	Codeine	1	40	46	02	54	49
46	Cyclomethycaine	1	67	68	16	–	–
47	Dextromethorphan	1	42	37	06	–	79
48	Diazepam	1	95	73	84	98	90
49	Dicyclomine	1	80	63	14	97	–
50	Diethylpropion	10	89	85	42	–	95
51	Dimethoxonate	1	43	48	27	–	–
52	Diphenhydramine	1	76	77	11	90	80
53	Diphenidol	1	68	71	16	–	–
54	Ethoheptazine	1	36	40	09	–	76
55	Halocaine	1	65	83	35	–	–
56	Heroin	1	58	54	08	80	77
57	Hydromorphone	5	30	45	02	–	–
58	Isopentylhydrocupreine	5	40	66	24	–	–
59	Isopropamide	5	14	15	00	–	–
60	Levallorphan	1	41	76	32	–	78
61	Lidocaine	10	95	73	71	–	–
62	Meperidine	2	71	64	16	–	79
63	Mepivacaine	10	87	74	49	–	90
64	Methadone	1	32	53	11	99	91
65	Methapyrilene	2	71	65	09	94	79
66	Methaqualone	5	96	75	86	–	86
67	Methixene	1	55	52	09	–	–
68	Methysergid	1	51	79	24	–	–
69	Morphine	3	21	46	01	32	21
70	Nicotine	1	68	60	09	90	78
71	Nikethamide	5	86	67	49	–	27
72	Nylidrin‡	10	25	69	55	–	–

Table 3 (Continued)

TERTIARY ANIMES REACTING WITH IODOPLATINATE*

Number	Compound	Minimum amount detected, μg	$R_f \times 100$				
			S-1	S-2	S-3	S-4	S-5
73	Orphenadrine	1	63	60	12	–	84
74	Papaverine	2	91	80	58	99	74
75	Pentazocine	2	43	75	60	–	72
76	Pentylenetetrazol	1	91	75	50	–	77
77	Phendimetrazine	10	92	66	21	–	80
78	Pheniramine	1	42	43	06	92	64
79	Phenmetrazine‡	1	61	64	11	–	54
80	Phenocaine	1	61	80	76	–	–
81	Phenyramidol	5	92	85	75	–	–
82	Physostigmine	1	56	68	12	–	–
83	Piperidolate	5	93	76	30	–	–
84	Piperilate	5	90	71	28	–	88
85	Piperocaine	1	68	67	13	–	–
86	Pramoxine	1	90	66	45	–	–
87	Procyclidene	1	49	51	15	–	80
88	Propoxyphene	1	95	74	60	90	90
89	Pyrilamine	1	51	60	10	90	–
90	Quinacrine†	1	25	50	05	97	–
91	Quinidine†	1	39	65	14	65	39
92	Quinine†	1	33	67	15	65	39
93	Scopolamine	1	52	27	100	–	59
94	Strychnine	1	44	29	03	63	33
95	Tetracaine	1	77	67	14	–	76
96	Theobromine	20	60	–	30	–	10
97	Theophylline	10	52	64	41	–	10
98	Thiothixene	1	56	51	07	–	66
99	Trimethobenzamide	1	46	58	06	–	–
100	Triprolidine	1	33	52	09	90	84
101	Yohimbine†	10	84	79	27	–	–
102	Zoxazolamine	10	78	84	87	–	–

*All compounds yield a blue to purple product. Drugs listed in Tables 1 and 2 also form colored products with the iodoplatinate.
†Fluorescence.
‡Not tertiary amines, but cannot be detected in amounts of 20 μg with the previous reagent sprays.

Some drugs and their metabolites may be tentatively identified by their R_f value in two developing systems and their reaction to the sprays. The R_f data reported in Tables 1 to 3 are illustrated in Figure 1. R_f values greater than 0.80 in the chloroform-methanol system were not plotted. The resolution of these substances is best achieved in System 3 (isopropyl ether-ethanol), as shown in Table 4.

If two or more positive reactions to the sprays are found on one chromatogram, two drugs may be present. Alternatively, if one of them is a tertiary amine with a high R_f and the other is a secondary or primary amine, a drug and its metabolites may be present. The relative intensity of each spot is significant. Sometimes higher concentrations of the metabolites are found and only small quantities of the unchanged drug. This is particularly

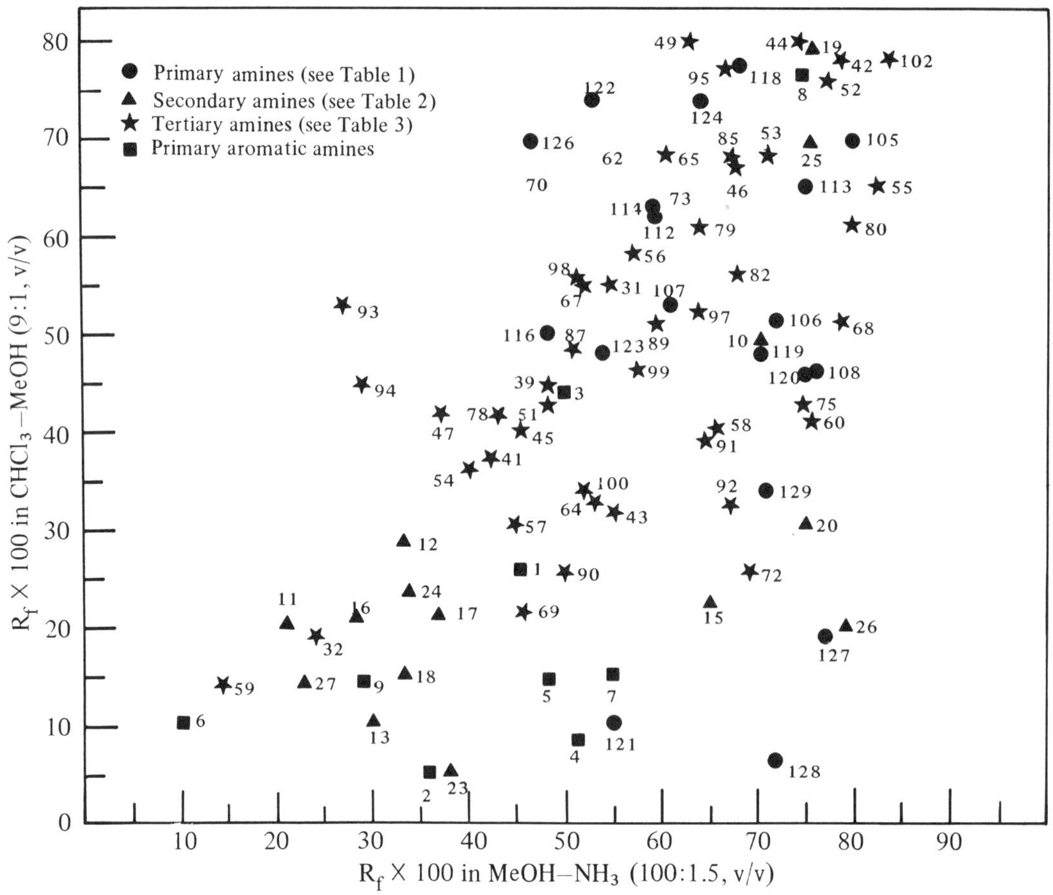

FIGURE 1. R_f of drugs in chloroform-methanol as compared with their R_f in methanol-ammonia. The numbers correspond to the numbers in Tables 1 to 3.

Table 4

R_f VALUES FOLLOWING DEVELOPMENT IN ISOPROPYL ETHER-ETHANOL (80:20)

Number	Compound	R_f	Number	Compound	R_f	Number	Compound	R_f
115	Metabutoxicaine	15	29	Aminophylline	41	88	Propoxyphene	60
132	Trifluoperazine	16	30	Aminopyrine	42	35	Benzphetamine	63
117	Methotrimeprazine	19	49	Diethylpropion	42	61	Lidocaine	71
110	Fluphenazine	19	111	Hydroxyzine	44	81	Phenyramidol	75
178	Phendimetrazine	21	85	Pramoxine	45	48	Diazepam	84
131	Thioridazine	21	37	Bupivacaine	46	66	Methaqualone	86
133	Trimeprazine	21	63	Mepivacaine	49	14	Isocarboxazid	87
130	Thiopropazate	23	71	Nikethamide	49	125	Propiomazine	87
38	Caffeine	24	76	Pentylenetetrazole	50	40	Chlordiazepoxide	91
101	Yohimbine	27	33	Benactyzine	52	104	Benzocaine	92
84	Peperilate	28	28	Adiphenine	55	103	Aminoglutethimide	93
83	Peperidolate	30	74	Papaverine	58	22	Phenothiazine	94
						109	Ethopromazine	94

true for meperidine and propoxyphene. Nicotine, caffeine, and metabolites of nicotine are usually found in the urine of smokers and coffee drinkers. Extracts of these urines yield spots that can be observed on plates developed in both Systems 1 and 2. Two metabolites appear after the iodoplatinate spray. The nicotine metabolites are only revealed when the iodoplatinate is oversprayed with concentrated hydrochloric acid. Identification of drugs whose R_f values are in these regions is, therefore, more difficult. Fortunately, drugs of primary interest in problems of drug abuse and drug misuse do not have R_f values in these regions. If a nonsmoker is involved, interpretation is simpler, because the nicotine spots are not found.

After becoming familiar with the pattern seen with normal urine, it is easier to distinguish small amounts of drug among the normal artifacts, but spraying and interpreting require experience and skill. However skillful, no one should positively identify any substance on the basis of an R_f value and the spray reactions. These are necessary, but not sufficient conditions for identification. Definitive proof requires substantiation by some other identification technique. Within the limits of the known sensitivity of the procedure, a negative result (no spot on a plate) is reasonably good evidence that the substance in question is not present.

For those who wish to refer to still another TLC system and for some drugs whose R_f values were not recorded in the preceding tables Dr. T. J. Siek* has supplied the following data (Table 5) which was obtained with solvent system 5.

*Dr. T. J. Siek, Northern Virginia Branch, Bureau of Forensic Science, P.O. Box 486, Merrifield, Va. 22116.

Table 5

THIN-LAYER CHROMATOGRAPHY OF BASIC DRUGS ON SILICA GEL G

Compound	$R_f \times 100$	Compound	$R_f \times 100$
Anileridine	90	Doxepin	87
Antazoline	69	Doxylamine	79
Antipyrine	62	Epinephrine	4
Apomorphine	33 str	Ethoheptazine	76
Bendroflumethiazide	31	Ethylmorphine	53
Benzocaine	83	Flurazepam	81
Biperiden	88	Haloperidol	93
Buclizine	92	Hydrochlorothiazide	12
Captodiamine	74	Hydroflumethiazide	13 str
Carbinoxamine	71	Hydroxyamphetamine	15
Chlorcyclizine	84	Hydroxychloroquine	72
Chlorpromazine	83	Hydroxyzine	18 str
Chlorprothixene	85	Iproniazid	50
Cotinine	58	Isoniazid	16 str
Cyclazocine	82	Isoproterenol	9
Cyclizine	79	Ketamine	85
Cyproheptadine	86	Levallorphan	78
Diethyltryptamine	73	Lysergic acid, diethylamide (LSD)	70
Dihydrocodeine	48	Meclizine	91
Dihydrocodeinone	51		
Dihydromorphinone	35	Mephentermine	66
Dimethindene	70	Mescaline	28 str
2,5-Dimethoxy-4-methylamphetamine	66	Methaqualone	86
Dimethyltryptamine	64	Methoxamine	26
Diphenoxylate	79	Methylenedioxyamphetamine (MDA)	49

Table 5 (Continued)

THIN-LAYER CHROMATOGRAPHY OF BASIC DRUGS ON SILICA GEL C

Compound	$R_f \times 100$	Compound	$R_f \times 100$
Methylphenidate	90	Procainamide	38
Methyprylon	68	Procaine	79
		Prochlorperazine	77
3-Monoacetylmorphine	60	α-Prodine®	71
6-Monoacetylmorphine	65	Promethazine	78
Nalorphine	35		
Naloxone	65	Propoxyphene	90
Nialamide	20	Proprandol	55
		Protriptyline	58
Nicotinamide	27	Pseudoephedrine	40
Norephedrine	40	Reserpine	74 str
Norisoephedrine	20		
Oxazepam	90	Sparteine	71
Oxycodone	79	Thioridazine	86
		Tolazoline	30
Oxymorphone	58	Trichlormethiazide	4
Perphenazine	62	Trifluperazine	69
Phencyclidine	95		
Phenelzine	85	Triflupromazine	84
β-Phenethylamine	44	Trihexphenidyl	91
		Trimeprazine	83
Phenformin	63	Tripelennamine	84
Phentermine	69	Triprolidine	84
Pilocarpine	37		
Piperilate	88	Tryptamine	27
Pipradrol	88	Tyramine	40
		Xylocaine®	83

REFERENCES

Bastos, M. L., Kananen, G. E., Young, R. M., Monforte, J. R., and Sunshine, I., Detection of basic organic drugs and their metabolites in urine, *Clin. Chem.*, 16, 931, 1970.

Beckett, A. H., Tucker, G. T., and Moffat, A. C., Routine detection and identification in urine of stimulants and other drugs, some of which may be used to modify performance in sport, *J. Pharm. Pharmacol.*, 19, 273, 1967.

Davidow, B., Petri, N. L., and Quame, B., A thin-layer chromatographic procedure for detecting drug abuse, *Am. J. Clin. Pathol.*, 50, 714, 1968.

Dole, V. P., Kim, V. K., and Eglitis, I., Detection of narcotic drugs, tranquilizers, amphetamines and barbiturates in urine, *JAMA*, 198, 349, 1966.

Fujimoto, J. M. and Way, E. L., Isolation and crystallization of bound morphine from urine of human addicts, *J. Pharmacol. Exp. Ther.*, 121, 340, 1957.

Mulé, S. J., Identification of narcotics, barbiturates, amphetamines, tranquilizers and psychotomimetics in human urine, *J. Chromatogr.*, 39, 302, 1969.

MODIFIED DAVIDOW TLC DRUG SCREENING PROCEDURE

Robert Forney, Jr.

Acid, basic, and neutral drugs are first separated from urine by extraction into organic solvent and then are separated from each other by thin-layer chromatography. Drugs are detected by spraying the plate with various reagents which produce visible spots if the drugs are present. The drugs are tentatively identified by the distance (R_f) which they migrate from the point of application and the colors of the spots produced by one or more of the spray reagents.

APPARATUS

1. Culture tubes, 35 ml, with Telflon®-lined screw caps
2. Bench top rotaters
3. Culture tubes, 15 X 75 mm
4. Small boiling chips (Prepare by crushing boiling chips with a hammer and sifting with mesh screens to obtain small chips.)
5. Hot water bath
6. Silica gel G thin-layer plates, 250μ
7. Electric oven
8. Reagent spray bottles

REAGENTS

Extraction

1. Ammonia buffer, pH 9.2
   Saturated ammonium chloride solution is adjusted to pH 9.2 with concentrated ammonium hydroxide.
2. Extraction solvent, chloroform-isopropanol (96:4)
3. H_2SO_4, 0.1*N*, in ethanol
4. Solid buffer, $NaHCO_3$:K_2CO_3 (3:1)
   Mix 30 g of $NaHCO_3$ with 10 g of K_2CO_3.
5. Absolute methanol

Spray Reagents

1. Ninhydrin®
   Dissolve 400 mg of Ninhydrin® in 100 ml of pH 10 phosphate buffer. The phosphate buffer is made by adjusting 0.1*M* K_2HPO_4 to pH 10 with 2*N* KOH.
2. Phenylacetaldehyde, 40 m*M*
   Dilute 4.8 ml of phenylacetaldehyde to one liter with ethanol.
3. Sulfuric acid, 3.6*N*
   Carefully add 10 ml of concentrated sulfuric acid to water and dilute the mixture to 100 ml with water.
4. Iodoplatinate
   Dissolve 1 g of $PtCl_6$ in 100 ml of water containing 10 g of KI. Dilute to 500 ml with water.
5. Mercuric sulfate
   Suspend 5 g of HgO in 100 ml of water. Add 20 ml of concentrated H_2SO_4 while cooling and stirring rapidly. Dilute to 250 ml with water.
6. Ammoniacal silver nitrate
   Mix 30 ml of 5*N* NH_4OH with 30 ml of 50% (w/v) $AgNO_3$. If the solution is cloudy, add 5*N* NH_4OH until it is clear. Protect this solution from light.
7. Potassium permanganate
   Dissolve 1.58 g of $KMnO_4$ in water and dilute to 500 ml.
8. Dragendorf's reagent
   (a) Dissolve 2.13 g of bismuth subnitrate in 25 ml of glacial acetic acid and 100 ml of water. (b) Dissolve 50 g of potassium iodide in 125 ml of water. Combine 10 ml each of solutions A and B, 20 ml of glacial acetic acid. and 100 ml of water.
9. Sodium nitrite, 5% (w/v), in water
   Dissolve 5 g in 100 ml of water.

Developing Solvents

1. Cyclohexane
   Mix 70 ml of ethyl acetate with 15 ml of cyclohexane, 8 ml of methanol, 0.5 ml of water, and 3 ml of concentrated ammonium hydroxide.
2. Modified Davidow
   Mix 80 ml of ethyl acetate with 15 ml of

methanol and 5 ml of water.

3. Davidow
   Mix 85 ml of ethyl acetate with 10 ml of methanol and 5 ml of ammonium hydroxide.
4. Barbiturate confirmation, isopropyl ether
5. Methaqualone and benzodiozepam confirmation
   Mix 90 ml of chloroform with 10 ml of acetone.

Urine Reference Solution

	Concentration, μg/ml
Amphetamine	5
Benzoyl ecgonine*	5
Ecgonine and cocaine	5
Codeine	5
Methadone	5
Methaqualone	5
Morphine	2.5
Librium®	5
Propoxyphene	5
Quinine	0.5
Pentobarbital	2.5
Valium®	5

* An ethanolic cocaine solution will spontaneously decompose in vitro upon standing at room temperature to benzoyl ecgonine and ecgonine, the two principle in vivo metabolites.

PROCEDURE

1. To a 35-ml culture tube with a Teflon®-lined screw cap, add 12 ml of sample (urine and reference solutions), 2.0 ml of pH 9.2 ammonia buffer, and 16.0 ml of the chloroform-isopropanol (9:1) extraction solvent.
2. Extract by rotating the capped tubes for 20 min. Centrifuge briefly to separate the phases.
3. Aspirate the upper (aqueous) layer to waste.
4. Filter the lower (organic) phase through Whatman #4 filter paper into a 15 X 75 mm culture tube containing a small boiling chip. Add 2 drops of ethanolic sulfuric acid to the extracts to prevent loss of amphetamine during evaporation.
5. Evaporate the filtered organic phase to dryness in a boiling water bath. Rinse the walls of the table with 1.0 ml of the extraction solvent and reevaporate to dryness.
6. Dissolve the residue in 3 drops of ethanol. Apply this solution to a silica gel G plate and allow the spots to dry.
7. Develop the plate first in the cyclohexane solvent for 12 min. Dry the plate for 10 min in an oven set at 85°C. Allow the plate to cool to room temperature. Develop the plate to the top in the Modified Davidow solvent. Dry the plate in the oven as before.

Spraying

1. Observe the plate under the 254-nm UV light and mark any blue fluorescence. Quinine emits a brilliant blue fluorescence; phenothiazines emit a less brilliant fluorescence in several spots lower on the column.
2. **Amphetamines and other primary amines** – Spray with Ninhydrin®, covering the plate about 4 times. Follow with a heavier spray of 40 m*M* phenylacetaldehyde, covering the plate 8 to 10 times. Heat the plate in the oven at 85°C for 10 min. Observe the plate under the 254-nm UV light and mark (⁝⁝) any spots which emit a green fluorescence.
3. **Quinine** – Spray lightly with 10% sulfuric acid, covering the plate 4 to 5 times. Observe the heightened fluorescence of quinine under the 254-nm UV light. Mark any new fluorescent bands which appear. Also, observe in visible light the colored spots for phenothiazines. Mark the bottom of the plate "Q" for quinine and "P" for phenothiazines.
4. **Tertiary amines** – Shield the upper 20% of the plate with a suitable clean glass plate and spray the lower portion of the plate with iodoplatinate until the background of the plate is pink. Mark any spots. Circle any unidentified spots. If a blue spot appears between the bands marked as possible quinines, mark a + at the bottom of the plate under Q. Spray the plate again with iodoplatinate and recheck the results.
5. **Barbiturates** – Spray only the upper fourth of the plate heavily with mercuric sulfate. A white band indicates the possible presence of a barbiturate. Mark these bands (=).
6. **Morphine** – (a) Spray lightly with ammoniacal silver nitrate over the "junkline" area at the morphine level. This bleaches the area, changing morphine and codeine spots to yellow. Dry plates in the oven for 10 min at 85°C. (b) Spray with potassium permanganate over the "junkline" area. Morphine, if positive,

produces a yellowish-brown spot against a purple background.

7. **Methaqualone** – Spray the upper fourth of the plate with Dragendorf to detect methaqualone, which turns bright orange.

CONFIRMATION

All positive results must be confirmed. Many prefer to use another procedure and details for recovering drugs from the chromatograms are given in the article following this material. Some prefer to confirm the original analysis by additional TLC procedures. Details for this follow.

1. **Barbiturates** – Place 12.0 ml of urine, 2.0 ml of phosphoric acid buffer, and 16.0 ml of chloroform in a 35-ml Teflon®-lined screw cap extraction tube. Extract and evaporate as before. Spot the residues on a silica gel GF 250-μ plate and develop in isopropyl ether. Dry the plate and observe any fluorescence under 254-nm UV light. Spray the plate with potassium permanganate and mark any spots which appear. Overspray the plate with mercuric sulfate until the silica gel is thoroughly saturated and wet. The dry white spots are barbiturates. Long acting barbiturates are found at the bottom of the plate, while the short acting ones migrate to the top.
2. **Methaqualone and the benzodiazepams** – Extract 12.0 ml of urine in the same way as described for the screening procedure. Spot the residues on a silica gel G 250-μ plate, dry, and develop in chloroform-acetone (90:10) solvent. Spray with the Dragendorf reagent after drying the plate. Bright orange spots indicate methaqualone; less bright spots indicate the benzodiazepams (Valium®, Librium®, Dalmane®, etc.). Overspray the plate with sodium nitrite to bleach the background. Methaqualone spots will become yellow-brown in color following this spray.
3. **Amphetamine and other primary amines, codeine, quinine, and morphine** – These can all be spotted on a silica gel G plate and developed in the Davidow solvent. Follow the regular spray sequence to verify the presence of these drugs.
4. **Cocaine and propoxyphene** – These can be spotted on a silica gel G plate and developed in cyclohexane solvent to *only* 5.0 cm. Dry the plate and develop again in the Modified Davidow solvent to the top of the plate to separate these two drugs. Spray the plate with sulfuric acid followed by iodoplatinate to identify the drugs.
5. **Methadone** – This can be spotted on a silica gel G plate and developed in cyclohexane solvent to 11 cm. After drying, the plate is developed to the top in the Modified Davidow solvent. Sulfuric acid spray followed with iodoplatinate identifies the methadone spot.
6. **Hydrolysis** – Hydrolysis will release morphine and other drugs, which are bound to glucuronic acid in urine, and increase the amount of drug available for extraction. In a 35-ml extraction tube, place 12.0 ml of urine and 2,0 ml of 6*N* HCl. Hydrolyze by putting the extraction tube in a boiling water bath for 30 min. Remove the tube and cool it to room temperature. Add 10 ml of ethyl acetate to the acidic solution, cap, and shake vigorously for about 1 min. Centrifuge and aspirate the top (ethyl acetate) layer to waste. Add 3.0 ml of 6*N* NaOH and 10.0 ml of ethyl acetate, cap, and shake vigorously as before. Again centrifuge and aspirate the top (ethyl acetate) layer to waste. Add 0.5 ml of 6*N* HCl and saturate the solution with the solid bicarbonate buffer. Add 16.0 ml of the extraction solvent (chloroform-isopropanol, 9:1) and follow the screening procedure for extraction development. Spray the developed plate only with iodoplatinate followed by the morphine sprays.

INTERPRETATION (see p. 7)

Thin-layer chromatography is a powerful qualitative urine-screening tool. The results of a single extraction, development, and spray should *not* be considered as conclusive when a spot is obtained. *An independent method of analysis must be utilized to confirm all positive identifications.* Also, it is very important that *both* blank and positive control urine reference solutions be included with each plate developed. The identification of drugs subject to abuse in urine is a serious matter. Thin-layer chromatography is an art which requires patient practice, careful work, and thoughtful consideration if its potential is to be realized.

A form such as shown in Figure 1, if printed on thin transparent paper, is well-suited for making a record of the TLC plate. On it can be noted the point of application, the height of solvent front, and the location and color of the spots.

Reproduction of Thin Layer Chromatograph

Specimen Blood ☐ Drug ☐ Urine ☐ Other ☐ ____________________

Composition of Thin Layer ____________________ Source ____________________ Time of run ________ Min.

Solvent Height ________ cm. Solvent used ____________________

Spray reagent ____________________

Date ____________ Run by ____________ Cuyahoga County Coroner's Laboratory (T50)

ELUTION OF IODOPLATINATE POSITIVE SPOTS FROM TLC PLATES

Philip Reynolds

Some analysts prefer to extract the material from the silica gel spot and characterize the eluted material by UV spectrophotometry, GLC, or immunoassay. An excellent procedure for this elution step follows.

CONFIRMATION

1. After the spraying of the plate is completed, scrape the spots of interest into separate small screw-capped test tubes. As a control also scrape a spot from an adjacent portion of the plate which gave no reaction to the spray reagent.
2. To each tube add 1 ml of H_2O, a pinch of sodium sulfite, and a pinch of sodium bicarbonate, or a drop of concentrated NH_4OH, and stir. **Note**: Use sodium bicarbonate for elution of suspected morphine or morphine-like compounds. Use concentrated NH_4OH for elution of spots from samples which have been originally extracted with ether.
3. Check the pH of all tubes. The tubes with sodium bicarbonate should have a pH of about 8. The tubes with concentrated NH_4OH should have a pH of about 11.
4. To each tube with sodium bicarbonate, add 4 ml of an ethanol in chloroform solution (90:10). Vortex the tube for 20 to 30 sec. Spin the tube for 5 min. To each tube with concentrated NH_4OH add 4 ml of ether. Vortex the tube for 20 to 30 sec, then centrifuge for 5 min. Set up a blank tube with either 4 ml of ether or 4 ml of the 10% ethanol in chloroform solution.
5. Set up a duplicate set of screw-capped test tubes. Aspirate off the water then filter the ethanol-chloroform solution through filter paper that has been wet with the solvent. Wash the respective filters with 1 to 2 ml of either ether or the ethanol-chloroform solution as indicated.
6. Add 1.2 ml of 0.5*N* HCl to the filtered solvent and blank. Vortex the mixture for 20 to 30 sec, then centrifuge for 5 min.
7. Read the acid extracts on the UV spectrophotometer vs their respective blanks.
8. Determine the UV absorption spectrum of the solutions using the solutions obtained from processing the control spots as the reference solution; or, make each solution alkaline, add 50 μl of chloroform, and vortex the mixture. Centrifuge the tubes and inject 3μl of the chloroform layer into a suitably prepared gas chromatograph.

GC FOR DRUGS OF ABUSE

Vijay Aggarwal and Phillip Santinga

Although many quantitative procedures require large volumes of organic solvent to separate drugs from various biological samples, the qualitative identification of most acidic, basic, or neutral drugs in urine can be accomplished by extraction with very small solvent volumes. Once the separation is performed, the extract may be analyzed by gas chromatography and/or thin-layer chromatography. Small volume extractions are very useful screening tools for several reasons: the required manipulations are minimal; there is no need to evaporate large solvent volumes, saving time and avoiding concentrating the contaminants in the extraction solvent; and the recovery, although inefficient, is sufficient to detect most drugs in concentrations greater than 1 μg/ml. The major limitation of this small volume extraction is that morphine and other amphoteric drugs are not adequately extracted.

APPARATUS

1. Conical centrifuge tubes (Pyrex® #8062), 15 ml
2. Vortex mixer (A. H. Thomas, Cat. #8294-F10)
3. Centrifuge
4. Gas chromatograph,* either one four column or two dual column instruments equipped with flame ionization detectors, on a column injection system, and (a) a glass column 3′ × 1/8″ i.d., packed with 5% OV-7 on Chromosorb WHP 80/100 mesh, and (b) another liquid phase such as OV-17 on Chromosorb WHP 80/100 mesh for GLC confirmation

   Operating Conditions

   Gas Flow Rates:
   - nitrogen – 30 ml/min
   - hydrogen – 30 ml/min
   - air – 350 ml/min

   Temperatures:
   - oven – 190°C
   - injection port – 260°C
   - detector – 260°C

REAGENTS

All chemicals should be analytical reagent grade.

1. Borate buffer

   Add 12*N* NaOH to a saturated solution of sodium borate to bring the pH to 9.9.
2. H_2SO_4, 0.5*N*

   Add 13.9 ml of concentrated sulfuric acid to approximately 500 ml of distilled water and dilute to one liter.
3. Extraction solvent

   Mix 95 ml of chloroform with 5 ml of isobutanol.
4. Stock control solution, 25 mg/100 ml

   To 100 ml of distilled water add the equivalent of 50 mg of free drug to be identified (e.g., 54.6 mg of the sodium salt of the barbiturates, 55.9 mg of methadone HCl, 68.1 mg of amphetamine sulfate, 56.1 mg of cocaine HCl, etc.). Dilute the mixture to 200 ml and store at 4°C.
5. Control solution, 0.3 mg/100 ml

   Dilute 0.6 ml of the stock control solution to 50 ml with fresh drug-free urine.

PROCEDURE

Basic Drugs

1. Pour 6 to 8 ml of sample (urine or control solution) into a centrifuge tube and add 3 ml of the buffer solution. The pH of the resulting solution should be 9.3 ± 0.3. A urine control sample must be analyzed along with each batch of samples.

*The GLC system listed is one of the many which are suitable for the analysis of the extract. The use of three isothermal columns is often superior to the use of one temperature programmed column when large numbers of samples are to be analyzed.

2. Add 100 μl of the extraction solvent and vortex for 20 sec.
3. Centrifuge the samples for 5 min to separate the phases.
4. Inject 3 μl of the solvent phase onto the OV-7 column to detect the organic bases and amphetamines, respectively.

Weak Acids and Neutrals

1. Pour 6 to 8 ml of sample (urine or control solution) into a centrifuge tube and add 0.5 ml of 0.5*N* H_2SO_4. The pH of the resulting solution should be less than 7. A urine control sample must be analyzed along with each batch of samples.
2. Add 100 μl of the extraction solvent and vortex for 20 sec.
3. Centrifuge the tubes for 5 min to separate the phases.
4. Inject a 3 μl-aliquot of the solvent phase onto the OV-7 column.

INTERPRETATION (see p. 7)

Using the stated GLC conditions, retention times approximating those listed in Table 1 should be obtained. Preliminary identification of known peaks can be made by reference to the standard retention time data reported by Finkle.[1] Any positive result should be confirmed by TLC or GLC analysis, using a column packed with another liquid phase. There are many liquid phases other than OV-7 that would be suitable for this analysis. The final choice of the column to use is a matter of personal experience and the availability of particular columns. If a large number of confirmation analyses are required, one important consideration is that the gas chromatograph used be able to rapidly (less than 1 min) return to baseline after injection of the sample. If this is not possible, the analysis time per sample may be increased, and this may make the GLC procedure unsuitable for the analysis of a large number of samples. This is only a problem for laboratories with a large throughput and would not vitiate the potential of this procedure if only a few samples are to be analyzed, as is usually the case in most clinical laboratories.

Table 1

Drug	R_t (min)
Amphetamine	0.9
Methamphetamine	1.2
Meperidine	2.0
Methadone metabolite	6.2
Methadone	7.0
Propoxyphene	7.7
Cocaine	8.2
Codeine	14.0
Amobarbital	1.8
Secobarbital	2.3
Phenobarbital	5.7

Although most of the acidic drugs could be analyzed on the same column that is used for analysis of the bases (5% OV-7) by lowering the temperature, in routine practice this has been found unwise. If many acidic extracts are injected onto a column, the organic bases do not chromatograph very well on that column, perhaps due to residual acid or the effects of small amounts of acid on the column. Thus, if a column has been used for analysis of many acid extracts, it should not be used for bases, and vice versa.

In routine use of the above procedure, it has been found possible to inject a sample into each column every 4 to 5 min. The use of a gas chromatograph in this fashion is possible because: (a) the use of small amounts of solvent keeps the amount of coextracted artifacts to a minimum, and (b) on any GLC column as a compound's retention time increases, the peak becomes broader and broader, and at very long retention times there is no noticeable peak at all. To identify quinine in the small volume extract, a higher temperature must be used. The analysis time per sample by GLC can be shortened by coinjecting aliquots of two or three samples.

TLC may be performed on an aliquot of the original small solvent extract to indicate if drugs are present. GLC results may be confirmed by spotting 30 to 40 μl of the extract on a TLC plate and developing and spraying the plate according to a TLC scheme similar to those described by Bastos[2] or Speaker.[3]

Other buffers may be substituted for the one recommended above. Aggarwal et al.[4] reported that small solvent extractions using a 3:2 w/w mixture of $NaHCO_3/K_2CO_3$ generally give more complete and reproducible recoveries of drugs, but this procedure is rather laborious if a large number of samples is to be analyzed.

REFERENCES

1. **Finkle, B., Cherry, E., and Taylor, D.**, A GLC based system for the detection of poisons, drugs, and human metabolites encountered in forensic toxicology, *J. Chromatogr. Sci.*, 9, 393, 1971.
2. **Bastos, M. L., Kananen, G. E., Young, R. M., Monforte, J. R., and Sunshine, I.**, Detection of basic organic drugs and their metabolites in urine, *Clin. Chem.*, 16, 931, 1970.
3. **Speaker, J.**, A single extraction thin layer chromatographic method in current use, *J. Chromatogr. Sci.*, 12, 297, 1974.
4. **Aggarwal, V., Bath, R., and Sunshine, I.**, Technique for rapidly separating drugs from biological samples, *Clin. Chem.*, 20(2), 307, 1974.

RETENTION INDICES FOR COMPOUND IDENTIFICATION

Leo Kazyak

Generally accepted practices for reporting GLC data do not permit easy comparison of results obtained in one laboratory with those obtained in another. Variations in operating conditions, however small, are the basis for the differences in the data. Since these are impossible to eliminate, it would be preferable to develop an index system that is independent of these variations; then one could make valid comparisons and tentative identifications based on the relative position of an unknown peak to those from known compounds. Data storage and retrieval systems could be developed to help do this more efficiently. Such an index system has been proposed by Kovats[1] and has been generally accepted. Regardless of liquid phase concentration, temperatures, or flow rates, retention data compiled according to this system are constant and can be standardized. If a substance's retention indices are obtained for more than one packing, the reliability of making an identification is enhanced. The following compilation provides data for three column packings in common use and should help the reader make tentative identification of substances whose GLC retention times are unfamiliar to the analyst.[2]

Table 1

Compound	Retention index		
	OV-1	OV-17	QF-1
Acetaminophen	1710	2150	2270
Acetophenetidin	1660	2035	2425
Acetylsalicylic acid	1260	1460	1800
Aconitine	2280	2650	3335
Aldrin (HHDN)	1950	2300	2150
Ambodryl®	2150	2465	2460
4-Aminoantipyrine	1950	2425	2830
Aminopyrine	1890	2300	2600
Amphetamine	1110	1300	1410
Amytal®	1725	1985	2350
Anileridine	2845	3410	3550
Antipyrine	1830	2310	2930

Note: "0" indicates retention index has not been determined. "33" indicates no retention time or retention index is below 1000.

Table 1 (Continued)

Compound	Retention index OV-1	OV-17	QF-1
Antistine®	2330	2820	3060
Artane®	2230	2590	2470
Atarax®	2840	3345	3110
Atropine	2175	2555	2700
Azacyclonol	2210	2700	2510
Barbital	1495	1780	2105
Benactyzine	2230	2645	2640
Benadryl®	1855	2135	2110
Benzylamine	33	1210	33
Brucine	3280	3740	4480
Buclizine	3285	3720	3630
Butisol	1780	1955	2280
Caffeine	1810	2265	2530
Cantharidin	1490	1870	2330
Captodiamine	2775	3210	3140
Carbromal	1500	1790	2020
Carphenazine (Proketazine®)	3590	4300	0
Celontin®	1595	1960	2260
Chlorbenside	2050	2440	2400
Chlorcyclizine	2215	2535	2240
Chlordane	2020	2180	2330
Chloroquine	2575	2885	3345
Chlorphentermine	1320	1530	1610
Chlorpromazine	2440	2890	3090
Chlor-Trimeton®	2000	2285	2315
Cinchonidine	2625	3065	3260
Cinchonine	2575	3070	3230
Cocaine	2180	2625	2800
Codeine	2385	2820	2890
Cotarnine	1780	2140	2110
Cyclizine	2010	2350	2240
Cyclohexylamine	33	1000	33
Dapsone (DDS)	2860	0	0
Darvon®	2180	2465	2400
DDT	2290	2705	2740
Demerol®	1740	2000	2015
Dieldrin (HEOD)	2110	2530	2560
Dihydroergotamine	2310	2870	3300
Dilantin®	2320	2920	3265
β-3,4-Dimethoxy-phenethylamine	1540	1850	2070
Dimethrin (isomers), *cis*	1953		
trans	1977	1430	1770
N,N-Dimethylaniline	1080	1260	1310
Dimethylphenethylamine	1160	1270	1350
Dionin®	2415	2900	2900
Diphenylpyraline	0	2765	0
Doriden®	1825	2235	2535
Ectylurea (Nostal®)	1360	1680	1820

Table 1 (Continued)

Compound	Retention index OV-1	OV-17	QF-1
Elavil (amitriptyline)	2200	2550	0
Ephedrine	1350	1590	1680
Ethoxyquin (Santoquin®)	2800	3260	3120
N-Ethylamphetamine	1210	1360	1390
N-Ethylbenzylamine	1120	1290	1300
Fluphenazine (prolixin)	3045	3525	0
Forhistal®	2220	2675	2620
Heroin	2615	3050	3135
Homatropine	2045	2440	2565
Hydrastine	2975	3680	4030
Hydrastinine	1590	2400	2790
Hyoscyamine	2225	2580	2695
Ipral®	1550	1850	2175
Iproniazid	1700	1890	0
Librium®	2780	3440	2735
Isoniazid	1630	1900	2305
Listica®	1740	2090	2245
Lobeline	1780	2090	2260
LSD (lysergide)	3445	0	0
Marplan® (isocarboxazid)	1960	2160	0
Mebutamate	1865	2310	2690
Meclizine (bonamine)	3050	3490	3425
Mellaril®	3110	3655	3595
Mepazine	2550	3040	2940
Mephenoxalone	2120	2680	3260
Mephentermine	1240	1400	33
Meprobamate	1790	2185	2630
Mesantoin®	1795	2185	2525
Mescaline	1690	2030	2290
Methadone	2170	2445	2465
Methamphetamine	1170	1340	1420
Methapyrilene	1970	2290	2300
Methaqualone	2117	0	0
Methopromazine	2500	3010	2990
Methoxychlor	2410	2850	2840
Methyl-dimethoxyamphetamine (STP)	1620	1900	2220
Methylenedioxyamphetamine (MDA)	1470	1760	2020
Methylparaben	1435	0	0
Methylphenidate (Ritalin®)	1780	2060	2700
Morphine	2435	2950	3015
Nalorphine (nalline)	2570	3100	2610
Nicotine	1340	1540	1620
Nikethamide	1500	1840	2200
Noludar®	1505	1840	2190
Normeperidine	1745	2075	2165
Nupercaine®	2690	3105	3485
Pargyline	1200	1400	1360
Pentazocine	2265	2620	2610

Table 1 (Continued)

Compound	Retention index		
	OV-1	OV-17	QF-1
Pentobarbital	1750	2030	2385
Pentothal® (thiopental)	1850	2185	2360
Perphenazine	2200	2730	2510
Phencyclidine (PCP)	1870	2140	2050
Phendimetrozine	1440	1660	1700
Phenelzine	0	1610	33
α-Phenethylamine	1010	1230	33
β-Phenethylamine	1120	1310	1450
Phenmetrazine	1430	1670	1720
Phenobarbital	1950	2365	2705
Phentermine	1130	1310	1390
Phenylpropanolamine	1310	1500	1670
Phenyl-2-propanone	1110	1340	1520
1-Phenyl-*N*-propylamine	1130	1305	1810
Phenyltoxalamine	2010	2250	2280
Physostigmine	1810	2270	2940
Picrotoxin	2205	2390	3840
Pipradrol	2150	2570	2470
Placidyl®	1030	1160	33
Plaquenil®	2860	3370	0
Primaquine	2105	2755	0
Primidone	2250	2815	3240
Procaine	1995	2410	2610
Promazine	2295	2765	2560
Promethazine	2260	2700	2680
Prominal	1920	2300	2530
N-Propylamphetamine	1330	1460	1490
Propylhexedrine	1170	1270	33
Pyribenzamine®	1960	2300	2290
Pyridoxamine	2000	2170	2405
Pyrimethamine (Daraprim®)	2140	2600	0
Pyrrobutamine	2430	2830	0
Quinidine	2760	3300	3490
Quinine	2755	3300	3500
Salicylamide	1460	1780	2070
Salicylic acid	1330	1550	0
Sanguinarine	2880	3990	3760
Santonine	1945	2640	3425
Scopolamine	2285	2440	3025
Seconal®	1775	2070	2420
Sevin®	1490	1780	1900
Soma® (carisoprodol)	1850	2250	2610
Sparteine	1765	1985	2785
Striatran®	33	1270	2000
Strychnine	3040	3760	3940
Surital®	1890	2240	2410
Tenuate®	1480	1705	1780

Table 1 (Continued)

Compound	Retention index		
	OV-1	OV-17	QF-1
Tetracaine	2215	2600	2915
Tetrahydrocannabinol (D-9)	2453	2854	0
Thebaine	2525	3085	2930
Thiantoin	2145	2900	3225
Thiopropazate	0	2845	0
Thonzylamine	2045	2585	2520
Tofranil®	2220	2605	2570
Trasentine®	2190	2580	2590
Tranylcypromine	1210	1430	1530
Tridione®	1100	1240	1570
Triflupromazine	2210	2580	0
Trimethylphenethylamine	1240	1390	1440
Triprolidine	2250	2715	2540
Tryptamine	1710	2140	2320
Tuamine®	33	960	1130
Valmid®	1360	1680	1770
Warfarin	1460	1630	1890
Xylocaine® (lidocaine)	1860	2175	0
Yohimbine	3290	3790	0

Table 2

Retention index			Compound
OV-1	OV-17	QF-1	
0	1610	33	Phenelzine
0	2765	0	Diphenylpyraline
0	2845	0	Thiopropazate
33	960	1130	Tuamine®
33	1000	33	Cyclohexylamine
33	1210	33	Benzylamine
33	1270	2000	Striatran®
1010	1230	33	α-Phenethylamine
1030	1160	33	Placidyl®
1080	1260	1310	*N,N*-Dimethylaniline
1100	1240	1570	Tridione®
1110	1300	1410	Amphetamine
1110	1340	1520	Phenyl-2-propanone
1120	1290	1300	*N*-Ethylbenzylamine
1120	1310	1450	β-Phenethylamine
1130	1305	1810	1-Phenyl-*N*-propylamine
1130	1310	1390	Phentermine
1160	1270	1350	Dimethylphenethylamine
1170	1270	33	Propylhexedrine
1170	1340	1420	Methamphetamine

Note: "0" indicates retention index has not been determined. "33" indicates no retention time or retention index is below 1000.

Table 2 (Continued)

Retention index			
OV-1	**OV-17**	**QF-1**	**Compound**
1200	1400	1360	Pargyline
1210	1360	1390	*N*-Ethylamphetamine
1210	1430	1530	Tranylcypromine
1210	1430	1770	Dimethrin
1240	1390	1440	Trimethylphenethylamine
1240	1400	33	Mephentermine
1260	1460	1800	Acetylsalicylic acid
1310	1500	1670	Phenylpropanolamine
1320	1530	1610	Chlorphentermine
1330	1460	1490	*N*-Propylamphetamine
1330	1550	0	Salicylic acid
1340	1540	1620	Nicotine
1350	1590	1680	Ephedrine
1360	1680	1770	Valmid®
1360	1680	1820	Ectylurea (Nostal®)
1430	1670	1720	Phenmetrazine
1435	0	0	Methylparaben
1440	1660	1700	Phendimetrazine
1460	1630	1890	Warfarin
1460	1780	2070	Salicylamide
1470	1760	2020	Methylenedioxyamphetamine (MDA)
1480	1705	1780	Tenuate®
1490	1780	1900	Sevin®
1490	1870	2330	Cantharidin
1495	1780	2105	Barbital
1500	1790	2020	Carbromal
1500	1840	2200	Nikethamide
1505	1840	2190	Noludar®
1540	1850	2070	β-3,4-Dimethoxy-phenethylamine
1550	1850	2175	Ipral®
1590	2400	2790	Hydrastinine
1595	1960	2260	Celontin®
1620	1900	2220	Methyl-dimethoxyamphetamine (STP)
1630	1900	2305	Isoniazid
1660	2035	2425	Acetophenetidin
1690	2030	2290	Mescaline
1700	1890	0	Iproniazid
1710	2140	2320	Tryptamine
1725	1985	2350	Amytal®
1740	2000	2015	Demerol®
1740	2090	2245	Listica®
1745	2075	2165	Normeperidine
1750	2030	2385	Pentobarbital
1765	1985	2785	Sparteine
1775	2070	2420	Seconal®

Table 2 (Continued)

Retention index			
OV-1	OV-17	QF-1	Compound
1780	1955	2280	Butisol
1780	2060	2700	Methylphenidate (Ritalin®)
1780	2090	2260	Lobeline
1780	2140	2110	Cotarnine
1790	2185	2630	Meprobamate
1795	2185	2525	Mesantoin®
1810	2150	2270	Acetaminophen
1810	2265	2530	Caffeine
1810	2270	2940	Physostigmine
1825	2235	2535	Doriden®
1830	2310	2930	Antipyrine
1850	2185	2360	Pentothal® (thiopental)
1850	2250	2610	Soma® (carisoprodol)
1855	2135	2110	Benadryl®
1860	2175	0	Xylocaine® (lidocaine)
1865	2310	2690	Mebutamate
1870	2140	2050	Phencyclidine (PCP)
1890	2240	2410	Surital®
1890	2300	2600	Aminopyrine
1920	2300	2530	Prominal
1945	2640	3425	Santonine
1950	2300	2150	Aldrin (HHDN)
1950	2365	2705	Phenobarbital
1950	2425	2830	4-Aminoantipyrine
1960	2160	0	Marplan® (isocarboxazid)
1960	2300	2290	Pyribenzamine®
1970	2290	2300	Methapyrilene
1995	2410	2610	Procaine
2000	2170	2405	Pyridoxamine
2000	2285	2315	Chlor-Trimeton®
2010	2250	2280	Phenyltoxalamine
2010	2350	2240	Cyclizine
2020	2180	2330	Chlordane
2045	2440	2565	Homatropine
2045	2585	2520	Thonzylamine
2050	2440	2400	Chlorbenside
2105	2755	0	Primaquine
2110	2530	2560	Dieldrin (HEOD)
2117	0	0	Methaqualone
2120	2680	3260	Mephenoxalone
2140	2600	0	Pyrimethamine (Daraprim®)
2145	2900	3225	Thiantoin
2150	2465	2460	Ambodryl®
2150	2570	2470	Pipradrol
2170	2445	2465	Methadone
2175	2555	2700	Atropine
2180	2465	2400	Darvon®

Table 2 (Continued)

Retention index			
OV-1	**OV-17**	**QF-1**	**Compound**
2180	2625	2800	Cocaine
2190	2580	2590	Trasentine®
2200	2550	0	Elavil (amitriptyline)
2200	2730	2510	Perphenazine
2205	2390	3840	Picrotoxin
2210	2580	0	Triflupromazine
2210	2700	2510	Azacyclonol
2215	2535	2240	Chlorcyclizine
2215	2600	2915	Tetracaine
2220	2605	2570	Tofranil®
2220	2675	2620	Forhistal®
2225	2580	2695	Hyoscyamine
2230	2590	2470	Artane®
2230	2645	2640	Benactyzine
2250	2715	2540	Triprolidine
2250	2815	3240	Primidone
2260	2700	2680	Promethazine
2265	2620	2610	Pentazocine
2280	2650	3335	Aconitine
2285	2440	3025	Scopolamine
2290	2705	2740	DDT
2295	2765	2560	Promazine
2310	2870	3300	Dihydroergotamine
2320	2920	3265	Dilantin®
2330	2820	3060	Antistine®
2385	2820	2890	Codeine
2410	2850	2840	Methoxychlor
2415	2900	2900	Dionin®
2430	2830	0	Pyrrobutamine
2435	2950	3015	Morphine
2440	2890	3090	Chlorpromazine
2453	2854	0	Tetrahydrocannabinol (D-9)
2500	3010	2990	Methopromazine
2525	3085	2930	Thebaine
2550	3040	2940	Mepazine
2570	3100	2610	Nalorphine (nalline)
2575	2885	3345	Chloroquine
2575	3070	3230	Cinchonine
2615	3050	3135	Heroin
2625	3065	3260	Cinchonidine
2690	3105	3485	Nupercaine®
2755	3300	3500	Quinine
2760	3300	3490	Quinidine
2775	3210	3140	Captodiamine
2780	2650	2735	Librium®
2800	3260	3120	Ethoxyquin (Santoquin®)
2840	3345	3110	Atarax®
2845	3410	3550	Anileridine

Table 2 (Continued)

Retention index			
OV-1	**OV-17**	**QF-1**	**Compound**
2860	0	0	Dapsone (DDS)
2860	3370	0	Plaquenil®
2880	3990	3760	Sanguinarine
2975	3680	4030	Hydrastine
3040	3760	3940	Strychnine
3045	3525	0	Fluphenazine (prolixin)
3050	3490	3425	Meclizine (bonamine)
3110	3655	3595	Mellaril®
3280	3740	4480	Brucine
3285	3720	3630	Buclizine
3290	3790	0	Yohimbine
3445	0	0	LSD (lysergide)
3590	4300	0	Carphenazine (Proketazine®)
9999	4300	0	Acetaminophen

REFERENCES

1. **Kovats, E.,** Gas-chromatographische charakterisierung organischer verbindung, *Helv. Chim. Acta,* 41, 1915, 1958.
2. **Kazyak, L. and Permisohn, R.,** Retention indices for compound identification by GC, *J. Forensic Sci.,* 15, 346, 1970.

ADSORPTION PROCEDURE USING A NONIONIC RESIN

S. Andryauskas and M. L. Bastos

The XAD-2 resin provides an excellent method for the rapid separation of organic poisons from a biological matrix into a small volume of organic solvents. Chloroform-isopropanol (3:1) is the eluant of choice. The residues from evaporation of the eluates are analyzed by standard TLC methods. Gas chromatography is not as suitable an identification method.

APPARATUS

1. Brinkmann* Drug-Skreen adsorbent cartridges†
2. Phase-separating filter paper for use in filter cartridge
3. Brinkmann* Drug-Skreen sample reservoirs
4. Filter cartridge, complete with phase-separating filter
5. Brinkmann* stainless steel aspirator
6. Water aspirator and rubber vacuum tubing, to supply vacuum to sample aspirator
7. Set of tools for replacing filter in filter cartridge
8. Stainless steel rack No. 1,* for holding assembled columns with filter cartridges
9. Stainless steel rack No. 11,* for use in conjunction with rack No. 1 to hold collected eluant in evaporation tubes
10. Evaporation tubes, 25 ml

REAGENTS

All chemicals should be analytical reagent grade.

1. Alkali mixture
   Mix 30 parts of anhydrous potassium carbonate with 20 parts of sodium bicarbonate.
2. Eluting solvent, chloroform-isopropanol, 3:1 (v/v)

PROCEDURE

Extraction of Urine

1. Adjust the urine to pH 8 to 9 with the alkali mixture.
2. Assemble the sample reservoir and the adsorbent cartridge. Wet the cartridge with 3 ml of distilled water.
3. Pour 20 ml of urine into a column and adjust the water aspirator so as to provide an appropriate flow rate (15 to 20 min total time for adsorption).
4. Remove the cotton plug (which may contain urine sediments above the resin), assemble the adsorbent cartridge, sample reservoir, and filter cartridge (wet filter with elution solvent), and place the complete unit in a suitable rack.
5. Elute the column twice using 10-ml portions of chloroform isopropanol (3:1) each time.
6. Add four drops of 6*N* HCl in methanol to the evaporation tube, and evaporate the organic solvent at 80°C under a stream of air. Brinkmann sells a special hot plate with air aspiration specially designed for this purpose.
7. Dissolve the residues in 100 μl of ethanol and use aliquots for TLC analysis.

Extraction of Blood

1. In a 250-ml Erlenmeyer flask dilute a 5-ml sample of blood to 20 ml with distilled water,

*The Brinkmann equipment is cited to illustrate the type required. Any other similar material may be used with equal success.

†These may be purchased from a commercial source or prepared in the laboratory. In the latter case, the adsorbent cartridges (#1) may be plugged with cotton and refilled with Amberlite XAD-2 resin (20 to 50 mesh) (Rohm and Hass Co., Philadelphia, Pa.). Prior to use, the resin is washed with stirring four times each with a four bed volume of acetone, three times each with a three bed volume of methanol, and three times each with a three bed volume of distilled water. The XAD-2 resin is then stored under distilled water in the refrigerator for at least 7 days. Finally, it is washed twice before use, each time with a two bed volume of distilled water. After the cartridge is filled, the resin is covered with a cotton plug which serves to regulate the flow rate of column.

and add 1.5 to 2.0 g of the previously washed XAD-2 resin.

2. Agitate the sample solution for 5 min on an Eberbach agitator.
3. After agitation pour the contents of the flask into a 250-ml separatory funnel. Wash the flask with approximately 20 ml of distilled water; pour this into the separatory funnel. The resin will settle to the bottom of the funnel, and the blood may easily be decanted and discarded through the top of the funnel. Disregard any minimal loss of resin.
4. Wash the resin twice with 25 ml of distilled water. The second 25 ml of wash water is left in the funnel to provide easier transfer of the resin to an empty cartridge.
5. Transfer the washed resin to a clean cartridge assembled as a reservoir. Aspirate the excess water from the cartridge.
6. Assemble the adsorbent cartridge sample reservoir and filter cartridge. Wet the filter with the eluting solvent and place the complete unit in the rack.
7. Follow Steps 5, 6, and 7 as described for the extraction of urine.

Extraction from Stomach Contents and Washing

1. Transfer the stomach contents to a 500-ml Erlenmeyer flask. Add sufficient water (up to 125 ml) to allow free movement of any suspended solid material. Adjust the pH to 8 to 9 with the alkali mixture.
2. Add 25 g of solid sodium chloride and 5 g of the previously washed XAD-2 resin. Shake the suspension for 5 min using an Eberbach agitator.
3. Decant the resin floating at the surface into a 250-ml separatory funnel with a portion of the liquid stomach contents. (Care should be taken at this point not to allow any large particles, which may clog the stopcock, to pass into the separatory funnel.)
4. Discard the stomach contents through the stopcock. (This fraction may be saved with the washings for analysis of salicylates, chloral hydrate, or ethchlorvynol.) Retain the resin in the separatory funnel.
5. Wash the resin two times with 50 ml of distilled water and transfer it to a cartridge, as described above (see Blood Extraction).
6. Follow steps 5, 6, and 7 as described for the extraction of urine.

TLC Analysis

Details for these procedures are not given here. Any one of the previously described systems may be used (see pp. 412, 434, and 443).

DISCUSSION

The use of Amberlite XAD-2 resin has been successfully applied to the extraction of drugs from urine. The advantages of this technique are the high recoveries obtainable, the elimination of emulsion problems, and the need for considerably smaller volumes of solvents than those required with the traditional solvent extraction methods, thereby requiring less time for evaporation of the solvent. Furthermore, volatile compounds (ethchlorvynol and chloral hydrate), water soluble drugs (quaternary ammonium compounds and glycosides), and metabolites (ecgonine, glucuromides of morphine, and other drugs) which are not extracted by the standard organic solvents (and hence are not routinely detected) are, by this procedure, adsorbed in significant quantities[1-3] by the resin. These may be partially recovered by elution of the column with methanol after the standard or differential type elution.[4] The application of XAD-2 resin, as a general method for the separation of drugs from biological material other than urine, may require a preliminary dilution so that the sample is suitable for passage through the resin columns. This solution must possess the proper flow characteristics and be free of suspended particles[5,6] unless the direct rapid methods described above are used. Drug recoveries from diluted blood (1:4) have been reported for amobarbital (81%), methaqualone (74%), and amitriptyline (61%), using a method[7] which is similar to that described above. The amount of drug present in the stomach of a victim of poisoning is usually sufficient to permit easy identification, even with the recommended rapid procedure involving poor recoveries for amphetamine (27%) and caffeine (29%).

REFERENCES

1. **Miller, W. L., Kullberg, M. E., Banning, M. E., Brown, L. D., and Doctor, B. P.,** Studies on the quantitative extraction of morphine from urine using nonionic XAD-2 resin, *Biochem. Med.*, 17, 145, 1973.
2. **Fujimoto, H. M. and Wang, R. I. H.,** A method of identifying narcotic analgesics in human urine after

therapeutic doses, *Toxicol. Appl. Pharmacol.*, 16, 186, 1970.

3. **Bastos, M. L., Jukofsky, D., Saffer, E., Chedekel, M., and Mulé, S. J.,** Modifications of the XAD-2 resin column method for the extraction of drugs of abuse from human urine, *J. Chromatogr.*, 71, 549, 1972.
4. **Bastos, M. L., Jukofsky, D., and Mulé, S. J.,** Routine identification of drugs of abuse in human urine. Differential elution, *J. Chromatogr.*, 81, 93, 1973.
5. **Osborne, D. N. and Gare, B.,** Improvement to drug screening with XAD-2 resin columns, *J. Chromatogr.*, 77, 223, 1973.
6. **Pranitis, P. A. F., Milzoff, J. R., and Stolman, A.,** Extraction of drugs from biofluids and tissue with XAD-2 resin, *J. Forensic Sci.*, 19, 917, 1974.
7. **Missen, A. and Lewin, J. F.,** A nonionic resin extraction of drugs in blood, *Clin. Chim. Acta,* 53, 389, 1974.

ADSORPTION PROCEDURE USING CHARCOAL*

John M. Meala and Michael Vanko

The drugs are adsorbed from urine onto charcoal, selectively eluted with small amounts of ethyl ether or chloroform-isopropanol, separated, and identified by thin-layer chromatography. The average detection limit for all drugs is 1.0 μg/ml of urine. The procedure is fast, economical, and adaptable to any urine screening program. No emulsions are formed and water washings are not required as with the use of resins. The preliminary charcoal-adsorption step permits excellent thin-layer chromatographic resolution of the drugs, with low background of interfering compounds.

APPARATUS

1. Thin-layer chromatographic equipment: (a) developing chamber, glass, 24-cm high, 8-cm wide, and 23-cm long; (b) "Chromato-vue," containing both short- (254 nm) and long- (365 nm) wavelength UV lamps (Model C-5, Ultra-Violet Products Inc.,); (c) capillary pipets, 75 × 1.1 to 1.2 mm i.d.; (d) reagent spray bottles; (e) silica gel G plates, 20 × 20 cm
2. Teflon®-lined screw-cap culture tubes, 16 × 150 mm (Kimble No. 45066-A)
3. Glass tubes, 10 × 75 mm (Kimble No. 73500)
4. Beaker, 5 ml

REAGENTS

All chemicals should be analytical reagent grade.

1. Charcoal, "Norit® A" neutral, pharmaceutical grade†
2. Carbonate buffer, pH 11.0
   Dissolve 21 g of sodium carbonate (Na_2CO_3) and 420 mg of sodium bicarbonate ($NaHCO_3$) in 700 ml of water. Adjust the pH to 11.0 ± 0.1 with 2*M* NaOH or 2*M* HCl. Dilute to one liter with water. Store at 4°C.
3. Diethyl ether
4. Chloroform:isopropanol, 50:10 (v/v)
   Mix 100 ml of chloroform and 20 ml of isopropanol.
5. Developing solvents: (A) chloroform:acetone (90:10, v/v); (B) chloroform:acetone: ammonium hydroxide (90:10:2, v/v); (C) chloroform:1-butanol:ammonium hydroxide (100:10:3, v/v); (D) ethyl acetate:methanol: ammonium hydroxide (85:10:5, v/v)
6. Fluorescamine reagent
   Dissolve 5 mg of fluorescamine‡ in 200 ml of acetone.
7. Diphenylcarbazone reagent
   Dissolve 10 mg of diphenylcarbazone‡ in 100 ml of acetone.
8. Mercuric sulfate reagent
   Dissolve 5 g of mercuric sulfate (AR; Matheson, Coleman & Bell) in 100 ml of water. Carefully add 5 ml of concentrated sulfuric acid and, when cooled to room temperature, dilute to 500 ml.
9. Iodoplatinate reagent
   Dissolve 2 g of potassium iodide (AR; Mallinckrodt®) in about 75 ml of water in a 100-ml volumetric flask. Add 2 ml of a 10 g/dl solution of chloroplatinic acid (platinic chloride, $PtCl_4 \cdot 2HCl \cdot 6H_2O$, AR, Mallinckrodt®). Dilute to the mark with water. Store at 4°C.
10. Reference stock control
    Drugs used as standards are USP grade. When a salt is used, the required amount is calculated from the desired amount of free drug. Dissolve 1.0 mg of quinine, 1.25 mg of morphine, 2.0 mg of codeine, 3.0 mg of chlorpromazine, and 4.0 mg each of methadone, cocaine, *d*-amphetamine, phenobarbital, secobarbital, and glutethimide in about 90 ml of methanol:

*Abridged from Meola, J. M. and Vanko, M., *Clin. Chem.*, 20(2), 184, 1974. With permission.
†Available from Amend Drug & Chemical Co., Irvington, N.J. 07111.
‡ Available from Roche Diagnostics, Division of Hoffman-La Roche, Inc., Nutley, N.J. 07110.
‡ Available form Matheson, Coleman & Bell, East Rutherford, N.J. 07073.

water (1:1, v/v) in a 100-ml volumetric flask. After the drugs are completely dissolved, dilute to the mark with methanol:water (1:1, v/v).

11. Reference working control
    Add 1.0 ml of the stock standard to 10 ml of normal, drug-free urine. This is analyzed in the same way as unknown urines.
12. Spotting standards
    Prepare solutions (1.0 mg/ml of methanol) to use as spotting standards. Prepare at least the following: (a) phenobarbital and secobarbital or amobarbital, glutethimide, and diazepam; (b) cocaine, methadone, morphine, codeine, quinine, *d*-amphetamine, and propoxyphene.

PROCEDURE

Adsorption of Drugs

1. Preparation of charcoal – To about 500 mg of charcoal add 200 ml of the carbonate buffer and mix thoroughly with a magnetic stirrer. Let the charcoal settle for about 10 min. Aspirate as much buffer as possible.
2. Into appropriately labeled 16 X 150 mm screw-cap culture tubes, add 10 ml of each sample (urine or working reference control), 5 ml of carbonate buffer, and 0.5 ml of the pretreated charcoal slurry.
3. Mix thoroughly by repeated gentle inversion, then allow to stand for a few minutes.
4. Centrifuge at about 2,000 rpm for 5 min.
5. Aspirate and discard as much of the supernate as possible.

Elution of Drugs

(A) Barbiturates, Glutethimide, Cocaine

1. To the extraction tube add 2.0 ml of ethyl ether (a glass syringe is helpful).
2. Shake vigorously by hand to ensure that the charcoal is dispersed and thoroughly extracted.
3. When the charcoal has settled, decant the ether into a 10 X 75 mm tube.
4. Add another 0.5 ml of ether to the tube containing the charcoal and shake again.
5. Pour the ether into the same 10 X 75 mm tube.
6. Evaporate to dryness at room temperature with the aid of compressed air or nitrogen.

(B) Amphetamines, Narcotic Alkaloids, and Other Drugs

1. To the same extraction tube that contained the charcoal, add 2.0 ml of the chloroform: isopropanol reagent.
2. Shake vigorously and filter through Whatman #1 paper, (5.5-cm diameter) into a 5-ml beaker. The filter paper should be pretreated with the solvent before adding the extract.
3. Add another 0.5 ml of chloroform:isopropanol to the charcoal, mix again, and add it to the same beaker with the filter paper.
4. Into another 10 X 75 mm tube, add a small drop of dilute HCl (0.1 mol/liter) and pour the contents of the beaker into it.
5. Use 2 to 4 drops of chloroform:isopropanol to rinse the beaker, and pour it into the same 10 X 75 mm tube.
6. Evaporate the mixture to dryness at room temperature under air or nitrogen.

Chromatography of Drugs

(A) Barbiturates, Glutethimide, Cocaine

1. Rinse the walls of the 10 X 75 mm tube from the ethyl ether extraction with 2 drops of methanol. Mix gently until the residue is dissolved.
2. Using a glass capillary tube, spot the methanolic solution on the chromatographic plate, a few microliters at a time, allowing to dry between applications.
3. The following two standard mixtures should also be applied to two spots on the same plate: (a) Overspot (i.e., spot on top of one another) phenobarbital, glutethimide, and secobarbital. (b) Overspot cocaine, propoxyphene, and methadone. (c) Any other single drug or combination of drugs, as required.
4. Using developing solvent A, allow the plate to develop for about 75 min.
5. Remove the plate and dry it under warm air from a hair dryer for 10 min.
6. Examine the plate under short-wavelength UV light. Make a light pencil mark where the phenobarbital absorbs, as well as any other barbiturates and glutethimide. Barbiturates

and glutethimide absorb 254-nm light, and they will be visible under the short UV lamp if their concentration is high enough.

7. Add 2.0 ml of ammonium hydroxide to the tank containing developing solvent A. Redevelop the plate using this system (which is developing solvent B), until the solvent front rises to the pencil mark (phenobarbital), and then remove the plate from the tank.
8. Let the plate dry overnight at room temperature or dry the plate in an oven at 90°C for 15 min.
9. Examine the plate under short-wavelength UV light and mark the spot where cocaine absorbs light.
10. Spray the lower part of the plate from cocaine down to the application point with dilute sulfuric acid (5 ml/liter).
11. Cover the upper portion of the plate from phenobarbital to glutethimide with paper or Parafilm, and spray the uncovered part with iodoplatinate.
12. Identify cocaine and propoxyphene, if present.
13. Uncover the plate and spray lightly with diphenylcarbazone.
14. Spray the plate with mercuric sulfate, lightly at first. Note if any of the barbiturates or glutethimide is present. Heavily respray the plate with mercuric sulfate, and note the chalky-white spots caused by these drugs (see Table 1 for R_f values).

(B) Chromatography of Narcotic Alkaloids and Amphetamines

1. To the 10 × 75 mm tube from the chloroform: isopropanol extraction, add 2 drops of methanol. Rinse the walls of the tube while adding the solvent. Mix gently until the residue dissolves.
2. Using a glass capillary tube, spot the methanolic solution on the chromatographic plate, a few microliters at a time, allowing to dry between applications.
3. After all the methanol solution is applied, rinse the tube with 4 to 5 μl of chloroform, and apply this wash on the same spot as before.
4. The following mixtures of standards should also be applied to two spots on the same plate: (a) Overspot chlorpromazine, codeine, and morphine. (b) Overspot amphetamine, propoxyphene, methadone, and quinine. Using developing solvent C, develop the plate for about 80 min.
5. Remove the plate and allow it to dry for at least 5 min at room temperature.
6. Examine under the short-wavelength UV light. Use a pencil to lightly mark chlorpromazine and any other fluorescent or UV light-absorbing spots.
7. Develop the plate with developing solvent D until the solvent rises only to the pencil mark where chlorpromazine was noted.
8. Dry the plate for 1 hr at room temperature.
9. Examine the plate under short- and long-wavelength UV light to detect quinine and its metabolites.
10. Spray the plate lightly with the fluorescamine reagent in the vicinity of quinine to detect amphetamine.
11. Place the plate in a chamber saturated with ammonia fumes for 5 min. Respray the plate with fluorescamine.
12. Examine the plate under long-wavelength UV light to see if *d*-amphetamine is present by comparison with the urine control and standards.
13. Let the plate dry overnight at room temperature and check with the long-wavelength UV

Table 1

APPROXIMATE R_f VALUES OF DRUGS

	R_f
In Solvent Systems A and B	
Cocaine	0.27
Propoxyphene	0.24
Methadone	0.21
Phenobarbital	0.47
Secobarbital	0.67
Amobarbital	0.60
Pentobarbital	0.60
Glutethimide	0.80
Ethchlorvynol	0.87
In Solvent Systems C and D	
Morphine	0.16
Codeine	0.38
Quinine	0.41
d-Amphetamine	0.57
Ephedrine	0.49
Meperidine	0.68
Methadone	0.72
Chlorpromazine	0.74
Propoxyphene	0.80
Cocaine	0.85

light for the greenish-yellow fluorescence of morphine.

14. Check for quinine and its metabolites under the long-wavelength UV lamp.
15. Spray the plate moderately with iodoplatinate reagent.
16. Examine the plate from the top down for the appearance of cocaine, propoxyphene, chlorpromazine, methadone, codeine, and morphine (see Table 1 for R_f values).
17. Compare any spot that appears with the urine control and standards.

INTERPRETATION (see p. 7)

Table 1 shows the approximate R_f values of the drugs. The ether elution also removes some methadone, cocaine, and propoxyphene, but they do not migrate far from the point of application in solvent systems A or B. If they are present, however, they are confirmed after the chloroform:isopropanol elution in solvent systems C and D.

Allowing the plate containing the narcotics and amphetamines to stand overnight at room temperature enhances the fluorescence of morphine under long-wavelength UV light, providing a valuable confirmatory test for this important drug. Allowing the plate to stand overnight seems to increase the sensitivity of the iodoplatinate reaction for some of the drugs.

Warning: Identifications based solely on thin-layer chromatography are not absolute. Other physical parameters may be required for certain applications. Should this be so, elution of the drug from the TLC plate may be a desirable isolation procedure. One such method is described by Reynolds (see p. 447).

REFERENCES

Berry, D. J. and Grove, J., Improved chromatographic techniques and their interpretation for the screening of urine from drug-dependent subjects, *J. Chromatogr.*, 61, 111, 1971.

Davidow, B., Petri, N., and Quame, B., A thin-layer chromatographic screening procedure for detecting drug abuse, *Am. J. Clin. Pathol.*, 50, 714, 1968.

Dole, V. P., Kim, W. K., and Eglitis, I., Detection of narcotic drugs, tranquilizers, amphetamines and barbitures in urine, *JAMA*, 198, 349, 1966.

Edwards, K. D. G. and McCredie, M., Studies on the binding properties of acidic, basic and neutral drugs to anion and cation exchange resins and charcoal in vitro, *Med. J. Aust.*, 1, 534, 1967.

Meola, J. and Vanko, M., A simple system for drug analysis, *Clin. Chem. Abstr.*, 17, 637, 1971.

Meola, J. and Vanko, M., The use of charcoal in the qualitative and quantitative analysis of drugs, *Clin. Chem. Abstr.*, 18, 713, 1972.

Mulé, S. J., Identification of narcotics, barbiturates, amphetamines, tranquilizers, and psychomimetics in human urine, *J. Chromatogr.*, 39, 302, 1969.

Oka, T. and Hosoya, E., Simple, sensitive and rapid methods for the detection of morphine in urine, *Keio J. Med.*, 16, 23, 1967.

Udenfriend, S., Stein, S., Bohlen, P., Dairman, W., Leingruber, W., and Weigele, M., Application of fluorescamine, a new reagent for assay of amino acids, peptides, proteins and other primary amines in the picomole range, *Science*, 178, 871, 1972.

INDEX

Column 1 indicates the primary substances of the methods described in the text. Some of the methods list certain substances as interfering substances. Theoretically, that method could be applied to the interfering substance if the original substance is not present; hence, it is listed in Column 2. Column 3 indicates any substance mentioned in the tables for whatever value it may have.

D

E

N

T